Artificial Intelligence Techniques for Sustainable Development

How can the efficiency of the algorithms be increased with a lesser number of computations as well as optimized with the resources for cost-effective solutions? *Artificial Intelligence Techniques for Sustainable Development* provides an answer. Further, it discusses important concepts such as green communication network design and implementation for the Internet of Things ecosystem, green computing in network security, and artificial intelligence models for remote sensing applications.

Key features:

- Presents the latest tools and techniques in developing solutions intended for resource utilization, energy efficiency, and human and environmental health.
- Highlights the advancement in electronics and communication technology for green applications.
- Covers smart energy harvesting/charging and power management techniques using machine learning.
- Explains green communication network design and implementation for the Internet of Things ecosystem, and green computing in network security.
- Illustrates prediction models for carbon emission and sequestration, environmental health, and climate change.

The book is aimed at senior undergraduates, graduate students, and academic researchers in the fields of electrical engineering, electronics, and communications engineering, computer science and engineering, environmental engineering, and biomedical engineering.

Smart Engineering Systems: Design and Applications

Series Editor – Suman Lata Tripathi

Internet of Things
Robotic and Drone Technology
Edited by Nitin Goyal, Sharad Sharma, Arun Kumar Rana, Suman Lata Tripathi

Smart Electrical Grid System
Design Principle, Modernization, and Techniques
Edited by Krishan Arora, Suman Lata Tripathi and Sanjeevikumar Padmanaban

Artificial Intelligence, Internet of Things (IoT) and Smart Materials for Energy Applications
Edited by Mohan Lal Kolhe, Kailash J. Karande and Sampat G. Deshmukh

Artificial Intelligence for Internet of Things
Design Principle, Modernization, and Techniques
Edited by N. Thillaiarasu, Suman Lata Tripathi and V.Dhinakaran

Machine Learning and Internet of Things in Solar Power Generation
Edited by Prabha Umapathy, Jude Hemanth, Shelej Khera, Abinaya Inbamani and Suman Lata Tripathi

Microgrid
Design, Optimization, and Applications
Edited by Amit Kumar Pandey, Sanjeevikumar Padmanaban, Suman Lata Tripathi, Vivek Patel, Vikas Patel

Artificial Intelligence Techniques for Sustainable Development
Edited by Deepika Ghai, Kirti Rawal, Kanav Dhir and Suman Lata Tripathi

For more information about this series, please visit: https://www.routledge.com/Smart-Engineering-Systems/book-series/CRCSESDA

Artificial Intelligence Techniques for Sustainable Development

Edited by
Deepika Ghai
Kirti Rawal
Kanav Dhir
Suman Lata Tripathi

CRC Press
Taylor & Francis Group
Boca Raton London New York

CRC Press is an imprint of the
Taylor & Francis Group, an informa business

Front cover image: metamorworks/Shutterstock

First edition published 2025
by CRC Press
2385 NW Executive Center Drive, Suite 320, Boca Raton FL 33431

and by CRC Press
4 Park Square, Milton Park, Abingdon, Oxon, OX14 4RN

CRC Press is an imprint of Taylor & Francis Group, LLC

ISBN: 978-1-032-77495-4 (hbk)
ISBN: 978-1-032-90161-9 (pbk)
ISBN: 978-1-003-54638-2 (ebk)

DOI: 10.1201/9781003546382

Typeset in Times
by SPi Technologies India Pvt Ltd (Straive)

Contents

Preface

In recent years, Artificial Intelligence (AI) has been considered the biggest game changer in developing new technologies for providing better healthcare, wildlife protection, pollution control, clean energy, waste management, and agriculture. In today's era, AI has achieved remarkable progress in a variety of applications such as the healthcare sector, speech recognition, image processing, object recognition, video processing, and robotics.

This new volume, *Artificial Intelligence Techniques for Sustainable Development*, offers a comprehensive overview of Introduction to AI, Green Electronic Technology, Green Energy Technology, Green Environmental Solutions, and Green Healthcare. Green AI covers a wide range of technologies that aid in reducing human interference on the environment and promoting long-term growth.

This book helps users to investigate, find, and implement novel AI-based solutions to green applications. It also emphasizes more on energy-efficient technologies and optimization of resources using green technology in real-life problems. Further, the fusion of artificial intelligence and green applications provides solutions to complex problems with minimum computational cost.

The chapters cover the fundamentals, significance, and advantages of green technology and its solutions focused on resource utilization; address the green applications for reliable IoT systems; and examine eco-friendly, energy-efficient solutions. This volume will serve as a valuable resource for individuals responsible for and engaged in technology and solutions focused on predicting climate change and enhancing environmental sustainability, including faculty and students specializing in this field.

About the Editors

Deepika Ghai has completed her PhD in the area of signal and image processing from Punjab Engineering College (Deemed-to-be University), Chandigarh. She did her MTech in VLSI Design & CAD from Thapar University, Patiala, and BTech in Electronics and Communications Engineering from Rayat Institute of Engineering and Technology, Ropar. She is associated with Lovely Professional University as an assistant professor with more than six years of experience in academics. She has received Dr. C.B. Gupta Award in 2021 at Lovely Professional University. She has published more than 40 research papers in refereed journals and conferences. She has worked as a session chair, conference steering committee member, editorial board member, and reviewer in international/national IEEE Journal and conferences. She has also published a number of edited books, *Health Informatics and Technological Solutions for Coronavirus (COVID-19)* in CRC Taylor & Francis, *Machine Learning Algorithms for Signal and Image Processing* with Wiley-IEEE Press, and *Multimodal Biometric and Machine Learning Technologies: Applications for Computer Vision* with Wiley Scrivener Publishing. She is associated as a life member of the Indian Science Congress. Her area of expertise includes signal and image processing, biomedical signal and image processing, and VLSI signal processing.

Kirti Rawal received her PhD degree in Electronics and Communication Engineering from Dr. B. R. Ambedkar National Institute of Technology Jalandhar in the area of Biomedical Signal Processing. Presently, she is working as a professor in the School of Electronics and Electrical Engineering at Lovely Professional University, Phagwara, Punjab, India.

She has published 16 research papers in reputed international journals and 12 papers in conferences. She is also guiding PhD scholars, MTech dissertation students, and BTech projects in the area of biomedical signals, medical imaging, and digital signal and image processing. She has 13+ years of rich experience in teaching and research and technical education management. Her areas of interest are digital signal processing, biomedical signal processing, medical imaging, artificial intelligence, image processing, machine learning, and healthcare services. She is a member of the Indian Science Congress, Calcutta. She is the reviewer of many SCI-indexed journals, Scopus-indexed journals, and conferences. She has also authored and reviewed diverse chapters in refereed books.

Kanav Dhir has completed his PhD in the area of inorganic and medicinal chemistry from Punjab Engineering College (Deemed-to-be University), Chandigarh. He did his MSc in chemistry from DAV College, Chandigarh, and BSc from A.S. College, Khanna. He is associated with DAV College, Chandigarh, as an assistant professor with more than five 10 years of experience in academics. He has published more than 12 research papers in refereed journals and conferences and four book chapters. He has published an edited book, *Health Informatics and Technological Solutions for Coronavirus (COVID-19)* in CRC Taylor & Francis. His area of expertise includes inorganic chemistry and bioinorganic chemistry. He is associated as a professional member of SESI.

Suman Lata Tripathi is working as Professor at Lovely Professional University with more than 22 years of experience in academics and research. She has completed her PhD in the area of microelectronics and VLSI Design from MNNIT, Allahabad. She did her MTech in Electronics Engineering from UP Technical University, Lucknow, and BTech in Electrical Engineering from Purvanchal University, Jaunpur. She has completed her remote post-doc from Nottingham Trent University, London, UK, in the year 2022–2023. She has published more than 125 research papers. She has also published 14 Indian patents and 4 copyrights. She has guided 6 PhD scholars and 3 are under submission stage. She has organized several workshops, summer internships, and expert lectures for students. She has worked as a session chair, conference steering committee member, editorial board member, and peer reviewer in international/national journals like IEEE, Springer, and Wiley and conferences. She has received the "Research Excellence Award" in 2019 and "Research Appreciation Award" in 2020, 2021, and 2023 at Lovely Professional University, India. She is recipient of the IGEN Women's for Green Technology "Women's Achievers Award" on International Women's Day, March 8, 2023. She received the best paper award at IEEE ICICS-2018. She has also received a funded project from SERB DST under the scheme TARE in the area of microelectronics devices. She has edited and authored more than 27 books in different areas of electronics and electrical engineering. She is also working as series editor for a book titled *Smart Engineering Systems* (CRC Press) and as conference series editor for "Conference Proceedings Series on Intelligent systems for Engineering designs" (CRC Press, Taylor & Francis). She is associated as senior member IEEE, Fellow IETE, and Life member ISC and is continuously involved in different professional activities along with academic work. Her area of expertise includes microelectronics device modeling and characterization, low-power VLSI circuit design, VLSI design of testing, and advanced FET design for IoT, embedded system design, reconfigurable architecture with FPGAs, biomedical applications, and so on.

Contributors

Manoj Singh Adhikari
School of Electronics and Electrical Engineering
Lovely Professional University
Phagwara, India

Naseer Ahmed
Department of Food Technology
Dr. Khem Singh Gill, Akal College of Agriculture
Eternal University
Baru Sahib, India

J. Anuradha
Department of Botany
NIMS Institute of Allied Medical Science and Technology
NIET, NIMS University Rajasthan
Jaipur, India

Rajni Aron
NMIMS University, India

Sandhya Avasthi
Department of Computer Science and Engineering
ABES Engineering College
Ghaziabad, India

E. Vijaya Babu
VNR Vignana Jyothi Institute of Engineering and Technology
Hyderabad, India

Indu Bala
School of Electronics and Electrical Engineering
Lovely Professional University
Phagwara, India

K. Baskaran
Department of Electrical and Electronics Engineering
ACGCET
Karaikudi, India

Ayush Behera
Department of Electrical Engineering
NIST Institute of Science and Technology (Autonomous)
Berhampur, India

Kanchan Bhatt
Department of Food Science and Technology
Dr Yashwant Singh Parmar University of Horticulture and Forestry
Nauni, Solan, India

Babji Prasad Chapa
Department of ECE
GMR Institute of Technology
Rajam, India

Priyanka Chauhan
Department of Fruit Science
Dr Yashwant Singh Parmar University of Horticulture and Forestry
Nauni, Solan, India

Deepika Ghai
School of Electronics & Electrical Engineering
Lovely Professional University
Phagwara, India

Sangita Gupta
Department of Chemistry
Poornima University
Jaipur, India

Hamid
Department of Food Technology and Nutrition
Lovely Professional University
Phagwara, India

Mamidipaka Hema
Department of ECE
JNTUGVCEV
Vizianagaram, India

J. Josalin Jemima
Department of Electrical and Electronics Engineering
Thiagarajar College of Engineering
Madurai, India

D. Nelson Jeyakumar
Department of Electrical and Electronics Engineering
Thiagarajar College of Engineering
Madurai, India

S. Ebenezer Juliet
Department of Computer Science and Engineering
Vellore Institute of Technology
Vellore, India

Gagandeep Kaur
Chitkara University Institute of Engineering and Technology
Chitkara University
Punjab, India

Mandeep Kaur
Chitkara University Institute of Engineering and Technology
Chitkara University
Punjab, India

Aruru Sai Kumar
Department of Electronics & Communication Engineering
VNR Vignana Jyothi Institute of Engineering & Technology
Hyderabad, India

Prasann Kumar
Department of Agronomy
School of Agriculture
Lovely Professional University
Phagwara, India

Sunita Kumari
Department of Chemistry
Poornima University
Jaipur, India

Jhansi Bharathi Madavarapu
Department of IT
University of the Cumberlands
Williamsburg, Kentucky

Kamalakanta Mahapatra
Department of Electronics and Communication Engineering
NIT Rourkela
Rourkela, India

Prajnyajit Mohanty
Department of Electronics and Communication Engineering
NIT Rourkela, India

K. Manimala
Department of Information Science & Technology
Anna University
Chennai, India

Manjushree Nayak
Department of Computer Science and Engineering
NIST Institute of Science and Technology (Autonomous)
Berhampur, India

N. Neelima
Department of Electronics & Communication Engineering
VNR Vignana Jyothi Institute of Engineering & Technology
Hyderabad, India

Naveen Palanichamy
Faculty of Computing and Informatics
Multimedia University
Cyberjaya, Malaysia

Balakumar Palaniyappan
School of Electrical Engineering
Vellore Institute of Technology
Chennai, India

Umesh C. Pati
Department of Electronics and Communication Engineering
NIT Rourkela, India

Pandiyan Pitchai
Department of Electrical and Electronics Engineering
KPR Institute of Engineering and Technology
Coimbatore, India

E. Fantin Irudaya Raj
Department of Electrical and Electronics Engineering
Dr. Sivanthi Aditanar College of Engineering
Tiruchendur, India

S. Charles Raja
Department of Electrical and Electronics Engineering
Thiagarajar College of Engineering
Madurai, India

G. Boopathi Raja
Department of Electronics and Communication Engineering
Velalar College of Engineering and Technology
Erode, India

Senthil Kumar Ramu
School of Electrical Engineering
Vellore Institute of Technology
Chennai, India

Rajeev
Department of Agronomy, School of Agriculture
Lovely Professional University
Phagwara, India

Shippu Sachdeva
School of Electronics and Electrical Engineering
Lovely Professional University
Phagwara, India

Indu Saini
Department of Electronics and Communication Engineering
Dr B R Ambedkar National Institute of Technology
Jalandhar, India

Lalit Saini
Department of Agronomy, School of Agriculture
Lovely Professional University
Phagwara, India

Ramandeep Sandhu
School of Computer Science & Engineering
Lovely Professional University
Phagwara, India

R. Sanjeevi
Department of Environmental Science
NIMS Institute of Allied Medical Science and Technology
NIET, NIMS University Rajasthan
Jaipur, India

Prashant Kumar B. Sathvara
Department of Environmental Science
NIMS Institute of Allied Medical Science and Technology
NIET, NIMS University Rajasthan
Jaipur, India

Manoj Kumar Shukla
Department of Robotics and Automation
Symbiosis Institute of Technology
Pune, India

Manoj Sindhwani
School of Electronics and Electrical Engineering
Lovely Professional University
Phagwara, India

Madhurima Sit
Department of Computer Science and Engineering
NIST Institute of Science and Technology (Autonomous)
Berhampur, India

Aditya Singh
Department of Civil Engineering
Amrita Vishwa Vidyapeetham
Coimbatore, India

Mayank Kumar Singh
Department of Electronics and Communication Engineering
Dr B R Ambedkar National Institute of Technology
Jalandhar, India

Neetu Sood
Department of Electronics and Communication Engineering
Dr B R Ambedkar National Institute of Technology
Jalandhar, India

Amit Srivastava
Department of Civil Engineering
Graphic Era Deemed to be University
Dehradun, India

Saravanan Subramani
Department of Electrical and Electronics Engineering
Amrita School of Engineering
and
Amrita Vishwa Vidyapeetham
Coimbatore, India

N. Sumalatha
Department of Electronics and Communication Engineering
ACGCET
Karaikudi, India

Jami Venkata Suman
Department of ECE
GMR Institute of Technology
Rajam, India

N. Sunanda
VNR Vignana Jyothi Institute of Engineering and Technology
Hyderabad, India

Righa Tandon
Chitkara University Institute of Engineering and Technology
Chitkara University
Rajpura, India

Srinivas Talasila
Department of Electronics & Communication Engineering
VNR Vignana Jyothi Institute of Engineering & Technology
Hyderabad, India

Tejas
Department of Agronomy, School of Agriculture
Lovely Professional University
Phagwara, India

Divya Shivani Thangi
Department of Genetics and Plant Breeding
Angrau, Bapatla, India

Sandeep Tripathi
Department of Environmental Science
NIMS Institute of Allied Medical Science and Technology
NIET, NIMS University Rajasthan
Jaipur, India

Suman Lata Tripathi
School of Electronics & Electrical Engineering
Lovely Professional University
Phagwara, India

Hina Upadhyay
Department of Agronomy, School of Agriculture
Lovely Professional University
Phagwara, India

M. Selva Vengatesh
Department of Electrical and Electronics Engineering
Thiagarajar College of Engineering
Madurai, India

Yogesh Kumar Verma
School of Electronics and Electrical Engineering
Lovely Professional University
Phagwara, India

Heena Wadhwa
Chitkara University Institute of Engineering and Technology
Chitkara University
Punjab, India

1 Introduction to Green and Red Artificial Intelligence

Indu Bala
School of Electronics and Electrical Engineering,
Lovely Professional University, Phagwara, India

1.1 INTRODUCTION

Green AI and Red AI are two emerging paradigms in the science of artificial intelligence, each with distinct roles in many aspects of human life. Green AI refers to the utilization of Artificial Intelligence (AI) to efficiently address environmental and sustainability concerns. This includes the optimization of energy consumption, the improvement of resource allocation, and the promotion of the preservation of natural ecosystems. The adoption of Green AI has demonstrated a substantial impact on the advancement of cleaner and more efficient technology, thereby playing a vital role in mitigating climate change and promoting environmentally friendly practices [1]. Nevertheless, it is important to acknowledge that the term "Red AI" is not widely recognized in the field of artificial intelligence and does not currently have a clear and universally acknowledged definition, according to the latest information at my disposal. The prospective applications of AI in the domains of healthcare, safety, and security are currently ambiguous due to the lack of a clear definition of its role and consequences in these areas. The ever-changing characteristics of AI paradigms emphasize the profound influence of AI on several facets of human existence, encompassing environmental preservation, advancements in healthcare, and security enhancements. This indicates a future in which artificial intelligence plays a vital role in addressing critical global challenges [2].

1.1.1 The Significance of Green and Red AI in Contemporary Society

The importance of Green and Red AI in modern society is of great significance and should not be underestimated. The implementation of Green AI, which prioritizes environmental sustainability, plays a crucial role in addressing urgent global issues. The optimization of energy usage, improvement of resource management, and advancement of clean energy technology are crucial factors in the mitigation of climate change. The use of Green AI has been found to significantly enhance the effectiveness of environmental monitoring and climate modeling, thereby playing

DOI: 10.1201/9781003546382-1

a crucial role in the preservation of the planet's overall well-being and long-term sustainability.

In contrast, Red AI pertains to matters concerning security and ethics, which are progressively gaining significance within the context of our interconnected digital society. This technology aids in the mitigation of cyber risks, safeguarding data privacy, and addressing ethical considerations about autonomous weaponry and deepfakes. In light of our society's increasing dependence on digital technologies, Red AI plays a crucial role in upholding the requisite security measures and ethical standards essential for a future characterized by safety and security. The dynamic relationship between Green and Red Artificial Intelligence (AI) underscores the imperative of adopting a well-rounded strategy that maximizes the advantages of AI while concurrently mitigating any hazards. The modern societal context highlights the crucial significance of these two artificial intelligence models, emphasizing the pressing need for both environmental stewardship and digital safeguarding [3].

1.1.2 Contribution of the Chapter

The main chapter contributions are highlighted below:

1. The definition, historical progression, and applications of Green AI are meticulously examined, providing a comprehensive understanding of its conceptual framework and practical implications.
2. The real-world case studies are enlisted to enhance the chapter's practicality, offering tangible examples that illustrate the implications and effectiveness of Green AI projects.
3. In-depth discussion is done on the negative aspects of AI, focusing on security-related concerns, cybersecurity risks, ethical dilemmas (privacy, misinformation, deepfakes), and the regulatory frameworks governing Red AI, supported by empirical case studies.
4. Commonalities Identification and Ethical Implications shared between Green AI and Red AI, fostering a nuanced understanding of the ethical landscape in artificial intelligence is explored.
5. The crucial role of policy and governance in managing and harmonizing AI paradigms, emphasizing the need for structured measures to guide the development and deployment of artificial intelligence is also highlighted.

1.1.3 Chapter Organization

This chapter provides a thorough examination of two nascent paradigms in the field of artificial intelligence (Figure 1.1). In Section 1.2, the concept of Green Artificial Intelligence (AI) is expounded upon, encompassing its definition, historical progression, and examination of its diverse range of applications, advantages, and obstacles. Real-world case studies serve as tangible examples that demonstrate the practical implications of Green AI projects. Section 1.3, titled "Red Artificial Intelligence," provides an in-depth exploration of the negative aspects associated with Artificial

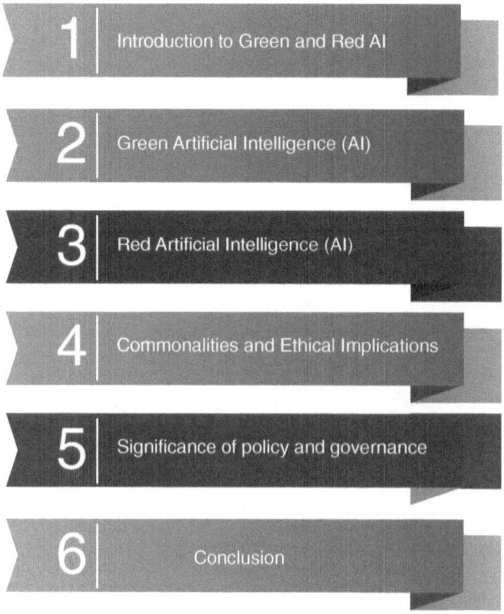

FIGURE 1.1 Chapter organization.

Intelligence (AI). This chapter specifically focuses on security-related apprehensions, including cybersecurity risks, as well as ethical quandaries about privacy, misinformation, and the emergence of deepfakes. This section additionally explores the regulatory frameworks and ethical principles governing Red AI, while also providing empirical case studies from real-world contexts. In Section 1.4, the author examines the commonalities and ethical implications that exist between Green AI and Red AI. Section 1.5 explores the significance of policy and governance in effectively managing and harmonizing various paradigms. In contrast, Section 1.6 provides the conclusion of the chapter with emphasis on the need for proactive measures to ensure a future for artificial intelligence that is both sustainable and secure.

1.2 GREEN ARTIFICIAL INTELLIGENCE

Green Artificial Intelligence, often abbreviated as Green AI, refers to the application of Artificial Intelligence (AI) techniques and technologies to address environmental and sustainability challenges [4, 5]. The primary goal of Green AI is to use AI in a way that reduces the negative impact of human activities on the environment and promotes sustainability. This can be achieved through various means (Figure 1.2), including:

1. ***Energy Efficiency*:** Green AI aims to make AI algorithms and hardware more energy-efficient. AI systems often require significant computational power, and optimizing them for lower energy consumption can reduce their carbon footprint.

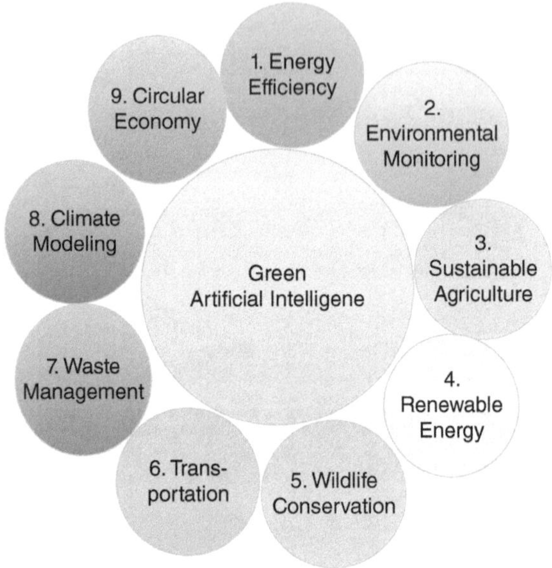

FIGURE 1.2 Various aspects of Green AI.

2. ***Environmental Monitoring*:** AI can be used to collect, analyze, and interpret data from various sensors and sources to monitor environmental conditions, such as air and water quality, climate change, and biodiversity. This information can inform decision-making and environmental conservation efforts.
3. ***Sustainable Agriculture*:** AI can help improve farming practices by optimizing crop management, resource allocation, and pest control, leading to more sustainable and efficient agriculture.
4. ***Renewable Energy*:** Green AI can be applied to enhance the efficiency and effectiveness of renewable energy sources like solar and wind power. It can also help in energy grid management to accommodate the intermittent nature of these energy sources.
5. ***Wildlife Conservation*:** AI-powered monitoring and tracking systems assist in protecting endangered species and natural habitats. AI can help in the analysis of camera trap images, satellite data, and audio recordings to monitor and protect wildlife.
6. ***Transportation*:** AI can be used to optimize transportation systems, reducing energy consumption and emissions. This includes applications in electric vehicle optimization, traffic management, and autonomous transportation.
7. ***Waste Management*:** AI can improve waste sorting and recycling processes, making them more efficient and reducing the environmental impact of waste disposal.
8. ***Climate Modeling*:** AI and machine learning are used in climate modeling and weather forecasting, which are crucial for understanding climate change and mitigating its effects.

9. ***Circular Economy*****:** AI can support the transition to a circular economy by optimizing resource use, reducing waste, and promoting recycling and reusing materials.

1.2.1 What is Green Artificial Intelligence?

Green AI is a developing field that investigates the intersection of artificial intelligence and environmental sustainability. The primary objective is to develop and employ AI technology in a way that minimizes ecological impact and effectively addresses pressing environmental concerns. The goal is to create AI systems that are energy-efficient, improve industries to support environmental sustainability and harness the powers of AI for monitoring, conservation, and sustainable practices. Green AI is a concept that aims to balance technology progress with environmental responsibility. Its objective is to utilize the revolutionary capabilities of AI to tackle urgent global issues, such as climate change and animal protection. Furthermore, Green AI aims to reduce the environmental impact linked to the implementation and functioning of AI technology.

1.2.1.1 Historical Development and Context

The origin of Green AI can be attributed to the growing awareness of the environmental consequences linked to artificial intelligence and the rising imperative to utilize AI's capacities to tackle these issues. Green AI has become increasingly important in recent years due to concerns about the significant energy usage and carbon emissions associated with AI, especially in the training of deep learning models. Scientists and institutions have made deliberate efforts to minimize the environmental consequences of AI by investigating energy-efficient algorithms and hardware remedies. Specialized technology, such as power-efficient Graphics Processing Units (GPUs), has played a substantial part in this effort. Furthermore, the use of Artificial Intelligence (AI) in environmental monitoring has improved accuracy in the observation of climate change, air and water quality, and deforestation. This is achieved by the analysis of data obtained from various sources such as satellites, drones, and Internet of Things (IoT) devices. AI is advantageous in sustainable agriculture as it optimizes resource management and encourages the use of environmentally friendly farming methods. While governments and regulatory authorities consider methods to promote the use of eco-friendly AI and address its environmental impact, the area of AI continues to evolve. This achievement entails promoting interdisciplinary collaboration and implementing creative ways that result in mutually advantageous consequences for both technology and the environment. Green AI is a recently popularized approach that harnesses artificial intelligence to tackle environmental problems and encourage ecological responsibility within the AI field. This strategy is seen as essential in the endeavor to achieve a sustainable future [6].

1.2.2 Applications of Green AI

1.2.2.1 Environmental Monitoring

The application of Green AI in environmental monitoring is of utmost importance, as it entails the utilization of artificial intelligence to gather, manipulate, and assess data about diverse environmental factors (Figure 1.3), and this application exerts a

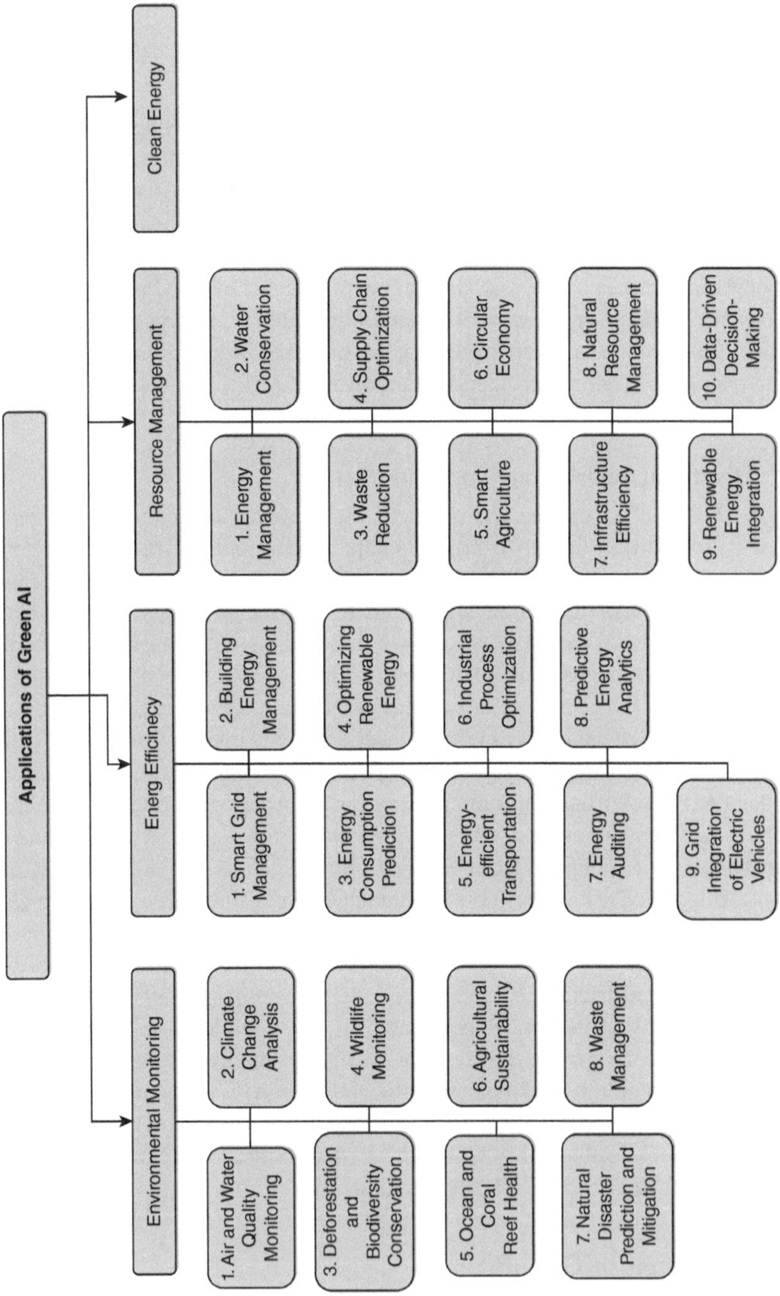

FIGURE 1.3 Applications of Green AI.

substantial influence on the preservation of the environment and the promotion of sustainability through the subsequent mechanisms:

1. ***Air and Water Quality Monitoring*****:** The application of Green AI involves the utilization of advanced computational techniques to analyze data collected from air quality sensors and water quality sensors. Machine learning algorithms possess the capability to discern patterns of pollution, ascertain the origins of contamination, and furnish timely alerts regarding prospective health dangers, thus facilitating prompt intervention by authorities to alleviate environmental hazards [7].
2. ***Climate Change Analysis*****:** Artificial intelligence (AI) is utilized in the field of climate modeling and analysis. The system utilizes extensive datasets, encompassing historical weather records and contemporary climate data, to enhance the precision of forecasts about climate change, extreme weather occurrences, and long-term environmental patterns [8]
3. ***Deforestation and Biodiversity Conservation*****:** The utilization of Green AI in the analysis of satellite imagery enables the monitoring of deforestation patterns and the tracking of ecosystem alterations. Machine learning models provide the capability to discern trends in illicit logging, habitat degradation, and the presence of endangered species, hence facilitating the advancement of conservation endeavors.
4. ***Wildlife Monitoring*****:** The monitoring of wildlife populations and behavior is facilitated through the utilization of AI-based camera traps and acoustic sensors. These systems can autonomously identify and categorize animals, monitor their migration patterns, and evaluate the well-being of diverse species, thereby providing valuable assistance to the field of wildlife conservation.
5. ***Ocean and Coral Reef Health*****:** The utilization of artificial intelligence (AI) systems in underwater robots enables the monitoring of coral reefs and marine ecosystems to assess their overall health. The utilization of AI-driven robots enables the analysis of photos and data to evaluate water quality and identify occurrences such as coral bleaching.
6. ***Agricultural Sustainability*****:** The application of Green AI in precision agriculture enables the efficient utilization of resources such as water and fertilizers. The utilization of AI-driven sensors enables the monitoring of soil conditions, crop health, and weather patterns, hence facilitating the implementation of real-time decision-making processes in the context of sustainable farming methods.
7. ***Natural Disaster Prediction and Mitigation*****:** Machine learning models possess the capability to assess data derived from many sources, including seismometers, weather radars, and satellite imaging, to predict natural calamities such as earthquakes, hurricanes, and wildfires. This facilitates the implementation of early warning systems and measures for catastrophe mitigation.
8. ***Waste Management*****:** Artificial intelligence (AI) has the potential to enhance waste management practices through the optimization of recycling and

garbage sorting procedures. Automated systems possess the capability to accurately detect and categorize recyclable items, hence enhancing the efficiency of trash sorting processes. Consequently, these systems contribute to the reduction of landfill waste and the facilitation of recycling practices.

1.2.2.2 Energy Efficiency

Green AI for energy efficiency is a crucial application that focuses on using artificial intelligence to optimize energy consumption and reduce the environmental impact of various energy-related processes. Following are several ways in which Green AI is applied to enhance energy efficiency [9, 10]:

1. ***Smart Grid Management*:** AI is used in smart grids to improve the efficiency of electricity distribution. Machine learning algorithms analyze data from smart meters and sensors to predict energy demand, identify faults, and optimize the grid's operation. This leads to reduced energy wastage and a more reliable energy supply.
2. ***Building Energy Management*:** AI-driven building management systems monitor and control energy usage in commercial and residential buildings. These systems adjust Heating, Ventilation, Air Conditioning (HVAC), lighting, and other building systems based on occupancy and weather conditions, resulting in lower energy consumption and cost savings.
3. ***Energy Consumption Prediction*:** AI can predict energy consumption patterns for specific industrial processes, allowing manufacturers to plan their production schedules to minimize energy usage during peak hours. Predictive maintenance powered by AI can also prevent unexpected energy-intensive equipment breakdowns.
4. ***Optimizing Renewable Energy*:** Green AI is applied to renewable energy sources like solar and wind. AI algorithms can predict renewable energy generation based on weather forecasts and adjust energy storage and distribution accordingly, making better use of clean energy sources.
5. ***Energy-Efficient Transportation*:** AI is used in transportation systems to optimize routes and schedules for public transit and delivery services, reducing fuel consumption and emissions. Autonomous vehicles are also being developed to drive more efficiently [11].
6. ***Industrial Process Optimization*:** AI systems analyze data from sensors in industrial settings to optimize manufacturing and production processes. This leads to energy-efficient operations and reduced waste.
7. ***Energy Auditing*:** AI-based tools are used for energy audits in homes and businesses, providing recommendations for energy-efficient improvements, such as insulation upgrades or equipment replacements.
8. ***Predictive Energy Analytics*:** Machine learning models can predict energy consumption and peak usage periods, allowing utility companies to plan their energy generation more efficiently, reducing the need for fossil fuel power plants during high-demand periods.
9. ***Grid Integration of Electric Vehicles*:** AI is used to manage the charging and discharging of electric vehicles (EVs) to ensure that they charge during periods of low electricity demand and help stabilize the grid during peak times.

1.2.2.3 Resource Management

Resource management using Green AI is a forward-thinking approach that utilizes artificial intelligence to optimize the allocation and utilization of various resources while minimizing waste and environmental impact. This encompasses a wide range of resources, including energy, water, materials, and more. Here's a comprehensive view of how Green AI is applied in resource management:

1. ***Energy Management*:** Green AI is instrumental in managing energy resources efficiently. It uses data analytics and predictive algorithms to optimize energy usage in buildings, industries, and transportation, reducing consumption and associated greenhouse gas emissions [12].
2. ***Water Conservation*:** AI-driven systems monitor and control water usage, detect leaks, manage irrigation, and enhance wastewater treatment processes. This not only conserves water but also reduces the energy needed for water-related operations.
3. ***Waste Reduction*:** AI systems optimize waste management processes by identifying recycling opportunities and suggesting efficient disposal methods. This reduces landfill waste and promotes recycling and reuse of materials.
4. ***Supply Chain Optimization*:** Green AI enhances supply chain management by predicting demand, optimizing transportation routes, and reducing excess inventory, ultimately minimizing resource consumption and emissions associated with logistics.
5. ***Smart Agriculture*:** AI technologies are applied in agriculture to optimize the use of water, fertilizers, and pesticides. This leads to increased crop yields with fewer resources and a reduced environmental impact.
6. ***Circular Economy*:** Green AI supports the transition to a circular economy by identifying opportunities for reusing, recycling, and repurposing materials. It helps industries design products for easy disassembly and recycling [13].
7. ***Infrastructure Efficiency*:** AI systems improve the efficiency of infrastructure, including buildings and transportation systems, by adjusting operations based on real-time data, reducing resource consumption.
8. ***Natural Resource Management*:** Green AI is used in forestry, fisheries, and wildlife conservation to monitor and manage the sustainable use of natural resources, reducing overexploitation and habitat degradation.
9. ***Renewable Energy Integration*:** AI optimizes the integration of renewable energy sources into the grid, ensuring a smooth transition to clean energy while reducing dependence on fossil fuels.
10. ***Data-Driven Decision-Making*:** AI provides data-driven insights for resource allocation and management, helping organizations make informed decisions that minimize resource waste and enhance sustainability [14].

Resource management using Green AI has the potential to significantly reduce resource consumption, promote sustainability, and mitigate environmental impacts. It enables more efficient use of resources and the development of strategies that benefit both the environment and economic prosperity. This approach is vital in addressing resource scarcity and environmental challenges in an increasingly resource-constrained world.

1.2.2.4 Clean Energy

The relationship between clean energy and Green AI is an integral part of our collective effort to combat climate change and create a more sustainable future. Green AI serves as a powerful ally to clean energy solutions, offering data-driven insights and optimization strategies that enhance the development and integration of renewable energy sources. It enables solar panels and wind turbines to generate power more efficiently, predicts energy production based on weather conditions, and manages the distribution of clean energy through smart grids, thus ensuring a stable and reliable energy supply. Additionally, Green AI plays a vital role in energy storage management, grid integration, energy efficiency, and predictive maintenance of clean energy infrastructure. Its capabilities are instrumental in reducing energy consumption, greenhouse gas emissions, and the environmental footprint of the energy sector as a whole. By combining the potential of clean energy with the intelligence of Green AI, we are advancing the transition to a more sustainable and eco-friendly energy landscape, where renewable energy sources are harnessed to their fullest potential, making clean energy a cornerstone of our environmental future.

1.3 BENEFITS AND CHALLENGES OF GREEN AI

1.3.1 Advantages of Green AI

Green AI offers numerous advantages that contribute to environmental sustainability, energy efficiency, and improved decision-making. Here are some key benefits of Green AI [15]:

1. ***Reduced Environmental Impact*:** Green AI focuses on minimizing the environmental footprint of AI and other technologies. This includes optimizing energy consumption, reducing carbon emissions, and conserving natural resources.
2. ***Energy Efficiency*:** Green AI promotes the development of energy-efficient AI algorithms and hardware, reducing the power consumption of AI applications, data centers, and devices.
3. ***Environmental Monitoring*:** Green AI enhances our ability to monitor and analyze environmental data, leading to better insights into climate change, air and water quality, deforestation, and wildlife conservation.
4. ***Sustainability*:** Green AI supports sustainable practices in agriculture, waste management, transportation, and renewable energy, making these sectors more environmentally friendly and economically efficient.
5. ***Cost Savings*:** Improved energy efficiency and resource management translate into cost savings for businesses and consumers, making it economically advantageous to adopt Green AI solutions.
6. ***Predictive Analytics*:** Green AI provides advanced predictive analytics for climate modeling, renewable energy forecasting, and natural disaster preparedness, helping communities and organizations plan and respond effectively.
7. ***Resource Optimization*:** Green AI optimizes the allocation and use of resources, reducing waste and promoting the circular economy, where

materials are reused and recycled, leading to a more sustainable resource management approach.

8. ***Conservation*:** Green AI plays a vital role in wildlife conservation and habitat preservation by automating the analysis of camera trap images, audio recordings, and satellite data, helping protect endangered species.
9. ***Improved Decision-Making*:** Data-driven insights from Green AI support better decision-making in areas such as energy management, infrastructure efficiency, and climate adaptation, enabling more sustainable policies and practices.
10. ***Technology Integration*:** Green AI seamlessly integrates with existing technology infrastructure, making it adaptable and accessible to a wide range of industries and applications, from smart grids to clean energy.
11. ***Circular Economy*:** It aids in the transition to a circular economy by promoting the reuse and recycling of materials, reducing waste, and lowering the ecological impact of manufacturing and consumption.
12. ***Regulatory Compliance*:** Green AI assists organizations in meeting environmental regulations and compliance standards by providing tools to reduce emissions and manage resources responsibly.

The advantages of Green AI extend beyond environmental benefits to encompass economic and societal advantages, creating a win-win situation by addressing environmental challenges while promoting innovation and efficiency in various sectors.

1.3.2 Challenges and Limitations of Green AI

Green AI, while offering significant advantages for environmental sustainability, faces several challenges and limitations [16, 17]:

1. ***Energy Consumption During Training*:** Training deep learning models, especially large ones, requires substantial computational power and energy, which can have a significant carbon footprint. Balancing AI model development with energy efficiency is a challenge.
2. ***Resource-Intensive Hardware*:** Specialized hardware like GPUs is often needed for AI training, and the production of such hardware can have environmental impacts. Additionally, not all organizations or individuals have access to energy-efficient AI hardware.
3. ***Data Quality and Availability*:** AI relies on high-quality data for training and decision-making. In environmental monitoring, data can be scarce, inaccurate, or biased, leading to less reliable AI-based analyses and predictions.
4. ***Complexity and Interpretability*:** AI models, especially deep neural networks, can be highly complex and challenging to interpret. This complexity can make it difficult to identify the reasoning behind AI-driven recommendations and decisions in environmental applications.
5. ***Lack of Universal Solutions*:** Environmental challenges can vary greatly by region and context. What works well in one location may not be directly applicable in another, making it challenging to develop one-size-fits-all Green AI solutions.

6. ***Initial Implementation Costs*:** Implementing Green AI solutions can require upfront investment in technology and infrastructure, which might deter organizations, particularly smaller ones, from adopting these practices.
7. ***Ethical Considerations*:** The use of AI in environmental monitoring and decision-making raises ethical concerns, such as privacy, data ownership, and potential biases in AI algorithms, which need to be carefully addressed.
8. ***Data Privacy*:** Collecting and analyzing environmental data, particularly in urban areas, can raise privacy concerns for individuals. Balancing the need for data with privacy rights is a challenge [18].
9. ***Algorithm Bias and Fairness*:** Biases in AI algorithms can affect the equitable distribution of environmental resources and benefits. Efforts are required to ensure AI solutions are fair and just.
10. ***Regulatory and Policy Hurdles*:** Developing and implementing policies and regulations to promote Green AI can be complex. Coordination among governments, industry stakeholders, and advocacy groups is needed to create effective frameworks.
11. ***Human Resistance to AI*:** There may be resistance to adopting AI-based recommendations in environmental decisions, as people might be uncomfortable ceding control to machines, particularly in matters related to the environment.
12. ***Technological Evolution*:** The rapid evolution of AI technologies requires continuous updates and adaptations, making it challenging for organizations to keep up with the latest advancements and remain environmentally responsible.

Green AI, while holding significant potential for addressing environmental challenges, requires a thoughtful and proactive approach to mitigate these challenges and limitations. Balancing the benefits of AI with its environmental impact and ethical considerations is an ongoing process that requires collaboration among stakeholders, innovation, and a commitment to sustainable practices.

1.4 REAL-WORLD EXAMPLES OF GREEN AI INITIATIVES

Several real-world examples of Green AI initiatives demonstrate how artificial intelligence is being applied to address environmental challenges and promote sustainability. These initiatives span various sectors and applications as described in Table 1.1.

1.5 RED ARTIFICIAL INTELLIGENCE

Red AI refers to the practice of creating more intricate and potent Artificial Intelligence (AI) models, disregarding efficiency and environmental consequences. These models typically need substantial quantities of data and computational resources for training and deployment, resulting in significant costs and adverse environmental impacts [19].

TABLE 1.1
Green AI Initiatives

Project Name	Description	Location
Solar Forecasting Systems	AI predicts solar energy generation for efficient grid integration.	United States, Europe, India, Australia
Smart-Grid AI	AI-based smart grids for real-time energy management and demand prediction.	South Korea, the United States, European countries
Precision Agriculture	AI-driven systems optimize irrigation, crop management, and pesticide use.	Global (various countries)
Wildlife Conservation AI	Camera traps and AI for wildlife monitoring and protection.	Various wildlife reserves and conservation areas worldwide
Waste Sorting Robots	AI-powered robots for efficient waste sorting and recycling.	Various recycling facilities globally
Climate Prediction	AI-enhanced climate modeling and prediction for better understanding of climate change.	Global, with a focus on climate research institutions
Autonomous Electric Vehicles	AI-driven electric vehicles for optimized transportation and reduced emissions.	Worldwide, including Tesla and other manufacturers
Disaster Prediction AI	AI models for earthquake, hurricane, and wildfire prediction and monitoring.	United States, Japan, and regions prone to natural disasters
Sustainable Building Systems	AI for smart buildings, optimizing energy use and climate control.	Various urban areas worldwide
Water Quality Management	AI systems to monitor and optimize water quality and distribution.	Various municipalities and regions globally
Ocean Health Monitoring	AI-equipped drones and boats for monitoring ocean health and biodiversity.	Various oceanic research institutions

The term “Red AI” was initially introduced by researchers at Google AI in 2019. It was noted that the computational expense of cutting-edge AI models had grown rapidly in recent years, although the performance improvements had been rather small. The driving force behind this trend is the aspiration of AI researchers to attain increasingly higher levels of accuracy and precision, although at a price. Several factors contribute to the increasing prevalence of Red AI. One factor contributing to this is the significant surge in data accessibility and computational capabilities in recent years. This advancement has enabled the training and implementation of artificial intelligence models that were previously impractical. Another factor contributing to the emergence of Red AI is the growing rivalry within the AI research community. Researchers face the demand to publish results that surpass the current highest level of achievement, which frequently results in the creation of more intricate and computationally demanding models. The utilization of Red AI presents several possible advantages. For instance, it can be utilized to cultivate AI models that exhibit unprecedented levels of accuracy and precision. This can be advantageous for endeavors such as medical diagnosis, financial forecasts, and scientific study [15]. Nevertheless, Red AI also possesses certain potential disadvantages. An inherent limitation is the considerable cost and time investment required for the development and implementation of Red AI models. Furthermore, Red AI models can exert a substantial ecological footprint. The training and deployment of these models necessitate a substantial amount of energy and result in significant greenhouse gas emissions. Before designing and implementing these models, it is crucial to carefully evaluate the potential advantages and disadvantages of Red AI. Occasionally, the advantages may surpass the disadvantages. Nevertheless, it is crucial to acknowledge the ecological repercussions of Red AI and implement measures to alleviate them.

1.5.1 Significance of Red AI

The significance of Red AI lies in its potential to profoundly transform numerous sectors and facets of human existence. Red AI has the potential to enhance the development of precise and efficient medical diagnostic tools, foster the creation of novel products and services, and automate work now performed by people. Nevertheless, it is crucial to acknowledge the possible disadvantages of Red AI, including its ecological footprint and the potential for malevolent utilization. Developing Red AI responsibly and ethically is crucial to ensure its beneficial application. Following are a few concrete instances illustrating the positive applications of Red AI [14]:

- Red AI has the potential to enhance the precision and efficiency of medical diagnostic instruments, including AI-driven cancer screening systems.
- Red AI has the potential to generate novel and cutting-edge products and services, such as AI-driven personal assistants and autonomous vehicles.
- Red AI can automate jobs that are presently performed by humans, like customer support and data entry.
- Crimson Artificial Intelligence (AI) is a prominent technology with the capacity to enhance all aspects of our lives. Nevertheless, it is crucial to employ it responsibly and ethically.

1.5.2 Historical Context and Emergence of Red AI

The historical origins of Red AI can be traced to the initial stages of artificial intelligence development. During the 1950s and 1960s, researchers in the field of artificial intelligence were primarily dedicated to the advancement of symbolic AI systems, which aimed to solve issues by employing logical reasoning. These systems were generally compact and effective; however, their powers were constrained.

During the 1970s, there was a transition toward connectionist artificial intelligence (AI), which is founded on the concept that intelligence arises from the interplay of numerous interconnected processing units. Connectionist AI systems, such as neural networks, exhibit greater complexity and computing demands compared to symbolic AI systems. However, they possess the ability to acquire knowledge and adjust their behavior in response to novel input [13].

The 1980s and 1990s witnessed a renewed fascination with symbolic AI, mostly driven by the emergence of novel methodologies like expert systems. Expert systems are specialized computer programs that possess extensive knowledge and expertise in a specific field, such as medical diagnosis or financial planning. Expert systems are generally characterized by their intricate nature and high computing cost, although they provide great utility in addressing particular challenges.

In the early 2000s, machine learning emerged as a subfield of artificial intelligence that specifically deals with the creation of algorithms capable of acquiring knowledge from data. Machine learning methods have superior computing efficiency compared to symbolic AI or connectionist AI algorithms, and possess the ability to acquire knowledge from vast quantities of data [15].

The ascent of Red AI has been propelled by the advent of machine learning. Over the past few years, there has been a significant surge in the accessibility of data and computational capabilities. This advancement has enabled the training and deployment of machine learning models that possess far greater complexity and potency compared to previous iterations.

The rise of Red AI can be attributed to several factors, including the growing accessibility of data and computing power, the advancement of more efficient and scalable machine learning algorithms, the intensifying competition within the AI research community, and the aspiration of AI researchers to attain higher levels of accuracy and precision [11].

It is crucial to acknowledge that Red AI is a relatively nascent phrase, and its definition is currently undergoing development. Nevertheless, it is commonly accepted to denote the inclination towards creating AI models that are progressively intricate and potent, but at the cost of efficiency and environmental consequences.

1.5.3 Importance of the Rise of Red AI

The advent of Red AI is noteworthy due to its capacity to profoundly transform several businesses and facets of human existence. Crimson Artificial Intelligence (AI) has the potential to enhance the precision and efficiency of medical diagnostic equipment, foster the creation of novel and inventive goods and services, and streamline the automation of jobs traditionally performed by people. Nevertheless, it is crucial to acknowledge the possible disadvantages of Red AI, including its ecological footprint and its susceptibility to malevolent intentions. Developing Red AI responsibly and ethically is crucial to ensure its beneficial utilization. The advent of Red AI represents a significant milestone in the AI field. It signifies a transition from a period of AI research that prioritized the creation of compact and effective systems to a period of AI research that prioritizes the development of expansive and robust systems. The advent of Red AI holds the capacity to drive substantial progress in various domains, such as medicine, finance, and transportation. Nevertheless, it is crucial to acknowledge the possible disadvantages of Red AI and implement measures to alleviate them [10–14, 20].

1.6 SECURITY CONCERNS

Crimson Artificial Intelligence (AI) presents several security apprehensions, which encompass:

1. Heightened susceptibility to hostile attacks. Crimson artificial intelligence models exhibit greater intricacy and present a higher level of challenge in terms of comprehension compared to conventional AI models. This renders

them more susceptible to adversarial attacks, wherein an assailant meticulously constructs inputs to the model to induce it to generate inaccurate or detrimental outputs.

2. Elevated susceptibility to data poisoning. Crimson artificial intelligence models are trained using enormous volumes of data. An attacker can manipulate this data to introduce inaccurate or dangerous patterns, thus compromising the learning process of the model.
3. Elevated susceptibility to model theft. Crimson artificial intelligence models possess significant value. A potential intruder could illicitly acquire a Red AI model to employ it for personal objectives, such as executing adversarial assaults or creating novel products or services.
4. Heightened susceptibility to prejudice and unfair treatment. Crimson artificial intelligence models are trained with data that accurately represents the actual world. This data has the potential to exhibit bias and discrimination. Consequently, Red AI models can acquire bias and engage in discriminating behavior [15, 16].

1.6.1 Cybersecurity Threats

Crimson Artificial Intelligence (AI) presents several cybersecurity risks, which include:

- ***Elevated Susceptibility to Hostile Attacks*:** Crimson artificial intelligence models exhibit greater intricacy and present a more formidable challenge in terms of comprehension compared to conventional AI models. This renders them more susceptible to adversarial attacks, wherein an assailant meticulously constructs inputs to the model to induce it to generate inaccurate or detrimental outputs. As an illustration, a malicious individual could generate a counterfeit image to deceive a Red AI model into incorrectly categorizing it as an authentic image [17].
- ***Elevated Susceptibility to Data Poisoning*:** Crimson artificial intelligence models undergo training using enormous volumes of data. An attacker can manipulate this data to introduce inaccurate or damaging patterns into the model's learning process. As an illustration, a malicious individual could introduce contaminated information into a Red AI model employed for disease diagnosis. This has the potential to result in the model making incorrect diagnoses for patients or perhaps recommending detrimental treatments [10].
- ***Elevated Susceptibility to Intellectual Property Theft*:** Crimson artificial intelligence models possess significant value. A potential assailant could pilfer a Red AI model to exploit it for their agenda, such as executing adversarial assaults or creating novel products or services. As an illustration, a malicious individual could unlawfully acquire a Red AI model employed for forecasting stock market fluctuations. This would enable individuals to generate profits by engaging in stock market trading based on the model's forecasts.
- ***Heightened Susceptibility to Partiality and Prejudice*:** Crimson artificial intelligence models are trained with data that accurately represents the actual world. This data may exhibit bias and discrimination. Hence, Red AI

models can acquire biases and exhibit discriminating behavior. For instance, a Red AI model employed to make hiring decisions might acquire the ability to exhibit bias against specific demographics, such as women or minority groups [12].

It is crucial to implement measures to counteract the cybersecurity risks presented by Red AI. The steps involve the development of adversarial training approaches to enhance the resilience of Red AI models against adversarial attacks.

- Creating data cleansing methodologies to eliminate contaminated data from training datasets.
- Designing novel watermarking approaches to enhance the security of Red AI models and deter theft.
- Creating auditing methodologies to detect and address bias and discrimination in Red AI models.
- Deploying security measures to safeguard Red AI models against illegal access and utilization.

Utilizing Red AI responsibly and ethically is of utmost importance. This entails utilizing Red AI to address practical challenges in a manner that is advantageous to the entirety of society. Furthermore, it entails refraining from employing Red AI for nefarious intentions, such as the creation of weaponry or systems capable of inflicting harm against others.

1.6.2 Misinformation and Deepfakes

Within the domain of Red AI, the combination of false information and sophisticated manipulated media known as deepfakes poses a significant and difficult obstacle. The field of Red AI, which specifically concentrates on the utilization of artificial intelligence in security and defense, is confronted with the potential danger of malevolent individuals exploiting these technologies to alter perceptions and undermine vital systems. Intentionally spreading false information, whether through manipulated data or stories, can be used to trick AI systems that make decisions in security situations. Deepfakes possess the capability to effectively generate counterfeit audio and video material, hence introducing an added level of intricacy since they have the potential to create misleading situations or falsified communications. With the increasing importance of Red AI in military and security contexts, it is crucial to have strong detection methods, ethical guidelines in AI development, and strict regulations. These measures are necessary to prevent deliberate manipulation of information and the creation of misleading stories, which could have significant impacts on national security and global stability [16].

1.6.3 ETHICS IN GREEN AI

Green AI, which focuses on the development and implementation of environmentally sustainable artificial intelligence technologies, is not exempt from ethical considerations. Ethical considerations in Green AI extend beyond environmental impact to encompass a range of issues, including fairness, transparency, and social responsibility [13].

1. ***Environmental Impact Assessment*:** Ethical Green AI requires a thorough examination of the environmental impact of AI systems. This assessment should consider not only energy consumption but also the entire life cycle of AI technologies, from manufacturing to disposal.
2. ***Equitable Access to Green AI*:** It is crucial to ensure that the benefits of Green AI are distributed equitably across different communities and regions. Ethical considerations include addressing potential disparities in access to environmentally sustainable technologies and preventing the creation of new digital divides.
3. ***Transparency and Accountability*:** Developers of Green AI should prioritize transparency in their processes. This includes providing clear information about the environmental benefits and limitations of AI technologies. Moreover, accountability mechanisms should be in place to address any unintended consequences or environmental trade-offs.
4. ***Data Privacy and Security*:** Ethical Green AI involves safeguarding the privacy and security of data used in environmental monitoring and decision-making. Striking a balance between collecting necessary data for sustainable practices and respecting individual privacy is a critical ethical consideration.
5. ***Long-Term Sustainability*:** Green AI solutions should be designed with long-term sustainability in mind. This includes considering the potential environmental impact of AI technologies over extended periods and developing strategies to adapt and minimize negative consequences.
6. ***Ethical Sourcing of Materials*:** The development of Green AI hardware should adhere to ethical sourcing practices, ensuring that materials used in manufacturing are obtained responsibly and do not contribute to environmental degradation or human rights violations.
7. ***Community Engagement*:** Engaging with local communities and stakeholders is an ethical imperative in Green AI. Understanding and addressing the concerns and needs of communities affected by the deployment of environmentally sustainable AI technologies is essential for responsible and ethical development.

As the field of Green AI continues to evolve, ethical considerations will play a pivotal role in shaping sustainable, responsible, and socially beneficial applications of artificial intelligence for the betterment of both the environment and society.

1.6.4 Ethics in Red AI

Red AI, centered on the use of artificial intelligence in security and defense applications, introduces a set of unique ethical considerations due to its potential impact on national and global security. The ethical dimensions of Red AI extend beyond technology development to encompass issues related to human rights, accountability, and the potential consequences of AI-enabled decision-making in conflict scenarios.

1. ***Human Rights and Warfare*:** Ethical considerations in Red AI involve addressing the potential impact on human rights during armed conflicts. Developers and users of AI technologies must ensure that these systems adhere to international laws and conventions, avoiding actions that could lead to indiscriminate harm or violate the principles of proportionality and distinction.
2. ***Bias and Discrimination*:** Red AI systems must be designed and trained with a commitment to fairness and non-discrimination. Biases in data or algorithms can have severe consequences, leading to unjust targeting or profiling. Ethical considerations in Red AI demand continuous efforts to identify and mitigate bias throughout the development life cycle.
3. ***Transparency and Accountability*:** Ethical Red AI requires transparency in the decision-making processes of AI systems used in security and defense. Clear accountability mechanisms must be established to address errors, malfunctions, or unintended consequences, ensuring responsible and accountable use in sensitive contexts.
4. ***Autonomous Weapons and Human Control*:** The development of autonomous weapons raises ethical questions about the level of human control over AI-enabled military systems. Maintaining meaningful human oversight and decision-making authority is crucial to prevent the indiscriminate use of force and to uphold ethical standards in warfare.
5. ***Dual-Use Technology*:** Red AI technologies often have dual-use potential, meaning they can be applied for both civilian and military purposes. Ethical considerations involve carefully managing the transition between civilian and military applications to prevent unintended consequences and ensure that the technology is used responsibly.
6. ***International Collaboration and Norms*:** Ethical Red AI involves fostering international collaboration to establish norms and guidelines for the responsible use of AI in security and defense. Multilateral efforts can help mitigate the risk of an AI arms race and contribute to the development of ethical frameworks that govern the use of AI technologies in a global context.
7. ***Privacy and Surveillance*:** Red AI applications may involve extensive surveillance capabilities, raising ethical concerns related to privacy. Striking a balance between security needs and individual privacy rights is essential, requiring careful consideration of the scope and limits of surveillance technologies.

As Red AI continues to advance, ongoing dialogue and collaboration among stakeholders, including policymakers, ethicists, and technologists, are essential to ensure that these technologies are developed and deployed in ways that prioritize ethical considerations, human rights, and global security.

1.7 BALANCING GREEN AND RED AI

Balancing Green AI, which focuses on environmentally sustainable artificial intelligence, with Red AI, centered on security and defense applications, necessitates comprehensive policy and governance frameworks. The following considerations outline the roles of governments and international bodies, as well as potential regulatory approaches:

1. ***Role of Governments and International Bodies*:** Coordination and Collaboration: Governments play a pivotal role in facilitating collaboration between stakeholders involved in Green AI and Red AI development. Establishing interdisciplinary task forces and international collaborations can foster the exchange of best practices and ensure a holistic approach to AI governance.
    a. ***Ethical Guidelines*:** Governments should actively contribute to the formulation of ethical guidelines specific to Green and Red AI applications. These guidelines should address environmental sustainability, human rights, and security concerns, striking a balance between innovation and responsible use.
    b. ***Research and Development Funding*:** Governments can incentivize research and development efforts that prioritize the convergence of Green and Red AI. Funding initiatives that support environmentally sustainable technologies within the defense sector can spur innovation while minimizing ecological impact.

2. ***Regulatory Approaches***
    a. ***Environmental Impact Assessments*:** Regulatory frameworks should mandate thorough environmental impact assessments for both Green and Red AI technologies. These assessments must evaluate the entire life cycle, from manufacturing to deployment, to identify and address potential environmental risks and consequences.
    b. ***Transparency Requirements*:** Regulations should enforce transparency in the development and deployment of both Green and Red AI systems. This includes disclosing information about the environmental impact, decision-making processes, and potential biases to ensure accountability and build public trust.
    c. ***Human Rights and Security Standards*:** Regulatory bodies should establish clear standards regarding the ethical use of Red AI in security and defense contexts. These standards should align with international human rights conventions and emphasize the importance of maintaining human control over AI-enabled decision-making in conflict scenarios.
    d. ***International Cooperation*:** Governments and international bodies should work collaboratively to establish common standards and norms for the responsible development and deployment of AI technologies. This can help prevent a fragmented regulatory landscape and promote global security and environmental sustainability.

Balancing Green and Red AI requires a nuanced approach that considers both ecological impact and security imperatives. Governments, in collaboration with international bodies, must adopt regulatory frameworks that promote innovation while addressing ethical concerns and ensuring the responsible use of AI technologies in diverse applications. By integrating environmental sustainability and security considerations into policy and governance, a harmonious coexistence between Green and Red AI can be achieved.

1.7.1 Responsible AI Development

Responsible AI development entails the incorporation of both Green and Red AI principles, ensuring that ethical and sustainable practices are at the forefront of technological advancement. Following are key considerations for responsible AI development:

1. ***Incorporating Green AI Principles***: Energy Efficiency: Developers should prioritize energy-efficient algorithms and hardware design to minimize the environmental impact of AI systems. This includes optimizing model architectures, using energy-efficient hardware, and implementing techniques like model quantization.
   a. ***Life Cycle Assessment***: Responsible AI development involves conducting comprehensive life cycle assessments for AI systems. This assessment should evaluate the environmental impact from raw material extraction and manufacturing to usage and disposal, ensuring a holistic understanding of the technology's ecological footprint.
   b. ***Renewable Energy Usage***: Emphasizing the use of renewable energy sources in data centers and AI infrastructure contributes to the overall sustainability of AI systems. Developers should explore ways to power AI applications with clean and renewable energy.
2. ***Incorporating Red AI Principles***
   a. ***Ethical AI Decision-Making***: Developers must embed ethical considerations into the decision-making processes of Red AI systems. This involves ensuring transparency, accountability, and adherence to human rights standards in the design and deployment of AI technologies in security and defense applications.
   b. ***Human Oversight***: Maintaining human control and oversight in Red AI systems is essential. Developers should design AI technologies to augment human decision-making rather than replace it entirely, particularly in sensitive contexts where the consequences of autonomous actions can be significant.
   c. ***Bias Mitigation***: Red AI developers need to actively address biases in data and algorithms. Robust measures should be implemented to identify and mitigate biases, ensuring fair and unbiased decision-making in security and defense applications.

3. ***Ensuring Ethical and Sustainable AI Practices***
   a. ***Interdisciplinary Collaboration*:** Responsible AI development requires collaboration between technologists, ethicists, environmental scientists, and other experts. Interdisciplinary teams can bring diverse perspectives to the table, fostering the development of AI systems that are both ethical and sustainable [21].
   b. ***Continuous Monitoring and Auditing*:** Developers should implement continuous monitoring and auditing mechanisms for AI systems. This includes regular assessments of environmental impact, ethical considerations, and potential biases, with a commitment to making necessary adjustments to enhance sustainability and fairness.
   c. ***Stakeholder Engagement*:** Engaging with diverse stakeholders, including communities, advocacy groups, and end-users, is crucial for responsible AI development. Incorporating feedback from various perspectives helps identify potential ethical concerns and ensures that AI systems align with societal values. By integrating Green and Red AI principles into the development process, responsible AI development aims to create technologies that not only advance innovation but also adhere to ethical standards and promote sustainability across diverse applications [22].

1.8 CONCLUSION

In conclusion, the intersection of Green and Red AI presents a dynamic landscape that requires careful consideration of environmental sustainability, ethical principles, and security imperatives. Responsible AI development involves balancing the advancements in technology with a commitment to minimizing ecological impact and ensuring ethical practices. Following are key takeaways and a summary of the ongoing evolution of Green and Red AI:

1. ***Balancing Act*:** Achieving a balance between Green and Red AI is crucial for a sustainable and secure AI future. This involves incorporating energy-efficient practices, ethical decision-making, and human oversight in the development of AI technologies.
2. ***Environmental Impact*:** Green AI emphasizes the importance of minimizing the ecological footprint of AI systems through energy efficiency, life cycle assessments, and the use of renewable energy sources.
3. ***Ethical Considerations*:** Red AI introduces unique ethical considerations, including human rights, transparency, and bias mitigation. Ethical AI development requires responsible decision-making in security and defense applications to ensure fairness and accountability.
4. ***Interdisciplinary Collaboration*:** Responsible AI development necessitates collaboration among diverse stakeholders, including technologists, ethicists, environmental scientists, policymakers, and communities. Interdisciplinary efforts contribute to well-rounded solutions that address both environmental and ethical concerns.

The evolution of Green and Red AI is an ongoing process that requires continuous innovation, adaptation, and ethical reflection. Technological advancements must align with environmental sustainability goals and ethical principles to meet the complex challenges posed by these two domains. As AI continues to evolve, the integration of responsible practices becomes integral to shaping a future where technology enhances human well-being without compromising the environment or ethical standards. Call to Action for a Sustainable and Secure AI Future: As we navigate the intricate landscape of Green and Red AI, a collective call to action is essential. This involves:

1. ***Regulatory Frameworks*****:** Governments and international bodies must collaborate to establish comprehensive regulatory frameworks that guide the responsible development and deployment of AI technologies. These frameworks should address environmental impact, ethical considerations, and security standards.
2. ***Industry Responsibility*****:** The tech industry should take a proactive role in adopting ethical and sustainable practices. This includes investing in research and development that prioritizes environmental sustainability, ethical AI principles, and the well-being of society.
3. ***Public Awareness*****:** Educating the public about the environmental and ethical implications of AI technologies fosters informed decision-making and encourages responsible AI use. Public awareness campaigns can drive demand for sustainable and ethical AI solutions.
4. ***Research and Innovation*****:** Encouraging ongoing research and innovation in AI technologies is crucial for finding new solutions that advance both environmental sustainability and security. Collaboration between academia, industry, and governments can drive breakthroughs in responsible AI development.

In the pursuit of a sustainable and secure AI future, the integration of Green and Red AI principles offers a pathway to harness the benefits of artificial intelligence while safeguarding the planet and upholding ethical standards. By embracing responsible AI development, we can shape a future where technology serves humanity and the environment in harmony.

REFERENCES

[1] Morrar, R., Arman, H., & Mousa, S. (2017). The fourth industrial revolution (Industry 4.0): A social innovation perspective. *Technology Innovation Management Review*, *7*(11), 12–20.
[2] Shukla, A. K., Janmaijaya, M., Abraham, A., & Muhuri, P. K. (2019). Engineering applications of artificial intelligence: A bibliometric analysis of 30 years (1988–2018). *Engineering Applications of Artificial Intelligence*, *85*, 517–532.
[3] Kassens-Noor, E., & Hintze, A. (2020). Cities of the future? The potential impact of artificial intelligence. *AI*, *1*(2), 12.

[4] Ortega-Fernández, A., Martín-Rojas, R., & García-Morales, V. J. (2020). Artificial intelligence in the urban environment: Smart cities as models for developing innovation and sustainability. *Sustainability*, *12*(19), 7860.

[5] Tiddi, I., Bastianelli, E., Daga, E., d'Aquin, M., & Motta, E. (2020). Robot–city interaction: Mapping the research landscape – A survey of the interactions between robots and modern cities. *International Journal of Social Robotics*, *12*, 299–324.

[6] Wirtz, B. W., Weyerer, J. C., & Geyer, C. (2019). Artificial intelligence and the public sector – Applications and challenges. *International Journal of Public Administration*, *42*(7), 596–615.

[7] Desouza, K. C., Dawson, G. S., & Chenok, D. (2020). Designing, developing, and deploying artificial intelligence systems: Lessons from and for the public sector. *Business Horizons*, *63*(2), 205–213.

[8] Yigitcanlar, T., & Cugurullo, F. (2020). The sustainability of artificial intelligence: An urbanistic viewpoint from the lens of smart and sustainable cities. *Sustainability*, *12*(20), 8548.

[9] Nishant, R., Kennedy, M., & Corbett, J. (2020). Artificial intelligence for sustainability: Challenges, opportunities, and a research agenda. *International Journal of Information Management*, *53*, 102104.

[10] Kuziemski, M., & Misuraca, G. (2020). AI governance in the public sector: Three tales from the frontiers of automated decision-making in democratic settings. *Telecommunications Policy*, *44*(6), 101976.

[11] Floridi, L., Cowls, J., Beltrametti, M., Chatila, R., Chazerand, P., Dignum, V., & Vayena, E. (2021). An ethical framework for a good AI society: Opportunities, risks, principles, and recommendations. In L. Floridi (Ed.), *Ethics, governance, and policies in artificial intelligence*, pp. 19–39. Cham: Springer.

[12] Yun, J. J., Lee, D., Ahn, H., Park, K., & Yigitcanlar, T. (2016). Not deep learning but autonomous learning of open innovation for sustainable artificial intelligence. *Sustainability*, *8*(8), 797.

[13] Mortoja, M. G., & Yigitcanlar, T. (2020). Local drivers of anthropogenic climate change: Quantifying the impact through a remote sensing approach in Brisbane. *Remote Sensing*, *12*(14), 2270.

[14] Gupta, S., Langhans, S. D., Domisch, S., Fuso-Nerini, F., Felländer, A., Battaglini, M., & Vinuesa, R. (2021). Assessing whether artificial intelligence is an enabler or an inhibitor of sustainability at indicator level. *Transportation Engineering*, *4*, 100064.

[15] Ye, Z., Yang, J., Zhong, N., Tu, X., Jia, J., & Wang, J. (2020). Tackling environmental challenges in pollution controls using artificial intelligence: A review. *Science of the Total Environment*, *699*, 134279.

[16] Haupt, S. E., Pasini, A., & Marzban, C. (Eds.). (2008). *Artificial intelligence methods in the environmental sciences*. Springer Science & Business Media.

[17] Jin, L., Duan, K., & Tang, X. (2018). What is the relationship between technological innovation and energy consumption? Empirical analysis based on provincial panel data from China. *Sustainability*, *10*(1), 145.

[18] Yigitcanlar, T., Mehmood, R., & Corchado, J. M. (2021). Green artificial intelligence: Towards an efficient, sustainable and equitable technology for smart cities and futures. *Sustainability*, *13*(16), 8952.

[19] Arshad, R., Zahoor, S., Shah, M. A., Wahid, A., & Yu, H. (2017). Green IoT: An investigation on energy saving practices for 2020 and beyond. *IEEE Access*, *5*, 15667–15681.

[20] Hornsey, M. J., & Fielding, K. S. (2020). Understanding (and reducing) inaction on climate change. *Social Issues and Policy Review*, *14*(1), 3–35.
[21] Van Wynsberghe, A. (2021). Sustainable AI: AI for sustainability and the sustainability of AI. *AI and Ethics*, *1*(3), 213–218.
[22] Attard-Frost, B., De los Ríos, A., & Walters, D. R. (2023). The ethics of AI business practices: A review of 47 AI ethics guidelines. *AI and Ethics*, 3(2), 389–406.

2 The Eco-Ethical Nexus
Convergence of Red and Green AI Paradigms

Srinivas Talasila, N. Neelima, Aruru Sai Kumar, E. Vijaya Babu, and N. Sunanda
VNR Vignana Jyothi Institute of Engineering & Technology, Hyderabad, India

2.1 INTRODUCTION TO ARTIFICIAL INTELLIGENCE

In recent years, there has been a remarkable surge in Artificial Intelligence, especially in the realm of deep learning. This advancement has ushered in transformative changes in our daily lives, exceeding what we could have envisioned just a few years ago. AI already proved its capability in various applications. One notable impact of AI is evident in the realm of autonomous vehicles, where cars are now capable of driving themselves. This breakthrough not only enhances convenience but also holds the potential to revolutionize transportation systems, making them safer and more efficient. Similarly, in the field of healthcare, machine learning and deep learning algorithms have become invaluable tools. Computer programs adeptly analyze complex medical images, such as X-rays, aiding in quicker and more accurate diagnoses. Amidst the challenges posed by pandemics, AI plays a pivotal role in forecasting disease outbreaks, supporting medical diagnoses, and influencing crucial healthcare decisions. Furthermore, the entertainment industry has witnessed significant changes with the integration of recommendation engines in video-on-demand services. These engines leverage machine learning algorithms to understand user preferences, providing personalized content suggestions. Especially during times when individuals find themselves confined to their homes, such services offer a welcome escape, allowing people to immerse themselves in entertainment and temporarily set aside their concerns [1–4].

The ongoing AI revolution has propelled us into an era where the applications of machine learning and deep learning extend far beyond our initial expectations. While the current landscape reflects impressive achievements, it is important to note that we are still far from reaching the culmination of the AI revolution. We are currently in the early stages of AI development, where the primary goal is to identify the architecture that yields the highest accuracy for a given task, essentially obtaining superior results by investing heavily in computational resources. The cost of conducting AI research is increasing due to the large models which increases

 DOI: 10.1201/9781003546382-2

computational requirements. This trajectory is unsustainable. There has been a lack of emphasis on prioritizing straightforward models, streamlined procedures, and results that can be easily reproduced [5]. Instead, researchers have directed their attention predominantly toward the pursuit of high accuracy in their findings. The call for a balance between the accuracy and simplicity of the models remains crucial for fostering a more robust and collaborative scientific landscape.

Figure 2.1 illustrates the evolution of the model size for several cutting-edge deep learning algorithms over time. Regardless of their diverse applications, these trends suggest that the expansion of deep learning theory and infrastructure—specifically, the accessibility of GPUs and TPUs for computing—has led to the development of exceptionally large models. Naturally, the next question to consider is whether increased computational requirements have led to improved accuracy. Figure 2.2 illustrates the relationship between accuracy and model size for a few widely used computer vision models. While some models show a slight increase in accuracy, the associated rise in computing resources is quite substantial. Popular benchmark leaderboards often showcase instances of heightened performance achieved by simply ramping up processing power, commonly referred to as Red AI. In Figure 2.2, the model's parameter count serves as a stand-in for its size. Typically, larger models are more realistic, as evident in the comparison above. However, it's worth noting that some of the smaller models exhibit nearly equivalent accuracy. What raises concerns here is that the bigger models require more electricity, putting a strain on our infrastructure. The size of the model not only has environmental implications but also comes with a hefty cost for those responsible for more power consumption.

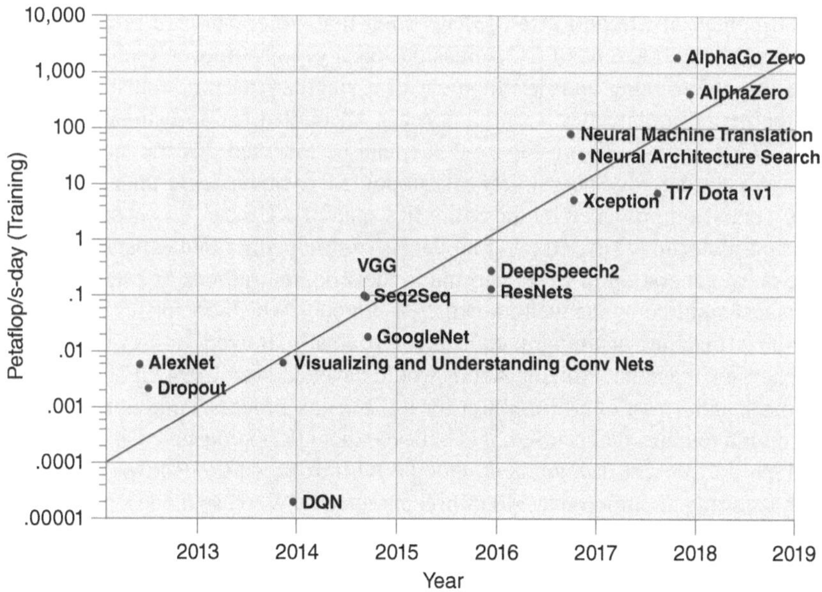

FIGURE 2.1 Petaflops/s-day required for training the state-of-the-art deep learning models [1].

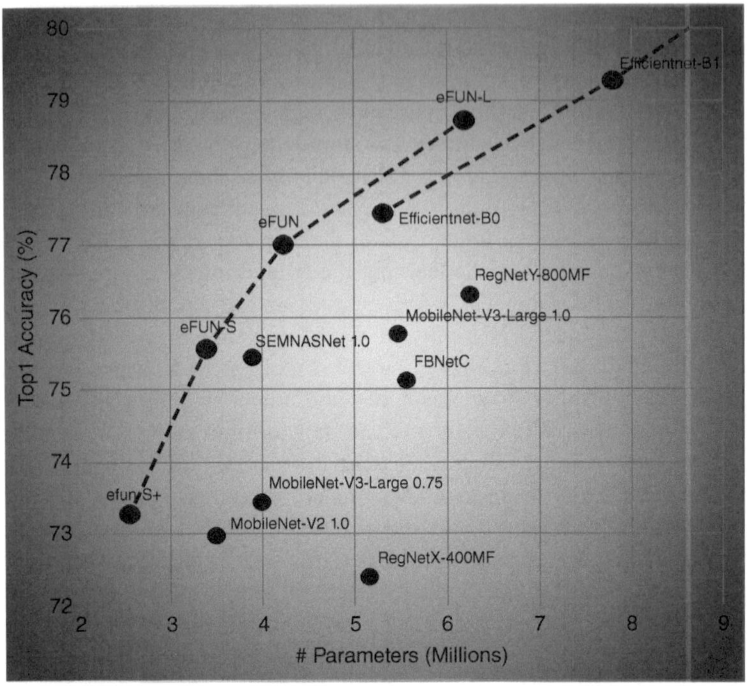

FIGURE 2.2 Accuracy versus parameters in deep learning models [2].

The findings of Strubell et al. [3] revealed that Americans are responsible for approximately 36,000 tons of CO_2 emissions each year. Moreover, their study highlighted that the training and development of a singular machine translation model using the neural architecture search approach accounted for an estimated 626,000 tons of CO_2 emissions. From Figure 2.3, it can be assessed that the environmental impact of a cutting-edge neural network model is five times larger than the cumulative CO_2 emission produced by the entire life span of a US car. It is noteworthy that the carbon footprint attributed to AI models is experiencing rapid expansion.

The latest generation of deep learning models boasts millions or even billions of weights, exemplified by the well-known GPT-3 model, which comprises a staggering 175 billion machine learning parameters. Originally trained on NVIDIA V100, researchers estimate that utilizing A100s would have required 1,024 GPUs, a duration of 34 days, and a cost of $4.6 million for the training process. Although the energy consumption remains undisclosed, it is believed that GPT-3 consumed approximately 936 MWh. In a recent development, Google AI introduced the Pathways Language Model, featuring an impressive 540 billion parameters. As these models grow in size, the demand for servers to process them increases exponentially, essential for handling progressively complex tasks.

Schwartz et al. [4] have proposed a classification framework distinguishing artificial intelligence into two categories: Red AI and Green AI. This categorization is based on the energy consumption characteristics of AI systems. In their model, Red AI

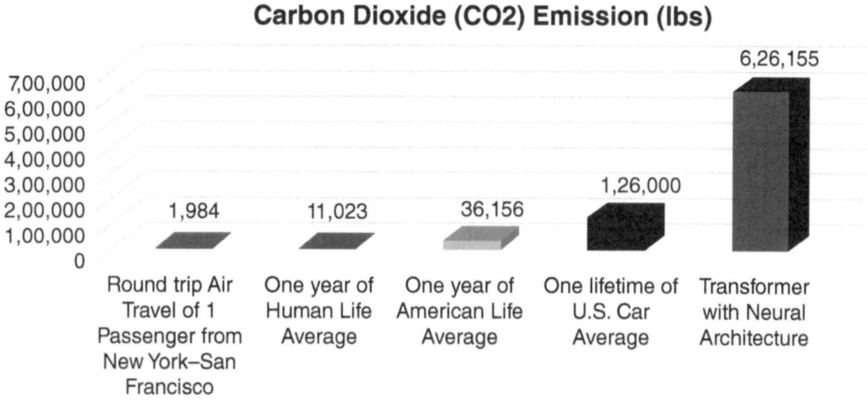

FIGURE 2.3 Carbon dioxide emission in lbs, based on data [3].

encompasses energy-intensive artificial intelligence applications, often referred to as Energy-Hungry AI. These systems typically demand significant computational resources and power to execute specific tasks. Examples of Red AI applications may include complex neural network training, large-scale data processing, and resource-intensive simulations. Conversely, Green AI, as identified by Schwartz et al. [4], represents energy-efficient artificial intelligence. This category is characterized by AI systems that prioritize resource optimization and reduce energy consumption. Green AI aims to develop intelligent algorithms and models that achieve high performance with minimal environmental impact. Applications falling under Green AI may include energy-efficient machine learning models, optimized algorithms, and approaches that prioritize sustainability in AI design.

The major contributions of this chapter include:

- Delves deeply into the nuanced aspects of Red AI, offering a comprehensive exploration of its ethical dimensions within the field of artificial intelligence.
- Examines how Green AI embodies sustainability by integrating principles of energy efficiency, renewable energy utilization, and environmental monitoring into the development of AI technologies.
- Discusses the intersection points between Red AI and Green AI, highlighting how ethical and ecological considerations are interrelated within the realm of artificial intelligence.
- Analyzes the implications of Red AI and Green AI on the broader landscape of AI development.

This chapter is designed to systematically navigate the intricate terrain of artificial intelligence (AI). Commencing with Section 2.1, it lays the groundwork by delivering a foundational introduction to AI. Sections 2.2 and 2.3 delve into the distinctive domains of Red AI, concentrating on ethical considerations, and Green AI, which revolves around sustainability. In Section 2.4, the chapter investigates the rationales behind the adoption of Green AI, providing insights into its motivations. Further,

Section 2.5 delineates the fundamental principles at the core of Green AI, serving as a guide for the development of environmentally conscious AI. Section 2.6 takes a pragmatic approach, exploring the crafting of efficient algorithms within the context of Green AI. Moving on to Section 2.7, the chapter scrutinizes the manifold applications of Green AI across diverse industries. Section 2.8 underscores pivotal factors crucial for the successful construction of Green AI, with an emphasis on practical considerations. Sections 2.9 and 2.10 furnish a framework for evaluating the performance, ethics, and environmental impact of both Green and Red AI. Finally, Section 2.11 concludes the chapter, by offering closing thoughts and summarizing the vital insights gleaned from the exploration of AI, ethics, and sustainability.

2.2 RED ARTIFICIAL INTELLIGENCE: RED AI

A broad range of AI-related tasks such as pattern recognition, object identification, classification, natural language processing, etc., have shown impressive advancements within the past decade. These advancements have been fueled by the development of increasingly larger and computationally demanding deep learning models. A substantial research effort that assessed the carbon emissions associated with various deep learning models argues that the current trajectory is economically and environmentally unsustainable, presenting obstacles to meaningful engagement in research. AI researchers are driven by the aspiration to foster creativity and advanced technology at the forefront. However, attaining these breakthroughs necessitates substantial computational resources, leading to an increased demand for additional resources to extract meaningful insights from data. Constructing larger deep learning models for significant performance, entailing exponential demands for computation, training data, time, and other costly inputs. An unfortunate consequence of these deep models is what they demand as substantial computational resources, leading to detrimental environmental effects. These resource-intensive AI systems are commonly labeled as "red AI."

The AI community's relentless focus on pushing the boundaries to achieve state-of-the-art results often prioritizes metrics like accuracy while neglecting important considerations such as cost and efficiency. This singular emphasis fails to account for the broader social, environmental, and economic impacts associated with pursuing these objectives. Despite the undeniable benefits of advancing model accuracy, the exclusive focus on this metric sidelines the crucial discussion about the overall costs and consequences involved. This gap in evaluation and discourse has spurred the emergence of the Red AI movement. The sustainability challenges and entry barriers associated with Red AI make it an impractical long-term solution, irrespective of its scientific merits. Looking ahead, the AI community must proactively focus on developing deep learning models that are energy-efficient to address environmental concerns.

2.3 GREEN ARTIFICIAL INTELLIGENCE: GREEN AI

"Green AI" refers to a well-established and broad interest in scientific research that prioritizes ecological sustainability. Artificial intelligence research can incur significant computational costs, but there are always avenues to improve efficiency. To set a standard for upcoming research aiming to use data more effectively, research publications might need to chart accuracy against computing cost and training set size.

A core principle of Green AI practices involves transparently disclosing the computing costs associated with model discovery, training, and operation.

Historically, the predominant focus in research has leaned toward Red AI, driven by the relentless pursuit of high accuracy levels. However, Green AI, despite not being a primary emphasis for most, addresses the computational costs linked to running deep learning algorithms, making it a noteworthy area deserving attention and support. Unlike Red AI, which contributes to atmospheric carbon emissions, Green AI prioritizes efficiency in its quest for accuracy. The financial barriers associated with achieving Green AI have made deep learning research inaccessible for stakeholders such as academics, researchers, and students. As a consequence, major corporations entrenched in the field of AI, such as Amazon, Google, and Microsoft, have taken the lead in embracing and advancing Green AI.

The research study conducted by Roy Schwartz et al. [4] for AI played a pivotal role in initiating conversation on Green AI. The report suggested prioritization of Green AI initiatives, specifically emphasizing the energy efficiency of AI systems. The motivation behind this study was the recognition that numerous significant advancements in artificial intelligence are accompanied by substantial carbon footprints. Despite the significant advancements expected in artificial intelligence during the 2020s, the development of infrastructure and energy efficiency in this field is still in its early stages.

Figure 2.4 provides a concise overview of the distinctions between Red AI and Green AI, highlighting their respective metric and measures [5]. Green AI places a primary emphasis on efficiency and cost reduction, aiming to optimize resource utilization. On the other hand, Red AI is oriented towards enhancing accuracy, prioritizing precision in its outcomes. Achieving a harmonious balance in systems requires careful consideration of how to seamlessly integrate heterogeneous components, ensuring that efficiency gains and accuracy improvements are realized cohesively. This emphasizes the importance of finding a middle ground between the efficiency-driven goals of Green AI and the accuracy-driven objectives of Red AI to create holistic and effective AI applications.

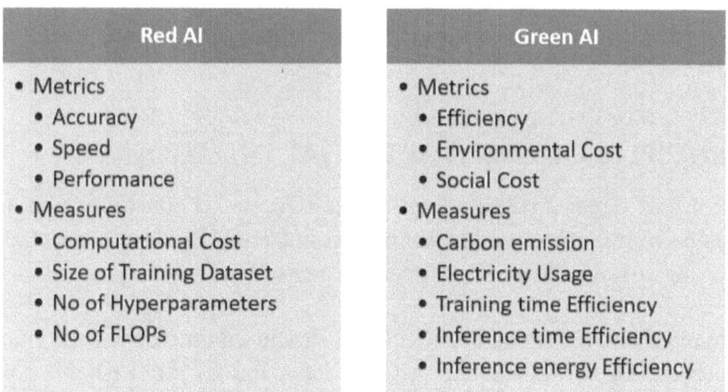

FIGURE 2.4 Comparisons between Red AI and Green AI.

2.4 REASONS FOR ADOPTING GREEN AI

The impact of Artificial Intelligence on the environment is currently a prominent and evolving topic of concern in contemporary discourse. AI can play a valuable role in advancing eco-friendly practices and solutions for climate mitigation, yet it is essential to acknowledge that harnessing its potential often demands substantial energy consumption. Understanding the evaluation of AI systems depends on the dataset size, with assessments conducted based on either energy consumption or carbon emissions. This is crucial because, unlike incremental improvements in accuracy, the complexity and computational demands of AI models increase exponentially. Achieving higher levels of accuracy and precision involves the development of larger, more intricate models, incurring costs associated with 1) model training; 2) dataset size; and 3) the number of trials required.

As per a blog article by OpenAI [1], there has been a staggering 300,000-fold increase in the computational power required for the most significant AI training operations from 2012 to 2018. This ongoing trend, which has been a pivotal driver of AI progress, underscores the need to prepare for the ramifications of systems that far surpass the capabilities of today's technology. The fervent focus of the AI community on attaining state-of-the-art results, often emphasizing accuracy and similar metrics while neglecting considerations of cost and efficiency, is the driving force behind the Red AI movement. The cumulative expenditure of time, energy, and finances in such projects significantly outweighs the cost of achieving the desired results. Consequently, this realization is driving the active promotion and expansion of "Green AI" practices that prioritize environmental sustainability.

The other three motives, beyond environmental sustainability, propel the advancement of green AI. Firstly, there is a noticeable decline in the performance of certain widely used models. To elaborate, as researchers strive for greater accuracy by increasing model and training data sizes, they encounter diminishing returns. In simpler terms, employing larger models no longer guarantees a proportional increase in accuracy. The second driver stems from the aspiration for inclusive AI development. When computational requirements become a barrier to entry, it becomes challenging for regular researchers to engage in AI research programs. The third motivation revolves around business considerations. While cloud AI services can be economically generated on the backend of a cloud infrastructure, edge AI products face limitations due to stringent energy efficiency requirements during deployment.

2.5 PRINCIPLES OF GREEN ARTIFICIAL INTELLIGENCE

The principles of Green Artificial Intelligence (Green AI) constitute a set of guidelines designed to minimize the environmental impact of AI development and usage while fostering sustainability. These principles encompass:

- ***Efficiency and Optimization***: Green AI should minimize the computational resources, energy consumption, and data storage requirements through techniques like model pruning, quantization, and hardware optimization.

- ***Sustainability and Circularity***: The entire AI lifecycle, from development and training to deployment and maintenance, should embrace sustainable practices. This involves utilizing renewable energy sources, reducing e-waste, and considering the environmental impact of data centers.
- ***Environmentally Beneficial Applications***: Green AI should prioritize applications that directly address environmental challenges and promote sustainability, including renewable energy optimization, smart grid management, precision agriculture, and environmental monitoring.
- ***Fairness and Equity***: Fair and equitable development and use of green artificial intelligence should take into account the possible social and environmental effects on various groups. This calls for guaranteeing broad benefits and eliminating biases in AI models.
- ***Transparency and Explainability***: Transparency and explainability are key components of green AI systems since they enable users to discern any biases and comprehend the decision-making processes involved. Establishing trust and promoting ethical AI development depends on this openness.
- ***Collaboration and Openness***: Supporting open-source AI initiatives, data-sharing agreements, and multi-stakeholder collaborations are a few examples of how collaborative and open green AI development should be to foster knowledge sharing and collective action.
- ***Lifelong Learning and Adaptation***: To ensure that green AI systems are effective in tackling environmental concerns over time, they need to continually learn from and adapt to new data as well as changing environmental circumstances.
- ***Ethical Considerations and Governance***: The development of green AI should take responsibility for matters like privacy, data security, and accountability while abiding by moral standards and strong governance structures.

Green AI may be a key player in solving environmental issues and advancing a sustainable future by adhering to these ideals.

2.6 DEVELOPMENT OF EFFICIENT GREEN AI ALGORITHMS AND HARDWARE

Efficiently developing AI algorithms and hardware with a focus on energy conservation is pivotal for realizing the full potential of Green AI. The following key strategies [6] outline comprehensive approaches in this endeavor:

1. ***Algorithm Optimization*:** Algorithmic improvements play a crucial role in energy-efficient AI. Model pruning involves the removal of redundant or insignificant connections in neural networks, reducing computational complexity. Quantization lowers the precision of data representation, thereby decreasing memory requirements and improving inference speed (for example: 64-bit floating-point model parameters as smaller ones, such as 32-bit and 16-bit). Knowledge distillation is a process of transferring insights from large, complex models to smaller, more efficient models [7].

2. ***Hardware Optimization*:** Tailoring hardware for AI workloads is essential for efficiency. Specialized AI accelerators, such as GPUs, TPUs, and FPGAs, are designed to enhance processing capabilities [8, 9]. Neuromorphic computing mimics the structure and function of the human brain, achieving energy-efficient computation [10]. Edge computing involves processing data closer to the source, reducing data transmission and energy consumption.
3. ***Data Optimization*:** Efficient data handling is crucial for energy-efficient AI. Data caching involves storing frequently accessed data in memory to reduce redundant data transfers. Data compression reduces the size of data without compromising its integrity. Data sampling selects a subset of representative data for training and inference, optimizing resource usage.
4. ***Software Optimization*:** Choosing energy-efficient algorithms and frameworks is vital in software optimization. Code optimization involves using compiler techniques to reduce code complexity and enhance performance. Efficient resource management, including CPU, memory, and power consumption, contributes to overall software optimization.
5. ***Infrastructure Optimization*:** Optimizing the infrastructure further enhances the energy efficiency of AI systems. Utilizing renewable energy sources, improving cooling efficiency, and employing virtualization techniques in data centers contribute to sustainability. Cloud computing involves leveraging energy-efficient cloud infrastructure and adopting cloud-native AI solutions. Edge devices benefit from employing low-power microcontrollers and optimizing AI applications for resource-constrained devices.

By implementing these strategies, we can create energy-efficient AI solutions that minimize the environmental impact of AI technologies and contribute to a more sustainable future.

2.7 GREEN AI IN VARIOUS INDUSTRIES

For the sake of environmental sustainability, Green Artificial Intelligence can be beneficial across a wide range of sectors. Some of them are:

2.7.1 Agriculture

Green AI has the potential to completely change agriculture by improving agricultural productivity, sustainability, and efficiency. Green AI enables precision agriculture by leveraging machine learning algorithms to analyze data from various sources such as satellites, sensors, and drones. This allows farmers to make data-driven decisions on irrigation, fertilization, and pest control, optimizing resource use and minimizing environmental impact [11]. By analyzing images of crops, Green AI systems can identify signs of diseases or nutrient deficiencies, enabling early intervention and reducing the need for excessive pesticide use [12]. Precisely delivering water to crops based on their actual needs, Green AI systems conserve water resources and reduce energy consumption [13]. These systems can be able to optimize planting strategies, manage inventory, and plan for market demand, thereby reducing waste and increasing overall productivity [14].

2.7.2 Energy

Green AI is making substantial strides in the energy sector, fostering sustainability and efficiency. In energy management, AI enables the optimization of consumption by analyzing historical and real-time data, leading to reduced waste and cost savings. Smart grids, powered by AI technologies, enhance grid stability and support demand response initiatives, contributing to a more resilient and efficient energy infrastructure [15]. AI plays a pivotal role in the integration of renewable energy sources, predicting production and managing intermittency for a smoother transition to cleaner energy. Predictive maintenance, facilitated by AI-driven analytics, prevents equipment failures and downtime, reducing the environmental impact of unplanned outages. Green AI also contributes to the optimization of energy-efficient buildings, controlling lighting, Heating, Ventilation, and Air Conditioning (HVAC) systems, and other utilities based on real-time data, leading to improved energy efficiency [16].

2.7.3 Medical

Green AI is making significant inroads in the medical field, contributing to enhanced healthcare practices and environmental sustainability. In medical imaging, AI applications are optimizing diagnostic processes by improving image analysis, aiding in early disease detection, and minimizing the need for resource-intensive procedures [17]. Additionally, AI-driven predictive analytics are streamlining patient care by analyzing vast datasets, identifying patterns, and assisting healthcare professionals in making informed decisions, ultimately improving efficiency and reducing unnecessary interventions [18]. By harnessing Green AI in medical practices, there is a dual benefit of advancing patient outcomes while also promoting environmentally conscious and resource-efficient healthcare solutions.

2.7.4 Transportation and Logistics

AI applications optimize route planning and traffic management, reducing fuel consumption and emissions by enhancing overall transportation efficiency [19]. Moreover, AI-driven predictive maintenance in logistics ensures the timely identification of potential equipment failures, reducing downtime and environmental impact [20]. In autonomous vehicles, Green AI focuses on optimizing energy efficiency, reducing emissions, and enhancing overall sustainability in transportation [21]. By leveraging Green AI in transportation and logistics, organizations can not only improve operational efficiency but also contribute to a more sustainable and environmentally conscious industry.

2.8 KEY FACTORS FOR BUILDING GREEN AI

Enhancing communication, advancing technology, and gaining a more profound understanding of deep learning are essential elements in constructing the future of Green AI. The first step toward developing AI that is more ecologically friendly is to have a suitable quantitative instrument. With the help of this tool, we can determine how much energy an AI model uses, describe it, compare it to other models, and look into more environmentally friendly variants. The number of floating-point operations is a statistic that the Allen Institute for AI recommends adopting and urges academics to include in their work. Additionally, a machine learning emissions calculator [22] is another tool that takes into account many parameters such as cloud providers, hardware kinds, and geographic locations [23]. Furthermore, OpenAI keeps a close eye on the most recent AI models' energy efficiency, concentrating on vision and translation applications in particular [24]. Encouraging the development and commercialization of environmentally friendly artificial intelligence can be achieved through the following methods (Figure 2.5):

- Researchers sometimes encounter difficulties in reproducing results, even with access to the code, and all too often, AI research is published without accompanying code. The act of making research publicly accessible may pose internal challenges for researchers. These factors, contributing to redundant efforts and impeding efficient sharing, are significant contributors to the challenges associated with Red AI today. Reforming the practice of publishing papers without accompanying code is crucial, as access to the source code is imperative for reproducing research results. All publishers need to adopt a policy requiring the submission of code along with research papers to ensure transparency and reproducibility in scientific endeavors.
- Improvements in hardware performance contribute to increased performance and more effective outcomes in handling deep learning workloads. Google introduced Tensor Processing Units (TPUs) in response to the AI community's demand for Graphics Processing Units (GPUs), prompting the entire semiconductor industry to shift towards more specialized products. Dedicated hardware tailored for AI workloads is what NVIDIA, Intel, and other chip industries need to concentrate on more.
- Researchers currently face a deficit in understanding deep learning. While the scientific community acknowledges the effectiveness of deep learning,

IMPROVING REPRODUCIBILITY AND SHARING INFORMATION
IMPROVING HARDWARE PERFORMANCE
UNDERSTANDING DEEP LEARNING
DEMOCRATIZATIO N OF DEEP LEARNING
AI PARTNERS

FIGURE 2.5 Key factors that need to be considered for building Green AI systems.

there remains an incomplete comprehension of how or why it achieves its outcomes. Providing detailed insights into the underlying science of deep learning and formally articulating its strengths and weaknesses can facilitate the development of more precise and efficient models.

- Exploring the democratization of deep learning in research is captivating, and existing models exhibit sufficient accuracy for versatile applications. Deep learning technologies have broad applicability across various business and scientific domains, and the likelihood of substantial enhancements in performance and energy efficiency increases when a diverse array of individuals engages in the development of the technology.
- Establishing partnerships is pivotal for AI development. While many executives at the world's largest firms may lack the skills required for effective AI development, they recognize the substantial role that deep learning and AI will play in future products and services. To initiate their AI strategy, companies should pursue collaborations with universities, accelerators, and startups instead of pursuing independent efforts.

2.9 PARAMETERS FOR EVALUATING GREEN AND RED AI

AI systems that are classified as Green AI or Red AI can be evaluated based on both system-specific criteria and the natural resources powering them. These factors encompass carbon emissions, data size, and training costs. Additionally, the evaluation includes an assessment of the resources expended in managing these costs, such as financial resources, carbon emissions, power consumption, model runtime, and other measurable inputs.

2.9.1 Carbon Emissions

The link between the calculation of carbon dioxide emissions and efficiency is significant. Efficiency plays a pivotal role in determining the environmental impact of algorithmic processes. A direct correlation exists between the efficiency of these processes and the amount of carbon released into the atmosphere. When an algorithm operates more efficiently, it signifies that it accomplishes its tasks with less waste and resource consumption, which in turn results in lower carbon emissions.

Enhanced efficiency contributes to a reduction in the overall carbon footprint in several ways. First and foremost, it leads to a shorter runtime for model training and testing. A more efficient algorithm can process and analyze data more quickly, requiring less time to complete its tasks. This reduced runtime is crucial because it directly translates to lower energy consumption during the computational processes. As a result, the overall carbon emissions associated with the energy-intensive tasks of model training and testing are diminished. Moreover, the improved efficiency also means that the algorithm utilizes computational resources more judiciously, requiring fewer computational cycles to achieve the same or even superior results. This optimized resource utilization further contributes to a decrease in energy consumption and, consequently, a reduction in the carbon footprint associated with the computational infrastructure supporting the AI system.

The quest for efficiency in algorithmic processes not only enhances the speed and effectiveness of AI models but also plays a vital role in minimizing their environmental impact. By reducing both runtime and energy consumption, efficiency becomes a key factor in mitigating the carbon emissions associated with the development and operation of AI systems.

2.9.2 Electricity

Carbon emissions and power usage in AI are indeed closely linked, and assessing the former can serve as evidence of the environmental impact of an AI system. The correlation between carbon emissions and power usage stems from the fact that the energy required to run AI algorithms often comes from power sources that emit carbon dioxide and other greenhouse gases.

The way an artificial intelligence algorithm works involves using electricity for its calculations and tasks. The type of energy used to generate this electricity has a direct impact on the carbon emissions associated with the AI's operation. When electricity comes from fossil fuels, like coal or gas, it contributes to climate change by releasing carbon dioxide into the air. In contrast, using renewable energy sources, such as wind or solar power, for electricity production is more environmentally friendly, as it results in lower carbon emissions. Measuring carbon emissions during each algorithm run provides a tangible indicator of how much carbon is released into the atmosphere as a direct result of the AI system's operation. This measurement helps quantify the environmental impact of the AI system and can be used to assess its overall sustainability and eco-friendliness. Reducing carbon emissions from AI operations involves not only optimizing the algorithms for efficiency but also sourcing energy from cleaner and more sustainable power options. Therefore, by monitoring and evaluating carbon emissions, stakeholders can gain insights into the environmental footprint of AI systems and make informed decisions to promote greener practices in AI development and deployment.

2.9.3 Runtime

The speed at which a model accomplishes its tasks is measured by its runtime. Runtime refers to the time it takes for the model to complete a specific operation or set of tasks. In the context of model performance, if all other factors remain constant, a model that operates more quickly is considered more efficient. Essentially, a shorter runtime implies that the model requires less computing time to process and analyze data, making the overall method more effective. This runtime efficiency is valuable as it indicates a quicker and more responsive performance, which can be crucial in various applications, from real-time decision-making to resource optimization in computational processes.

2.9.4 Parameter Count

The number of parameters in an algorithm serves as a metric for gauging its computational cost. Parameters, or weights, are values learned or initially set during the training process of a system. As each parameter contributes to the calculation of other parameters or influences the model's output, there is a significant correlation between the count of parameters and the computational workload.

In essence, a higher number of parameters implies more calculations and updates are required, particularly in deeper layers of the model. The method incurs higher computing demands, leading to increased resource requirements and higher operational costs throughout its lifespan. Therefore, the number of parameters serves as an indicator of the computational effort and complexity associated with running the algorithm. It provides insights into the algorithm's effectiveness and resource utilization.

2.9.5 Floating Point Operations

One useful indicator to evaluate a model's implementation cost is the number of floating-point operations (FPO) required to produce an output. FPO offers a comprehensive perspective on the computational burden that includes both addition and multiplication operations. It is possible to create a weighted index of computational complexity by giving cost values to each operation. This index considers both the total number of operations and the proportionate contribution of each operation to the overall computing burden.

Gaining a deeper understanding of the computational demands of a system is facilitated through the utilization of the weighted complexity index. This index elucidates the relative significance of various types of operations, allowing for a more nuanced evaluation of the computational intensity of the model. Such insights are crucial for accurately estimating the processing power necessary for training and executing the model, presenting a more precise and informed perspective on associated costs. Therefore, a thorough comprehension of floating-point operations (FPO) and the weighted complexity index significantly simplifies the assessment of computing resources required for the successful implementation of a model. This knowledge proves invaluable for budgeting and resource allocation, offering a clearer insight into the implementation costs associated with specific machine learning or artificial intelligence models.

2.10 METRICS FOR ESTIMATION OF GREEN AI MODELS

Accuracy has been the focus of machine learning and deep learning modes that belong to Red AI, and for good reason. A model cannot be used in production if it is not accurate enough for the intended applications. When it comes to Green AI, it's not just about getting high accuracy but also considering efficiency. Assessing the performance of Green AI models involves the calculation of specific efficiency metrics. These metrics serve as quantitative measures to evaluate how well a model strikes a balance between delivering accurate results and minimizing resource consumption. Some key efficiency metrics are shown in equations (Eqs. (2.1)–(2.6)) in this context may include aspects like energy consumption, computational speed, and overall resource utilization [25]. By analyzing these metrics, researchers and practitioners can gain insights into the environmental impact and sustainability of

AI models, thereby promoting the development of more eco-friendly and resource-efficient artificial intelligence solutions:

$$\text{Energy Efficiency} = \frac{\text{Work Done}}{\text{Energy}} \tag{2.1}$$

$$\text{Model Size Efficiency} = \frac{\text{Accuracy}}{\text{Model Size}} \tag{2.2}$$

$$\text{Training Time Efficiency} = \frac{\text{Accuracy}}{\text{Training Time}} \tag{2.3}$$

$$\text{Training Energy Efficiency} = \frac{\text{Accuracy}}{\text{Training Energy}} \tag{2.4}$$

$$\text{Inference Time Efficiency} = \frac{\text{Accuracy}}{\text{Inference Time}} \tag{2.5}$$

$$\text{Inference Energy Efficiency} = \frac{\text{Accuracy}}{\text{Inference Energy}} \tag{2.6}$$

2.11 FUTURE DIRECTIONS OF GREEN AI AND RED AI

As Artificial Intelligence (AI) progresses, the once clear distinction between Green AI and Red AI is gradually fading. Green AI emphasizes the creation of environmentally friendly and sustainable solutions, while Red AI prioritizes performance and accuracy, often overlooking environmental considerations. The future trajectory of AI appears to involve a convergence of these approaches, where AI systems aim to be both efficient and powerful. This convergence is anticipated to be fueled by several factors.

Firstly, ongoing advancements in hardware, such as neuromorphic computing and specialized AI accelerators, are expected to enable more efficient AI algorithms. Simultaneously, software improvements, including enhanced optimization techniques and algorithm design, will further contribute to AI efficiency. Second, the escalating need to address environmental challenges is anticipated to drive demand for AI solutions that minimize their environmental impact, fostering the development of Green AI technologies and eco-friendly practices.

Moreover, as AI becomes increasingly integrated into society, ethical considerations and societal expectations will play a pivotal role. The demand for AI systems that are not only high-performing but also ethical, fair, and transparent will necessitate the infusion of Green AI principles into Red AI development. Data availability and quality remain crucial, with Green AI benefiting from increased access to environmental data, and Red AI leveraging the growing volume and diversity of data across various domains.

Collaboration between Green AI and Red AI researchers is identified as a key factor in driving innovation and accelerating progress. The exchange of knowledge and cross-pollination of ideas is expected to bridge the gap between these approaches, leading to more sustainable and powerful AI solutions. Looking ahead, the vision for AI systems encompasses energy efficiency and environmental friendliness through algorithmic optimization and power-conscious hardware design. Renewable energy sources are anticipated to play an increasingly prominent role in powering AI infrastructure. Simultaneously, AI systems are expected to maintain and enhance their high performance and accuracy levels, enabling them to address complex problems and achieve groundbreaking results.

Ethical considerations will remain paramount, with future AI systems being developed with principles that ensure fairness, transparency, and accountability. This ethical foundation is seen as instrumental in building trust and acceptance of AI within society. Additionally, AI systems are anticipated to exhibit adaptability and resilience, capable of responding to changing environments and new data, ensuring their long-term viability and effectiveness.

A forward-looking approach envisions AI as a force for societal benefit, addressing challenges such as climate change, healthcare, and education. By integrating Green AI principles into Red AI development, the goal is to create AI systems that are not only powerful but also responsible and sustainable. The future of AI lies in striking the right balance between efficiency and performance, sustainability, and societal impact.

2.12 CONCLUSION

In summary, the comparison between Red Artificial Intelligence (Red AI) and Green Artificial Intelligence (Green AI) underscores a profound shift in the discourse surrounding AI, highlighting the critical importance of harmonizing ethical considerations with ecological sustainability. Green AI propels us into an era where technological advancement is synonymous with environmental responsibility, achieved through the shared goals of optimizing energy usage, incorporating renewable resources, and actively monitoring environmental impacts. Concurrently, the ethical principles embedded in Red AI lay the foundation for responsible AI development, ensuring that the deployment and governance of AI technologies carefully consider the broader societal and individual implications. This dual approach not only seeks to maximize efficiency but also strives to uphold ethical standards, marking a transformative step forward in our collective journey toward a future where AI serves as a force for positive change while respecting both ethical principles and environmental well-being.

REFERENCES

[1] Amodei, D., & Hernandez, D. (2018). AI and compute. *OpenAI*.

[2] Goldberg, K., Shapiro, S., Richardson, E., & Avidan, S. (2020). Rethinking fun: Frequency-domain utilization networks. arXiv preprint arXiv:2012.03357.

[3] Strubell, E., Ganesh, A., & McCallum, A. (2019). Energy and policy considerations for deep learning in NLP. arXiv preprint arXiv:1906.02243.

[4] Schwartz, R., Dodge, J., Smith, N. A., & Etzioni, O. (2020). Green AI. *Communications of the ACM*, 63(12), 54–63.

[5] Kim, H., Ben-Othman, J., & Mokdad, L. (2023). Intelligent terrestrial and non-terrestrial vehicular networks with Green AI and Red AI perspectives. *Sensors*, 23(2), 806. doi: 10.3390/s23020806

[6] Lin, H.-Y. (2021). Colors of artificial intelligence. *Computer*, 54(11), 95–99. doi: 10.1109/MC.2021.3102359

[7] TinyML brings AI to smallest arm devices. *Arm Blueprint*. https://www.arm.com/blogs/blueprint/tinyml (accessed May 16, 2021).

[8] Feng, X., Jiang, Y., Yang, X., Du, M., & Li, X. (2019). Computer vision algorithms and hardware implementations: A survey. *Integration*, 69, 309–320. doi: 10.1016/j.vlsi.2019.07.005

[9] Lee, J., Kang, S., Lee, J., Shin, D., Han, D., & Yoo, H.-J. (2020). The hardware and algorithm co-design for energy-efficient DNN processor on edge/mobile devices. *IEEE Transactions on Circuits and Systems I, Regular Papers*, 67(10), 3458–3470. doi: 10.1109/TCSI.2020.3021397

[10] Kulkarni, S. R., Kadetotad, D. V., Yin, S., Seo, J.-S., & Rajendran, B. (2019). Neuromorphic hardware accelerator for SNN inference based on STT-RAM crossbar arrays. In *Proceedings of the 2019 26th IEEE International Conference on Electronics, Circuits and Systems (ICECS)* (pp. 438–441). doi: 10.1109/ICECS46596.2019.8964886

[11] Saxena, R., Joshi, A., Joshi, S., Borkotoky, S., Singh, K., Rai, P. K., … Sharma, R. (2023). The role of artificial intelligence strategies to mitigate abiotic stress and climate change in crop production. In Srivastav, A., Dubey, A., Kumar, A., Narang, S. K., & Khan, M. A. (Eds.), *Visualization Techniques for Climate Change with Machine Learning and Artificial Intelligence* (pp. 273–293). Elsevier.

[12] Talasila, S., Rawal, K. & Sethi, G. (2023). Black gram disease classification using a novel deep convolutional neural network. *Multimedia Tools and Applications*, 82, 44309–44333. doi: 10.1007/s11042-023-15220-4

[13] Haghverdi, A., & McCabe, M. F. (2019). Improving operational land surface temperature estimation from geostationary satellites with machine learning. *Remote Sensing of Environment*, 233, 111379.

[14] Kowalska, A., & Ashraf, H. (2023). Advances in deep learning algorithms for agricultural monitoring and management. *Applied Research in Artificial Intelligence and Cloud Computing*, 6(1), 68–88.

[15] Khan, M. A., Saleh, A. M., Waseem, M., & Sajjad, I. A. (2022). Artificial intelligence enabled demand response: Prospects and challenges in smart grid environment. *IEEE Access*, 11, 1477–1505.

[16] Xiang, Y., Chen, Y., Xu, J., & Chen, Z. (2022). Research on sustainability evaluation of green building engineering based on artificial intelligence and energy consumption. *Energy Reports*, 8, 11378–11391.

[17] McKinney, S. M., Sieniek, M., Godbole, V., Godwin, J., Antropova, N., Ashrafian, H., … Takats, Z. (2020). International evaluation of an AI system for breast cancer screening. *Nature*, 577(7788), 89–94.

[18] Rajkomar, A., Dean, J., & Kohane, I. (2019). Machine learning in medicine. *New England Journal of Medicine*, 380(14), 1347–1358.

[19] Bansal, S., Khandelwal, A., & Kapoor, A. (2020). An approach towards sustainable urban logistics using artificial intelligence: A review. *Sustainable Cities and Society*, 55, 102041.

[20] Merdivan, E., & Hopoglu, H. (2021). Artificial intelligence in predictive maintenance and its impact on sustainable logistics: A review. *Sustainable Production and Consumption*, 26, 307–321.

[21] Chen, Y., Gao, B., & Qin, R. (2021). Sustainable development of artificial intelligence in autonomous vehicles. *IEEE Transactions on Intelligent Transportation Systems*. doi: 10.1109/TITS.2021.3075115

[22] Machine learning emissions calculator. *GitHub*. https://mlco2.github.io/impact/#compute (accessed May 16, 2021).

[23] Lacoste, A., Luccioni, A., Schmidt, V., & Dandres, T. (2019). Quantifying the carbon emissions of machine learning. arXiv:1910.09700.

[24] Hernandez, D., & Brown, T. AI and efficiency. *OpenAI*. https://openai.com/blog/ai-and-efficiency/ (accessed May 16, 2021).

[25] Eriksson, O. (2021). Moving from Red AI to Green AI, Part 1: How to save the environment and reduce your hardware costs. *Blog Spot*, DataRobot.

3 Impact of Artificial Intelligence Techniques and Green AI Applications

Aditya Singh
Amrita Vishwa Vidyapeetham, Coimbatore, India

Amit Srivastava
Graphic Era Deemed to be University, Dehradun, India

3.1 INTRODUCTION

Green Artificial Intelligence is also known as Green AI, which includes several AI technology applications that could directly solve concerns as well as issues related to the environment. At present, it is a developing branch of Artificial Intelligence technology to reduce the impact of human activities as well as technological development on the environment, in addition to helping in the mitigation of climate change up to a certain extent. Based on Ecomena.org, Green Artificial Intelligence includes developing in addition to designing algorithms that are considered to be sustainable or eco-friendly. So, Green AI has the aim to work on the maximum efficient way to obtain energy optimization, decrease the release of Greenhouse Gases (GHGs), as well as to encourage and support practices that are sustainable. It is believed that for businesses as well as policymakers across the globe, Green Artificial Intelligence could help in solving sustainability problems because of its massive potential. However, Artificial Intelligence also has its challenges regarding the environment, which need to be overcome [1, 2]. In the current scenario, AI technology is expected to proceed with an increase in its reputation in the tech world, as well as this trend is not going to stop in the coming years at the least. This is because Artificial Intelligence technology has helped in several ways to all types of individuals, industries as well as businesses, from the time it became functional. Then, last year, that is, in 2022, ChatGPT 2.0 was launched, which made the AI's growth even more clear, and based on the data provided by Statista, the market of Artificial Intelligence reached around five hundred billion USD in the year 2023. In simple words, humans have benefitted in several ways from the increase in the popularity of Artificial Intelligence. Therefore, this is the reason behind the extraordinary acceleration of the demand for

DOI: 10.1201/9781003546382-3

AI app development services. Nevertheless, as earlier mentioned the advancement of Artificial Intelligence, is also harming the environment in various ways. These environmental problems which are even caused by AI itself, could be solved with the assistance of Green AI, apart from the harms caused by human activities. The computational techniques are being controlled by Green AI in such a way that the risk of any ecological harm is reduced completely. For instance, a robot is being created to receive orders from the user and accomplish those tasks, but with Green AI's assistance, the robot will be built in such a way that it consumes as little energy as possible and performs those same tasks. This makes a big difference when considering it on a large scale, which could have a major impact on the environment. Green AI has not only the ability to make energy-efficient Artificial Intelligence systems but also decreases wastage significantly which decreases the carbon footprint, as well as the electricity cost and so on [3–5]. There are several benefits for businesses with the implementation of Green AI, which are:

3.1.1 Cost Savings
3.1.2 Regulatory Compliance
3.1.3 Optimization of Resources
3.1.4 Long-Term Predictability
3.1.5 Sustainability as well as Reputation of Brands
3.1.6 Improved Innovation
3.1.7 Efficiency Improvement
3.1.8 Improvise Reproducibility
3.1.9 Enhanced Hardware Performance
3.1.10 Democratize as well as understand deep learning

3.1.1 Cost Savings

Implementing Green AI practices in businesses will help in obtaining considerable savings in terms of cost. Companies can decrease the bills for electricity consumption of Artificial Intelligence interference as well as training, with the incorporation of Green Artificial Intelligence hardware as well as algorithms, which are highly energy efficient. If Artificial Intelligence Infrastructure is energy efficient then this can help in attaining lower costs for maintenance as well as for cooling in the case of data centers.

3.1.2 Regulatory Compliance

At present, many industries are going with severe sustainability reporting necessities as well as environmental regulations. Accepting Green AI features will assist businesses in complying with various regulations which will prevent possible fines or legal problems for businesses.

3.1.3 Optimization of Resources

If Green AI techniques are leveraged then it is possible to optimize the computing resources of businesses. So, with way fewer computational resources, it will be possible to attain the same Artificial Intelligence results, which will permit the deployment of supplementary Artificial Intelligence solutions in addition to the allocation of resources to further important jobs.

3.1.4 Long-Term Predictability

To power Green Artificial Intelligence Infrastructure, generally renewable energy sources like wind as well as solar power are utilized, which frequently comes with steady as well as foreseeable costs. This helps give businesses better defense against unstable energy prices in addition to higher anticipation of cost.

3.1.5 Sustainability as Well as Reputation of Brands

To exhibit a promise of environmental responsibility as well as sustainability is possible by implementing Green Artificial Intelligence. This improves not only the brand reputation of a particular company but also entices investors who are socially responsible, in addition to pleas to eco-conscious customers.

3.1.6 Improved Innovation

To encourage motivation within any company, investment in Green AI can be one of the ways to achieve it. With higher efforts in research as well as development, it is possible to achieve the making of highly energy-efficient Artificial Intelligence technologies in addition to algorithms, which has the potential to open up novel market prospects.

3.1.7 Efficiency Improvement

The implementation of Green Artificial Intelligence also helps in increasing the efficiency of individuals as well as companies or businesses. This improvement in efficiency doesn't have any drawbacks, so it is a sustainable as well as eco-friendly process that helps in financial gains at the same time.

3.1.8 Improvise Reproducibility

Sharing in addition to the reproducibility of intermediary info is important to raise the development efficiency of Artificial Intelligence. Very frequently, research on Artificial Intelligence is published with the absence of source code. Also, researchers at times face internal hindrances while making their own as open source. Such factors promote Red Artificial Intelligence, as they help in stopping effective sharing as well as replication of efforts.

3.1.9 Enhanced Hardware Performance

At present, there is an overabundance of advanced hardware which gives enhanced performance on tasks based on deep learning as well as improves dependability. To decrease the cost as well as usage of energy, it is important to either upgrade to hardware that is performance-based or to have such hardware in the first place.

3.1.10 Democratize as Well as Understanding Deep Learning

Since deep learning is effective as well as efficient, so revealing its fundamental science in addition to officially describing the inadequacies as well as strengths of deep learning will be helpful in the making of highly practical and dependable models. Outspreading deep learning's precision is still a study area with high optimism. The precision of the current models is sufficient enough to be utilized in several applications. The tools of deep learning can assist nearly any science domain as well as business. In case the people from various industries who are willing to work on this technology, increase in number, then it is possible for unforeseeable enhancements in the consumption of energy as well as performance to occur.

3.2 GREEN ARTIFICIAL INTELLIGENCE VERSUS CONVENTIONAL ARTIFICIAL INTELLIGENCE FOR SUSTAINABLE DEVELOPMENT

Unlike conventional Artificial Intelligence, Green Artificial Intelligence prioritizes making sure AI technology remains eco-friendly. It focuses on decreasing carbon emissions, improving energy efficiency as well as supporting sustainable practices. Conventional Artificial Intelligence systems consume huge amounts of energy, especially while training deep neural networks. Artificial Intelligence operations supported by Data Centers are big consumers of electricity, and the source of this electricity generally comes from a non-renewable source, which further leads to a higher amount of carbon footprint. All such problems caused by conventional AI on the environment have negative effects, particularly in the long run, and are solved by Green AI. Green Artificial Intelligence is giving several benefits to businesses like as decreasing their consumption of energy which leads to significant savings in terms of cost of energy and electricity bills. Plus, the Green AI Infrastructure normally, uses renewable sources of energy, which not only saves energy but also is safe in the long run. This makes the businesses using Green AI save money in incorporating any supplementary sustainable schemes or plans. Since the whole thing is sustainable and eco-friendly, it also prevents any legal actions against the businesses as well as improves the businesses or a particular company's image in the market if they are implementing Green AI. Then, Green AI could also help in the Digitalization and Digital Transformation of the construction sector in a sustainable manner. Further, it supports the development of an Intelligent Transport System which will advance Traffic and Transportation Engineering.

3.2.1 Objectives

There are various objectives of this book chapter, which are:

- To understand the basic concept of Green AI and how it works.
- To understand the difference between traditional AI and Green AI.
- To understand the benefits and applications of Green AI.
- To understand the gaps in the research on Green Artificial Intelligence.
- To understand the market and trend of Green AI.

3.2.2 Motivation

The authors performed the study on Green AI because the market of Artificial Intelligence has been growing at a rapid rate but there are also harmful impacts on the environment caused by Artificial Intelligence. So, the authors felt the need to look into the emerging Green Artificial Intelligence, which is a part of AI technology but has a positive impact on the environment. Through this study, the authors covered the benefits that could be attained with the implementation of Green AI and its impact on the promotion of eco-friendly as well as sustainable practices, which would be helpful in the long run.

3.3 LITERATURE REVIEW

Tian et al. [1] in 2023 studied artificial intelligence and they worked on inspecting how its application is affecting the green technology innovation performance of Chinese manufacturing enterprises. They considered listed manufacturing companies in China from the year 2014 to the year 2020 for their study and they constructed a multi-period difference in differences model to obtain results that displayed that AI considerably made a positive impact on the innovation performance of the studied enterprises in association to the green technology's development in addition to its decomposition variables.

Chang et al. [2] in 2023 studied AI and they worked on finding its role in green economic development through their study. They proposed a two-way influence of the market of natural resources, in addition to AI on green total factor productivity. They systematically calculated artificial intelligence's effects on green economic development with the assistance of a relevant mathematical model as well as an example of China in their study.

Liu [3] in 2023 studied green supply chain management and he worked on incorporating a new uncertainty model to construct it, which was intended for medium as well as small-sized enterprises with the assistance of AI. This paper integrated deep learning technology as well as AI to construct the above-mentioned green supply chain management system to not only make an intelligent model but also to enhance an intelligent algorithm.

Rodriguez-Gracia et al. [4] in 2023 studied smart or green buildings and they worked on a review paper on using AI techniques in them. They found that incorporating Artificial Intelligence techniques in green as well as smart buildings has an outstanding perspective, which could make sure to not only decrease the negative ecological impacts on the society as well as environ, but also aid in obtaining higher structural stability. Since the understanding of people on these aspects is still fragmented, so they utilized a bibliometric analysis to support their study.

Azhar et al. [5] in 2023 studied AI as well as optimization of green synthesis to perform them on the framework of copper gallic acid metal organic in addition to its application particularly in the removal of dye from wastewater, where they proposed a novel method so that they can extend Artificial Intelligence's application. Through their study, they explored the hyperdimensional relationship which was complex, between the chosen synthesis parameters as well as the qualities of their resulting product to obtain the desired study outcomes.

Zhao et al. [6] in 2022 studied green economic growth and they worked to find out how AI could affect it, by taking the case of China in their study. They created an appropriate mathematical model to propose Artificial Intelligence's two-way impact, especially on green total factor productivity to find that Artificial Intelligence has a major U-shaped effect on the latter.

Elouariaghli et al. [7] in 2022 studied Life Cycle Management as well as Environmentally friendly design and they worked on two life cycle evaluation methods which were Life Cycle Assessment—Consequential in addition to Life Cycle Assessment—Attributional. In the field of eco-design, they brought novel perspectives through their study, which was intended for dissimilar kinds of product applications especially in the information technology area, on a conceptual as well as macroscopic scale.

Xiang et al. [8] in 2022 studied energy consumption as well as AI and they selected them as the basis of their research to work on sustainability assessment of green building engineering to suggest an AI-based energy management model that could be used in green buildings. They stated that Long Short Term Memory models were utilized to improve the consumption of energy.

Wang and Li [9] in 2023 studied natural resource management as well as AI, and they worked on their role in sustainable development in addition to the economic growth in China. They considered the country's economic growth from the year 1981 till the year 2021, as well as other explanatory variables which comprised inflation, interest rate, government expenditures in addition to trade openness to obtain desired results.

Pan and Nishant [10] in 2023 studied digital sustainability and they worked to find out how AI could be used for it. They stated that research on digital sustainability has the potential to help in accomplishing the Sustainable Development Goals of the United Nations, where AI will play a major role.

Bermejo and Juiz [11] in 2023 studied AI and they worked on enhancing edge or cloud sustainability through it. Through their systematic review study, they clarified the uncertainty of AI's application to enhance the sustainability of edge, cloud, Internet of Things, or fog ecosystems to obtain the preferred study outcomes.

Wang et al. [12] in 2023 studied AI as well as natural resource management, and they used them to perform economic analysis in the case of value addition of sustainable exports. They considered the economy of China from the year 1980 till the year 2020 and they examined the asymmetric role of their studied area on sustainable export value embedment, with the assistance of a Nonlinear Autoregressive Distributed Lag model to accomplish their study.

Sipola et al. [13] in 2023 studied sustainable businesses and worked on using AI in them. They stated that considerably less research was done on the sustainable implementation of artificial intelligence in comparison to other industries. So, through their study, they examined Artificial Intelligence benefits in the case of sustainable businesses, where they performed quality content analysis to get the desired results.

Cheng et al. [14] in 2023 studied sustainability performance and they worked on finding out how it is affected by green knowledge management, big data analytics capability, in addition to business intelligence. They accomplished their study to understand the determinants that could affect sustainability performance, particularly in the case of manufacturing companies, for which they conducted an online questionnaire survey in the country Malaysia to test their developed framework.

Samadhiya et al. [15] in 2023 studied sustainable competitiveness and they worked on AI partner relationships management which was intended for climate management in business-to-business firms to attain them. They claimed that, through their research, they furthermore discovered the impact of several other dimensions which are considered necessities to incorporate Artificial Intelligence-based partner relationship management.

Al-Sharafi et al. [16] in 2023 studied environmental sustainability and they worked to find out how Generation Z's utilization of AI products impacted it, by performing a cross-cultural comparison through their research. They developed their theoretical model by combining two famous theories which were PMT as well as UTAUT, to clarify the determinants that influence Generation Z's utilization of AI products as well as the way they affect environmental sustainability.

Sanchez et al. [17] in 2022 studied sustainable agriculture and they performed a bibliometric analysis of publications to discuss the utilization of AI technique agent-based models in it. They consulted Web of Science in addition to SCOPUS as scientific databases as well as PRISMA methodology to find 86 publications that matched their insertion standards to accomplish their study.

Kar et al. [18] in 2022 studied AI and they worked on a systematic literature review to find out how it affects sustainability. They applied the Preferred Reporting Items for Systematic Reviews and Meta-Analyses (PRISMA)-based method to select 287 manuscripts out of over 8300 search results, and they paid attention to dissimilar usage cases in industries such as transportation, agriculture, construction, water, manufacturing as well as healthcare, to obtain favorable results.

Zhang et al. [19] in 2023 studied biohydrogen production and they worked on finding out the newest possibilities as well as methods for it, particularly from algal, which could be used in the direction of optimizing energy sustainably. They found that AI is a technology that could aid in achieving such goals with time as observed in research, through their study.

Sachithra and Subhashini [20] in 2023 studied agricultural sustainability and they worked on the way AI utilization could help in accomplishing it through their systematic review study. They stated that the nonstop improvement of Artificial Intelligence especially in the field of agriculture, several agricultural models were proposed like weed control, advanced care of crops, prediction, resource management, etc., where they assessed such models in agriculture functions to understand the limitations which needs to overcome in the future.

Liu et al. [21] in 2023 studied biofuel production and they worked on macroalgae which could be used as a possible source of biomass intended for it. They concentrated on studies as well as approaches performed on the production of energy from various species of macroalgae, in addition to the development of numerous AI applications to help in the generation of biofuel from a particular kind of algae, along with the detection of challenges in the direction of sustainable environs.

Calabrese et al. [22] in 2023 studied the human AI method and they worked on using it to understand the way Industry 4.0 as well as sustainability are tangled with each other. They inspected 1501 reports on sustainability with the assistance of mixed human AI method based on text mining libraries of Python, to obtain their study outcomes.

Dadebo et al. [23] in 2023 studied AI and they worked on social as well as economic viewpoints to incorporate it in drinking water treatment systems to detect the dosage of coagulants, which could be a shift in the direction of sustainability. They used a particular AI technique, which is Artificial Neural Network (ANN), to proceed with their study and developed prediction models to obtain the desired results.

Saheb et al. [24] in 2022 studied sustainable energy and they worked on AI which was intended to help in achieving it, by performing content analysis as contextual topic modeling through their research. They presented an innovative contextual topic modeling by merging Clustering, Bidirectional Encoder Representations for Transformers (BERT) as well as Latent Dirichlet Allocation (LDA), to get the preferable study outcomes.

Cai et al. [25] in 2023 studied environmental externalities and they worked on applying denoising-based AI to predict it. They considered the case of Saudi Arabia for their study and they compared various hybrid AI models as well as found that Compressed Sensing-based Denoising (CSD)-based denoising has outclassed. They claimed that their study findings could be beneficial in reaching sustainable development goals.

Debrah et al. [26] in 2022 studied green buildings and worked on using AI in them. They used a bibliometric systematic analysis method and they worked to expose the synthesis between green building as well as Artificial Intelligence. They then detected three hundred eighty-three research publications from the database of Scopus for their quantitative bibliometric analysis and they selected 76 research publications on Artificial Intelligence in green buildings to perform their qualitative systematic analysis, to improve not only the efficiency but also the sustainability of Architecture, Engineering and Construction sector.

Konig et al. [27] in 2023 studied AI and they worked to understand its sustainability challenges as well as the regulatory preferences of the citizens through their research. They considered the population of Germany which was represented by survey data to display total moderate to strong backing in the case of Artificial Intelligence being regulated by the government.

Aniza et al. [28] in 2023 studied environmental sustainability and they reviewed bio-waste valorization as well as remediation which was intended for it. To proceed with their study, they used the AI method to overcome various problems and they analyzed 118 works where numerous Artificial Intelligence algorithms were applied to the valorization as well as remediation of bio waste-related published studies from the year 2007 till the year 2022, to accomplish their study [28].

Singh [29] in 2023 studied Artificial Intelligence and worked on how AI could help support sustainable practices. They found the gaps in the current research and performed graphical analyses to support their study on applying AI in the construction sector.

3.4 RESEARCH GAPS

After considering numerous scientific and research publications, the ones published in recent years were selected further. It was found that most of the research on Green AI regarding sustainability, is related to green buildings, economic growth, or agriculture, but there was a lack of research or insufficient research in recent years on implementing Green AI in Traffic and Transportation Engineering, Water Resource Engineering, Waste Water Engineering, and Smart Cities. Then, most of the research on Green AI regarding sustainability was done in China, some from European countries, and some from India. However, sustainable development is a global issue and the decrease of carbon footprint is a major problem in almost every country in the world, so other countries also need to do more research on incorporating Green AI in various ways to promote sustainability, as their advancement should be in a sustainable manner [30–36].

3.5 MAJOR CONTRIBUTION OF CHAPTER

The book chapter focused on Green AI and how it is different from traditional AI technology. It also pointed out the reason behind the importance of Green AI as well as how sustainability and sustainable development could be achieved through the implementation of Green AI. Then, some gaps in the current research were also talked about in this chapter. Some major problems and benefits along with the applications of Green AI were also focused on in the chapter. Further, supporting graphical analyses were performed in the book chapter to understand the status of Green AI and its scope.

3.6 ISSUES, CONTROVERSIES, AND PROBLEMS

There are numerous benefits of incorporating Green AI to promote sustainable development. However, there are also some problems, and issues, which can't be ignored. With more development, there will be an increase in the generation of electronic waste, which will create environmental issues. Then, the data storage problems in the future will increase even further, as the population and demand for Green AI technology will only be more with time. Then, even Green AI will have a carbon footprint if used for unnecessary tasks that could be handled by humans. The amount of energy and water which are precious resources will be consumed even way more in the future by the development of Green AI technology. Of course, these problems and issues will be way less than the use of conventional AI, but that doesn't eliminate the problems. Quality of data, limited expertise, in addition to privacy as well as security, will also remain a major concern. So, it will be a big challenge to minimize or eliminate such problems and issues associated with the future development of Green AI. The design and proper use of Green AI will be a major hurdle along with technological constraints.

3.7 APPLICATIONS OF ARTIFICIAL INTELLIGENCE IN DIFFERENT SECTORS

Various applications of Green AI are presented in Table 3.1.

TABLE 3.1
Applications of Green Artificial Intelligence in Different Sectors

Major Sectors of AI	Technological Intervention	Advantages	References
Waste Management & Recycling	Smart Bins; Waste Sorting Robots; Waste Monitoring and Tracking; Pyrolysis of Plastic Waste; Waste Logistic Model; Sensor-based Waste Monitoring; Waste to Energy; Waste Identification (Biological and Fossil Carbon)	36.8% reduction in waste transportation distance; 13.35% cost saving; 28.22% Time Saving	Fang et al. [35], 2023
Smart Buildings	Expert systems; Fuzzy Logic; Genetic Algorithms; Machine Learning; Machine Vision; Natural Language Processing; Neural Networks; Pattern Recognition	Improving the efficiency of a building's operation and management thereby reducing energy consumption through better automation and control apart from improving the safety and comfort level of the occupant	Panchalingam and Chan [36], 2021
Infrastructure Systems	Artificial Neural Networks (ANN); Support Vector Machines (SVMs); Random Forests (RFs); Fuzzy Logic	Applied in Energy Infrastructure, Water and Waste Water, Transport and Telecommunication for forecasting, routing, maintenance, and security, as well as network quality management	McMillan and Varga [37], 2022
Smart Cities	AI algorithms, such as ANN, RNN/LSTM, CNN/R-CNN, DNN and SVM/LS-SVM for intelligent decision-making to ensure safety and improve the comfort level with reduced cost	Sectors like healthcare (23% impact), the energy sector (10% impact), education, environment, waste management agriculture, transportation, mobility (19% impact), risk management, and security systems (11% impact) highly benefited	Herath and Mittal [38], 2022

(Continued)

TABLE 3.1 (Continued)

Major Sectors of AI	Technological Intervention	Advantages	References
Transport	Artificial Neural Networks (ANN); Genetic Algorithms (GA); Simulated Annealing (SA); Artificial Immune system (AIS); Ant Colony Optimizer (ACO); Bee Colony Optimization (BCO); Fuzzy Logic Model (FLM)	To address issues related to traffic management, traffic safety, public transportation, and urban mobility. Relieving traffic congestion, improving travel time, reducing CO_2 emission, handling safety and security concerns, improving upon economics and productivity	Abduljabbar et al. [39], 2019
Data Management of Smart Cities	Holistic Big Data Integrated Artificial Intelligent Modelling (HBDIAIM)	To meet the challenges of urbanization, such as privacy, security, confidentiality, and authenticity that play a vital role in smart city infrastructure's data management interface	Chen et al. [40], 2021
Manufacturing	Image processing technique—for defect detection; Machine Learning (ML) and Deep Learning (DL) neural networks—for data analysis and decision-making; AI for predictive maintenance; ML for generative design to produce design options for a product; Machine vision technology for quality control; Robotics to automate monotonous operations; Digital Twin for improving shop floor performance; AIOPs—for IT operations; IoT with AI to improve precision and output; Augmented Reality (AR) and Virtual Reality (VR) for product development; Computer vision for quality assurance	Predictive Maintenance; Quality Control; Inventory Management; Customer Relationship Management; Predictions; Demand Planning; Digital Twins; Robotics; Factory Automation Safety; Supply chain management Troubleshooting; Hidden cost elimination; cyber security	Arinez et al. [41], 2020
Energy	Machine learning methods; Metaheuristic algorithms; Intelligent fuzzy inference systems	Cybersecurity; Smart Grid management; Energy Saving; Power loss minimization; Fault diagnosis; Renewable energy sources	Szczepaniuk H and Szczepaniuk EK [42], 2022

Agriculture and Farming	Management Oriented Modeling (MoM); Fuzzy Logic: Soil Risk Characterization-Decision Support System (SRC-DSS); ANN combined with Digital Elevation Models (DEM); PROgramming in LOGics (PROLOG) for logic programming; Robotics- Demeter, Computer Vision; Genetic Algorithm; Web Geographic Information Systems (Web GIS); Unmanned Aerial Vehicle (UAV) Drone; SVM; GPS; Learning Vector Quantization (LVQ)-ANN; Digital Image Analysis (DIA); Sensors with ML	Soil Management; Crop Management; Weed Management; Disease Management	Bannerjee et al. [43], 2018 and Eli-Chukwu [44], 2019
Water and Waste Water Treatment	Artificial Intelligence; Machine Learning model integrated with IoT and sensor Technologies; ANN; CNN; k-NN; Random Forest (RF); SVM/SVR; Fuzzy Interference System; Genetic Algorithm-Genetic Programming (GA-GP)	Source Water Quality Determination; Coagulation and Flocculation; Disinfection; Membrane Filtration; Desalination; Heavy metal removal; Biochemical Oxygen Demand (BOD) and Chemical Oxygen Demand (COD) levels	Lowe et al. [45], 2022 and Safeer et al. [46], 2022

3.8 RESULTS AND DISCUSSION

In this section, data from different sources were collected to perform a graphical analysis representation [47–56]. The data source of Figures 3.1 and 3.2 is taken from BCG Analysis and AIMultiple. The data source of Figure 3.3 is taken from PwC, Google, and AIMultiple. The data source of Figure 3.4 is taken from the US Renewable Energy Factsheet, Universal workflow of artificial intelligence for energy saving, DeepMind, and AIMultiple. The dataset source of Figures 3.5 and 3.6 is taken from Statista. Figure 3.1 shows the impact of green artificial intelligence on climate control.

Figure 3.2 shows the contribution of green artificial intelligence to corporate sustainability.

Figure 3.3 shows the impact of green artificial intelligence on flood warnings.

Figure 3.4 shows the impact of green artificial intelligence on sustainable energy systems.

Figures 3.5 and 3.6 show the international share of organizations using green artificial intelligence and artificial intelligence's market revenue, respectively.

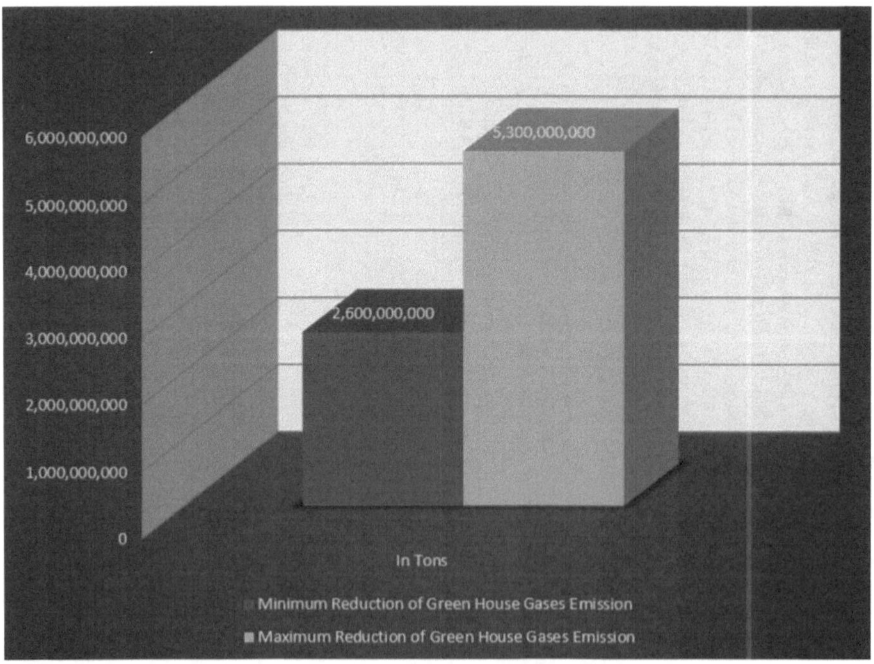

FIGURE 3.1 Impact of Green artificial intelligence on climate control.

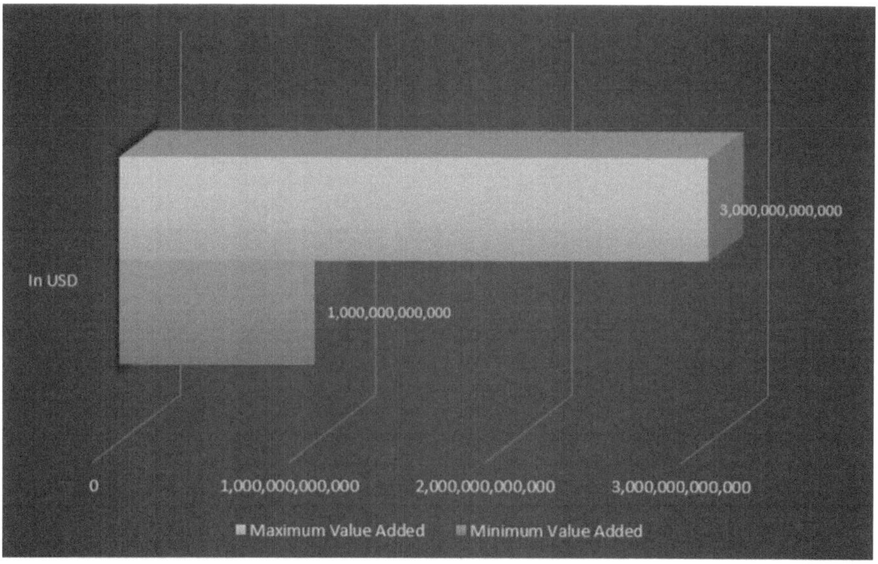

FIGURE 3.2 Contribution of Green artificial intelligence to corporate sustainability.

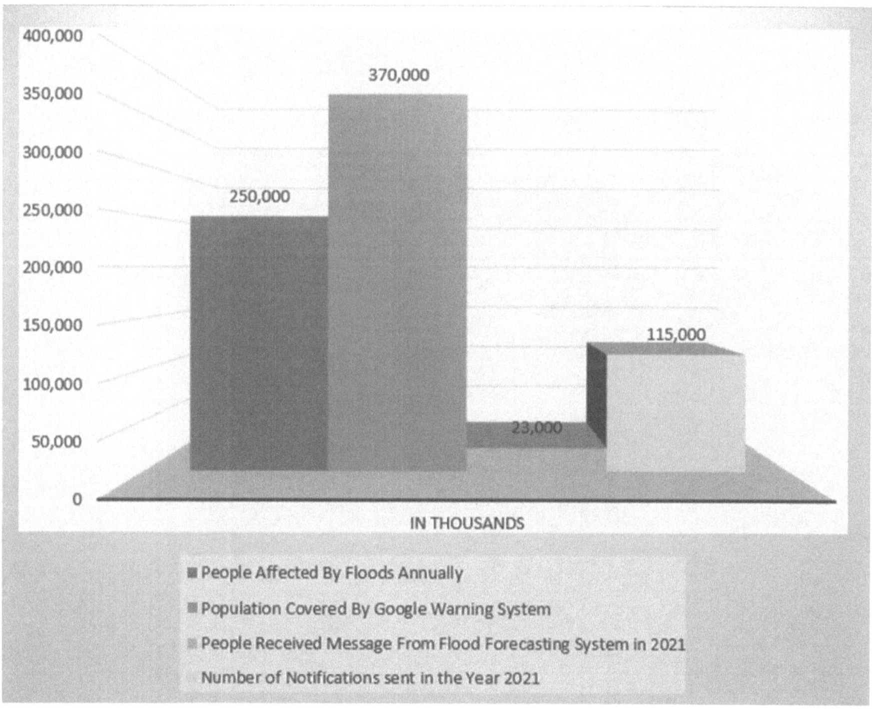

FIGURE 3.3 Impact of Green artificial intelligence on flood warnings.

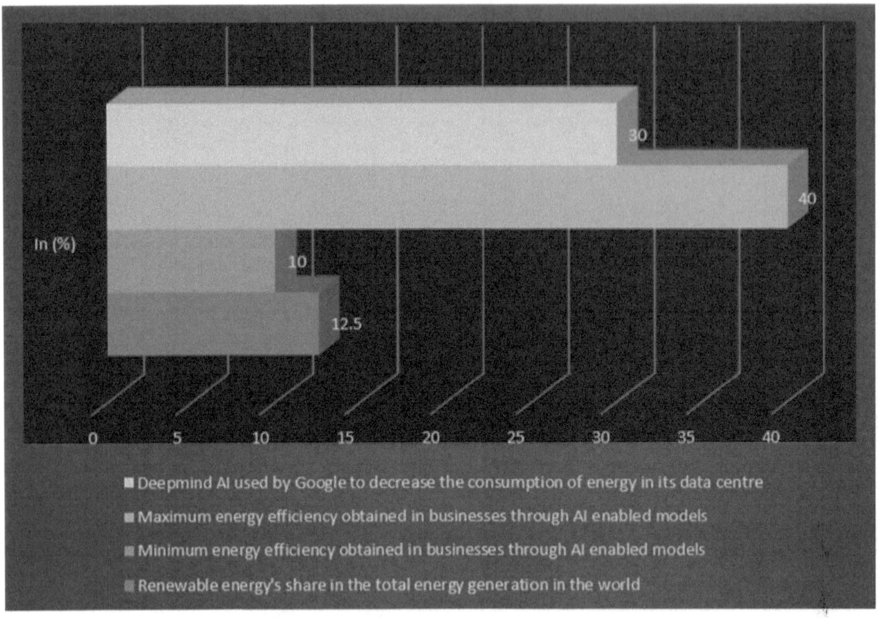

FIGURE 3.4 Impact of Green artificial intelligence on sustainable energy systems.

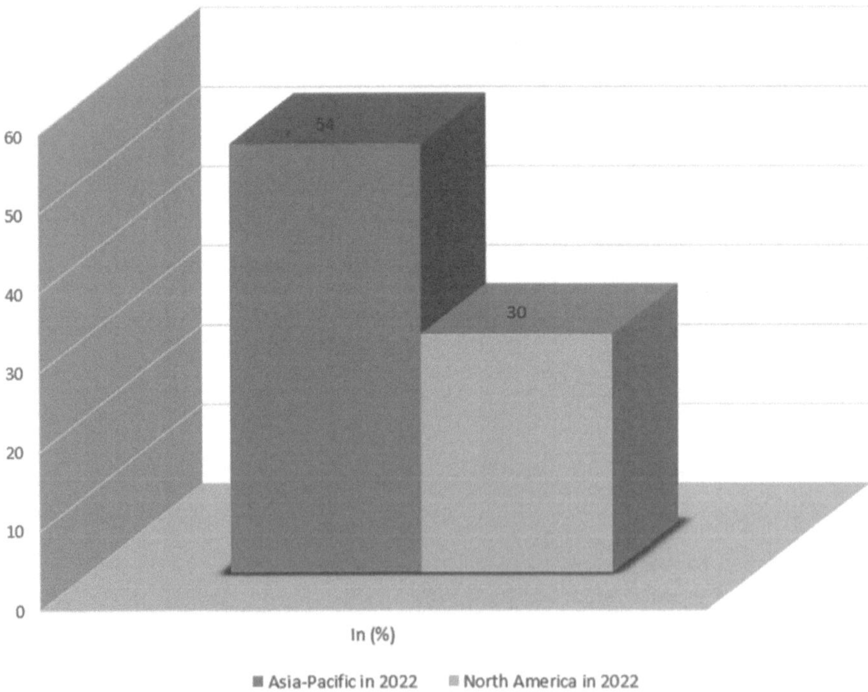

FIGURE 3.5 International share of organizations using Green artificial intelligence.

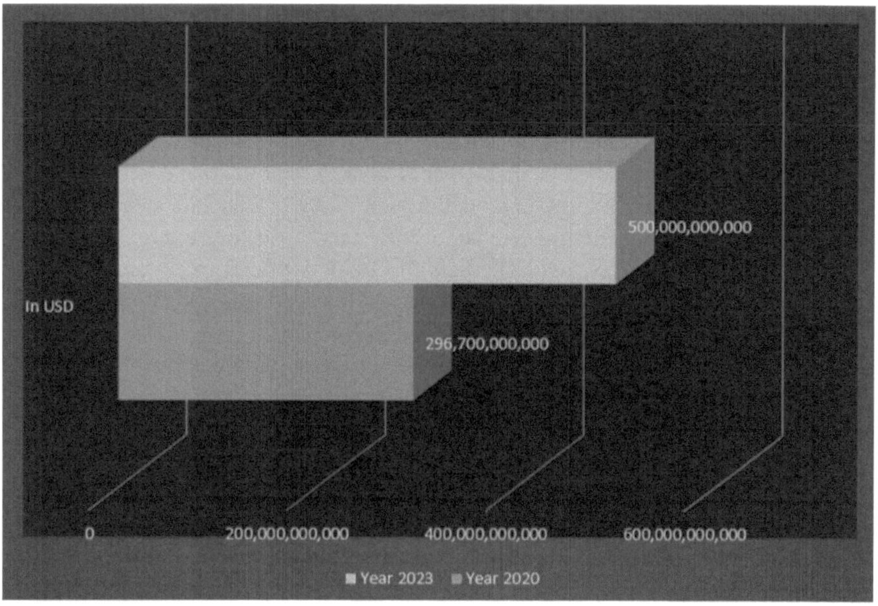

FIGURE 3.6 Artificial intelligence's market revenue.

3.8.1 Advantages and Challenges of Implementing Green AI

Based on the graphs from Figures 3.1–3.6, the focus is given to understanding the advantages as well as challenges of implementing Green Artificial Intelligence:

- According to Figure 3.1, with the assistance of Green AI, the minimum reduction of Green House gas emissions by the year 2030 is expected to be 2.6 billion tons whereas the maximum reduction of Green House gas emissions is expected to be over 5 billion tons. It is safe to say that within the next 7 years, Green AI could reduce Carbon Footprint significantly if applied properly all over the world.
- Based on Figure 3.2, by applying Green AI in corporate sustainability the minimum value added by the year 2030, is expected to be USD 1,000,000,000 but the maximum value added is expected to be USD 3,000,000,000. It indicated that Green Artificial Intelligence has the potential to increase the economic value of corporate sustainability significantly, which will be useful for corporate sustainability in the future.
- According to Figure 3.3, every year on average 250,000,000 people are affected by floods all over the world, whereas Google Warning System can cover a population of 370,000,000; then in the year 2021, 23 million people received messages from the Flood Forecasting System and 115 million notifications were sent by Google in that year. This shows the importance of Green Artificial Intelligence to prevent the loss of human lives before a natural disaster like a flood comes. Of course, it also allows the prevention of loss of valuables by giving alert notifications and allowing the user to

have sufficient time to decide his or her appropriate measures to deal with the impending problems.

- Based on Figure 3.4, renewable energy's share in the total energy generation in the world is just 12.5%, but the minimum, as well as maximum, energy efficiency obtained in businesses through AI-enabled models are 10% and 40%, respectively, then DeepMind AI used by Google to decrease the consumption of energy in its data center is 30%. This indicates that the share of renewable energy is nowhere sufficient in the total energy generation internationally, but with the help of Green Artificial Intelligence, it is possible to reduce the carbon footprint and increase energy efficiency as well as energy saving which will also save cost.
- According to Figure 3.5, the international share of organizations using Green Artificial Intelligence in the Asia-Pacific Region is 54% in the year 2022, but in the North American continent, it is 30% in the same year. This shows that organizations in developing countries are using Green AI more than in developed countries, which also means that developing countries are taking sustainable practices more seriously while developing themselves.
- Based on Figure 3.6, Artificial Intelligence's market revenue was close to three hundred billion USD in the year 2020, but by the year 2023, AI's market revenue reached five hundred billion USD. This shows the rapid increase in market revenue of Artificial Intelligence in just 3 years. It is safe to say that the market revenue of Artificial Intelligence will increase further in the coming years which also shows its increasing future demand.

3.9 CONCLUSION

This chapter reviews the application of Artificial Intelligence (AI) and specifically Green Artificial Intelligence in various sectors like smart cities, infrastructure, agriculture and farming, water and wastewater treatment, energy, etc., for sustainable development. Technological interventions like ANN, Robotics, Computer Vision, AR/VR, Sensor Technology, IoT, GIS, and GA/GP, when integrated with AI-ML have huge potential to improve upon systems and processes thereby improving productivity, Efficiency, Safety, and cyber security, and benefitting the nation with huge profit and high satisfaction level.

REFERENCES

[1] Tian, H., Zhao, L., Li, Y., and Wang, W. "Can enterprise green technology innovation performance achieve "corner overtaking" by using artificial intelligence?—Evidence from Chinese manufacturing enterprises," *Technological Forecasting and Social Change*, 194, 122732, 2023.

[2] Chang, L., Taghizadeh-Hesary, F., and Moshin, M. "Role of artificial intelligence on green economic development: Joint determinates of natural resources and green total factor productivity," *Resources Policy*, 82, 103508, 2023.

[3] Liu, B. "Integration of novel uncertainty model construction of green supply chain management for small and medium-sized enterprises using artificial intelligence," *Optik*, 273, 170411, 2023.

[4] Rodriguez-Gracia, D., Capobianco-Uriarte, M.D.L.M., Teran-Yepez, E., Piedra-Fernandez, J.A., Iribarne, L., and Ayala, R. "Review of artificial intelligence techniques in green/smart buildings," *Sustainable Computing: Informatics and Systems*, 38, 100861, 2023.
[5] Azhar, B., Avian, C., and Tiwikrama, A.H. "Green synthesis optimization with artificial intelligence studies of copper–gallic acid metal–organic framework and its application in dye removal from wastewater," *Journal of Molecular Liquids*, 389, 122844, 2023.
[6] Zhao, P., Gao, Y., and Sun, X. "How does artificial intelligence affect green economic growth?—Evidence from China," *Science of The Total Environment*, 834, 155306, 2022.
[7] Elouariaghli, N., Kozderka, M., Quaranta, G., Pena, D., Rose, B., and Hoarau, Y. "Eco-design and life cycle management: Consequential life cycle assessment, artificial intelligence and Green IT," *IFAC-PapersOnLine*, 55(5), 49–53, 2022.
[8] Xiang, Y., Chen, Y., Xu, J., and Chen, Z. "Research on sustainability evaluation of green building engineering based on artificial intelligence and energy consumption," *Energy Reports*, 8, 11378–11391, 2022.
[9] Wang, Y., and Li, Y. "Chinese economic growth and sustainable development: Role of artificial intelligence and natural resource management," *Resources Policy*, 85(Part B), 103996, 2023.
[10] Pan, S.L., and Nishant, R. "Artificial intelligence for digital sustainability: An insight into domain-specific research and future directions," *International Journal of Information Management*, 72, 102668, 2023.
[11] Bermejo, B., and Juiz, C. "Improving cloud/edge sustainability through artificial intelligence: A systematic review," *Journal of Parallel and Distributed Computing*, 176, 41–54, 2023.
[12] Wang, F., Wong, W.-K., Ortiz, G.G.R., Shraah, A.A., Mabrouk, F., Li, J., and Li, Z. "Economic analysis of sustainable exports value addition through natural resource management and artificial intelligence," *Resources Policy*, 82, 103541, 2023.
[13] Sipola, J., Saunila, M., and Ukko, J. "Adopting artificial intelligence in sustainable business," *Journal of Cleaner Production*, 426, 139197, 2023.
[14] Cheng, J., Singh, H.S.M., Zhang, Y.-C., and Wang, S.-Y. "The impact of business intelligence, big data analytics capability, and green knowledge management on sustainability performance," *Journal of Cleaner Production*, 429, 139410, 2023.
[15] Samadhiya, A., Kumar, A., Yadav, S., Luthra, S., Jabbour, C.J.C., and Agrawal, R. "Artificial intelligence – partner relationships management for climate management in B2B firms to achieve sustainable competitiveness," *Industrial Marketing Management*, 115, 510–525, 2023.
[16] Al-Sharafi, M.A., Al-Emran, M., Arpaci, I., Iahad, N.A., AlQudah, A.A., Iranmanesh, M., and Al-Qaysi, N. "Generation Z use of artificial intelligence products and its impact on environmental sustainability: A cross-cultural comparison," *Computers in Human Behavior*, 143, 107708, 2023.
[17] Sanchez, J.M., Rodriguez, J.P., and Espitia, H.E. "Bibliometric analysis of publications discussing the use of the artificial intelligence technique agent-based models in sustainable agriculture," *Heliyon*, 8(12), e12005, 2022.
[18] Kar, A.K., Choudhary, S.K., and Singh, V.H. "How can artificial intelligence impact sustainability: A systematic literature review," *Journal of Cleaner Production*, 376, 134120, 2022.
[19] Zhang, G., Liu, J., Pan, X., Abed, A.M., Le, B.N., Ali, H.E., and Ge, Y. "Latest avenues and approaches for biohydrogen generation from algal towards sustainable energy optimization: Recent innovations, artificial intelligence, challenges, and future perspectives," *International Journal of Hydrogen Energy*, 48(55), 20988–21003, 2023.

[20] Sachithra, V., and Subhashini, L.D.C.S. "How artificial intelligence uses to achieve the agriculture sustainability: Systematic review," *Artificial Intelligence in Agriculture*, 8, 46–59, 2023.
[21] Liu, J., Zhou, F., Abed, A.M., Le, B.N., Dai, L., Ali, E., Khadimallah, M.A., and Zhang, G. "Macroalgae as a potential source of biomass for generation of biofuel: Artificial intelligence, challenges, and future insights towards a sustainable environment," *Fuel*, 336, 126826, 2023.
[22] Calabrese, A., Costa, R., Tiburzi, L., and Brem, A. "Merging two revolutions: A human-artificial intelligence method to study how sustainability and Industry 4.0 are intertwined," *Technological Forecasting and Social Change*, 188, 122265, 2023.
[23] Dadebo, D., Obura, D., Etyang, N., and Kimera, D. "Economic and social perspectives of implementing artificial intelligence in drinking water treatment systems for predicting coagulant dosage: A transition toward sustainability," *Groundwater for Sustainable Development*, 23, 100987, 2023.
[24] Saheb, T., Dehghani, M., and Saheb, T. "Artificial intelligence for sustainable energy: A contextual topic modeling and content analysis," *Sustainable Computing: Informatics and Systems*, 35, 100699, 2022.
[25] Cai, D., Aziz, G., Sarwar, S., Alsaggaf, M.I., and Sinha, A. "Applicability of denoising-based artificial intelligence to forecast the environmental externalities," *Geoscience Frontiers*, 15, 101740, 2023.
[26] Debrah, C., Chan, A.P.C., and Darko, A. "Artificial intelligence in green building," *Automation in Construction*, 137, 104192, 2022.
[27] Konig, P.D., Wurster, S., and Siewert, M.B. "Sustainability challenges of artificial intelligence and Citizens' regulatory preferences," *Government Information Quarterly*, 40, 101863, 2023.
[28] Aniza, R., Chen, W.-H., Petrissans, A., Hoang, A.T., Ashokkumar, V., and Petrissans, M. "A review of biowaste remediation and valorization for environmental sustainability: Artificial intelligence approach," *Environmental Pollution*, 324, 121363, 2023.
[29] Singh, A. "The present and future role of artificial intelligence in the promotion of sustainable practices in the construction sector," In: Kahraman, C., Sari, I.U., Oztaysi, B., Cebi, S., CevikOnar, S., and Tolga, A.Ç. (Eds.), *Intelligent and Fuzzy Systems. INFUS 2023*. Lecture Notes in Networks and Systems, Vol. 59, Springer, Cham, 2023. https://doi.org/10.1007/978-3-031-39777-6_2
[30] Singh, A. "The significance of digitalization of the construction sector," In: Vasant, P., Weber, G.W., Marmolejo-Saucedo, J.A., Munapo, E., and Thomas, J.J. (Eds.), *Intelligent Computing & Optimization. ICO 2022*. Lecture Notes in Networks and Systems, Vol. 569, Springer, Cham, 2023. https://doi.org/10.1007/978-3-031-19958-5_100
[31] Singh, A. "Importance of fuzzy logic in traffic and transportation engineering," In: Vasant, P., Zelinka, I., and Weber, G.W. (Eds.), *Intelligent Computing & Optimization. ICO 2021*. Lecture Notes in Networks and Systems, Vol. 371, Springer, Cham, 2022. https://doi.org/10.1007/978-3-030-93247-3_10
[32] Bhowmik, S., Singh, A., and Misengo, C. "A case study on intelligent transport system using traffic lights," *Our Heritage*, 67(7), 96–110, 2019.
[33] Singh, A. "Use of geographical information system in intelligent transport system," *International Journal of Research and Analytical Reviews*, 5(4), 882–890, 2018.
[34] IMI, https://www.global-imi.com/blog/what-green-ai-and-how-do-we-benefit#:~:text=Its%20goal%20is%20to%20optimize,and%20businesses%20around%20the%20world
[35] Fang, B., Yu, J., Chen, Z. et al. "Artificial intelligence for waste management in smart cities: A review," *Environmental Chemistry Letters*, 21, 1959–1989, 2023. https://doi.org/10.1007/s10311-023-01604-3

[36] Panchalingam, R., and Chan, K.C. "A state-of-the-art review on artificial intelligence for smart buildings," *Intelligent Buildings International*, 13(4), 203–226, 2021. https://doi.org/10.1080/17508975.2019.1613219
[37] McMillan, L., and Varga, L. "A review of the use of artificial intelligence methods in infrastructure systems," *Engineering Applications of Artificial Intelligence*, 116, 105472, 2022.
[38] Herath, H.M.K.K.M.B., and Mittal, M. "Adoption of artificial intelligence in smart cities: A comprehensive review," *International Journal of Information Management Data Insights*, 2(1), 100076, 2022.
[39] Abduljabbar, R., Dia, H., Liyanage, S., and Bagloee, S.A. "Applications of artificial intelligence in transport: An overview," *Sustainability*, 11(1), 189, 2019.
[40] Chen, J., Ramanathan, L., and Alazab, M. "Holistic big data integrated artificial intelligent modeling to improve privacy and security in data management of smart cities," *Microprocessors and Microsystems*, 81, 103722, 2021.
[41] Arinez, J.F., Chang, Q., Gao, R.X., Xu, C., and Zhang, J. "Artificial intelligence in advanced manufacturing: Current status and future outlook," *Journal of Manufacturing Science and Engineering*, 142(11), 110804, 2020.
[42] Szczepaniuk, H., and Szczepaniuk, E.K. "Applications of artificial intelligence algorithms in the energy sector," *Energies*, 16(1), 347, 2022.
[43] Bannerjee, G., Sarkar, U., Das, S., and Ghosh, I. "Artificial intelligence in agriculture: A literature survey," *International Journal of Scientific Research in Computer Science Applications and Management Studies*, 7(3), 1–6, 2018.
[44] Eli-Chukwu, N.C. "Applications of artificial intelligence in agriculture: A review," *Engineering, Technology & Applied Science Research*, 9(4), 4377–4383, 2019.
[45] Lowe, M., Qin, R., & Mao, X. "A review on machine learning, artificial intelligence, and smart technology in water treatment and monitoring," *Water*, 14(9), 1384, 2022.
[46] Safeer, S., Pandey, R.P., Rehman, B., Safdar, T., Ahmad, I., Hasan, S.W., and Ullah, A. "A review of artificial intelligence in water purification and wastewater treatment: Recent advancements," *Journal of Water Process Engineering*, 49, 102974, 2022.
[47] Ghai, D., Tripathi, S.L., Saxena, S., Chanda, M., and Alazab, M. (Eds.). *Machine Learning Algorithms for Signal and Image Processing*, John Wiley & Sons, 2022.
[48] Appventurez, https://www.appventurez.com/blog/green-ai-for-sustainable-future#:~:text=Green%20AI%20focuses%20on%20algorithm,a%20vast%20amount%20of%20data
[49] Accubits, https://blog.accubits.com/what-is-green-ai/
[50] TechTarget, https://www.techtarget.com/searchenterpriseai/feature/Green-AI-tackles-effects-of-AI-ML-on-climate-change
[51] EcoMENA, https://www.ecomena.org/everything-you-need-to-know-about-green-ai/#google_vignette
[52] Vegavid, https://vegavid.com/blog/what-is-green-ai/#
[53] PWC UK, https://www.pwc.co.uk/services/sustainability-climate-change/insights/how-ai-future-can-enable-sustainable-future.html
[54] AIMultiple, https://research.aimultiple.com/sustainability-ai/#:~:text=Reduced%20energy%20consumption,Even%20though%20investments&text=Therefore%2C%20saving%20energy%20is%20an,not%20compromising%20the%20company%27s%20productivity
[55] Statista, https://www.statista.com/statistics/1384656/sustainability-ai-use/
[56] Statista, https://www.statista.com/statistics/694638/worldwide-cognitive-and-artificial-intelligence-revenues/#:~:text=Artificial%20Intelligence%20market%20size%20worldwide%202020%2D2023&text=In%202022%2C%20revenues%20from%20the,trillion%20U.S.%20dollars%20by%202023

4 Impact of Artificial Intelligence Techniques on Green Applications

Mandeep Kaur
Chitkara University Institute of Engineering and Technology, Chitkara University, India

Rajni Aron
NMIMS University, India

Righa Tandon, Heena Wadhwa, and Gagandeep Kaur
Chitkara University Institute of Engineering and Technology, Chitkara University, India

Ramandeep Sandhu
School of Computer Science and Engineering, Lovely Professional University, Phagwara, India

Deepika Ghai
School of Electronics and Electrical Engineering, Lovely Professional University, Phagwara, India

4.1 INTRODUCTION

Technology progress and global environmental problems have come together in a way that has never been seen before in the 21st century, forcing a move toward more sustainable practices. The use of Artificial Intelligence (AI) in green uses has become a source of hope in this situation, offering new ways to solve important environmental problems. The idea behind this chapter comes from realizing how closely technology and ecology are connected, as well as the urgent need for new ways to stop climate change, protect natural resources, and restore ecological balance.

To balance technological growth with environmental responsibility, it is now more important than ever to look into how AI can be used in green applications. This is because they think AI could completely change how we do sustainable

DOI: 10.1201/9781003546382-4

development. After all, it can look at huge amounts of data, make processes more efficient, and make smart predictions. This chapter explores the complex connection between the current state of the environment and the driving force of AI, imagining a world where technological progress and environmental responsibility work hand in hand [1].

Using AI has had a big effect on green applications, starting a new age of sustainability and caring for the environment. In the field of energy control, AI has made important improvements that stand out. AI systems use complex algorithms and machine learning to look at huge amounts of data and find ways to save energy, make things more efficient, and offer changes that will make things more eco-friendly. In agriculture, AI is very important for precision farming, which uses resources more efficiently and has less of an effect on the environment. Systems that are driven by AI can look at data from sensors, satellites, and other places to give farmers useful information about the health of their crops, the best times to water them, and how to keep pests away. In line with environmental goals, this not only increases crop yields but also cuts down on the use of water and pesticides [2].

Also, AI has changed the way trash is managed by making predictive modeling and optimization possible. AI is used in smart garbage management systems to predict how much trash will be made, plan more efficient collection routes, and find recycling opportunities. By making it easier to get rid of trash, AI helps cut down on the carbon emissions that come from using old-fashioned ways of waste management. Technologies that are based on AI are helping to make green uses for transportation. AI algorithms power intelligent traffic control systems that help improve traffic flow, lower congestion, and use less fuel. The development of self-driving cars also opens the door to more fuel-efficient driving habits, which could reduce the environmental impact of transportation. It's important to note, though, that the widespread use of AI in green uses also brings up ethical and environmental issues. Making and throwing away the electronic parts that make up AI systems add to electronic waste. Also, if AI operations aren't powered by renewable sources, the energy they use may cancel out any good effects.

To sum up, artificial intelligence methods have many effects on green applications. AI is a big part of making many areas more sustainable, but it's important to deal with the environmental problems that come with using it to make sure that these technologies are properly integrated and good for the environment. There are many objectives for this chapter. In the first place, it wants to give a full picture of how AI is being used in green technology right now. The second goal is to describe the difficulties and chances that come with using AI in environmentally friendly ways of doing things. This research looks into a lot of different areas, from managing energy and keeping an eye on the environment to healthy farming and getting rid of trash. The chapter tries to give a complete picture of the various methods AI can help change the course of sustainable development by focusing on these specific areas [3].

As we begin, the chapter's structure shows how complicated the subject is by building on itself in a way that makes sense. This section will look at how green technology and sustainable development work together. It will also look at AI's role in managing energy, how it can be used to protect and monitor the environment, how it can help with sustainable farming, and how it affects the management of waste and recycling. Case studies, ethical and social effects, and predictions for the future will add to the story even more. It will all come together in a full conclusion that summarizes the main points and suggests possible directions for more research and use. This chapter offers advice for those who want to understand and use AI's transformative power to work towards a better and more sustainable future.

4.1.1 Major Contributions

The major contributions of this chapter as given below:

- The chapter mainly focuses on green technology and sustainable development. It discusses the challenges and opportunities in Sustainable Development. Along with this it also focuses on the role of Artificial Intelligence in Green Technology.
- Secondly, it explains AI-Based Energy Management which mainly focuses on smart grids, renewable energy sources, and load management.
- The chapter also covers Environmental Monitoring which mainly focuses on remote sensing and wildlife conservation.
- Moreover, it covers sustainable agriculture and food production. Along with this the chapter also covers smart waste management using AI.

4.1.2 Chapter Organization

The further sections of the chapter are organized as follows: Section 4.2 covers green technology and sustainable development. Section 4.3 explains AI-based energy management. This section is further divided into sub-sections: smart grids and energy efficiency, predictive maintenance for renewable energy sources, and demand response and peak load management. Section 4.4 covers environmental monitoring and conservation. Section 4.5 covers sustainable agriculture and food production. Its sub-sections cover precision agriculture and crop management, AI in aquaculture and livestock farming, and supply chain optimization for sustainable food distribution. Section 4.6 covers waste management and recycling. Section 4.7 covers ethical and social implications. Section 4.8 covers future prospects and challenges of Artificial Intelligence techniques on green applications. Section 4.9 concludes the chapter and provides future directions.

4.2 GREEN TECHNOLOGY AND SUSTAINABLE DEVELOPMENT

The idea of "green technology," which is the same thing as "clean" or "sustainable" technology, changes the way we think about progress and invention. It means committing to using science and technology to create goods, systems, and processes that not only meet our needs but also care deeply about how they affect the environment. The main goal is to do as little damage to the environment as possible by using eco-friendly products, saving energy, and reducing waste. Green technology is important for both human progress and environmental protection because it helps with everything from making and using energy to dealing with trash and farming.

However, sustainable growth goes beyond just technology and includes a view of the whole world. As a philosophy, it looks to the future and tries to meet the urgent needs of the present while also making sure that resources and landscapes are protected for the benefit of future generations. The idea of sustainable development isn't just about the environment; it also includes economic, social, and cultural aspects, to achieve a balance that promotes well-being around the world. This approach looks at many areas of life and the environment as being linked, focusing on responsible actions that encourage resilience, fairness, and inclusion [4].

When we look at how technology and sustainability are related, we see how complex the relationships are between new technologies and the natural world. This intersection is a moving place with a lot of possibilities for good things to happen, but it's also very complicated. In one way, technology helps the environment by giving people the tools and knowledge they need to deal with problems like climate change, resource loss, and pollution. However, technology can also be bad for the earth because it can lead to problems like electronic waste and using too much energy.

If you look closely at how this crossing works, you can see both problems and chances. The problems are reducing the bad effects of technology on the environment, like pollution, over-consumption, and using resources in ways that aren't sustainable. However, these problems also present chances for new ideas, better ways of doing things, and better ways of thinking. Sustainable technologies can help the economy grow, create jobs, and make businesses that are strong and care about the environment. Sustainable living is not only the right thing to do, it's also the way to a better, more fair future.

This intersection is already complicated and exciting, but the role of Artificial Intelligence (AI) in supporting green technology makes it even more so. The way we deal with environmental problems could be completely changed by AI, which can analyze data, spot patterns, and make decisions. It can help farms do better, make waste handling easier, and use energy more efficiently. But using AI also brings up moral questions and problems linked to its effect on the environment. Finding the right mix between using AI's benefits for sustainable development and reducing its possible downsides is an important part of making sure that technology and sustainability can live together in peace. As we move through this changing world, we need to be careful and encourage responsible innovation that fits with the ideas of both caring for the earth and making progress for people [1–4].

4.2.1 The Intersection of Technology and Sustainability

There is a dynamic space where innovation and environmental duty meet at the point where technology and sustainability meet. Using technology to solve important environmental problems is a great way to work toward sustainable growth. We are using fewer fossil fuels and climate change is being slowed down by improvements in renewable energy systems like solar and wind power. It's also possible to make eco-friendly goods with smaller impacts on the environment thanks to progress in materials science and manufacturing methods. It is better to use energy and resources efficiently when smart technologies are built into city planning and structures. People who live in smart towns use technology to make their lives better by using less energy, better managing trash, and living in a smart city. At this point, the goal is not just to lessen the damage to the environment, but to make sure that human growth and environmental well-being are in balance [5, 6].

4.2.2 Challenges and Opportunities in Sustainable Development

Given its many objectives, sustainable development faces several difficulties that need new answers. In particular, these problems are resource shortage issues, where the growing needs of a growing world population put unimaginable stress on limited resources. These factors need to be carefully balanced, and plans need to be made to meet current needs while also making sure that important resources will be available in the future. Navigating this complexity takes a deep understanding of how people's actions affect the environment in many complex ways. Losing biodiversity is another big problem. Invasions of invasive species are speeding up, which is putting ecosystems' delicate balance at risk and affecting their ability to recover and provide benefits to people. Promoting sustainable development means protecting different kinds of life, understanding how species are linked, and the important part they play in keeping ecosystems stable.

Human actions are causing climate change, which is one of the world's biggest problems. Adapting to and lowering the effects of climate change, extreme weather events, and rising sea levels requires quick and organized action. Climate-resilient practices and innovations that lower greenhouse gas pollution and make communities better able to deal with a changing climate must be part of effective strategies for sustainable development. There are, however, amazing chances for innovation and imagination hidden in these problems. Startup owners, scientists, and policymakers are all working hard to find and adopt ways to balance economic growth with environmental responsibility. Sustainable farming methods, like agroecology and precision farming, minimize damage to the environment while increasing food security. Beyond raising yields, these methods also help keep the soil healthy and protect wildlife [1].

Thinking about a circular economy is a big change in how we think about trash and using resources. In contrast to a linear approach of using things and throwing them away, circular economy projects focus on recycling and reusing materials. This keeps the world cleaner and creates jobs by turning trash into useful materials. Therefore, sustainable development turns into an active way for the economy to grow which is also good for the earth. Clean energy investments are a great example of a way that economic growth and chances for sustainable development can come together. In addition to reducing our reliance on fossil fuels, the move towards green energy sources like solar and wind power also encourages new ideas and jobs. These businesses help the economy grow while also lowering carbon emissions, showing that everyone can benefit from working towards sustainability [7].

There is a delicate balance between human progress and environmental protection that is shown by the challenges and possibilities in sustainable development. Dealing with these problems needs a complete strategy that includes new ideas, careful handling of resources, and a dedication to balance the needs of today with the need to protect tomorrow. The road to a more resilient, fair, and prosperous global society is through sustainable development.

4.2.3 Role of Artificial Intelligence in Green Technology

To make green technology better and help with sustainable growth, artificial intelligence (AI) is very important. Machine learning and data analytics are two examples of AI technologies that are used to improve efficiency, make processes run more smoothly, and reduce damage to the environment. Artificial Intelligence (AI) can be used in many areas of green technology, including transportation, waste reduction, energy control, and farming. Analytics that use AI looks at trends of energy use in energy management to help better allocate resources and use energy more efficiently. Precision farming, making the best use of resources, and less damage to the environment are all helped by AI in agriculture. The use of AI in garbage management makes predictive modeling possible, which makes recycling and collecting trash more efficient. Artificial intelligence is also a big part of making smart transportation systems that use less gas and make traffic flow more smoothly [1].

However, it is important to think about the moral issues and possible environmental effects of making and using AI systems, even though AI has a lot of potential to help green technology. Another important part of the ongoing conversation about technology and sustainability is finding a balance between using AI to help sustainable development and reducing the bad things that could happen as a result.

4.3 AI-BASED ENERGY MANAGEMENT

Automated intelligent energy management is a revolutionary way to improve the creation, distribution, and use of energy resources. Increasing global energy demand and the need to switch to more environmentally friendly methods make artificial intelligence a strong tool to improve efficiency and lower environmental impact. AI-based energy management is highly effective at looking at very large and complicated data sets. Intelligent computer programs called machine learning algorithms can handle real-time data from smart grids, weather forecasts, and trends in energy use. This study helps make more accurate predictions about how much energy will be needed, which makes it easier to make decisions that match supply with demand in a reactive and changing way. Incorporating sustainable energy sources like solar and wind power, which are naturally variable, this ability to predict the future is especially important.

Artificial intelligence also helps make energy sharing and grid stability better. Some sophisticated computer programs can find possible inefficiencies and weak spots in the energy system's construction, letting people act quickly to stop power outages or system breakdowns. Artificial Intelligence (AI) systems make energy grids more reliable by changing how energy is distributed based on real-time conditions. This makes the energy environment more resilient and flexible. Energy conservation is an area where AI-based systems can help by reducing waste and increasing

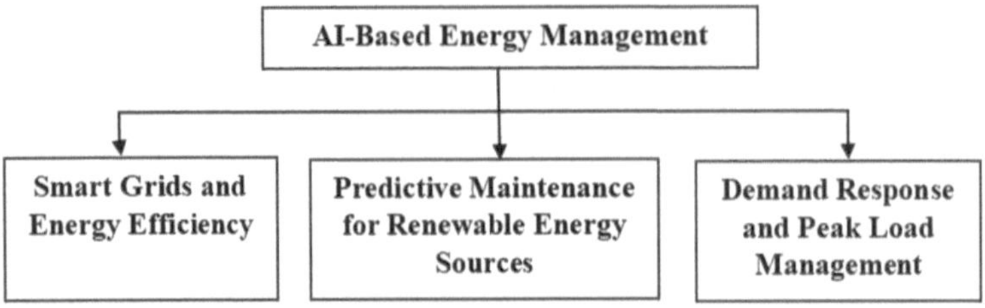

FIGURE 4.1 AI-based energy management.

total efficiency. AI technology in smart buildings lets the lighting, heating, and cooling systems change on their own based on how many people are in the building and the weather. In addition to using less energy, this helps companies and homeowners save money [8, 9].

Artificial Intelligence (AI)-powered demand-response systems also let people take an active role in saving energy. Offering real-time details on energy costs and usage patterns helps people and businesses choose when to use energy-consuming appliances, lowering peak demand and easing the strain on the energy grid. Although AI-based energy management has a lot of possible benefits, there are still some problems that need to be solved. It is important to think carefully about AI infrastructure's ethical effects, data protection, and environmental impact. A safe and reliable energy future depends on finding a balance between using AI to save energy and reducing its possible negative effects. Artificial Intelligence (AI) is at the forefront of new technologies that are transforming the energy scene into one that is more intelligent and sustainable. Figure 4.1 represents various types of AI-Based Energy Management.

4.3.1 Smart Grids and Energy Efficiency

Smart grids are a big step forward in managing electricity. They aim to make the transfer of energy more efficient, reliable, and environmentally friendly. Smart grids are different from standard power grids because they use advanced information and communication technologies. These grids let power providers and customers talk to each other back and forth, so energy flow can be tracked and controlled in real time. Smart grids use automation, sensors, and data analytics to improve how power is distributed, lower transmission losses, and make it easier for renewable energy sources to be added. By making the electrical infrastructure more responsive and adaptable to changing demand trends and changing energy inputs, smart grids help make energy use more efficient [10, 11].

4.3.2 Predictive Maintenance for Renewable Energy Sources

When used on green energy sources like solar and wind installations, predictive maintenance is a proactive way to make sure that these systems work well and last a long time. Predictive maintenance systems use sensors and data analytics to check the health of machines and see what problems might happen before they do. This lets people step in at the right time, cutting down on downtime and making the most of the performance of renewable energy sources. For example, predictive maintenance can find and fix problems like dust buildup or broken parts in solar panels, which increases their energy output and lowers the cost of repairs. The main goal is to make green energy generation more efficient and long-lasting, and this use of predictive maintenance fits in with that [12].

4.3.3 Demand Response and Peak Load Management

Consumers change how much energy they use in reaction to signals that tell them when electricity demand is high or low. This is called demand response. The goal of this plan is to keep the supply and demand of energy in balance and make the power grid less stressed, especially during times of high demand. People and businesses can make smart choices about when to use energy-hungry equipment or cut back on overall energy use thanks to demand response programs. These programs give people real-time information about energy prices and grid conditions. Demand response is a good way to handle peak loads, which not only makes the power supply more stable but also helps people use less energy and save money for both energy providers and consumers. The main goal is to make the energy infrastructure more responsive and resilient, and this method fits with that [13].

4.4 ENVIRONMENTAL MONITORING AND CONSERVATION

Maintaining the planet's biodiversity, ecosystems, and general environmental health is hard, but environmental monitoring and conservation are important places where technology and good ecological management come together. To study, protect, and observe the natural world, this broad area includes a wide range of technologies and methods. Using technologies for remote sensing is an important part of keeping an eye on the world. Science and environmentalists can keep an eye on changes in land cover, deforestation, and the health of ecosystems around the world using satellites with high-tech sensors that take high-resolution pictures. You can use these facts to make smart decisions about conservation efforts because they show how human actions and natural processes affect the environment.

Ground-based sensor networks make it even easier to keep an eye on the surroundings. Data is collected in real time from specific places by these networks, which are made up of sensors like weather stations, water quality sensors, and biodiversity trackers. The data collected helps in tracking changes or oddities in the environment that could mean pollution or damage is happening. Combining information from satellites and sensor networks on the ground gives us a full picture of ecosystems, which helps us make better plans for protecting them. AI has made environmental tracking much more accurate and efficient. Huge amounts of data can be analyzed by machine learning algorithms, which can then find patterns and predict future changes in the environment. Artificial intelligence is used in conservation to look at satellite images, find species that are in danger of going extinct, and guess where ecosystem loss might happen. By combining AI with environmental tracking, we can not only quickly look at large amounts of data, but we can also find small

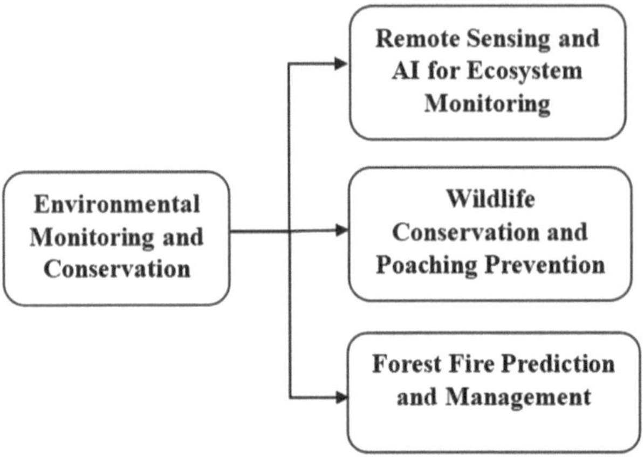

FIGURE 4.2 Environmental monitoring and conservation.

changes in the environment that might be missed by older methods [14]. Figure 4.2 represents various types of environmental monitoring and conservation.

Additionally, keeping an eye on the surroundings is very important for protecting different kinds of life. Tracking the movements and behavior of wildlife is possible with the help of acoustic sensors, cameras, and other tracking tools. Finding out how populations change, how people move around, and how changes in the environment affect different species is made much easier with this information. To protect habitats, keep endangered species safe, and increase biodiversity, conservationists use this knowledge to plan and carry out their plans. Geographic Information System (GIS) systems, which use spatial data to make accurate maps and models, are also very important for conservation efforts. The GIS lets us see trends in the environment, find important habitats, and make plans for protected areas. Geography is used by conservationists to figure out how ecosystems are connected, to plan wildlife corridors, and to decide which places need to be fixed up first for habitat restoration. When planning how to use resources for conservation projects, this spatial viewpoint makes it easier to do so [15].

Climate change and other world problems can't be solved without combining technologies for protecting and monitoring the environment. Climate change effects can be tracked by scientists by keeping an eye on changes in temperature, rainfall, and sea levels. This helps them come up with ways to adjust. It is becoming more and more important for conservation efforts to make environments more resilient, help species adapt to changing conditions, and lessen the effects of change caused by climate. In conclusion, monitoring and protecting the environment is an area that is always changing and growing. It uses technology to conserve nature. A wide range of tools, such as satellites, ground-level sensor networks, AI, and geographic information systems, collect and analyze data to help people and the planet live together in harmony for a long time. To make the future more resilient and environmentally balanced, we need to keep coming up with new technologies and working to protect the environment.

4.4.1 Remote Sensing and AI for Ecosystem Monitoring

Artificial Intelligence (AI) and remote sensing have become a strong combination for monitoring ecosystems, giving us new insights into the Earth's many landscapes. Satellites and other aerial platforms used for remote sensing collect a lot of data, such as temperature, spectral information, and topographical features. Amazingly accurate identification of ecosystem changes, land cover dynamics, and environmental trends is made possible by AI programs that process and analyze this huge dataset. Through this integration, ecosystems can be monitored in real time around the world, giving conservationists, policymakers, and academics important data.

By automating the study of remote sensing data, AI is a key part of making ecosystem monitoring more accurate and efficient. Classifying land cover types, finding deforestation, and noticing changes in vegetation trends are all things that machine learning algorithms can do. Integration of AI and remote sensing allows the tracking of environmental factors like water quality and soil health, which helps us fully comprehend how ecosystems work. Early detection of environmental threats is made possible by this excellent mix of technologies. This allows proactive conservation measures to be taken to safeguard biodiversity, protect habitats, and deal with the effects of climate change on ecosystems [16].

4.4.2 Wildlife Conservation and Poaching Prevention

Conservation of wildlife faces many problems, such as ecosystem loss, climate change, and poaching, which is against the law. Remote sensing and AI are now very important for protecting rare species and the places where they live. With its high-resolution sensors, satellite imagery helps plan and keep an eye on wildlife habitats. This helps conservationists find places that need to be protected and figure out how human activities affect ecosystems. AI algorithms make this process better by automatically analyzing big datasets. This lets scientists find out about the movements of animals, changes in population trends, and possible threats.

To stop poaching, AI and remote sensing tools offer new ways to do things. Thermal imaging cameras on drones can keep an eye on large areas, finding illegal activity and following poachers' moves, especially at night. Machine learning algorithms look at this data in real time, telling the difference between people and animals and pointing out actions that might be suspicious so that they can be looked into further. Smart sensor networks on the ground, along with AI, can also pick up gunshots or strange moves, which makes the police respond right away. Using technology in wildlife conservation not only makes the work more effective but also stops people from poaching animals, leading to a stronger and more technologically driven approach to saving endangered species [17].

4.4.3 Forest Fire Prediction and Management

The use of remote sensing and AI together has changed how forest fires are predicted and managed, giving us ways to prevent them before they happen and lessen their destructive effects. Remote sensing systems based on satellites give real-time data on temperature, moisture levels, and the health of plants. This helps find places that might be prone to fire early on. This information is processed by AI systems, which figure out how likely it is that fires will start and how vulnerable different areas are. When trained on past fire data, machine learning models can find patterns and factors that can help start a fire. This lets us make more accurate predictions and act more quickly when needed.

During a blaze, AI-driven systems are very important for improving how people respond and handle the situation. Infrared cameras on drones can be used to look over the affected areas and give specific information about how the fire is spreading and where the hotspots are. AI algorithms look at this information to figure out where the fire will go, which helps the officials decide how to best use their resources. Also, sensor networks on the ground can pick up on changes in weather and air quality, giving real-time information that can help people and animals get out of harm's way. The use of AI and remote sensing in forest fire management is a big step towards more proactive and effective ways to stop, watch, and fight wildfires, which will reduce their negative effects on society and the environment [18].

4.5 SUSTAINABLE AGRICULTURE AND FOOD PRODUCTION

Sustainable agriculture is one of the most important ways to solve the difficult problems that come up when you try to produce food, protect the environment, and improve people's health. Sustainable agriculture is a method that looks at the whole picture and tries to meet today's food needs without making it harder for future generations to do the same. It's different from normal farming methods, which depend on using a lot of chemicals, growing only one type of plant, and using a lot of resources. Instead, sustainable agriculture is based on principles that put caring for the earth, fairness for everyone, and making money first. Promoting soil health and fertility is one of the most important ideas behind sustainable agriculture. Healthy soils are important for plant growth, making sure nutrients are available, and encouraging variety. The use of cover crops, crop rotation, and agroforestry are examples of sustainable farming methods that improve and protect soil health, cutting down on the need for synthetic fertilizers and preventing soil loss. Sustainable agriculture improves the long-term output and sustainability of farmlands by creating soil ecosystems that are strong and full of different kinds of life [19].

Smart use of water resources is another important part of healthy farming. When you use efficient watering methods like drip irrigation and collecting rainwater, you waste less water and help protect it. Sustainable agriculture also stresses how important it is to choose crops based on the climate and water supply in the area, encouraging the growth of drought-resistant varieties. Sustainable agriculture solves the urgent problem of water shortage by improving how water is used and managed. It also makes farming more resilient to changes in the weather. Protecting biodiversity is an important part of sustainable farming because it helps ecosystems stay strong and lets bugs and diseases be controlled naturally. To make agricultural systems more stable, it is important to grow a wide range of crops, including both traditional and locally adapted varieties. This increases crop variety. The addition of natural habitats to or near farming landscapes also helps organisms like pollinators and predators, which helps keep the ecosystem balanced.

Organic and agroecological practices are very important in sustainable agriculture, and industrial pesticides and herbicides are used very little. Agroecological approaches use ecological ideas to create farming systems that protect biodiversity, increase soil health, and lessen their negative effects on the environment. With its focus on natural pesticides and fertilizers, organic farming is in line with sustainable agriculture's goal of using as few chemicals as possible and protecting the health of the environment. Sustainable agriculture also takes into account the whole food supply line, not just what happens on the farm. This includes treating workers fairly, responsibly getting food, and wasting less food. Local and community-based food systems are emphasized in sustainable agriculture. Shorter supply lines improve food security and lower the carbon footprint of transportation. When it comes to making food, sustainable agriculture tries to find a balance between meeting the wants of a growing world population and protecting natural resources. Sustainable food production is helped by new ideas like precision farming, which uses technology to make the best use of resources, and vertical farming, which makes farming more efficient in cities. Using technology, data analytics, and artificial intelligence together also makes it easier to keep an eye on and handle crops, which saves time and money and is better for the environment [20].

In conclusion, sustainable agriculture and food production is a big step toward meeting the world's nutritional needs in a way that is more adaptable, fair, and eco-friendly. Sustainable agriculture focuses on healthy soil, protecting wildlife, using water efficiently, and doing the right thing throughout the food supply chain. This leads to a safer and more secure global food system that is good for everyone.

4.5.1 Precision Agriculture and Crop Management

A big part of modern farming is precision agriculture, which uses technology and data-driven methods to improve crop management and farming efficiency generally. Precision agriculture uses many technologies, like Global Positioning System (GPS), sensors, and data analytics, to gather and study detailed information about the environment, crop health, and soil health. These large amounts of data help farmers make very specific choices, adjusting their actions to meet the needs of each field.

Managing crops precisely is an important part of precision agriculture. Using real-time data and differences in space within a field to precisely apply resources like water, fertilizers, and chemicals. Soil wetness levels can be measured by sensors, which lets farmers only water crops when they need to and avoid waste. Additionally, using GPS-guided tools for planting and harvesting allows for exact work, which increases crop yields and reduces the use of resources. By employing precision agriculture methods, farmers can make better use of resources, have less of an effect on the environment, and increase crop yields generally [21].

4.5.2 AI in Aquaculture and Livestock Farming

Agriculture and fishing have both been greatly affected by Artificial Intelligence (AI), which has completely changed how these fields work and how their resources are managed. For smart monitoring and control of aquatic environments in aquaculture, AI is used. Within aquaculture sites, sensors and cameras gather information about the temperature, quality of the water, and health of the fish or prawns. By analyzing this data in real time, AI algorithms can make instant changes to feeding schedules, water conditions, and the search for diseases. In addition to making aquatic life healthier, this also increases the total productivity of farms [22].

Using AI for predictive analytics and health tracking is very important in livestock farming. Wearable sensors and devices collect information about an animal's behavior, health, and the surroundings it lives in. After this data is collected, AI algorithms look for trends that could mean someone is sick or stressed. Soon after, farmers can step in and provide tailored care, which will lower the need for broad-spectrum medications. Additionally, AI helps improve feed mixes, oversee breeding programs, and guess market trends, which makes farming animals more safe, effective, and financially viable.

4.5.3 Supply Chain Optimization for Sustainable Food Distribution

Optimization of the supply chain is a key part of ensuring sustainable food distribution, which gets food to people quickly while having the least amount of effect on the environment. The goal is to make different parts of the supply chain more efficient by using technology and data analytics. This includes production, shipping, distribution, and retail. Route planning and transportation are two areas where supply chain optimization can be used. For example, advanced algorithms look at things like delivery times, fuel efficiency, and transportation costs to find the best ways to get food from fields to distribution centers and then to stores. While lowering the cost of shipping, this also lowers the amount of greenhouse gases released when food is moved.

Managing inventory and predicting demand are two more areas where supply chain optimization is exceptionally important. With the help of historical data, market trends, and outside factors, AI algorithms can more correctly predict what consumers will want. By keeping the right amount of goods on hand, retailers and distributors can cut down on food waste and make sure that products are available when and where they are needed. In addition, supply chain optimization helps make the food system more transparent and easier to track. A good example of Blockchain technology is how it can safely record every trade or movement of food along the supply chain. Improving food safety and giving customers knowledge about where the food they buy comes from and how it got there builds trust and accountability in the food distribution system. Implementing supply chain optimization for sustainable food distribution involves using technology, data analytics, and smart logistics to make sure that food is grown, transported, and distributed with the least amount of damage to the environment and the most efficiency. To solve problems like food waste, lower carbon footprints, and build a stronger and longer-lasting food supply chain, this optimization is imperative [23, 24].

4.6 WASTE MANAGEMENT AND RECYCLING

The growing amount of trash that people make means that garbage management and recycling are important parts of sustainable environmental practices. The starting point is organized waste collection systems that encourage proper sorting by separating trash into recycling, organic materials, and things that can't be recycled. For best resource recovery and fast recycling processes, this first sorting is necessary. As a basic principle of trash management, recycling means turning things that would otherwise be thrown away into new things. To make new goods, materials like metals, glass, plastic, paper, and glass are collected, sorted, cleaned, and processed. In addition to protecting natural resources, recycling lowers the amount of energy used and climate gases released when new materials are made.

Utilizing waste-to-energy technologies, certain kinds of trash, mostly organic and non-recyclable trash, can be used to make energy. Various processes, including burning, gasification, and anaerobic digestion, turn trash into energy in the form of electricity, heat, or biogas. This helps reduce the amount of trash that ends up in landfills and supports the production of green energy. Liquid garbage disposal in landfills needs to be managed properly, which includes engineering and environmental concerns to reduce the damage to the environment. This includes steps to keep the soil and water from getting dirty, limit gas emissions, and encourage the ultimate improvement or reuse of landfills. Although there are problems with waste management and recycling, like not enough infrastructure and public knowledge, these activities also present chances for new ideas, job creation, and economic growth. For example, using artificial intelligence to sort trash and promoting the idea of a circular economy can help make garbage management more effective and long-lasting. In the end, recycling and garbage management are very important for moving towards a more sustainable and circular economy, which helps the environment and encourages smart resource use [25, 26]. Figure 4.3 provides different aspects of waste management.

4.6.1 AI-Enabled Waste Sorting and Recycling

AI-powered recycling and sorting of trash is a completely new way to deal with the growing problem of trash in our towns. Sorting trash the old-fashioned way

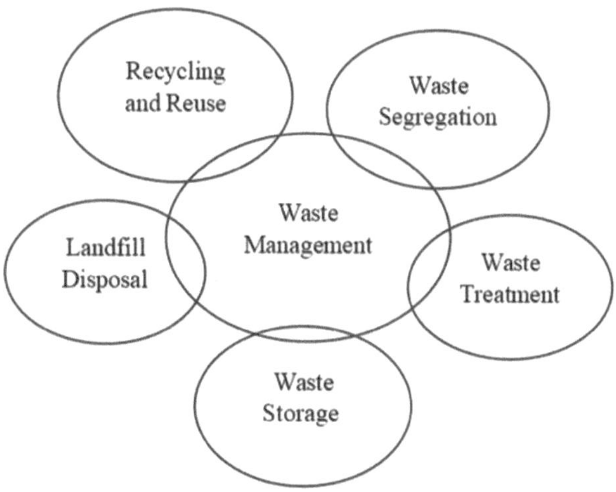

FIGURE 4.3 Different aspects of waste management.

often requires a lot of work and doesn't always work well. But the use of Artificial Intelligence (AI) technologies has caused a big change in how trash is managed. AI-enabled systems with advanced sensors and machine learning algorithms can quickly and correctly sort different kinds of trash, like metals, plastics, paper, and glass.

Sensors sort and label things as they move along conveyor belts in AI-enabled trash sorting. By looking for trends in data, machine learning algorithms keep getting better at what they do. This technology makes it easier to sort trash accurately, which leads to more recycling and less pollution of materials that can be recycled. So, AI not only makes recycling more efficient, but it also helps cut down on trash in landfills and encourages a more circular and healthy way of using resources [26].

4.6.2 Circular Economy and Resource Recovery

The circular economy idea is very different from the usual one-way model of production and consumption. Its goal is to reduce waste and make the best use of resources. A circular economy makes sure that resources are recovered, used again, and recycled as much as possible throughout a product's life cycle. Taking a whole-systems approach makes sure that goods and materials stay in the economy for as long as possible, which cuts down on the need to take raw materials and protects the environment.

Resource recovery in a cyclical economy means collecting materials, processing them, and putting them back into the production cycle in a planned way. Recycling plants are very important because they take useful things out of trash and keep them out of landfills. In addition, tactics like reusing, reconditioning, and extending producer responsibility help the circular economy reach its goal of promoting sustainability and lowering the environmental impact of human activities [4].

4.6.3 Waste-to-Energy Solutions

Waste-to-energy options are a new way to deal with the environmental and energy problems that come with managing waste. In these systems, trash, mostly biological and non-recyclable trash, is turned into energy by burning, gasifying, or anaerobic digestion, among other methods. Not only do these technologies cut down on the amount of trash that ends up in dumps, but they also use the energy potential that some types of trash have. By burning trash to make heat, for example, incineration can be used to make power or heat buildings. Gasification is the process of turning trash into a gas that can be used to make energy. In anaerobic digestion, microorganisms break down organic garbage to make biogas, which can be used as a source of clean energy. Waste-to-energy solutions not only help handle waste more sustainably, but they also help spread out energy sources, which means we use fewer fossil fuels and put out fewer greenhouse gases [27].

While waste-to-energy solutions can help restore resources and make energy, they also bring up new environmental and social issues, such as air pollution and possible health effects. So, putting these technologies into use needs careful planning, close monitoring by regulators, and input from the public to make sure that the result is good for the environment and the communities concerned.

4.7 ETHICAL AND SOCIAL IMPLICATIONS

Many ethics and social issues need to be carefully thought through when new technologies like AI, biotechnology, and automation come out. Questions about privacy, security, and fair access come up as these tools are used more and more in different parts of daily life. There are ethical worries about the proper growth and use of AI, especially in areas like autonomous systems, algorithmic decision-making, and facial recognition. Concerns about ethics are also raised by the effect on jobs and the chance of making social problems worse. It is important to find a balance between new ideas and morals, which means that technological growth must be open and responsible. Furthermore, conversations about the morality of bio-technologies, like genetic editing, and their effects on society show how important it is to have strong moral guidelines to lead scientific progress. Because these technologies will affect the future, it is important to start a conversation in society that promotes responsible, inclusive, and moral technological growth [28].

4.7.1 Environmental Ethics in AI Applications

Environmental ethics in AI look into how to use AI to solve environmental problems in a way that is responsible and long-lasting. As AI technologies become more important in areas like climate modeling, managing energy resources, and making the best use of resources, ethics concerns rise to the surface. It's important to ask about the environmental effect of AI infrastructure, how to use data responsibly, and how AI affects ecological systems as a whole. The main idea in environmental ethics in AI is to find a balance between using AI to help protect the environment and reducing the negative effects it might have. To do this, AI applications must be made that prioritize energy efficiency, reduce electronic waste, and help the world as a whole [28].

4.7.2 Equity and Access in Green AI Technologies

Equity and access to green AI technologies are all about making sure that people from all walks of life can benefit from artificial intelligence innovations that are good for the environment. Although green AI technologies are meant to help the environment, they mustn't make social problems worse. Concerns include making sure that underrepresented groups can equally benefit from sustainable technologies and are not unfairly affected by any bad effects. Concerning green AI, ethical frameworks should put inclusion first, taking into account things like economic differences, location, and cultural contexts to make sure that everyone can enjoy the benefits of being environmentally friendly and that no group is left out [29].

4.7.3 Job Displacement and Reskilling in Sustainable Industries

It looks at the effects of new technologies on society, especially when it comes to switching to practices that are better for the environment. This is called the ethical side of job displacement and reskilling in sustainable industries. Businesses that use environmentally friendly technologies may lose jobs in traditional areas as these technologies become more popular. Making plans to reskill the workforce to adapt to the changing job environment is an ethical thing to think about. Taking proactive steps like educational programs, skill-building efforts, and policies that help workers move from industries that are going out of business to those that can grow in the sustainable sector are examples of this. To make sure that everyone has a fair and easy transition to a more sustainable and technologically advanced economy, ethical frameworks try to reduce the bad effects of technological progress on society [30].

4.8 FUTURE PROSPECTS AND CHALLENGES

As society learns more about new technologies and how they affect the world, the opportunities and problems that come with protecting the environment and using them in a good way are linked. On the plus side, the future could bring about groundbreaking new technologies, AI uses, and environmentally friendly ways of doing things. As more eco-friendly solutions, renewable energy sources, and moral AI frameworks are created, they could help solve important world problems like climate change and resource loss. Some prospects of artificial intelligence techniques on green applications are explained as follows:

1. ***Advanced Waste Management Technologies*:** Artificial intelligence, robotics, and data analytics will be used in more advanced garbage management technologies in the future to make sorting, recycling, and turning trash into energy better. Smart sensors, automatic sorting systems, and new ways to turn trash into energy could help restore resources much more efficiently and have less of an effect on the environment [26].
2. ***Adopting the Circular Economy*:** The circular economy concepts are becoming more and more popular. Going forward, businesses and industries are likely to focus on more circular and sustainable practices, like reusing, refurbishing, and returning products. As a result of this change, less trash might be made, resources might be used more efficiently, and production and consumption processes might be more environmentally friendly [4].
3. ***Precision Agriculture Advancements*:** In the future of farming, precision farming tools may get even better. Putting together artificial intelligence, the Internet of Things (IoT), and data analytics can help make better use of resources, protect the environment, and boost food yields [27].
4. ***Sustainable Urban Movement*:** Solutions for sustainable urban movement will be widely used in the future. Electric cars, smart transportation systems, and eco-friendly city planning can all help cut down on carbon pollution, make the air cleaner, and make cities more sustainable overall [3].
5. ***Innovation in Renewable Energy*:** New developments in renewable energy technologies, like better solar and wind power options, could completely change the way energy is used. Better energy storage systems and more efficient renewable energy sources could speed up the move to a world with less carbon emissions [31].

6. ***Closed-Loop Supply Chains*:** In the future, many goods may be made with recycling and reusing in mind, which is called a closed-loop supply chain. This might mean less trash being made and a more environmentally friendly way of using resources [32].
7. ***Green Building Technologies*:** Improvements in green building technologies, such as designs that use less energy, long-lasting materials, and systems that use renewable energy, could completely change the building industry. In theory, this could make buildings and equipment much less harmful to the environment [29].

4.9 CHALLENGES OF GREEN ARTIFICIAL INTELLIGENCE

Various challenges faced by Green AI are represented in Figure 4.4 and explained in this section.

1. ***Plastic Pollution*:** Plastic pollution is still a big problem, especially in seas and other bodies of water. To solve this issue, people all over the world need to work together to cut down on single-use plastics, make recycling better, and support alternatives [26].
2. ***Cutting Down Trees*:** Increasing farming, logging, and building new roads and bridges are all things that cause trees to be cut down. This is very bad for wildlife and makes climate change worse. Deforestation must be stopped by sustainably using land and protecting it [17].
3. ***Degradation of Soil*:** Pollution, heavy farming, and cutting down trees all damage soil, which threatens food security and the health of ecosystems. To deal with this problem, it is important to use sustainable farming methods and take steps to protect the land [33].

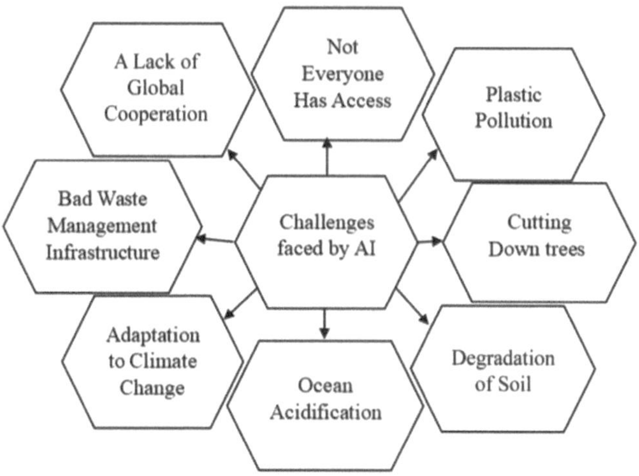

FIGURE 4.4 Various challenges faced by Green AI.

4. ***Ocean Acidification*:** Aquatic ecosystems are in danger because the seas are becoming more acidic because they are absorbing more carbon dioxide. Cutting down on carbon emissions and taking steps to protect marine life are needed to slow down ocean acidification [34].
5. ***Adaptation to Climate Change*:** It is very hard to get used to the effects of climate change, such as extreme weather, rising sea levels, and changes in ecosystems. To make communities more climate-resilient, it's important to come up with and use effective adaptation methods [35–40].
6. ***Bad Waste Management Infrastructure*:** Many places are still having problems with bad waste management infrastructure, which causes trash to be thrown away in the wrong way and pollutes the environment. To deal with this problem, we need to make waste management methods stronger around the world [25].
7. ***Not Everyone has Access to Sustainable Technologies*:** The fact that sustainable technologies and innovations are not spread out equally is a problem for global attempts to be more sustainable. For global sustainability, closing the technological gap and making sure everyone has equal access to long-term answers are musts.
8. ***A Lack of Global Cooperation*:** To solve global environmental problems, countries must work together and coordinate their efforts. The lack of broad global agreements and cooperation makes it harder to solve problems like pollution, climate change, and the loss of biodiversity. Improving unity between countries is necessary to deal with these problems in a complete way [32].

4.10 CONCLUSION AND FUTURE DIRECTIONS

Artificial Intelligence (AI) in the context of green uses shows how it can change things and how hard it can be to use. The list of important results brings together a lot of useful information, covering topics like how AI can help make technologies more environmentally friendly and how to use AI ethically. AI is especially important because it helps with precise resource management, energy saving, and making decisions that are good for the environment. It creates a world where technology and environmental responsibility work well together.

The last call to action fits with the idea that we all must ethically use AI's promise. Concerned parties are urged to deal with problems, encourage everyone to use technology, and push people all over the world to work together. This chapter imagines a future where AI is a big part of environmentally friendly practices. The call to action encourages more study, new ideas, and teamwork, paving the way for a more eco-friendly and technologically advanced era.

In the future, there are a few key areas that will make it possible for artificial intelligence (AI) and green applications to work together. AI programs should be improved in the future so that resources can be managed more accurately, allowing for the best use of energy and the least damage to the environment. By working together across different fields, experts can find new ways to make AI models more flexible in dealing with different environmental problems. This helps us understand complex ecosystems as a whole.

Furthermore, creating and using strong ethical standards are very important. Setting global guidelines for responsible AI use, making sure everyone has equal access, and reducing bias should be top priorities for the future. Promoting educational programs that bring together AI developers, policymakers, and the public can also help people have a better conversation about the moral, social, and environmental effects of AI in the framework of sustainability. You can steer the progress of AI in green applications in these ways. This will lead to a future of technological progress that works well with protecting the environment.

REFERENCES

[1] A. Srivastava, M. S. Gupta, and G. Kaur, "Impact of Artificial Intelligence on Future Green Communication," in *Artificial Intelligence to Solve Pervasive Internet of Things Issues*, pp. 1–12, 2021, doi: 10.1016/B978-0-12-818576-6.00001-0

[2] C. Prabha, M. Malik, S. Kumari, N. Sharma, A. Sharma, and M. S. Khan, "A Review on Sensors and Technologies in Smart Farming Using AI and IoT Perspective and Their Challenges," in *2023 IEEE 2nd International Conference on Industrial Electronics: Developments & Applications (ICIDeA)*, pp. 322–327, 2023, doi: 10.1109/ICIDeA59866.2023.10295251

[3] T. Yigitcanlar, R. Mehmood, and J. M. Corchado, "Green Artificial Intelligence: Towards an Efficient, Sustainable and Equitable Technology for Smart Cities and Futures," *Sustainability (Switzerland)*, vol. 13, no. 16, pp. 1–14, 2021, doi: 10.3390/su13168952

[4] M. Guo, J. Nowakowska-Grunt, V. Gorbanyov, and M. Egorova, "Green Technology and Sustainable Development: Assessment and Green Growth Frameworks," *Sustainability (Switzerland)*, vol. 12, no. 16, 2020, doi: 10.3390/su12166571

[5] L. Mesjar, K. Cross, Y. Jiang, and J. Steed, "The Intersection of Fashion, Immersive Technology, and Sustainability: A Literature Review," *Sustainability (Switzerland)*, vol. 15, no. 4, 2023, doi: 10.3390/su15043761

[6] S. Harnal, G. Sharma, S. Malik, G. Kaur, S. Khurana, P. Kaur, S. Simaiya, and D. Bagga, "Bibliometric Mapping of Trends, Applications and Challenges of Artificial Intelligence in Smart Cities," *EAI Endorsed Transactions on Scalable Information Systems*, vol. 9, no. 4, 2022, doi: 10.4108/eetsis.vi.489

[7] S. D. Sasmito, M. Basyuni, A. Kridalaksana, M. F. Saragi-Sasmito, C. E. Lovelock, and D. Murdiyarso, "Challenges and Opportunities for Achieving Sustainable Development Goals Through Restoration of Indonesia's Mangroves," *Nature Ecology and Evolution*, vol. 7, no. 1, pp. 62–70, 2023, doi: 10.1038/s41559-022-01926-5

[8] S. U. Khan, N. Khan, F. U. M. Ullah, M. J. Kim, M. Y. Lee, and S. W. Baik, "Towards Intelligent Building Energy Management: AI-Based Framework for Power Consumption and Generation Forecasting," *Energy Build*, vol. 279, 2023, doi: 10.1016/j.enbuild.2022.112705

[9] M. Kaur and R. Aron, "A Novel Load Balancing Technique for Smart Application in a Fog Computing Environment," *International Journal of Grid and High-Performance Computing*, vol. 14, no. 1, pp. 1–19, 2022, doi: 10.4018/IJGHPC.301583

[10] J. Control, T. Vinothkumar, S. S. Sivaraju, A. Thangavelu, and S. Srithar, "An Energy-Efficient and Reliable Data Gathering Infrastructure Using the Internet of Things and Smart Grids," no. May, 2023, doi: 10.1080/00051144.2023.2205724

[11] M. Kaur, R. Aron, H. Wadhwa, R. Tandon, H. N. Oo, and R. Sandhu, "A Comprehensive Exploration of Machine Learning and IoT Applications for Transforming Water Management," In *Innovations in Machine Learning and IoT for Water Management*, pp. 25–50, IGI Global, 2024, doi: 10.4018/979-8-3693-1194-3.ch002

[12] L. B. Bosman, W. D. Leon-Salas, W. Hutzel, and E. A. Soto, "PV System Predictive Maintenance: Challenges, Current Approaches, and Opportunities," *Energies*, vol. 13, no. 6, 1398, 2020.

[13] D. Yu, H. Liu, and C. Bresser, "Peak Load Management Based on Hybrid Power Generation and Demand Response," *Energy*, vol. 163, pp. 969–985, 2018, doi: 10.1016/J.ENERGY.2018.08.177

[14] H. Pakdel, M. Jahanshahi, and R. Fotohi, "An Approach to Environmental Monitoring in Sparse Linear Wireless Sensor Networks for Energy Conservation Using Dual Sinks," *Wireless Personal Communications*, vol. 126, no. 1, pp. 635–663, 2022, doi: 10.1007/s11277-022-09763-2

[15] F. Danielsen, H. Eicken, M. Funder, N. Johnson, O. Lee, I. Theilade, D. Argyriou, and N. D. Burgess, "Community Monitoring of Natural Resource Systems and the Environment," *Annual Review of Environment and Resources*, vol. 47, pp. 637–670, 2022, doi: 10.1146/annurev-environ-012220-022325

[16] R. Sandhu, P. Kumar, C. Bhasin, N. Fatima, and A. Pal, "Resnet-34 Model for Human Activity Recognition on Smartphone Sensor Data," *International Journal of Intelligent Systems and Applications in Engineering*, vol. 11, no 9s, pp. 644–652, 2023.

[17] A. K. Rana and N. Kumar, "Current Wildlife Crime (Indian Scenario): Major Challenges and Prevention Approaches," *Biodiversity and Conservation*, vol. 32, no. 5, pp. 1473–1491, 2023, doi: 10.1007/s10531-023-02577-z

[18] J. Ananthi, N. Sengottaiyan, S. Anbukaruppusamy, K. Upreti, and A. K. Dubey, "Forest Fire Prediction Using IoT and Deep Learning," *International Journal of Advanced Technology and Engineering Exploration*, vol. 9, no. 87, pp. 246–256, 2022, doi: 10.19101/IJATEE.2021.87464

[19] A. Sridhar, A. Balakrishnan, M. M. Jacob, M. Sillanpää, and N. Dayanandan, "Global Impact of COVID-19 on Agriculture: Role of Sustainable Agriculture and Digital Farming," *Environmental Science and Pollution Research*, vol. 30, no. 15, pp. 42509–42525, 2023, doi: 10.1007/s11356-022-19358-w

[20] A. Persiani, M. Diacono, and F. Montemurro, "Agroecological Practices in Organic Fennel Cultivation to Improve Environmental Sustainability," *Agroecology and Sustainable Food Systems*, vol. 47, no. 5, pp. 668–686, 2023, doi: 10.1080/21683565.2023.2180699

[21] K. Lakhwani, G. Sharma, R. Sandhu, N.K. Nagwani, S. Bhargava, V. Arya, and A. Almomani, "Adaptive and Convex Optimization-Inspired Workflow Scheduling for Cloud Environment," *International Journal of Cloud Applications and Computing (IJCAC)*, vol. 13, no. 1, pp. 1–25, doi: 10.4018/IJCAC.324809

[22] J.-J. Seok, S. D. Ho, and J. Kim, "Factors Affecting Intention to Accept Artificial Intelligence-based Smart Aquaculture System," pp. 304–313, 2023, doi: 10.46254/sa04.20230091

[23] D. G. Mogale, A. Ghadge, N. Cheikhrouhou, and M. K. Tiwari, "Designing a Food Supply Chain for Enhanced Social Sustainability in Developing Countries," *International Journal of Production Research*, vol. 61, no. 10, pp. 3184–3204, 2023, doi: 10.1080/00207543.2022.2078746

[24] M. Abbasian, Z. Sazvar, and M. Mohammadisiahroudi, "A Hybrid Optimization Method to Design a Sustainable Resilient Supply Chain in a Perishable Food Industry," *Environmental Science and Pollution Research*, vol. 30, no. 3, pp. 6080–6103, 2023, doi: 10.1007/s11356-022-22115-8

[25] D. Sengeni, G. Padmapriya, S. S. Imambi, D. Suganthi, A. Suri, and S. Boopathi, "Biomedical Waste Handling Method Using Artificial Intelligence Techniques," in *Handbook of Research on Safe Disposal Methods of Municipal Solid Wastes for a Sustainable Environment*, no. July, pp. 306–323, 2023, doi: 10.4018/978-1-6684-8117-2.ch022

[26] B. Fang, J. Yu, Z. Chen, A. I. Osman, M. Farghali, I. Ihara, E. H. Hamza, D. W. Rooney, and P.-S. Yap, "Artificial Intelligence for Waste Management in Smart Cities: A Review," *Environmental Chemistry Letters*, vol. 21, no. 4, pp. 1959–1989, 2023, doi: 10.1007/s10311-023-01604-3

[27] J. Zhao, D. Liu, and R. Huang, "A Review of Climate-Smart Agriculture: Recent Advancements, Challenges, and Future Directions," *Sustainability (Switzerland)*, vol. 15, no. 4, pp. 1–15, 2023, doi: 10.3390/su15043404

[28] M. C. Fritzsche, K. Akyüz, M. C. Abadía, S. McLennan, P. Marttinen, M. T. Mayrhofer, and A. M. Buyx, "Ethical Layering in AI-Driven Polygenic Risk Scores—New Complexities, New Challenges," *Frontiers in Genetics*, vol. 14, no. January, pp. 1–11, 2023, doi: 10.3389/fgene.2023.1098439

[29] B. X. Huang, W. Y. Li, W. J. Ma, and H. Xiao, "Space Accessibility and Equity of Urban Green Space," *Land (Basel)*, vol. 12, no. 4, 2023, doi: 10.3390/land12040766

[30] G. V. Auktor, "Green Industrial Skills for a Sustainable Future," United Nations Industrial Development Organization ..., no. November, p. 50, 2020.

[31] M. K. Hasan, A. A. Habib, S. Islam, M. Balfaqih, K. M. Alfawaz, and D. Singh, "Smart Grid Communication Networks for Electric Vehicles Empowering Distributed Energy Generation: Constraints, Challenges, and Recommendations," *Energies (Basel)*, vol. 16, no. 3, 2023, doi: 10.3390/en16031140

[32] M. Javaid, A. Haleem, R. P. Singh, R. Suman, and E. S. Gonzalez, "Understanding the Adoption of Industry 4.0 Technologies in Improving Environmental Sustainability," *Sustainable Operations and Computers*, vol. 3, no. May, 2021, pp. 203–217, 2022, doi: 10.1016/j.susoc.2022.01.008

[33] R. Sandhu, A. Singh, M. Faiz, H. Kaur, and S. Thukral, "Enhanced Text Mining Approach for Better Ranking System of Customer Reviews," in *Multimodal Biometric and Machine Learning Technologies: Applications for Computer Vision*, pp. 53–69, 2023.

[34] A. D. Apa, R. Boenish, and K. Kleisner, "Effects of Climate Change and Variability on Large Pelagic Fish in the Northwest Atlantic Ocean: Implications for Improving Climate-Resilient Management for Pelagic Longline Fisheries," no. September, pp. 1–30, 2023, doi: 10.3389/fmars.2023.1206911

[35] L. Manny, "Socio-Technical Challenges Towards Data-Driven and Integrated Urban Water Management: A Socio-Technical Network Approach," *Sustainable Cities and Society*, vol. 90, no. December 2022, p. 104360, 2023, doi: 10.1016/j.scs.2022.104360

[36] D. Ghai, S. L. Tripathi, S. Saxena, M. Chanda, and M. Alazab (Eds.), *Machine Learning Algorithms for Signal and Image Processing*, John Wiley & Sons, 2022.

[37] V. K. Somayajula, D. Ghai, and S. Kumar, "Land Use/Land Cover Change Analysis using NDVI, PCA," in *2021 5th International Conference on Computing Methodologies and Communication (ICCMC)*, 2021 April 8 (pp. 849–855). IEEE.

[38] V. K. Somayajula, D. Ghai, S. Kumar, S.L. Tripathi, C. Verma, C.O. Safirescu, and T.C. Mihaltan, "Classification and Validation of Spatio-Temporal Changes in Land Use/Land Cover and Land Surface Temperature of Multitemporal Images," *Sustainability*, vol. 14, no. 23, p. 15677, 2022.

[39] P. R. MahiDar and D. Ghai, "Bio-Inspired Optimization Algorithms for Machine Learning in Agriculture Applications," in *Smart Agriculture: Emerging Pedagogies of Deep Learning, Machine Learning and Internet of Things*, 2021 February 10 (pp. 53–60). CRC Press.

[40] V. Kiranmai, D. Ghai, and S. Kumar, "A Review on Classification of Land Use/Land Cover Change Assessment Based on Normalized Difference Vegetation Index," *Journal of Critical Reviews*, vol. 7, pp. 2416–2431, 2020.

5 Green Communication Technologies and Protocols

G. Boopathi Raja
Velalar College of Engineering and Technology, Erode, India

5.1 INTRODUCTION

Wireless networks will alter when computers, phones, cars, and gadgets are instantly and intelligently linked for pervasive services. In a smart home, sensors on appliances and systems enable monitoring and control. Embedded body sensors and actuators can assess patient data and respond intelligently [1]. Sensors that detect temperature, humidity, and toxicity have been used to evaluate pesticides and fertilizers in agriculture [2, 3]. Machine-to-machine (M2M), Cloud Computing (CC), Wireless Body Area Networks (WBAN), Wireless Sensor Networks (WSN), Home Area Networks (HAN), Wireless Personal Area Networks (WPAN), Neighborhood Area Networks (NAN), and data centers are wireless networks. Technologies for communication and information simplify data access, storage, transit, and modification. Energy efficiency and data transport need green technologies. These wireless network methods may deactivate unnecessary facilities, transfer only critical data, decrease wireless transmission data route, emphasize processing over communications, and use sophisticated communication methods [4]. Data transmission solutions for green wireless networks must enhance energy efficiency, throughput, and performance. Eco-friendly wireless network transmission methods are available at the network layer and above.

Most protocols are for transmission or network implementation and cannot handle wireless network physical constraints. When sensor networks are homogeneous and have uniform processing delay, bundle protocols may not improve transmission speed. Bundle protocols seldom need physical connections despite their extensive use in unpredictable and dynamic wireless contexts. Sensor network applications experience unexpected delays due to wireless channel instability. Furthermore, sensor network energy savings reduce channel and transmission reliability. Intermittent connections and unexpected delays make data transfers harder with sensors that deactivate or enter sleep mode for energy savings. Green wireless networks emphasize energy savings above throughput, channel utilization, and reliability. Green wireless networks have limitations, hence transmission methods beyond bundle protocols have been devised.

DOI: 10.1201/9781003546382-5

Medium Access Control (MAC) layer solutions may help green wireless networks. Energy and physical channels are managed at the MAC layer in green wireless networks. The MAC layer controls power, scheduling, rate adaptation, channel access, energy detection, and error correction. The MAC layer offers numerous methods to increase channel utilization, data transmission rate, energy efficiency, and dependability for green wireless networks. Network connections are enabled by the MAC layer, which manages throughput, congestion, and delay among physical and network levels. MAC transmission methods operate with bundle protocols in many wireless networks. Thus, researchers have studied MAC transmission methods to improve eco-friendly wireless network transmission efficiency.

5.2 CHALLENGES IN DESIGNING PROTOCOLS FOR GREEN WIRELESS NETWORKS

Green wireless network features impact MAC layer designs and data delivery techniques across sensors and interfaces. The primary characteristics of green wireless networks show MAC protocol application needs and design issues. Figure 5.1 shows the structure of the reservation-based MAC Solution frame.

5.2.1 Limitations on Energy and Resources

Most sensors use battery power, which has restricted memory and computing capabilities to save money. Applications utilizing permanent or mobile sensors in distant regions with a 15–20-year lifetime include energy constraints. Sensor energy use influences sensor network lifespan [5]. Health monitoring sensors in nearby businesses must be economical and durable to provide data to the central data center. These cheap, compact sensors have limited processing power and memory, limiting their calculation and data storage capabilities.

5.2.2 Dynamic Topology and Traffic Patterns

The majority of sensor networks consist of quantitative fixed or mobile sensors that use comparable transmission techniques on a significant scale. The interconnections among sensors exhibit dynamism and intermittency, leading to diverse viewpoints on the network structure and traffic patterns. When building elegant schemes for MAC

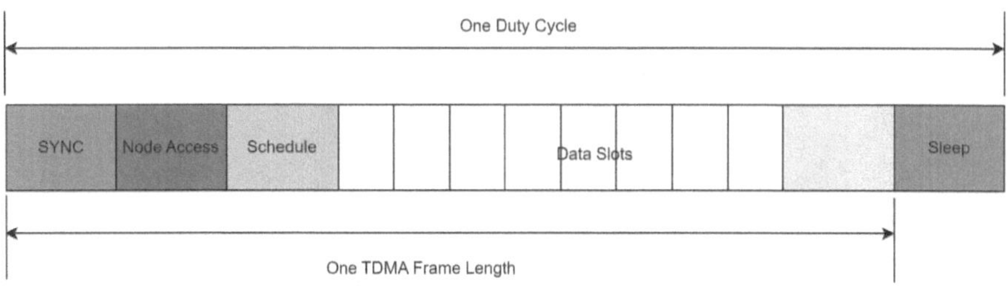

FIGURE 5.1 Reservation-based MAC solution frame structure.

transmissions, it is necessary to take into account both fixed and dynamic topologies as well as traffic circumstances.

5.2.3 Topology

Sensor networks primarily exhibit self-organizing topologies that can flexibly adjust to meet data transmission needs. Based on sensor locations or logical connections, MAC protocols classify dynamic topologies as star, peer-to-peer, or hybrid. Figure 5.2 shows different types of topologies and associated traffic of the Green wireless network.

1. ***Peer-to-peer connection***: Sensors provide data packets to the right partners. They are causally linked and may become disconnected as a result of mobility or collisions. There is no predetermined or specifically assigned means of communication between sensors. In sensor communications, MAC protocols struggle with access contentions, concealed terminals, and collisions. Peer-to-peer transmission methods may be scaled up and used in non-stationary cases.
2. ***Star-connected***: Sensors are organized into clusters based on their geographical position or logical links in a star-connected architecture. The clusterheads can manage and arrange the transmissions of other sensors. They also collect and deliver cluster sensor data to data sinks. Under high traffic, this design provides better energy and throughput efficiency. This design offers direct, obvious links that improve transmission efficiency.
3. ***Mixed-connected***: Few sensors can create star-connected data connections in densely populated areas. The others can create one peer-to-peer connection during extended searches. When designing media access techniques and MAC frame structure, MAC protocols should take into account different topologies.

5.2.4 Traffic

The flow of data inside sensor networks is frequently subject to change, and the directions in which the data travels might vary as a result of the distinct needs for

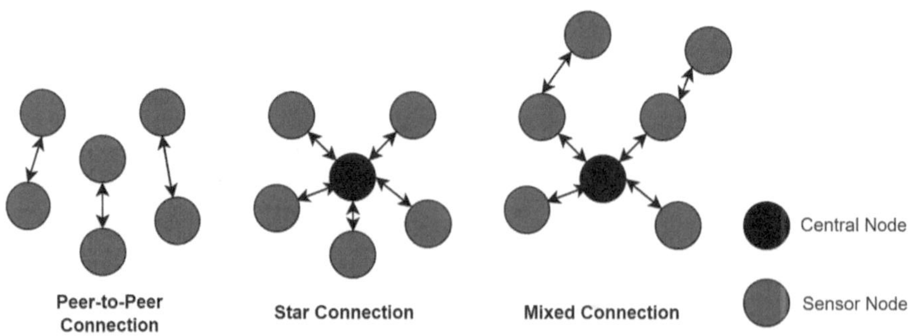

FIGURE 5.2 Types of Green wireless network topology.

data gathering by the sensors. The traffic flows may exhibit either unidirectional or bidirectional patterns. Sensors monitor the environment and traffic and provide data to the data center at regular intervals or when prompted. This traffic usually targets data center drains or routers. Bi-directional traffic allows data sinks to send control and data messages to sensor nodes. Sensor placement and timing greatly impact traffic. Sensor mobility impacts green wireless network traffic.

5.2.5 Mobile Sensors

Mobile sensors are increasingly being used in sensor networks for dynamic and evolving situations. Examples include road-detecting sensors installed in automobiles, body sensors embedded in humans, migratory birds, and animals, as well as temporary sensors deployed in disaster relief operations. Mobility affects MAC design in several ways.

1. ***Topology Changes***: Mobile topological changes will interrupt present connections, requiring new ones to transfer data packets. MACs must provide sensor mobility and data transfer across topologies. The act of departing sensors might potentially degrade the integrity of an established connection, hence leading to a higher frequency of packet retransmission. The collision possibilities may be heightened when unanticipated terminals attempt to access the current connections, resulting in an elongation of the connection establishment operations.
2. ***Contention Changes***: Ad-hoc networks with moving sensor nodes have more hidden terminals and contentions. Collision avoidance strategies are anticipated, and there may be an increase in retransmissions in mobile contexts.
3. ***Synchronization and Schedule Changes***: Since node synchronization depends on location and speed, central nodes or sinks find it more difficult to manage. The central nodes have the responsibility of identifying the newly incoming sensors and promptly recalculating the planned list.

MAC designers must take into account the rigorous mobility of application needs to enhance performance at the MAC layer. MAC layer duty cycles may be changed to enable more mobile nodes. Unpredictable sensor motion causes collisions and hidden terminal issues. The transmission schedules of MAC frames may undergo frequent modifications, resulting in the introduction of additional overhead messages. Ensuring the ability to move about in environmentally friendly wireless networks is another obstacle in the design of MAC protocols.

5.2.6 Delay Tolerance

Green wireless networks include delay tolerance, resulting in Medium Access Control (MAC) protocol creation being challenging since it affects other performance parameters including latency optimization. MAC designers must analyze the reasons for delays and identify the parameters that may be adjusted to improve other aspects of performance in green wireless networks. The factors contributing to delays in MAC protocols may be categorized at the MAC layer based on many considerations.

- ***Processing Delay***: Latency of nodes in detecting and processing the packet header.
- ***Queueing Delay***: Buffer residency time of MAC packets in sensor node buffers.
- ***Accessing Delay***: After packet processing and queueing, nodes link to physical channels with node delay.
- ***Propagation Delay***: Latency refers to the duration needed for a wireless communication to attain its designated destination.
- ***Transmission Delay***: Quantifying the duration required for nodes to transmit MAC data packets onto channels.

The oscillating physical channels of sensor networks are the root cause of the substantial delay that has been seen in green wireless networks. This fluctuation leads to unexpected delays in queueing, access, and transmission at the MAC layer. Additionally, the processes provide chances to enhance efficiency in terms of throughput, energy savings, and dependability. There are certain sensor networks in which the primary source of latency is propagation delay, and this delay may be predicted. Agile MAC methods may be devised to increase particular performance in green wireless networks. This is possible whenever applications are not real-time and carry a variety of delays in data transfers that are either unexpected or predictable.

There is a possibility that applications for green wireless networks would encounter energy limits, dynamic topologies and traffic, mobility requirements, and many delay features. When these qualities are taken into account as the primary problems, designers of MACs can choose a variety of performance measures to develop or optimize data transmissions along with media access control functions.

5.3 METRICS FOR EVALUATING THE PERFORMANCE OF GREEN WIRELESS NETWORKS

Performance indicators influence MAC protocol design. They assess protocol effectiveness in ecologically friendly wireless network applications. Energy economy, mobility, data transmission rate, and dependability become the important parameters for developing and analyzing MAC schemes in green wireless networks when the time limitation is lifted.

5.3.1 Energy Conservation

In tough and isolated locations, battery-powered sensors must save energy to last longer. MAC protocols must consider energy use during data delivery. Three primary concerns affect energy saving at the MAC layer:

- ***Collisions***: Collisions may happen when many nodes broadcast at the same time within their transmission range. When transmissions collide, they are stopped, and new transmissions might be planned.

- ***Overhearing and Idle Listening***: Sensors can remain in a state of readiness and actively monitor the communication channels. Sensors sometimes detect extraneous packets. This superfluous hearing or redundant listening may deplete the energy of sensors.
- ***Overhead***: The Medium Access Control (MAC) layer uses control messages to synchronize and organize sensors for transmission. The use of more resources by MAC protocols leads to increased energy consumption during a single transmission.

The implementation of MAC protocols has been significantly influenced by the need to adhere to energy-saving regulations. Wireless sensor networks use duty cycles to hold energy and prolong longevity. A sensor plays a major role in the transition between gearbox, reception, listening, and a low-power resting mode that uses one-tenth of the energy used during gearbox [5]. Several MAC protocols are intentionally designed to balance the length of network operation with characteristics such as latency, reliability, scalability, and data transmission rate.

5.3.2 Throughput

Green wireless networks may not necessarily prioritize throughput as their primary concern. To conserve energy, MAC techniques sometimes compromise throughput or capacity. In green wireless networks, monitoring or recording tasks in sensor networks have highlighted the necessity for throughput. Video sensors embedded inside automotive networks have the potential to detect and monitor road surfaces as well as individual cars. In these situations, the balance between energy saving and dependability might be adjusted in favor of throughput to meet the specific needs of the application.

Enhancing data transfer rates in environmentally friendly wireless networks is a difficult task. Wireless channel status is negatively affected by duty cycle, fault nodes, and mobility, resulting in reduced capacity of physical channels. MAC protocols are designed to enhance the sharing of wireless channels among several nodes by scheduling their broadcasts and preventing collisions and retransmissions.

5.3.3 Mobility

Sensor mobility might be classified by speed and pattern. The sensor's velocity may vary between 0 and 150 kilometers per hour, resulting in an extremely brief contact period for data transfer between sensors. Furthermore, the constant movement of sensors leads to the dynamic alteration of the structure of the current network, which consequently leads to heightened intricacy in the development of MAC protocols. MAC protocols in Wireless Sensor Networks (WSN) include sensor mobility patterns, especially the distinct movement patterns of sensors. The categorization of mobility patterns might be determined by several characteristics such as dimension, velocity, group orientations, predictability of movement, and limitations. Green wireless network scenarios typically include three primary mobility patterns:

- ***Random Walk Mobility Pattern***: Mobile organisms and people may have sensor nodes linked to their organs. The sensors move randomly or predetermined along pedestrian pathways at a limited pace.

- ***High-Speed Mobility Pattern***: Vehicle sensors may shift quickly over two-dimensional pathways or highway trajectories. The mobility trend associated with highway traffic conditions might involve collective data.
- ***Dynamic Medium Mobility Pattern***: Sensors deployed in natural habitats may be transported by several carriers, including birds, water, and dirt. The movement patterns of these sensors are mostly influenced by the characteristics of the carriers.

Designers of MAC systems may use these common speeds and trends as scenarios for applications to create and assess transmission methods in environmentally friendly wireless networks. Wireless networks are influenced by three interconnected performance metrics: latency, throughput, and mobility. According to reference [6], the time it takes for a single packet to be sent in a wireless network decreases as the rate of movement of the mobile nodes increases. The overall data transfer rate of this network is unaffected by the speed at which the mobile nodes are moving. As stated in reference [7], the amount of data that can be sent within a given time frame may be increased in mobile contexts where meeting time limitations are flexible. However, the potential for boosting data throughput is restricted in stationary circumstances. Nevertheless, the constant rise in node mobility does not guarantee an improvement in data throughput beyond a certain delay requirement, known as the critical delay.

5.3.4 Reliability

Data transmission reliability is a key factor in the expectations regarding applications in green wireless networks. In some contexts, such as situations involving environmental monitoring, the importance of dependability might be seen to be as lenient as the importance of delay. Nevertheless, in some contexts, such as automobile number identification and tracking situations, it is essential that the collected data be precise, and a high level of dependability is necessary for transmitting the data. Furthermore, the use of robust MAC protocols might lead to a decrease in retransmissions at the upper layers, resulting in enhanced efficiency of end-to-end transmission. Diverse techniques are used to attain reliability in the MAC layer.

- ***Forward Error Control***: Error management is a very efficient method for enhancing the dependability of transmission and minimizing the need for retransmissions. To improve reliability, it is advisable to provide more space in every frame for error control purposes.
- ***ARQ and Retransmissions***: The error control technique Automatic Repetition Request (ARQ) employs confirmations and time-outs to decide packet transmission. Upon receiving a negative acknowledgment, it is necessary to transmit further retransmissions, hence causing an increase in packet latency.
- ***Redundant Transmissions***: The receiver may recover the original data packet without any retransmissions by combining several copies or versions sent across various channels, paths, or distinct MAC frames. The technique exchanges various resources, such as channels or pathways, to achieve both strong dependability and decreased latency.

MAC protocols strive to meet performance objectives by effectively managing the trade-offs between dependability, overhead expenditure, and latency.

5.3.5 Delay Trade-Off

When latency is decreased in green wireless networks, numerous MAC layer methods may be used to meet performance goals.

- ***Flexible Resource Allocation and Scheduling***: Green wireless networks benefit from a relaxed latency, which enables the use of flexible channel access strategies for sharing wireless channels. In green wireless networks, MAC protocols may use greater resource allocation and scheduling techniques in comparison to situations that prioritize minimizing latency.
- ***Contention Relief***: Green wireless networks may reduce transmission frequency conflicts. Various tactics may be used to prevent or manage conflicts.
- ***Extra Energy Consumption***: Increased transmission length results in higher energy usage. There exists an equilibrium between energy consumption and delay in efficiency, dependability, and throughput.

Green wireless networks promote low-latency MAC protocols to conserve energy and improve mobility, throughput, and reliability. Green wireless networks have intricate characteristics and many sensor application performance criteria; hence, MAC transmission techniques are distinct.

5.4 TECHNIQUES FOR MAC TRANSMISSION IN WSN

Wireless data transfers in sensor networks can encounter significant delays as a result of challenging environmental conditions and resource constraints. Several sensor applications need reduced transmission latency and enhanced performance in energy efficiency, data transfer rate, dependability, and mobility [8]. Delay-Tolerant Sensor Networks (DTSN) use the MAC layer to identify shaky wireless channels and improve transmission efficiency. This chapter discusses a variety of MAC designs for DTSN and their protocols for unexpected and predicted delays. Our focus is on MAC protocols that prioritize energy saving, mobility, throughput, and/or dependability above minimizing delays in data transfers. Additionally, DTSN MAC protocols change access control and transmission operations depending on predicted delays. The chapter evaluates the delay tolerance of various MAC protocols, weighing latency against other performance parameters. The chapter introduces and examines DTSN-appropriate MAC techniques and explores possible topics for future research to develop new DTSN-specific MAC protocols.

5.4.1 MAC Protocols for Sensor Networks

MAC protocols manage MAC layer communication and allocate wireless channels among sensor nodes. Two primary MAC methods are contention-based and reservation-based [5]. Nodes provide synchronization and scheduling packets to peers in reservation-based systems to report frame length, scheduling list, address, time cycle, and more. The nearby nodes watch the channel for synchronization packets, then send, receive, and sleep. The listener may determine a sender's transmission slot and the coordinator's reception slot by studying synchronization as well as scheduling frames.

Senders may send data frames within a specified time interval. The recipient can acknowledge the sender within a designated time frame for receipt. If the transmitter has several data frames for transmission, it must await an additional planned transmission slot inside the subsequent duty cycle. The channel access mechanism is collision-free as a result of the scheduling list. By reducing control frames, carrier identification, and collision avoidance time, non-coordinator sensor nodes save energy and data transmission latency. Within densely populated regions, the central nodes can efficiently coordinate numerous data transfers between sensors, hence enhancing the overall network throughput. The central nodes, also known as coordinators within clusters, use additional energy during the transmission of synchronous and scheduling frames.

Sensor nodes that rely on unsynchronized contention contest for shared wireless channels, with the first node that can use the channel being granted permission to broadcast. Carrier Sense Multiple Access (CSMA) is a contention-based MAC protocol. A node listens for carrier sensing on the wireless channel after a transmission request. When the channel is identified as occupied, the node will delay its broadcast until a vacant channel is available, to prevent any conflicts.

Once the channel is determined to be unoccupied, the node commences data transmission following a randomly chosen delay period. This situation is a common occurrence in which trading occurs between sensing and waiting periods to prevent collisions and get access to the wireless channel. Since they are topologically free, contention-based MAC techniques scale well in big networks. Transmission requests determine sensor node energy allocation. This saves energy in low- and moderate-traffic circumstances without slowing data delivery. Nevertheless, the occurrence of access collisions rises as the level of traffic is elevated In contention-based MAC protocols. The presence of extra control frames and retransmissions leads to a deterioration in both throughput and energy-saving performance. Contention-based MAC protocols with concealed terminal concerns will worsen throughput along with access performance.

By easing latency, the DTSN environment allows the design of MAC settings, procedures, and algorithms to improve sensor application performance metrics. Delay-tolerant sensor networks use several MAC protocols for different reasons. Within Delay-Tolerant Sensor Networks (DTSNs), some applications can relax the restrictions on delay to prioritize enhanced performance in terms of throughput, mobility, or dependability. Nevertheless, many applications encounter significant delays in transmitting data in certain situations that use MAC layer methods. The MAC protocols examined in this research are categorized based on the factors that contribute to latency and the performance metrics in DTSNs, including MAC solutions that address propagation delay and MAC solutions that address accessing and transmission delay.

5.4.2 MAC Solutions for Propagation Delay

Propagation delay is the duration needed for wireless communications to reach their intended destination. In transmission over long distances and underwater circumstances, the propagation delay is much greater. Electromagnetic signals serve as the typical transmission medium for carrying data in terrestrial contexts. Due to the almost instantaneous speed of these signals in the air, the time it takes for them to travel is not significant when compared to the time it takes for processing and queuing. Propagation delay may impact transmission scheduling and access control when two nodes are far away, especially in satellite communications [9]. Underwater wireless propagation delays are another key issue. The transmission time for a signal is five orders of magnitude greater in underwater acoustic settings compared to terrestrial radio environments, even when the distance is the same [9]. Conventional media access control techniques exhibit reduced performance in terms of throughput, energy efficiency, and channel utilization. Consequently, there has been a significant increase in research focused on the MAC layer to accommodate or exploit propagation delay.

5.4.2.1 Methodology to Improve Channel Utilization

The transmission distance predicts propagation delay, which rises with distance. Thus, the MAC scheduler can handle further data transmissions while waiting for the propagation to finish within a single data transmission cycle [9]. To enhance the efficiency of data frame transmission, the MAC layer may use the RTS-CTS-DATA-ACK method to arrange the transmission of control frames and data frames sequentially. Due to the significant propagation delay, the sender has the opportunity to transmit additional frames during the interval between sending and receiving frames. Following the delivery of the Request to Send (RTS) and awaiting the Clear to Send (CTS), this gap in communication takes place. According to [9], a method known as the parallel algorithm of instructions was implemented at the MAC layer. It was discovered that an increase in the utilization of simultaneously managed MAC broadcasts led to an increase in the ability of the wireless channel.

Underwater acoustic sensor networks also use similar tactics to increase channel utilization. Wireless broadcasting and underwater audio channel propagation delay were employed in the investigation. The MAC technique allows a single sensor node to communicate with several nodes via RTS/CTS. The system uses Multiple Access with Collision Avoidance (MACA) protocols [10]. For several synchronous nodes underwater, it was created. Local nodes' busy signals are used to estimate transmission time. The gadget then broadcasts control or data frames at intervals when its neighbors are not broadcasting. The approach described in [11] improved channel utilization and network performance while reducing conflict from hidden and exposed endpoints. The research properly predicted propagation delay using stationary underwater nodes. Due to ocean motion, propagation delay estimates may not be adequate to correctly time a broadcast.

5.4.2.2 Methodology for Collision-Avoidance

The underwater collision-avoidance method promotes systems that enable collision-free access and dependable gearbox. Cluster-based Delay-Tolerant Protocol (CBDTP) uses reservation-based MAC [12]. This method selected a cluster head for a central controller to coordinate all cluster node data transfers. The cluster head distributes a preset order for each node to all nodes. Each sensor schedules data transmission via the central unit or sleeps to preserve energy. This approach improves transmission efficiency by reducing node communication after the sensor produces data. Nodes must remain stationary for clusters to identify communication connections and estimate propagation round trip latency during registration. Furthermore, the cluster head may experience energy depletion due to its extensive processing of computations and buffer use, hence impacting the overall transmission throughout the cluster.

A node's information was included in the longer propagation delay to avoid collisions and improve throughput [13]. The procedure requires no handshaking but does not require reservations. Sensor nodes intercept and analyze data frames from nearby nodes. By taking into account the time it takes for the signals to propagate, the sensor nodes create a local database that records the periods when neighboring sensor nodes are occupied. The sensor nodes may additionally transmit a concise preliminary notification packet (NTF), enabling neighboring sensors to compute the timing of incoming data frames. This approach has the potential to decrease the occurrence of collisions in underwater sensor settings that have modest movement or are stationary, without the need for any extra synchronous conditions. The process is straightforward and economical.

5.4.2.3 Methodology for Energy Conservation

Underwater sensor networks might use energy-efficient MAC [14]. Instead of using a sleep state, handshaking frames, and transmission time scheduling, this solution reduced physical layer transmission power to save power. Propagation delays classify sensor nodes by their proximity to the sink node. As a result, nodes within the same group have comparable propagation delays. A unique frequency band is subsequently adopted by members of a specific group. An energy-saving lower frequency band may be used for a bigger group. Based on this configuration, the extended time it takes for signals to travel does not necessitate any specific precautions when operating within the same frequency range among a given set of devices. Sensor nodes receive such frequency bands as channels from the central sink node via propagation delays. The sink node then notifies all cluster sensor nodes about the sub-channel allocation. Subsequently, every node can transmit a data packet via a specifically assigned sub-channel. This sensor group channel assignment may cut transmission power and save sensor energy by matching underwater signal-to-noise ratio (SNR) standards.

5.4.3 Energy-Saving MAC Protocols

The motivation for building a MAC protocol in sensor networks is mostly driven by the need to save energy. Sensors that are turned off reduce network longevity and performance. Several DTSN MAC protocols emphasize energy savings to extend network life. The duty cycle is a method for conserving energy by frequently alternating between the active and sleep modes of sensors, hence reducing power consumption during transmission and reception. Extended delays during transmission might lead to increased energy use.

General Energy Conservation Solutions: The MAC layer can identify the energy usage throughout the operations of access, transmission, and reception. Recent sensor networks often use three primary MAC techniques to minimize the energy consumption of sensors [5, 15].

- ***Reducing Collisions***: Collisions result in the inefficient use of data transfers and the unnecessary expenditure of energy. Implementing Agile Medium Access Control (MAC) techniques may effectively prevent or minimize collisions, resulting in energy conservation. Reservation-based MAC approaches synchronize sensors and assign data transmission and reception times to avoid collisions. Collision-free channels need trade-offs in synchronization and scheduling. To establish sensor communication channels, contention-based MAC protocols such as MACA and Carrier Sense Multiple Access/Collision Avoidance (CSMA/CA) [16] exchange short control packets like RTS and CTS before sending data. Transmissions often take place between two nodes, and collisions may occur when hidden terminals are involved. Collisions may grow with node density. Protocols including Sensor-MAC (S-MAC) and Timeout-MAC (T-MAC) do not need time synchronization. These protocols establish time slots among nearby neighbors as virtual clusters, resulting in a reduced collision risk compared to CSMA or MACA techniques.
- ***Reducing Overhead***: Preambles, scheduling packets, acknowledgment packets, and interactive message synchronization are the focus of most packet research. FlexiMAC [17] and other reservation-based MAC protocols leverage tree topologies or position-based knowledge to reduce synchronization costs. Some protocols break preambles into fragments and distribute them at intervals because the brief prelude uses less energy. These protocols use methods borrowed from Berkeley MAC (B-MAC) [18]. Utilizing data aggregation algorithms may effectively minimize the number of RTS/CTS and header broadcasts in asynchronous MAC communications [19].
- ***Minimizing Idle Listening and Overhearing***: Energy is saved with efficient scheduling solutions that reduce overhearing and idle listening. Preamble address information prevents untargeted receivers from intercepting incoming packets [20]. Frame header transmission time avoids idle listening by non-participating receivers. Reservation-based techniques only activate potential recipients within scheduled time windows. Nevertheless, asynchronous request messages have the potential to activate several senders and recipients, resulting in the inefficient use of energy. The time information sent by RTS/CTS signals serves to notify other receivers about the duration of the communication, hence preventing unnecessary idle listening and inadvertent eavesdropping. 802.11 used the Network Allocation Vector (NAV) to signify the length of MAC frame transmission for listeners, allowing them to remain in a sleep state until the designated period had elapsed [21].

The majority of MAC protocols used in DTSNs utilize hybrid techniques to save energy. Asynchronous and Synchronous MAC techniques use distinct approaches to energy conservation in DTSNs. Four distinct techniques on the MAC layer are outlined below to optimize energy consumption in DTSN scenarios.

5.4.3.1 Synchronous Transmissions

Synchronous MAC approaches synchronize sensors and data flow using a global or local clock from central nodes. By using a synchronous frame originating from the central nodes, it is possible to arrange data transfers using various time slots, hence reducing the occurrence of collisions throughout the access period. Table 5.1 is a compilation of synchronous MAC protocols that have been chosen based on their diverse performance objectives [28].

Wireless Sensor Networks with significant traffic use Crankshaft, a Time Division Multiple Access (TDMA) synchronous MAC technology. Crankshaft sensor nodes engage at a predetermined duty cycle to collect signals. Broadcast and unicast channels are created for MAC frames by this protocol. To receive packets via unicast slots and monitor broadcast slots for common data within each frame, every node is synchronized. The sender nodes engage in competition for packet transmissions during the designated time windows while their recipients are actively listening. The average message delay grows in congested traffic because nodes must wait for another duty cycle to resend their messages. This happens when center nodes do not choose the node in the current duty cycle or when its receiver does not acknowledge it. Crankshaft simplifies sender-receiver communication linking compared to contention-based MAC techniques. Nevertheless, the TDMA-based approach limits

TABLE 5.1
Synchronous Transmissions for Energy Saving MAC

Protocols	Crankshaft [22], O-MAC [23], PMAC [24]	S-MAC [25]	T-MAC [26]	LTM-MAC [27]
Scenario	Static nodes, centralized topology, and intensive traffic.	Mobile or stationary, local or centralized, low or medium.	Traffic load might be static, mobile, local, centralized, or fluctuating.	The network is centralized and has little urgent traffic.
Strategies	Data transmission is centralized to save costs.	Local synchronous MAC with a defined duty cycle.	Local synchronous MAC with configurable duty cycle.	Fixed nodes communicate in a pre-defined sequence, whereas mobility nodes prioritize data transfers.
Performance Improvement	Reduce contentions and overhead to save energy.	Local control reduces overhead and enhances scalability.	Reduce overhead via local control; High traffic load.	Improve throughput and energy efficiency.

the capacity of the networks to scale and accommodate mobility. Prioritized Medium Access Control (PMAC) [23] and Optimized-MAC (O-MAC) [24] use similar methods. Scalability and no central nodes are the major features of S-MAC [25], a loosely synchronized MAC system. If a sensor receives no SYNC frame from other nodes within a certain period, it may transmit its schedule using the SYNC packet. S-MAC enables a more relaxed synchronization among neighboring nodes in comparison to TDMA methods.

TDMA necessitates the allocation of predetermined, brief time intervals for synchronization, scheduling, transmission, and reception. Random access and SYNC have a time limit in S-MAC. Therefore, further delays are added to degrade synchronization. All nodes may pick their own sleeping and listening habits. Multiple nodes compete for data transfers to an individual node by sending RTS messages. The winning node is determined by the CTS message sent by the receiver. The process necessitates a greater amount of time to guarantee the transmission of data between senders and receivers compared to TDMA. To build communication linkages, weakly synchronized nodes increase the delay. If no relevant information is received, a potential receiver announces its schedule and remains inactive. The sender might exceed its deadline and must wait for a new cycle. Several repeats may bring the transmitter and receiver together. This is the cost of a delay from central synchronization failure. S-MAC adapts to topology changes since it lacks clustering and core nodes. Listening and connection scheduling take longer than reservation-based MAC techniques.

S-MAC has a constant duty cycle, whereas T-MAC [26] adapts to traffic flow. Due to duty cycles, all nodes wake up to listen to broadcasting neighbors. Energy may be saved throughout this duty cycle. Some nodes queue messages. To manage queued packets, duty cycle active time varies. When the center node arranges queue data transfers, an active node observes and sends data frames. T-MAC solution duty cycle varies. Dynamically finding an ideal active time under changeable load improves the greatest projected traffic load. It also delays node transmission and network joining. In underwater sensor networks, Local Traffic Manager-MAC (LTM-MAC) [27] transmits mobile to stationary nodes via a single-hop, location-based TDMA MAC protocol. Fixed nodes transmit data less than mobile nodes. It takes a long time for stationary sensors to detect no mobile nodes. This architecture enables mobile nodes to send urgent data to static sensors at short contact intervals. During urgent data transfers with short contact intervals, LTM-MAC enhances energy efficiency relative to data speed.

5.4.3.2 Asynchronous Transmissions

Without synchronization, asynchronous MAC protocols allow transmitters and receivers to communicate directly. BMAC [18] recommends preamble sampling and low-power listening to activate receivers. In preamble sampling, data frames follow. Nodes close may detect the initial signal and receive subsequent data frames.

To prolong the preamble, asynchronous MAC protocols may sample non-data, address, time, and data. Long introductions need more energy and close attention. As a result, MAC designers segment a lengthy preface into many smaller preambles to reduce the amount of time spent on listening. An example of this is Enhanced BMAC

[29], which configures the time information in such a way that the receivers may return to an energy-saving mode after they have decoded the information from the preambles. The receivers activate depending on the time to receive data. MFP [30], B-MAC [31], SpeckMAC [32], DPSMAC [33], and SyncWUF [34] employ similar methods. From the preambles, receivers may obtain the broadcast time and conserve energy by sleeping until data frames are received. Carrier Sense Multiple Access-Minimum Preamble Sampling (CSMA-MPS), TICER, X-MAC, and Mobile Hash-Based Message Authentication Code (MHMAC) have a preamble architecture [35–38].

In MX-MAC [39] and SpeckMAC-D [32], data packets may be preambles to repeat data packets. Receivers may receive data packets immediately without preambles or data frames. Implementing this method may reduce energy usage throughout the process of preamble detection. Nevertheless, the recipients are required to decipher the data packet preambles to ascertain the intended recipients based on the destination address. Consequently, the period of channel sampling and energy usage both rise. Optimizing the length and timing of data packets as preambles is crucial for energy conservation.

Duty cycle and Low-Power Listening minimize mesh network waking up in Asynchronous Scheduled-MAC (AS-MAC) [40]. The sensor nodes collect surrounding node wake-up schedules. Consequently, the nodes are unable to intercept any packets due to the presence of individualized wakeup offsets for each receiver. This allows senders to use the channel during receiver wake-up. Asynchronous MAC uses more energy and has more collisions and overheating than AS-MAC. Wakeup offset only works for non-moving sensors. AS-MAC cannot handle DTSN mobility and dynamic change.

The majority of asynchronous solutions are appropriate for settings with modest traffic flow. In such cases, preambles and channel avoidance methods prove to be effective due to the negligible overhead messages required for channel detections. Table 5.2 lists energy-efficient asynchronous transmission MAC techniques.

5.4.3.3 Methodology for Cross-Layer Designs

Various methodologies are being developed to enhance energy efficiency in cross-layer designs, since these designs can minimize the transmission of control signals across layers in DTSN. Network-Coding-based Cooperative ARQ-Medium Access Control (NCCARQ-MAC) [41] is a collaborative ARQ MAC protocol for mobile networks. It combines network coding with ARQ messaging. The technique uses neighboring nodes between source and destination stations to send erroneously acquired packets to the destination. Intermediary nodes send redundant data between source and destination to execute network coding. Reduce the amount of control packets and contention process in a transmission to save energy. The NCCARQ-MAC demonstrates an energy efficiency that is 80 percent higher than the standard ARQ MAC, as determined via rigorous research and simulations.

Cuomo and colleagues [42] introduced a ZigBee sensor network architecture that is both energy-efficient and cross-layered. Using network topology information, this paper developed a central coordinator election process for self-organized ZigBee networks. Reduce the average hops among sensor nodes and the coordinator to save energy.

TABLE 5.2
Asynchronous Transmissions for Energy Saving MAC

Protocols	X-MAC [37], MHMAC [38], TICER [36], CSMA-MPS [35]	BMAC [31], DPS-MAC [33], SyncWUF [34], Enhanced BMAC [29], MFP [30]	MX-MAC [39], SpeckMAC [32]	AS-MAC [40]
Scenario	For low to medium traffic, use a static or mobile ad-hoc network.	For low to medium traffic, use a static or mobile ad-hoc network.	For low to medium traffic, use a static or mobile ad-hoc network.	Low-to-medium traffic, static mesh network structure.
Strategies	Start with time information to lengthen sleep time.	A slotted preamble reduces idle listening.	Preamble data repetition reduces idle listening.	Use wake-up offset and schedule to identify receivers and minimize collisions and overhearing.
Performance Improvement	Save energy by prolonging sleep duration.	Transmission length reduction for energy conservation.	Energy-efficient and fast data decoding.	Reduced energy consumption in fixed networks.

TABLE 5.3
Cross-Layer Designs for Energy-Saving MAC

Protocols	NCCARQ-MAC [41]	Cuomo et al. [42]	Luca Catarinucci [43]
Scenario	Mobile or static, ad-hoc, low or medium	Centralized static PAN, low or medium	Mobile, ad-hoc, and diverse traffic loads
Strategies	Asynchronous MAC	Synchronous MAC	Asynchronous MAC
Performance Improvement	Employing network coding to minimize retransmissions and contentions.	Choose center nodes using hop counts.	Wake up radios for transmission detection.

An alternate cross-layer technique to minimize sensor network energy utilization was proposed by Luca Catarinucci [43]. An energy-efficient wakeup radio locates top-layer data streams. Adjusting wake-up radio-equipped sensor nodes' duty cycle saves energy. Table 5.3 displays a comprehensive collection of energy-saving strategies for cross-layer MAC architecture [28].

5.4.3.4 Technique for Improving Traffic-Adaptive and Throughput with MAC Solutions

Traffic adaptation is often used to increase throughput in DTSNs with restricted physical channels. Traffic adaptability optimizes the allocation of resources to nodes that experience high demand, resulting in enhanced functional throughput in sensor networks. In crowded traffic locations, the MAC layer scheduling mechanism may spread channel resources between nodes due to greater transmission, enhancing network efficiency. Nodes with less traffic may have slower data transfers. MAC protocols provide the ability to adjust the rate at which data is sent based on the patterns of network traffic. Recent MAC protocols have recently been developed for sensor networks with changing traffic loads.

5.4.3.4.1 Methodology 1: Dynamic Resource Allocation

Traffic-Adaptive Medium Access Protocol (TRAMA) [44], a novel MAC protocol, conserves sensor network energy via traffic-adaptive algorithms. TRAMA avoids network collisions by scheduling access. This strategy is comparable to Sensor-MAC (S-MAC) and includes local synchronization. A selection process is used to choose receivers based on the broadcast schedules and traffic loads in the following manner: Every sensor collects data from its surrounding area and determines its transmission schedule. This metadata delineates the prospective recipients of its traffic. Subsequently, the nearby central node can allocate time intervals for the transmission or reception of packets by these adjacent nodes. When receiving the schedule in this period, certain nodes may convert to energy-saving mode. However, traffic adaption is confined to a high-traffic area. The process of local synchronizing and scheduling in TRAMA may deplete the resources of local center nodes and result in significant energy consumption, particularly when the traffic volume is low. Consequently, there has been an increase in the development of MAC protocols to accommodate various traffic conditions.

Traffic-adaptive Medium Access Control (TaMAC) [45] is a MAC system with a star topology designed specifically for Wireless Body Area Networks. In this arrangement, a central coordinator assumes the responsibility of overseeing the organization and coordination of network operations, including scheduling and synchronizing. The TaMAC protocol handles normal and urgent traffic with two-channel access methods. The wake-up radio concept focuses on allocating resources for immediate and requested communication. Traffic-based wakeup manages regular traffic requests that are not urgent. In this mechanism, the coordinator allocates and distributes channel resources to nearby nodes depending on their traffic patterns. The technique efficiently divides the present traffic into several categories depending on priority, leading to decreased power use and the capability to provide a particular Quality of Service for different kinds of traffic using TDMA.

Prioritized Medium Access Control (PMAC) [23], a TDMA-based protocol, adapts to traffic circumstances using neighborhood traffic information like TRAMA. Power Adapted MAC (PAMAC) sets sensor wake-up and sleep timings depending on local traffic, unlike TRAMA. These patterns allow sensor nodes to sleep while MAC Synchronization or broadcast frames save energy while the network is idle. After each frame, sensors share their patterns, which are then used to update the node pattern. This revised pattern provides local traffic information. The pattern information is sent by either increasing or reducing the awake and sleep duration in a multiplicative or additive manner. The rate at which sleep time increases may either be acute, meaning it is multiplied, or sluggish, meaning it is added. The specific situation of the application determines which kind of rise occurs. PMAC is designed to optimize energy consumption during low traffic loads and improve data transmission efficiency during high traffic loads. However, it fails to tackle the problem of passive listening that occurs between consecutive periods of active engagement. Additionally, using a pre-established time duration for the wake-up phase might result in heightened probabilities of crashes during times characterized by high traffic volume.

A Traffic Load Aware Sensor (ATLAS) [46] uses the IEEE 802.15.4 superframe structure with contention, specified, and sleeping periods. According to traffic volume, contention, allocated, and sleep periods may be changed. ATLAS may raise contention and dedicated periods to accommodate more data transfers in high-volume network environments. Sleeping longer saves energy with low traffic. ATLAS enhances the efficiency of traffic load management by optimizing network capacity, resulting in improved energy efficiency and channel utilization. The Priority-based Load Adaptive MAC (PLA-MAC) [47] employs a superframe architecture dependent on traffic demand to save power use. ATLAS and PLA-MAC are constrained to Delay-Tolerant Sensor Networks (DTSN) applications due to the Wireless Personal Area Network (WPAN) design of IEEE802.15.4. Table 5.4 displays a collection of strategies for dynamically allocating resources in MAC protocols, intending to improve traffic adaptability and throughput.

TABLE 5.4
Dynamic Resource Allocation

Protocols	TRAMA [44]	TaMAC [45]	PMAC [23]	ATLAS [46], PLA-MAC [47]
Scenario	Local centralized networks have low to medium traffic, sluggish, and static mobility.	Centralized, static network with low-to-medium load.	Static, centralized, adaptable traffic.	Slow, static mobility, Local centralized, WPAN Low to medium, adaptable.
Strategies	Set nodes to sleep based on traffic patterns, and choose receivers based on traffic load.	Dual channel access, central node resource allocation based on traffic patterns, emergency wake-up radio.	Neighborhood traffic affects node wakefulness patterns.	Adjust MAC 802.15.4 superframe for traffic volume.
Performance Improvement	Medium traffic loads are energy-efficient, whereas low traffic loads have significant energy costs.	Enhanced energy efficiency and service quality.	Energy conservation during a traffic-free time.	Save energy and boost output.

5.4.3.4.2 Methodology 2: Hybrid Access

Many MAC protocols allow mobile sensor networks with hybrid architectures. While adapting to traffic and loads, this may employ contention-based or reservation-based MAC protocols. Contention-based MAC protocols such as slotted CSMA/CA save energy and improve efficiency in low-traffic areas. Due to overhead and collisions from many transmission requests in a brief contention time, they degrade network throughputs in high-traffic locations. Reservation-based MAC protocols like TDMA provide high throughput under heavy traffic. However, they place a significant burden on central coordinating nodes and use substantial energy during scheduling and synchronization operations when the traffic is less. Consequently, the combination of these two systems promotes versatile traffic adaptation at the MAC layer.

Gilani et al. [48] introduced an IEEE 802.15.4-based TDMA-CSMA hybrid MAC scheme. This method uses the data frame's reserved bits to retrieve network node queue status information. The central coordinator identifies network collisions and monitors surrounding node data queues. It causes traffic congestion. The coordinator assigns CSMA/CA and TDMA Contention Access Periods (CAP) using this data. TDMA uses a short CAP to minimize collisions and access overhead from heavy traffic. Low traffic may cause a lengthy CAP utilizing CSMA/CA to minimize scheduling and synchronization. Thus, this hybrid technique reduces energy use and boosts data throughput.

iQueue-MAC [49] uses CSMA for minimal usage and TDMA for high loads. Based on queue length, iQueue-MAC allocates the sender's time slots in synchronous mode under high traffic. Queue-MAC uses a low-duty-cycle CSMA MAC protocol under light traffic to conserve electricity. Sensor movement is ignored by the protocol.

Zebra-Media Access Control (Z-MAC) [50] improved collision resolution using CSMA MAC and a timeline as a TDMA mechanism. During deployment, Z-MAC uses Distributed Randomized (DRAND) to allocate time slots to every node, like TDMA. This operation consumes energy and additional messages, but it prioritizes preset users over randomly accessed nodes for these slots. Like CSMA, carrier sensing and data transport may randomly access each period. Establishing a beginning contention window gives the specified user priority over other users. This architecture prevents slot access collisions, saving energy and increasing throughput. CSMA and TDMA are combined in Funneling MAC [51]. WSN multi-layer sink data collecting funnels. The sensors near the washbasin are suited for TDMA due to heavy usage. However, sensors further away from the washbasin have limited usage and are ideal for CSMA. Funneling MAC-like protocol Multimode Hybrid-MAC (MH-MAC) [38]. Traffic may switch nodes among asynchronous and synchronous modes. For heterogeneous traffic in stationary sensor nodes, these three hybrid MAC approaches function effectively. However, mobile nodes cause frequent network structure changes and assignment process recalculations, which increase energy consumption and overhead messages, making these protocols difficult. Figure 5.3 shows the illustration of hybrid access methods.

Table 5.5 displays a set of hybrid access strategies for MAC protocols that aim to increase traffic adaptability and throughput.

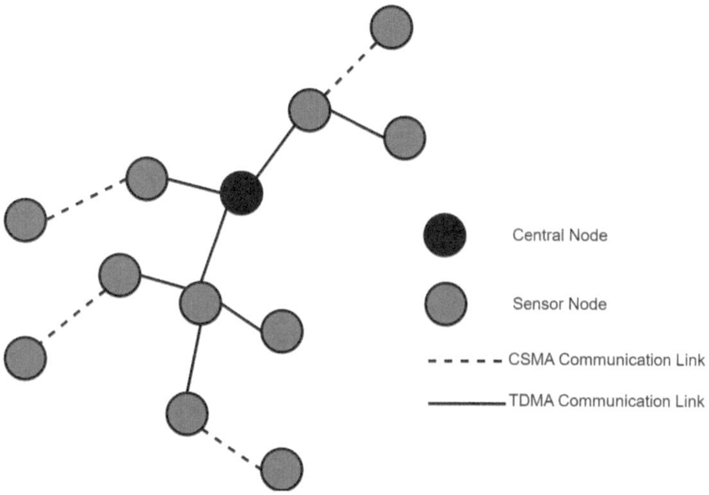

FIGURE 5.3 Hybrid access methods.

TABLE 5.5
Hybrid Access Methods

Protocols	Hybrid CSMA/ TDMA [48]	iQueue-MAC [49]	MH-MAC [38], Z-MAC [50], Funneling MAC [52]
Scenario	Slow, static mobile, Local centralized, WPAN Low to medium, adaptable	Local centralized, Low to medium, adaptable	Ad-hoc static Low to moderate adaptability
Strategies	CSMA and TDMA combined, resource reserved based on queue status.	CSMA and TDMA coupled, buffer queue length determines resource reservation.	Switch between TDMA and CSMA based on traffic.
Performance Improvement	Boost throughput and keep energy.	Improve the throughput and preserve energy.	Boost throughput and preserve energy.

5.4.3.4.3 Methodology 3: Block and Aggregated Transmission

Burst transmissions [53] provide body sensor networks with an auto-adaptive methodology. To handle burst transmissions, the algorithm adjusts sample time and preamble based on traffic patterns. The protocol also provides energy-efficient sink node communication. This method is energy-efficient during burst transmissions because it dynamically adjusts to network traffic.

Adaptive Frame Length Aggregation Scheme (AFLAS) [19] is a wireless delay tolerance MAC 802.11 adaptive aggregation. Figure 5.4 shows an integrated AFLAS frame with many small MAC sub-frames. AFLAS combines tiny MAC frames into big ones. The aggregated frame length depends on higher layer needs

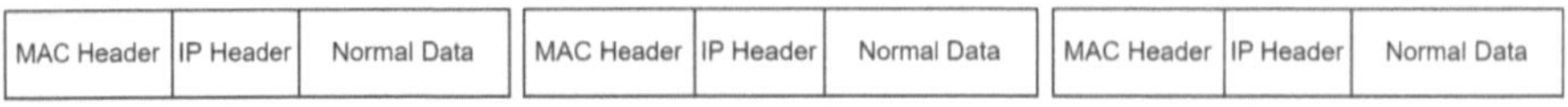

FIGURE 5.4 MAC protocol aggregation frames.

TABLE 5.6
Block and Aggregated Transmission

Protocols	Burst Transmissions [53]	AFLAS [19]
Scenario	Static or low mobile traffic, ad hoc traffic, low to medium traffic, adaptive traffic	Ad-hoc, mobile, low to high-traffic
Strategies	Adjust the sample duration and preamble length based on traffic trends.	Depending on the traffic load and wireless channels, combine several MAC frames into a bigger one.
Performance Improvement	Improve throughput and energy efficiency	Reducing overhead and improve throughput

and wireless channel state [54]. This method lowers transmissions and overhead. Under dynamic channel conditions, AFLAS improves energy efficiency and transmission throughput.

Table 5.6 shows the MAC protocol block along with aggregated transmission choices for improving traffic flexibility and throughput.

5.5 MOBILITY SUPPORT MAC PROTOCOLS

The structure and traffic of sensor networks change as they move. These changes have an impact on MAC designs in terms of connection connectivity, collision avoidance, as well as access control. Cluster and ad hoc linked MAC systems connect and manage resources for incoming and outgoing mobile sensors differently. Hybrid and cross-layer systems regulate traffic density to save energy and increase throughput.

1. ***Cluster-based MAC Technique***: The Mobile-aware TDMA (M-TDMA)-based MAC protocol [51] separates superframe cycles among control and data. The first slot comprises head transmission cluster data for mobility-management control, the second slot access data for additional nodes, and the third slot broadcast information. Free spaces for additional nodes and node transmission slots are in the data section. Clusterheads schedule and allot slots to each node in each cluster. Extra slots are shared between clusters and open for future allocation to control mobility. Mobility in this TDMA protocol takes time due to these additional slots. The control component of an incoming sensor's MAC frame delivers access data to a clusterhead. It checks unassigned data slots and provides spaces for this node. If TDMA superframe control area conflicts occur, fresh incoming nodes retransmit access requests using a randomized back-off timer. The protocol

allocates resources based on mobility and flexible slot access contentions. However, outgoing sensor slots are not reconfigured quickly to conserve energy. This protocol is only utilized in low-speed mobility when clusterhead can synchronize nearby sensors along with reserve slots for them while moving.

2. ***Ad-Hoc Connected MAC Technique***: In MS-MAC, nodes monitor SYNC messages with predetermined schedules for a certain time, similar to S-MAC, [55]. If no SYNC packets are received, the node will compute its duty cycle and send it as a packet before entering sleep mode. Nodes engage on both schedules if they receive multiple SYNC messages. MS-MAC's SYNC message comprises transmitter scheduling, neighboring device mobility, and sensor velocity estimates. The transient central node may recognize a busy region and schedule data transmission based on mobility data and surrounding node velocity. It may also create new connections for incoming mobile nodes and alter them as they move to different clusters. A fast-moving node cannot receive SYNC data from adjacent nodes or adhere to a broadcasting schedule. The MS-MAC protocol dynamically adapts the frequencies of the synchronization period based on the speed of the nodes. This ensures that the SYNC information, either from neighboring nodes or the node itself, may be effectively received. Mobile nodes can quickly connect to new neighbors and conserve energy during idleness because of the variable duty cycle.

   The Mobility adaptive MAC (MMAC) [56] algorithm takes into account the changes in physical connections between nodes caused by their movement and changes in topology. It allocates data transfers to sensors dynamically and establishes a customizable duration inside a superframe. The protocol has the potential to enhance both energy efficiency and throughput in circumstances involving mobility. Nevertheless, the availability of location information from sensors has often been unattainable in the majority of sensor networks, hence restricting the potential uses of this protocol.
3. ***Hybrid MAC Technique***: FlexiMAC is also known as Flexible MAC. This protocol is synchronized and based on TDMA. It has a flexible slot structure that enables it to accommodate node mobility and network dynamics. Sinks capture neighbor exchange packets during competition to construct a data tree. FlexiMAC's slot designs are divided into two types: data-gathering and multi-functional. The created tree provides data-gathering spaces for sinks to collect uplink traffic. Multi-functional slots are used to carry downlink traffic and synchronization. Fault Tolerant Slot (FTS) contention periods allow new mobile nodes to make transmission requests for inclusion in the existing data-gathering tree.
4. ***Cross-layer Designs for Mobile Sensors***: In a cluster-tree topology, a hybrid design comprising fixed and mobile nodes is employed [57]. Mobile nodes communicate with immobile nodes through multi-channel communications and rapid cluster hand-off, while clusterheads provide a durable and effective backbone having a high data transfer rate. Topology information and network and MAC layer access requests may be used to modify the contention

window to reduce collisions. MobiSense achieves high throughput through multi-channel at the MAC layer. While the cross-layer architecture of MobiSense enables mobility support and high throughput, it is limited in fixed topology and scalability when dealing with unique combined static and mobile sensor applications. When a significant influx of mobile nodes occurs in a given network, the hand-off and scheduling method may not be executed quickly, thereby compromising transmissions [58–61].

5.6 MAC PROTOCOLS FOR RELIABILITY

MAC methods provide robust dependability by using two approaches: retransmission and redundant transmissions. Retransmission methods in sensor networks sacrifice latency and energy to enhance dependability. Redundant solutions, on the other hand, often result in increased resource consumption.

1. ***Retransmission-based Solutions***: Retransmission is a commonly used technique in data communication networks to ensure the dependability of data transmission. A packet is sent again until the permitted retransmission limit has been reached if it is not received correctly owing to a NACK message or ACK time-out. Retransmission is a commonly used technique in sensor networks to retrieve lost data, particularly when there are limitations in energy and memory resources. Routing Enhanced MAC protocol (RMAC) [62] represents a multi-hop CSMA/CA MAC that acknowledges the sender with explicit ARQ messages for error control. Sensor nodes placed at the intermediate level can transmit data packets to the next hop immediately after receiving a packet, without having to wait for the back-off time [28, 63–67]. The sender interprets the transmitted message as confirmation that the intermediary nodes were reached. RMAC uses both explicit and implicit acknowledgments to maintain dependability. RMAC dynamically adjusts the permitted amount of retransmission attempts based on packet defects to improve node-to-node reliability. A similar retransmission method may be seen in other dependable MAC systems as E2RMAC [63].
2. ***Redundant-based Solutions***: Sending multiple packets improves reliability. The packet duplicate may be broadcast by various channels, networks, radios, or pathways. To recover corrupted packets, the receiver may use agreed-upon methods. Frequency channel shifting separates channels to reduce fading and interference. The wireless channels may be used for transmitting duplicate packets to improve the dependability of Alert [58–60]. The energy-efficient strategy prevents the implementation of redundant-based MAC solutions because of limitations in resources such as channels, routes, and radios.

The Random Backoff MAC [61] protocol leverages the inherent broadcast nature of wireless network data transmissions over numerous channels and receivers. This allows for duplicate transmissions to occur without any additional energy usage. One multicast receiver should convey the packet to the next node with the exactly obtained broadcast message, according to the protocol. PFR is used to distribute data across numerous channels in the Random Backoff MAC protocol, picking pathways with a better chance of success without flooding the network over broadcast messages. This step guarantees that at least one recipient can accurately receive the packets. Multiple receivers may relay the information, and three collision avoidance algorithms reduce energy and interference. The Simple Random Backoff Protocol (SRBP) controls receiver forwarding using an equally distributed and randomly generated backoff timer. This stochastic backoff time depends on application delay and energy needs. Network traffic and density determine the time range for the Adaptive Random Backoff Protocol (ARBP). Range Adaptive Random Backoff Protocol (RARBP) dynamically adjusts time dependent on message transmission line distance. To prevent collisions, Random Backoff MAC trades latency for dependability. among many downstream devices in multipath transmission networks. Nevertheless, the use of the multipath method in Backoff MAC is limited to unidirectional or sparsely populated network traffic scenarios. During instances of high transmission demand, there is a risk of message overload, which may destroy data connections.

5.7 CONCLUSION

This chapter discusses three data transmission strategies for green wireless networks to improve throughput, energy economy, and overhead performance. CPMAC seems to be an effective MAC solution for weakly coupled vehicle networks. The presented sensor-sink contact interval guides three transmission algorithms to effectively transfer data to the sink, balancing data throughput and energy. The MAC technique operates two standard protocols in sparse vehicular network data throughput, transmission delay, and power-saving simulations. AFLAS examines the relationship between SNR and MAC layer frame length and recommends the cumulative frame length based on current SNR using priority queues to account for collision and transmission fault. AFLAS simulations demonstrate that the adaptive frame length strategy outperforms non-adaptive alternatives in data throughput, repeated transmissions, and effectiveness of transmission. Energy efficiency is essential for MAC transmission development and evaluation. The energy efficiency of MAC protocols is measured by comparing data packets to energy consumption. We study energy-efficient MAC features to construct green wireless networks. TREE MAC optimizes energy efficiency and traffic demand via reservation and contention modes. TREE simulations demonstrate that high-traffic green wireless networks are more energy efficient than MAC approaches.

REFERENCES

[1] Y. Ren, R. Werner, N. Pazzi, and A. Boukerche, "Monitoring patients via a secure and mobile healthcare system," *IEEE Wireless Communications*, vol. 17, no. 1, pp. 59–65, 2010.

[2] A. Camilli, C. E. Cugnasca, A. M. Saraiva, A. R. Hirakawa, and P. L. Correa, "From wireless sensors to field mapping: Anatomy of an application for precision agriculture," *Computers and Electronics in Agriculture*, vol. 58, no. 1, pp. 25–36, 2007.

[3] J. Burrell, T. Brooke, and R. Beckwith, "Vineyard computing: Sensor networks in agricultural production," *IEEE Pervasive Computing*, vol. 3, no. 1, pp. 38–45, 2004.
[4] C. Zhu, V. C. Leung, L. Shu, and E. C.-H. Ngai, "Green internet of things for smart world," *IEEE Access*, vol. 3, pp. 2151–2162, 2015.
[5] A. Bachir, M. Dohler, T. Watteyne, and K. K. Leung, "MAC essentials for wireless sensor networks," *IEEE Communications Surveys & Tutorials*, vol. 12, no. 2, pp. 222–248, 2010.
[6] N. Bansal and Z. Liu, "Capacity, delay and mobility in wireless ad-hoc networks," *INFOCOM 2003. Twenty-Second Annual Joint Conference of the IEEE Computer and Communications*. IEEE Societies, vol. 2, pp. 1553–1563, 2003.
[7] M. Grossglauser and D. Tse, "Mobility increases the capacity of ad-hoc wireless networks," *INFOCOM 2001. Twentieth Annual Joint Conference of the IEEE Computer and Communications Societies. Proceedings*. IEEE, vol. 3, pp. 1360–1369, 2001.
[8] A. E. Gamal, J. Mammen, B. Prabhakar, and D. Shah, "Throughput-delay trade-off in wireless networks," *INFOCOM 2004. Twenty-third Annual Joint Conference of the IEEE Computer and Communications Societies*, vol. 1, 2004.
[9] A. Markhasin, "Performance analysis of the delay-tolerant satellite distributed MAC reservation protocols," *Satellite and Space Communications, 2009. IWSSC 2009. International Workshop on*, pp. 376–380, 2009.
[10] V. Bharghavan, A. Demers, S. Shenker, and L. Zhang, "Macaw: A media access protocol for wireless LAN's," *ACM SIGCOMM Computer Communication Review*, vol. 24, no. 4, pp. 212–225, 1994.
[11] Y. Zhong, J. Huang, and J. Han, "A delay-tolerant MAC protocol with collision avoidance for underwater acoustic networks," *Wireless Communications, Networking and Mobile Computing, 2009. WiCom'09. 5th International Conference on*, pp. 1–4, 2009.
[12] Z. Zhang, "A cluster based delay tolerant mac protocol for underwater wireless sensor network," *Proceedings of the International Conference on Wireless Networks (ICWN)*, p. 1, 2013.
[13] N. Chirdchoo, W.-S. Soh, and K. C. Chua, "Aloha-based mac protocols with collision avoidance for underwater acoustic networks," *INFOCOM 2007. 26th IEEE International Conference on Computer Communications*. IEEE, pp. 2271–2275, 2007.
[14] J. Cheon and H.-S. Cho, "A delay-tolerant ofdma-based mac protocol for underwater acoustic sensor networks," *Underwater Technology (UT), 2011 IEEE Symposium on and 2011 Workshop on Scientific Use of Submarine Cables and Related Technologies (SSC)*, pp. 1–4, 2011.
[15] A. Boukerch, L. Xu, and K. El-Khatib, "Trust-based security for wireless ad hoc and sensor networks," *Computer Communications*, vol. 30, no. 11, pp. 2413–2427, 2007.
[16] P. Karn, "Maca-a new channel access method for packet radio," *ARRL/CRRL Amateur Radio 9th Computer Networking Conference*, vol. 140, pp. 134–140, 1990.
[17] W. L. Lee, A. Datta, and R. Cardell-Oliver, "Fleximac: A flexible TDMA-based MAC protocol for fault-tolerant and energy-efficient wireless sensor networks," *Networks, 2006. ICON'06. 14th IEEE International Conference on*, vol. 2, pp. 1–6, 2006.
[18] A. Woo and D. E. Culler, "A transmission control scheme for media access in sensor networks," *MobiCom '01: Proceedings of the 7th Annual International Conference on Mobile Computing and Networking*, pp. 221–235, 2001.
[19] X. Zhou and A. Boukerche, "Aflas: An adaptive frame length aggregation scheme in vehicular networks," *IEEE Transactions on Vehicular Technology*, vol. PP, no. 99, pp. 1–1, 2016.
[20] A. Bachir, D. Barthel, M. Heusse, and A. Duda, "Micro-frame preamble MAC for multihop wireless sensor networks," *Communications, 2006. ICC'06. IEEE International Conference on*, vol. 7, pp. 3365–3370, 2006.

[21] "IEEE draft standard for information technology – telecommunications and information exchange between systems – local and metropolitan area networks – specific requirements – part 11: Wireless LAN medium access control (MAC) and physical layer (PHY) specifications," IEEE P802.11-REVmb/D10.0, pp. 1–3026, August 2011.
[22] G. P. Halkes and K. Langendoen, "Crankshaft: An energy-efficient MAC protocol for dense wireless sensor networks," In: Langendoen, K., Voigt, T. (eds), *Wireless Sensor Networks*, pp. 228–244, 2007. https://doi.org/10.1007/978-3-540-69830-2_15
[23] T. Zheng, S. Radhakrishnan, and V. Sarangan, "PMAC: An adaptive energy efficient MAC protocol for wireless sensor networks," *Parallel and Distributed Processing Symposium, 2005. Proceedings. 19th IEEE International*, pp. 8–pp, 2005.
[24] H. Cao, K. W. Parker, and A. Arora, "O-mac: A receiver centric power management protocol," *Network Protocols, 2006. ICNP'06. Proceedings of the 2006 14th IEEE International Conference on*, pp. 311–320, 2006.
[25] W. Ye, J. Heidemann, and D. Estrin, "An energy-efficient MAC protocol for wireless sensor networks," *INFOCOM 2002. Twenty-First Annual Joint Conference of the IEEE Computer and Communications Societies. Proceedings*. IEEE, vol. 3, pp. 1567–1576, 2002.
[26] T. Van Dam and K. Langendoen, "An adaptive energy-efficient MAC protocol for wireless sensor networks," *Proceedings of the 1st International Conference on Embedded Networked Sensor Systems*, pp. 171–180, 2003.
[27] J. Mao, S. Chen, J. Yu, Y. Gu, R. Yu, and Y. Xu, "LTM-MAC: A location-based TDMA MAC protocol for mobile underwater networks," *OCEANS 2016*, Shanghai, pp. 1–5, 2016.
[28] X. Zhou, "Green communication protocols for mobile wireless networks," Doctoral dissertation, Université d'Ottawa/University of Ottawa, 2017.
[29 S. Lim, S. Kim, J. Cho, and S. An, "Medium access control with an energy efficient algorithm for wireless sensor networks," *IFIP International Conference on Personal Wireless Communications*, pp. 334–343, 2006.
[30] A. Bachir, D. Barthel, M. Heusse, and A. Duda, "Micro-frame preamble MAC for multihop wireless sensor networks," *Communications, 2006. ICC'06. IEEE International Conference on*, vol. 7, pp. 3365–3370, 2006.
[31] M. Avvenuti, P. Corsini, P. Masci, and A. Vecchio, "Increasing the efficiency of preamble sampling protocols for wireless sensor networks," *Mobile Computing and Wireless Communication International Conference, 2006. MCWC 2006. Proceedings of the First*, pp. 117–122, 2006.
[32] K.-J. Wong and D. Arvind, "Speckmac: Low-power decentralised MAC protocols for low data rate transmissions in specknets," *Proceedings of the 2nd International Workshop on Multi-hop Ad Hoc Networks: From Theory to Reality*, pp. 71–78, 2006.
[33] S. Lim, Y. Ji, J. Cho, and S. An, "An ultra low power medium access control protocol with the divided preamble sampling," *Ubiquitous Computing Systems*, pp. 210–224, Springer, 2006.
[34] X. Shi and G. Stromberg, "Syncwuf: An ultra low-power MAC protocol for wireless sensor networks," *IEEE Transactions on Mobile Computing*, vol. 6, no. 1, pp. 115–125, 2007.
[35] S. Mahlknecht and M. Bock, "CSMA-MPS: A minimum preamble sampling MAC protocol for low power wireless sensor networks," *Factory Communication Systems, 2004. Proceedings. 2004 IEEE International Workshop on*, pp. 73–80, 2004.
[36] E.-Y. Lin, J. M. Rabaey, A. Wolisz, et al., "Power-efficient rendezvous schemes for dense wireless sensor networks," *Communications, 2004 IEEE International Conference on*, vol. 7, pp. 3769–3776, 2004.
[37] M. Buettner, G. V. Yee, E. Anderson, and R. Han, "X-MAC: A short preamble MAC protocol for duty-cycled wireless sensor networks," *Proceedings of the 4th International Conference on Embedded Networked Sensor Systems*, pp. 307–320, 2006.

[38] L. Bernardo, R. Oliveira, M. Pereira, M. Macedo, and P. Pinto, "A wireless sensor MAC protocol for bursty data traffic," *Personal, Indoor and Mobile Radio Communications, 2007. PIMRC 2007. IEEE 18th International Symposium on*, pp. 1–5, 2007.

[39] C. Merlin and W. Heinzelman, "Network-aware adaptation of MAC scheduling for wireless sensor networks," *Proceedings of the Conference on Distributed Computing in Sensor Systems (Poster Session)*, pp. 24–28, 2007.

[40] B. Jang, J. B. Lim, and M. L. Sichitiu, "An asynchronous scheduled MAC protocol for wireless sensor networks," *Computer Networks*, vol. 57, no. 1, pp. 85–98, 2013.

[41] A. Antonopoulos, C. Verikoukis, C. Skianis, and O. B. Akan, "Energy efficient network coding-based MAC for cooperative ARQ wireless networks," *Ad Hoc Networks*, vol. 11, no. 1, pp. 190–200, 2013.

[42] F. Cuomo, A. Abbagnale, and E. Cipollone, "Cross-layer network formation for energy-efficient IEEE 802.15. 4/zigbee wireless sensor networks," *Ad Hoc Networks*, vol. 11, no. 2, pp. 672–686, 2013.

[43] L. Catarinucci, R. Colella, G. Del Fiore, L. Mainetti, V. Mighali, L. Patrono, and M. L. Stefanizzi, "A cross-layer approach to minimize the energy consumption in wireless sensor networks," *International Journal of Distributed Sensor Networks*, vol. 10, no. 1, 2014. https://doi.org/10.1155/2014/268284

[44] V. Rajendran, K. Obraczka, and J. J. Garcia-Luna-Aceves, "Energy-efficient, collision-free medium access control for wireless sensor networks," *Wireless Networks*, vol. 12, no. 1, pp. 63–78, 2006.

[45] S. Ullah and K. S. Kwak, "An ultra low-power and traffic-adaptive medium access control protocol for wireless body area network," *Journal of Medical Systems*, vol. 36, no. 3, pp. 1021–1030, 2012.

[46] M. O. Rahman, C. S. Hong, S. Lee, and Y.-C. Bang, "ATLAS: A traffic load aware sensor MAC design for collaborative body area sensor networks," *Sensors*, vol. 11, no. 12, pp. 11560–11580, 2011.

[47] I. Anjum, N. Alam, M. A. Razzaque, M. Mehedi Hassan, and A. Alamri, "Traffic priority and load adaptive MAC protocol for QOS provisioning in body sensor networks," *International Journal of Distributed Sensor Networks*, vol. 9, no. 3, 2013. https://doi.org/10.1155/2013/205192

[48] M. H. S. Gilani, I. Sarrafi, and M. Abbaspour, "An adaptive CSMA/TDMA hybrid MAC for energy and throughput improvement of wireless sensor networks," *AdHoc Networks*, vol. 11, no. 4, pp. 1297–1304, 2013.

[49] S. Zhuo, Z. Wang, Y.-Q. Song, Z. Wang, and L. Almeida, "IQueue-MAC: A traffic adaptive duty-cycled MAC protocol with dynamic slot allocation," *Sensor, Mesh and Ad Hoc Communications and Networks (SECON), 2013 10th Annual IEEE Communications Society Conference on*, pp. 95–103, 2013.

[50] I. Rhee, A. Warrier, M. Aia, J. Min, and M. L. Sichitiu, "Z-MAC: A hybrid MAC for wireless sensor networks," *IEEE/ACM Transactions on Networking (TON)*, vol. 16, no. 3, pp. 511–524, 2008.

[51] A. Jhumka and S. Kulkarni, "On the design of mobility-tolerant TDMA-based media access control (MAC) protocol for mobile sensor networks," *Distributed Computing and Internet Technology*, pp. 42–53, Springer, 2007.

[52] G.-S. Ahn, S. G. Hong, E. Miluzzo, A. T. Campbell, and F. Cuomo, "Funnelingmac: A localized, sink-oriented MAC for boosting fidelity in sensor networks," *Proceedings of the 4th International Conference on Embedded Networked Sensor Systems*, pp. 293–306, 2006.

[53] R. Kuntz, A. Gallais, and T. Noel, "Auto-adaptive MAC for energy-efficient burst transmissions in wireless sensor networks," *Wireless Communications and Networking Conference (WCNC), 2011 IEEE*, pp. 233–238, 2011.
[54] Y. Zhao, C. Miao, and M. Ma, "An energy-efficient self-adaptive duty cycle MAC protocol for traffic-dynamic wireless sensor networks," *Wireless Personal Communications*, vol. 68, no. 4, pp. 1287–1315, 2013.
[55] H. Pham and S. Jha, "An adaptive mobility-aware MAC protocol for sensor networks (MS-MAC)," *Mobile Ad-hoc and Sensor Systems, 2004 IEEE International Conference on*, pp. 558–560, 2004.
[56] M. Ali, T. Suleman, and Z. A. Uzmi, "MMAC: A mobility-adaptive, collision-free MAC protocol for wireless sensor networks," *Performance, Computing, and Communications Conference, 2005. IPCCC 2005. 24th IEEE International*, pp. 401–407, 2005.
[57] A. Gonga, O. Landsiedel, and M. Johansson, "Mobisense: Power-efficient micromobility in wireless sensor networks," *Distributed Computing in Sensor Systems and Workshops (DCOSS), 2011 International Conference on*, pp. 1–8, 2011.
[58] V. Namboodiri and A. Keshavarzian, "Alert: An adaptive low-latency event driven MAC protocol for wireless sensor networks," *Proceedings of the 7th International Conference on Information Processing in Sensor Networks*, pp. 159–170, 2008.
[59] J. So and N. H. Vaidya, "Multi-channel MAC for ad hoc networks: Handling multi-channel hidden terminals using a single transceiver," *Proceedings of the 5th ACM International Symposium on Mobile Ad hoc Networking and Computing*, pp. 222–233, 2004.
[60] R. Maheshwari, H. Gupta, and S. R. Das, "Multichannel MAC protocols for wireless networks," *Sensor and Ad Hoc Communications and Networks, 2006. SECON'06. 2006 3rd Annual IEEE Communications Society on*, vol. 2, pp. 393–401, 2006.
[61] I. Chatzigiannakis, A. Kinalis, and S. Nikoletseas, "Wireless sensor networks protocols for efficient collision avoidance in multi-path data propagation," *Proceedings of the 1st ACM International Workshop on Performance Evaluation of Wireless Ad Hoc, Sensor, and Ubiquitous Networks*, pp. 8–16, 2004.
[62] R. Biswas, V. Jain, C. Ghosh, and D. P. Agrawal, "On-demand reliable medium access in sensor networks," *Proceedings of the 2006 International Symposium on World of Wireless, Mobile and Multimedia Networks*, pp. 251–257, 2006.
[63] V. Jain, R. Biswas, and D. P. Agrawal, "Energy-efficient and reliable medium access in sensor networks," *World of Wireless, Mobile and Multimedia Networks, 2007. WoWMoM 2007. IEEE International Symposium on a*, pp. 1–8, 2007.
[64] D. Ghai, S. L. Tripathi, S. Saxena, M. Chanda, and M. Alazab (Eds.), *Machine Learning Algorithms for Signal and Image Processing*, John Wiley & Sons, 2022.
[65] G. B. Raja, "Impact of internet of things, artificial intelligence, and blockchain technology in Industry 4.0," In *Internet of Things, Artificial Intelligence and Blockchain Technology*, pp. 157–178, 2021. https://doi.org/10.1007/978-3-030-74150-1_8
[66] G. B. Raja, "Impact of IIOT in future industries: Opportunities and challenges," *Internet of Things*, pp. 101–112, 2021.
[67] G. B. Raja, "Effective waste management system for smart cities," *Intelligent Green Technologies for Sustainable Smart Cities*, pp. 33–52, 2022. https://doi.org/10.1002/9781119816096.ch3

6 EnSlight
Energy Autonomous LoRaWAN-Based, IoT-Enabled, Real-Time Street Light Management System for Smart Cities and Smart Villages

Prajnyajit Mohanty, Umesh C. Pati, and Kamalakanta Mahapatra
NIT Rourkela, Rourkela, India

6.1 INTRODUCTION

The ever-evolving landscape of modernization ushers a continuous wave of progress, particularly the ingenious design of smart cities and villages using digital technology. According to reports, it is anticipated that a significant proportion of the global population, approximately 68%–70%, will undergo a transition from rural to urban regions by 2050 [1]. Similarly, the villages and rural areas have attracted researchers' attention to turn them into smart villages nowadays. There have been significant developments over the years in various applications associated with smart cities and smart villages, such as smart healthcare, smart transportation, smart governance, smart energy, smart education, smart building and infrastructure, etc. Street lighting is a prominent application among others, which affects the day-to-day life in cities and villages. Currently, cities account for 75% of global energy consumption, with street lights alone using around 30%–40% of total electricity consumption in a city [2]. Hence, the consideration of energy efficiency is of paramount importance when designing street lights. There have been continuous and persistent efforts in the recent past to integrate the Internet of Things (IoT) into this application to incorporate smart features. The rise in the number of IoT nodes has experienced exponential growth due to its integration into a diverse array of applications. The number is reportedly anticipated to surpass 30 billion by 2025 [3]. Most of the existing IoT devices are

 DOI: 10.1201/9781003546382-6

powered by primary and secondary batteries. The replacement or recharge of these batteries is not practically feasible or cost-effective as well. Powering such a large number of IoT nodes has emerged as a formidable challenge, which may hinder the widespread adoption of IoT globally. Thus, unfeigned efforts are being made to design energy-autonomous IoT devices to replace conventional battery-powered ones. The ultimate way to provide energy sustainability is to incorporate an energy harvesting framework in IoT devices, which enables them to harness energy, manage it, and utilize it for the operation of the device. As a result, it makes them truly *plug and forget*-devices. Energy can be harvested from diverse renewable sources such as sunlight, mechanical vibration/movement, kinetic energy, radiofrequency (RF), heat, etc. The widespread adoption of solar energy as the primary energy source in outdoor applications can be attributed to its high power density and ubiquitous nature. Similarly, RF energy is stable which makes it widely adopted in indoor applications. The source of energy can be selected based on a few criteria, such as the characteristics of the device, the location of the targeted device, and the application requirements.

6.1.1 Contributions of the Proposed Work

The major contributions of the work are outlined as follows:

- In this work, a self-powered, energy-autonomous Street Light Management System (SLMS) has been proposed, which can be integrated with street lights to manage their operation energy-efficiently.
- The device harvests energy using a small monocrystalline solar cell having a surface dimension of 4.5 cm × 3.0 cm integrated with an ultralow-power management circuit. It harvests energy from sunlight and powers the management system during the night.
- It is IoT-enabled and incorporated with a Long Range Wide Area Network (LoRaWAN) for long-range wireless communication.
- The power consumption of the device has been optimized to enhance the lifetime of the storage element.
- In the pursuit of advancing sustainable IoT technologies, the proposed work is a self-powered, IoT-enabled, low-power, portable device that requires ultra-low maintenance.

6.1.2 Prior Research Work

The global smart street lighting market is expected to experience significant growth. It is estimated to increase from \$2.41 billion in 2022 to \$8.23 billion by 2029 [4]. Extensive research and development efforts have been carried out over the past decade to enhance the energy efficiency of street lights using various techniques. In [5], a system has been proposed to adjust the brightness of street lights based on the volume of traffic throughout the day. Weather-adaptive smart LED street light systems are designed in [6, 7]. These systems can enhance visibility in various weather conditions and effectively reduce the occurrence of road accidents. Energy-saving methods to conserve electricity in smart cities have been proposed in [8, 9]. The illuminance of LED street lights can be regulated based on the occupancy of pedestrians and vehicles around the road. In [10], attempts have been made to regulate the illumination levels of street lights by implementing the Artificial Bee Colony (ABC) algorithm. In [11], illumination has been controlled using Received Signal Strength (RSS) from the movements of vehicles and pedestrians on roads. In [12], illuminance has been controlled based on the presence of objects around the road detected by the Artificial Intelligence (AI) technique. Subsequently, a secure cloud-based street lighting management system has been proposed in which a Secure Shell (SSH) based encryption technique is implemented to secure the communication between edge node and cloud [13]. In [14], a system has been proposed that enables the street lights to adjust their intensity according to scheduled timings, traffic conditions, and weather conditions.

The utilization of communication technology is a fundamental component of the SLMS and substantially influences the overall management process. In [14], a wireless smart SLMS has been proposed incorporating a Digital Addressable Lighting Interface (DALI) protocol. The systems can be considered as a low-cost solution to control and monitor the public lights. ZigBee has been implemented in SLMS [15, 16] to enable a remote control feature. However, the communication range of ZigBee is reported to be short, thus General Packet Radio Service (GPRS) along with ZigBee has been used as a communication system in SLMS to enhance the communication range [17]. Further attempts to enhance the communication range are achieved by incorporating Wireless Fidelity (Wi-Fi) in street lights. LoRaWAN has been widely adopted in IoT and Wireless Sensor Network (WSN) devices for featuring a long communication range at the cost of low power consumption. Thus, it has also incorporated many energy-autonomous devices to validate its performance in various applications in real-world scenarios [18–20]. A health monitoring solution based on LoRaWAN has been developed for soldiers stationed in adverse environmental circumstances, aiming to enhance the response time of the system [21]. A LoRaWAN-based energy-efficient smart metering system has been designed that is capable of selecting the appropriate spreading factor to transmit compressed time series data to the operator [22]. The low-power consuming feature of LoRa technology has been leveraged in [23–34] to design a battery-less air quality monitoring system.

This chapter is organized as follows: Section 6.2 presents the issues in the existing SLMS, proposed solutions, and novel contributions of the proposed work. The proposed system architecture has been discussed in Section 6.3. Prototyping and Deployment in Real-World Testbed is explained in Section 6.4. The discussion on experimental results is depicted in Section 6.5. The chapter concluded by narrating the future scope of research in Section 6.6.

6.2 ISSUES IN EXISTING WORKS AND NOVEL CONTRIBUTION

Though the existing works have been practically deployed on the field and tested its performance, there are still a few lacks that need to be addressed.

1. Issues Identified in the Existing Works: The issues in the existing solutions are listed as follows:
   - Most of the existing solutions rely on either grid power or conventional batteries to meet their energy needs. In [5–7, 9, 10, 14, 24, 33] the proposed management systems have been powered from the 220V AC power line, which is used for powering the street lights. These systems are designed explicitly for grid-powered street lights because obtaining the necessary amount of energy for the management system from the grid is easier. However, these systems may not be considered suitable solutions for off-grid street lights, primarily standalone or split-type solar street lights that lack a management system, unlike all-in-one solar street lights. The solar panels in existing standalone solar street lights are designed to match the energy consumption of the LED light and its associated circuits. Therefore, adding the management system to the same solar panel of a street light can disrupt the design balance of the street light, resulting in a reduction in lighting hours. To power both the management system and LED lights from a single panel, it is necessary to replace the solar panels of street lights with slightly larger ones. However, this replacement would disrupt the entire infrastructure of standalone solar streetlights [35–45].
   - In [8, 25], the designed devices are powered from rechargeable batteries which implies the requirement of frequent maintenance, specifically recharge or replacement of batteries. The battery charging schemes are not addressed in the aforementioned works. Replacing dead batteries from every SLMS is not a practical or cost-effective solution.
   - In [42], a supercapacitor-based SLMS has been proposed that harvests energy from the street light. However, the low energy density of supercapacitors can cause power failure in the management system during adverse weather conditions such as fog or heavy rain. In [43, 46–48], attempts have been made to design an SLMS system, however, a much bigger size solar cell has been used and the systems have not been fully deployed on the field.
   - The power consumption in the related works is not optimized and ranges from 350 mW to 4.13 W, which is relatively high. This power consumption level makes them unsuitable to be used with solar-powered street lights.
2. Motivation of the Proposed Work and Our Vision on SLMS:
   - Reports indicate that less than 18% of 350 million street lights around the globe are currently LED-based, and less than 2% are IoT-enabled [26]. This presents a significant future perspective of research and development. It has been projected that approximately 15% of streetlights worldwide are going to be IoT-enabled by 2023. This would result in the connection of at least 50 million additional street lights.
   - The number of IoT-connected smart streetlights is estimated to reach 41 million by 2023 [27].

- According to the report issued by the Ministry of New and Renewable Energy (MNRE), 9 lakh solar street lights have been successfully deployed across India as of 2021. These installations have been implemented under the off-grid and decentralized solar application scheme [28].
- As reported in [29], it is essential to address the issue regarding the short lifespan of batteries unless about 78 million batteries used in IoT devices are estimated to be discarded worldwide daily by 2025. Optimization of power consumption and enabling energy harvesting schemes in IoT devices has been regarded as a prominent method to enhance the lifetime of batteries.
- Our vision for SLMS is shown in Figure 6.1. In this work, a portable, low-power, IoT-enabled, energy-autonomous SLMS has been designed considering the aforementioned issues, motivation, and vision. It can be retrofitted to any existing LED-based street light. It indicates seamless integration of the system to existing LED-based street lights introducing smart features and IoT connectivity to it. It possesses all the necessary features aimed at reducing the energy budget associated with the street light.
- This can be particularly useful in the case of standalone solar streetlights. The energy-autonomous capability of the system would benefit the users or consumers to retrofit it to the standalone solar street lights without disturbing its design equations.

3. Novel Contributions: The novel contributions of the proposed work are written as follows:
    - The proposed work presents an SLMS that exhibits complete energy autonomy promoting Sustainable Development Goals (SDG), that is, SDG7 and SDG9 of the United Nations (UN). In furtherance of the existing advancements in the existing solutions, the chapter proposes a technique to introduce energy autonomy to the SLMS, which possesses the

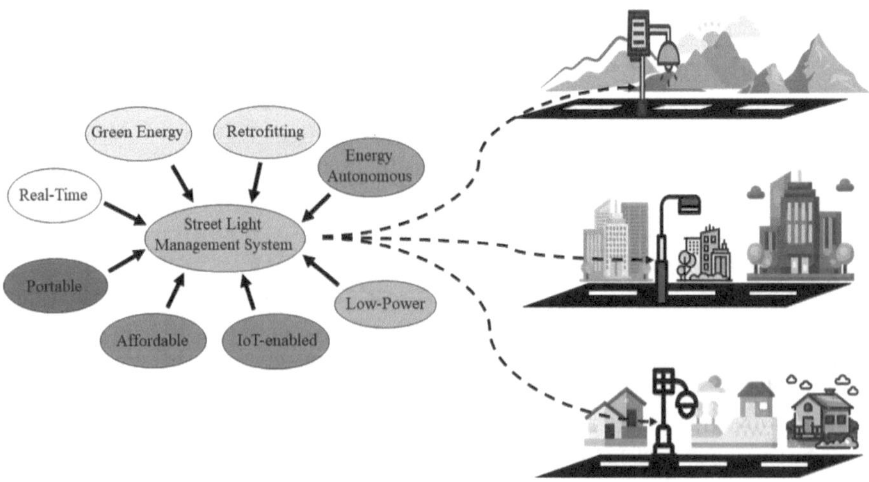

FIGURE 6.1 Our vision for SLMS.

necessary features to operate the street light to reduce the energy budget associated with it.

- The optimization of power consumption in the system has been achieved by implementing the duty cycle technique. It is reported to be minimal compared to state-of-the-art technologies.
- The proposed system operates with more than three times the percentage of duty cycle compared to state-of-the-art solar energy powered energy autonomous LoRaWAN systems despite having the smallest size of the solar cell.
- The proposed system is a real-time, energy-autonomous, IoT-enabled, portable system that can be integrated or retrofitted into any existing LED-based street light to make it work energy-efficiently indicating its high adaptability. It has been manufactured at an affordable price. The proposed device is incorporated with a rechargeable battery, which is expected to have a prolonged lifespan without the need for battery replacement. It highlights the low maintenance requirement of the device.

6.3 PROPOSED SYSTEM ARCHITECTURE

The block diagram of the proposed system has been shown in Figure 6.2. It is comprised of several subunits, which are discussed as follows:

1. ***Power Management Unit (PMU)***: It is responsible for several vital functions, including harnessing solar energy, optimizing the harvested power, storing energy, and regulating the output voltage of the battery following the specification of the sensor node, ensuring that the power supply is efficiently managed and utilized. The unit incorporates a small mono-crystalline type

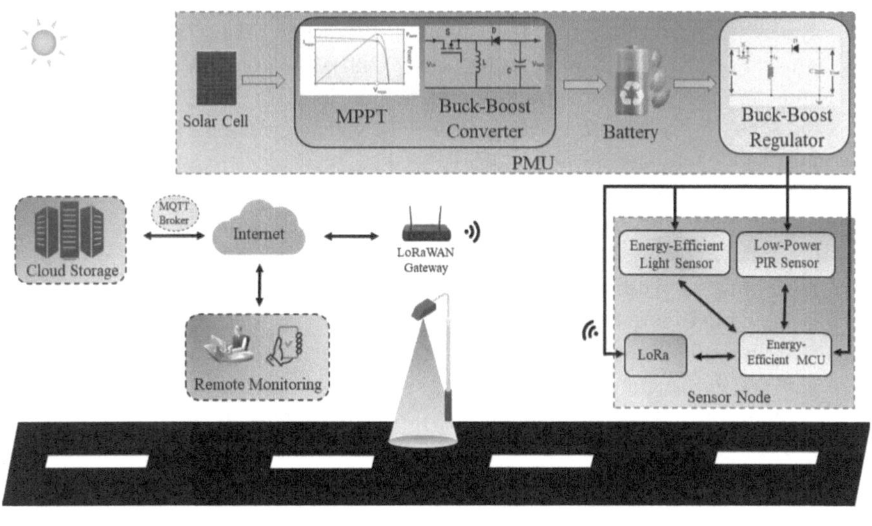

FIGURE 6.2 Block diagram of the proposed system.

solar cell with a dimension of 45 mm × 36 mm, exhibiting efficiency up to 18%–25% as per the manufacturer [31]. It can produce maximum power (P_{max}) of 307 mW with open circuit voltage (V_{oc}) ranging from 0 V–6.91 V and short circuit current (I_{sc}) ranging from 0 mA to 58.6 mA. An off-the-shelf ultralow Power Management Integrated Circuit (PMIC) has been incorporated which can enhance the efficiency of input power derived from a solar cell. The PMIC is comprised of the below modules which are responsible for managing the power management operation of the device.

- ***Buck-Boost Converter***: The PMIC has an input voltage range (V_{in}) from 0 V to 18 V. The buck-boost converter can start operating subject to V_{in} lies in the range of 2.6 V to 18 V. The primary function of the buck-boost converter is to step up and step down V_{in} to maintain the Maximum Power Point (MPP) ratio.
- ***MPPT Module***: It provides PMIC the capability of extracting maximum power from the harvesting source. The solar cell can deliver an MPP voltage (V_{MPP}) of 5.58 V and an MPP current (I_{MPP}) of 55.1 mA as per the datasheet provided by the manufacturer. Thus, MPPT module regulates its impedance in a way to delivers maximum power at load conditions (P_{MPP}).
- ***Battery Voltage Control***: The PMIC can provide the battery with a maximum voltage (V_{BATT}) of 4.25 V with a maximum current (I_{BATT}) of 70 mA. This module keeps V_{BATT} within a safe range by comparing it with the over-voltage protection threshold (V_{EOC}) and under-voltage protection threshold (V_{UVP}) to ensure safety in battery health.

2. ***Sensor Node***: It is primarily responsible for coordinating sensing, controlling, and communication tasks associated with the system. All the components are chosen critically to ensure optimum performance at low power consumption. There are two sensors integrated with the sensor node which are the motion sensor and the light sensor. An energy-efficient high-performance microprocessor specifically designed for low-power real-time systems has been employed for computing tasks as per the framework of the sensor node. It is a 32-bit microprocessor with ARM cortex M4 architecture and can operate at a maximum frequency of 80 MHz. The components in the sensor node can be operated in several software-defined modes, ensuring their energy efficiency. LoRaWAN has been incorporated to achieve long-range communication at low power consumption.
3. ***Energy Efficient Framework for Sensor Node***: The sensor node performs the following set of tasks implementing the duty cycle technique to optimize power consumption. The flowchart of the energy-efficient framework is shown in Figure 6.3.
   - It measures light intensity "L_{DN}" to decide if it is day hours or night in every 900-second interval. It keeps the MCU and PIR sensor in sleep mode to meanwhile to minimize power consumption. It turns off the street light during day hours.
   - The system continuously detects occupancy and adjusts the brightness of the street light based on the movement of pedestrians and vehicles. It can operate in either high light mode or low light mode. The illuminance level is set to 100% in high light mode and 50% in low light mode.

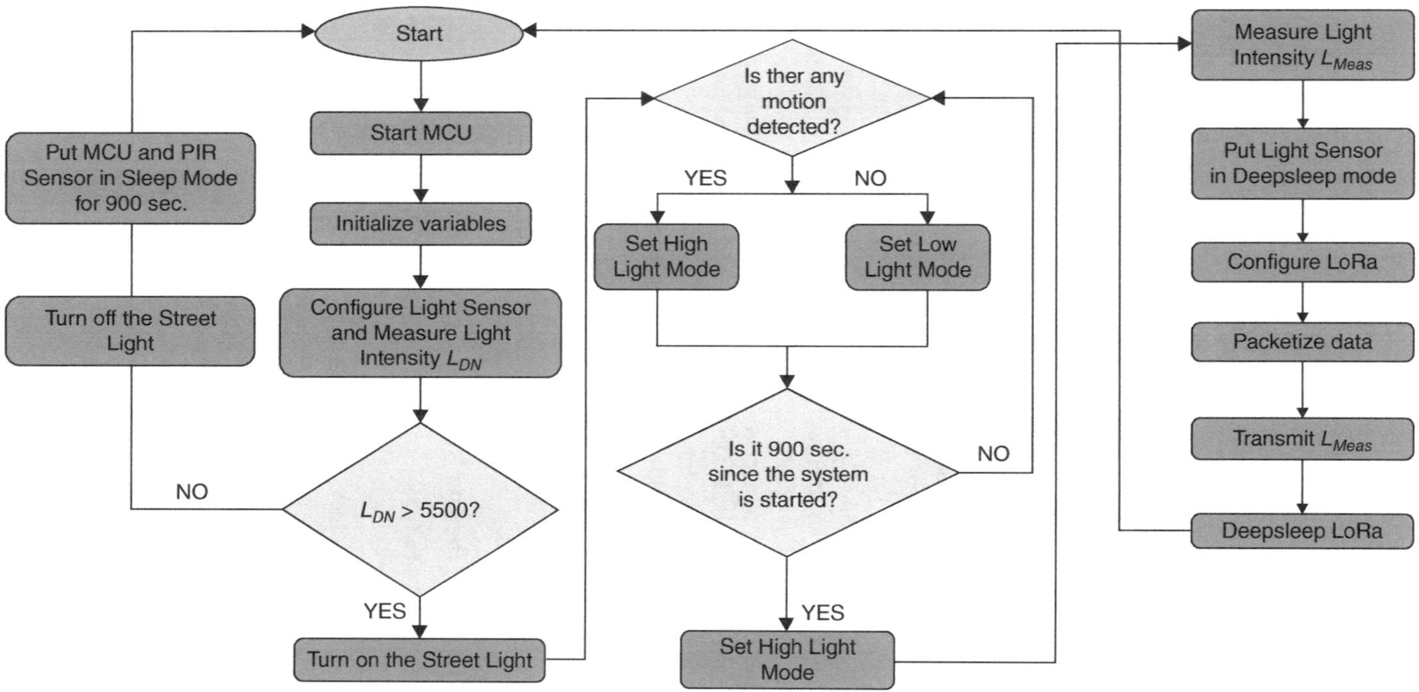

FIGURE 6.3 Framework of the sensor node.

- It measures the light intensity of the street light at 100% illuminance every 900 seconds to help the authority identify faulty lights based on their prescribed illuminance level during night hours.

4. ***LoRaWAN Gateway Node***: It is designed to receive the necessary signal from the sensor node of the system. It can be placed at a central location to ensure seamless communication with all sensor nodes. It further uploads the data received from sensor nodes to the cloud server through the Message Queuing Telemetry Transport (MQTT) protocol. The data gets stored in a cloud server and subsequently displayed on a Graphical User Interface (GUI). Therefore, the administrator can remotely monitor the operational status of each street light at any given time.

6.4 PROTOTYPING AND DEPLOYMENT IN REAL-WORLD TESTBED

The components detail of the prototype has been presented in Table 6.1. In the first step of prototyping, the PMU has been configured. A highly efficient off-the-shelf PMIC has been implemented for efficient power management which is configured as per the system requirement. The external components are calculated as per the design rules explained in the datasheet of the PMIC [30]. The schematic diagram of the PMU is shown in Figure 6.4. The PMIC includes a pass transistor between the STORE and BATT pins to accomplish both V_{UVP} and V_{EOC} safety levels. These thresholds are regulated via the Under Voltage Protection (UVP) and End-of-Charge (EOC) pins, which are generally linked to the STORE pin through a resistor divider. The operating voltage of the battery lies in the range of 2.75 V–4.2 V, as per the manufacturer of the battery.

TABLE 6.1
Component Details of the End Node Installed at the Street Light

Component	Part	Key Specification	Approximate Cost (USD)
Solar cell	SM141K10LV	Maximum output: 307 mW	6.1
PMIC	SPV1050	Input: 0.15–18 V, Output: 4.2 V	2.1
Buck-boost regulator	MAX77827	Input: 1.8–5.5 V, Output: 3.3 V	1.3
Battery	Lithium-ion	Capacity: 600 mAh	2
PIR sensor	EKMB1103111	Range: 12–14.5 m	9
Micro controller	STM32L476	Architecture: ARM cortex M4	8.19
Light sensor	VEML7700	Range: 0–120 klx	9.9
LoRa	RFM95	Frequency Band Range: 868 MHz or 915 MHz	15.57
Total			53.16

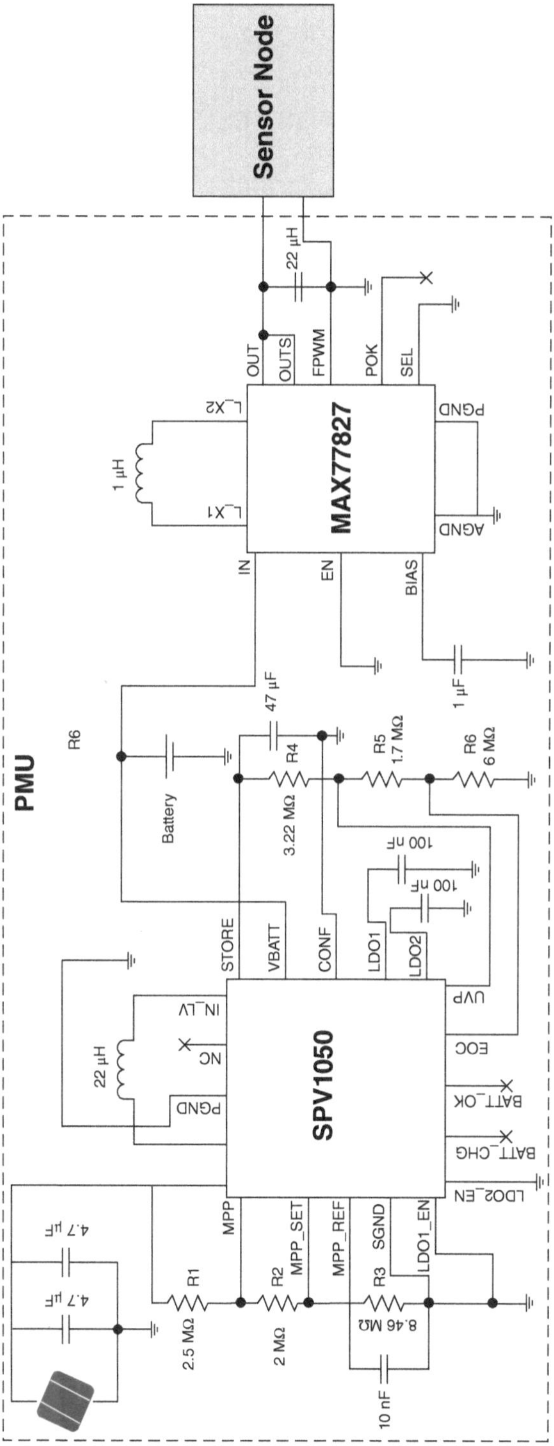

FIGURE 6.4 Schematic of the power management unit of the proposed system.

Thus, V_{EOC} of the PMIC should be configured at 4.2 V. Subsequently, V_{UVP} is set to 2.75 V. These parameters have been set to solve the design expressions (Eqs. (6.1)–(6.5)).

$$R_{OUT} = R_4 + R_5 + R_6 \tag{6.1}$$

$$10M\Omega \leq R_{OUT} \leq 20M\Omega \tag{6.2}$$

$$R_6 = \left(\frac{V_{BG}}{V_{EOC}}\right) \times R_{OUT} \tag{6.3}$$

$$R_5 = \left(\frac{V_{BG}}{V_{UVP}}\right) \times R_{OUT} - R_6 \tag{6.4}$$

$$R_4 = R_{OUT} - (R_5 + R_6) \tag{6.5}$$

where R_{OUT} represents the total external resistance and V_{BG} depicts the internal reference voltage which has been considered as 1.23 as per the datasheet of the PMIC [30]. The calculated values of the external output resistors responsible for setting these two parameters are R4, R5, and R6 which are calculated as 6.08 MΩ, 1.7 MΩ, and 3.22 MΩ, respectively. The internal logic of the PMIC guarantees tight monitoring of both V_{EOC} and V_{UVP} by opening the pass transistor at the triggering of the V_{EOC} threshold or triggering the V_{UVP} threshold to preserve the battery life. The MPPT controller in the PMIC periodically wakes up to calculate the V_{MPP}. V_{MPP} and V_{OC} of the solar cell are observed as 5.5 V and 6.91 V, according to the manufacturer [31]. The MPP ratio has been calculated as 0.8. Thus, the resistors responsible for setting up the MPP can be calculated following the below expressions (Eqs. (6.6)–(6.10)).

$$R_{in} = R_1 + R_2 + R_3 \tag{6.6}$$

$$R_{in} \geq \left(\frac{V_{OC}}{I_{lkg}}\right) \times MPP_{Ratio} \tag{6.7}$$

$$R_1 = R_{in} \times \left(1 - \frac{V_{MPP}}{V_{OC}}\right) \tag{6.8}$$

$$R_2 = R_{in} \times \left(\frac{V_{MPP}}{V_{OC}}\right) \times (1 - MPP_{Ratio}) \tag{6.9}$$

$$R_3 = R_{in} \times \left(\frac{V_{MPP}}{V_{OC}}\right) \times MPP_{Ratio} \tag{6.10}$$

where R_{in} represents the total input resistance of the PMIC. The calculated values of the input resistors are 2.5 MΩ, 2 MΩ, and 8.46 MΩ. I_{lkg} refers to the permissible amount of leakage that can occur through the resistors in the input stage. It has been considered approximately 0.5 μA as it lies in the range of 0.1 μA to 1 μA in most of the applications [30]. A 600-mAh Lithium-ion (Li-ion) battery has been used to store the harvested energy. V_{BATT} is observed to be approximately 4.2 V when it reaches its maximum capacity, which exceeds the input supply voltage capacity of a few components of the sensor node. Thus, a highly efficient buck-boost regulator with ultralow quiescent current (I_Q) is incorporated to solve this issue which provides a constant 3.3 V supply to the sensor node. The prototype has been fabricated in a suitable form factor as shown in Figure 6.5.

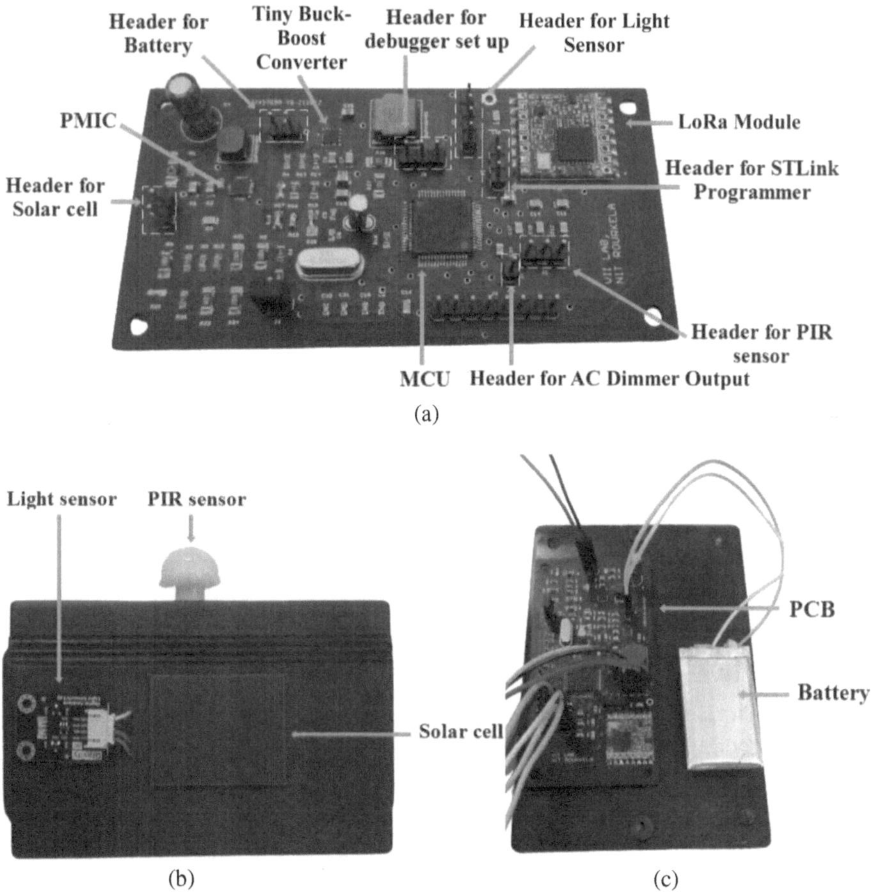

FIGURE 6.5 Designed prototype of the system in the total dimension of 12.5 cm × 8.5 cm × 3.5 cm: (a) fabricated PCB of the device, (b) outer casing of the proposed device, and (c) inner view of the proposed device.

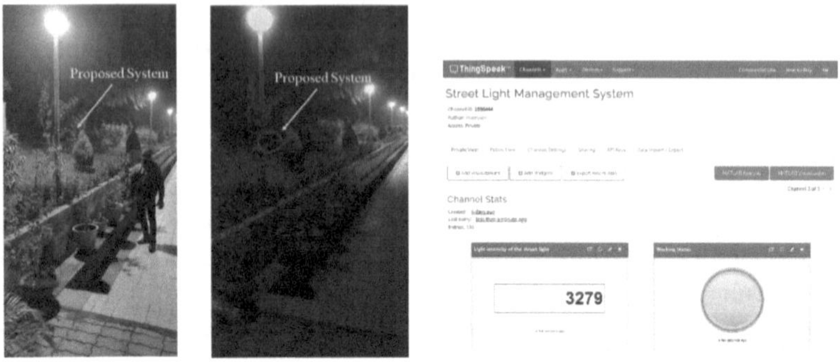

(a) (b) (c)

FIGURE 6.6 Deployment of the system with a street light: (a) illuminance level is 100% in the presence of a pedestrian, (b) illuminance level is 50% in the absence of any movement, and (c) operating status of the street light showing on cloud GUI.

Further, the system is deployed outdoors, as shown in Figure 6.6. It has been deployed with an LED-based street light in the garden area of a hostel. Upon detection of the pedestrian, the illuminance level is set at 100% as shown in Figure 6.6(a). The illuminance level is 50%, while no movement is detected around the road as shown in Figure 6.6(b). The availability of sunlight varies from season to season and is found to be minimal during the rainy season. Therefore, there is a high chance of power failure in the system during the rainy season. To ensure that the system can work during rainy days, the system has been deployed in the field for more than 70 days. It is tested under sunny weather during autumn and fully cloudy as well as rainy weather during the rainy season. The data from the installed device is uploaded to the cloud through the LoRaWAN gateway. The authority can monitor the working status of each street light through the GUI. Figure 6.6(c) shows the operating status and light intensity of the street light when the illuminance level is 100%.

The light intensity at this particular illuminance level is measured as 3279 lux. The working status is indicated using a virtual lamp indicator. The indicator would glow red at any time if the intensity is measured below the mentioned threshold.

6.5 EXPERIMENTAL RESULTS AND ANALYSIS

The experimental results obtained during the duration of deployment of the system have been reported in the following sub-sections.

6.5.1 Electrical Characteristics of the Harvester

Figure 6.7 shows the VI characteristics of the solar cell in different irradiance under sunlight. The solar cell is tested through various weather conditions. Different irradiances are taken into consideration in various weather conditions such as sunny day noon (852 W/m^2), partly cloudy (470 W/m^2), and mostly cloudy (276 W/m^2) to observe the MPP point during various conditions. The irradiance has been measured by Metravi 207 Solar Power Meter. The maximum power obtained from the

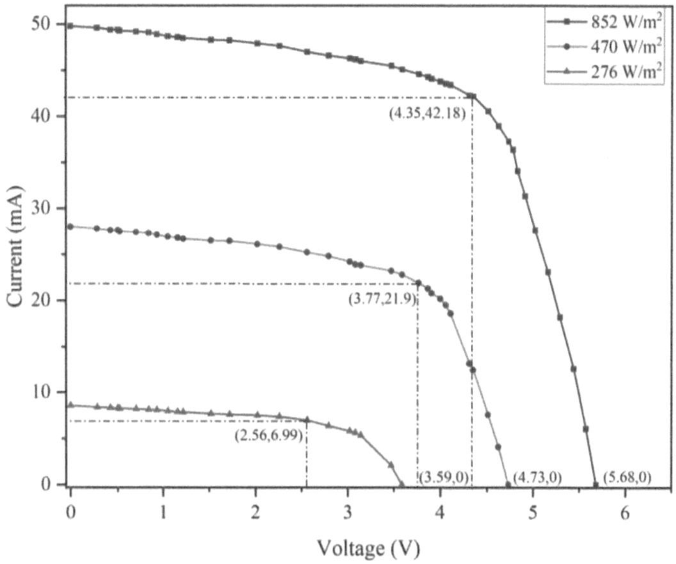

FIGURE 6.7 VI characteristics of the solar cell under direct sunlight.

solar cell at 276 W/m^2 is 17.89 mW. The output voltage is 2.56 V, and the V_{oc} is 3.59 V. The MPPT ratio can be calculated as 2.56/3.59 = 0.71. At 470 W/m^2, the solar panel can result in a maximum of 82.56 mW while the output voltage is 3.77 V. The corresponding V_{oc} is measured as 4.73 V. Thus, the MPP ratio is 3.77/4.73 = 0.79. At 852 W/m^2, the maximum output power is 183.48 mW with an output voltage of 4.35 V. The corresponding V_{oc} is 5.68 V. Subsequently the MPP ratio is 4.35/5.68 = 0.76.

6.5.2 Energy Harvesting and Storage

The device has been deployed on the field, and the charging curve of the battery is shown in Figure 6.8. The sensor node is disconnected in this condition.

The voltage level of the battery is 2.7 V at the beginning. The voltage level gradually increases and reaches 4.2 V, which is the maximum output voltage of the battery. Further, the PMU cuts the supply to the battery once the battery reaches 4.2 V due to the EOC feature. The system has been tested under two weather conditions, such as the rainy season and autumn season, during which ambient solar energy availability is generally low. It has been observed that the battery takes around 39 hours and 66 hours to get fully charged during the autumn and rainy seasons, respectively. In the application, the battery gets charged during the day hours and discharged during the operation of the sensor node during the night. The charge rate of the battery depends on the availability of ambient sunlight during a particular day and the discharge rate for one-day operation lies between 45 mV and 54 mV. The result is shown in Figure 6.9. The battery takes 14 days during the spring season to get fully charged with the load connected to it. It takes 19 days during the rainy season.

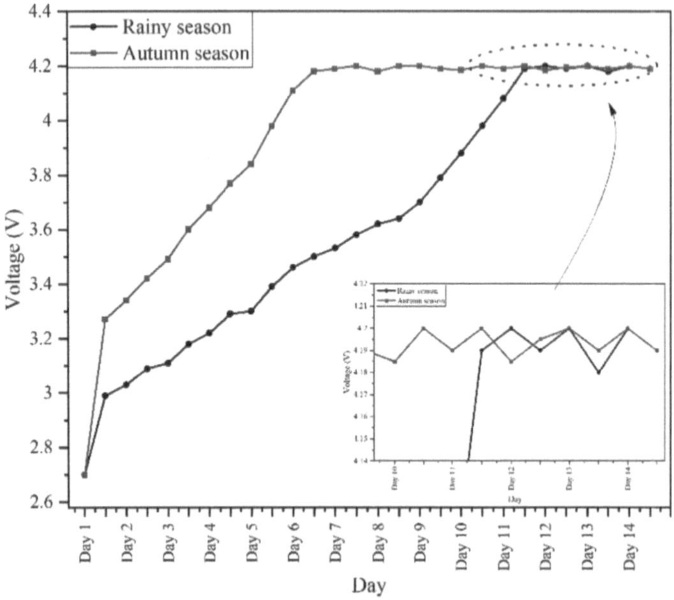

FIGURE 6.8 Output voltage of the battery when the solar cell is harvesting energy and the sensor node is disconnected.

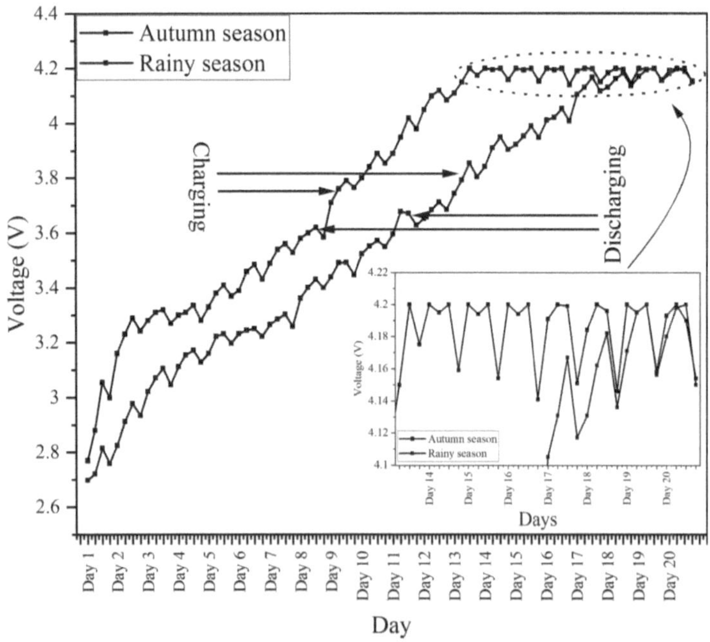

FIGURE 6.9 Output voltage of the battery during deployment and testing of the system.

6.5.3 Supply to Sensor Node

The buck-boost regulator effectively maintains a stable voltage of 3.3 V to power the sensor to facilitate its optimal functioning. The battery has been purposefully discharged with a current of approximately 1 A to observe the output voltage of the regulator, as depicted in Figure 6.10. The battery voltage exhibits a discernible fall from 4.2 V to 2.4 V during this experiment. It can be noted that the buck-boost regulator exhibits an output voltage of approximately 3.3 V, maintaining this level until the battery output voltage reaches 2.6 V. Further drop in battery output voltage results in a significant fall in the output voltage of the regulator that lies below the voltage threshold required by the sensor node. This is evident that the sensor node can only be operated till the battery output voltage ranges from 4.2 V to 2.6 V.

6.5.4 Energy Consumption of the System

The energy consumption of the system can be calculated using Eq. (6.11).

$$E_{sys} = E_{PMIC} + E_{BBReg} + E_{SN} \tag{6.11}$$

where E_{sys} represents the energy consumption of the system. E_{PMIC}, E_{BBReg}, E_{SN} denote the energy consumption by PMIC, buck-boost regulator, and sensor node, respectively, in a complete day, that is, 24 hours duration.

The current consumption of the sensor node in 900 seconds has been measured and presented in Figure 6.11. The average current consumption of different components

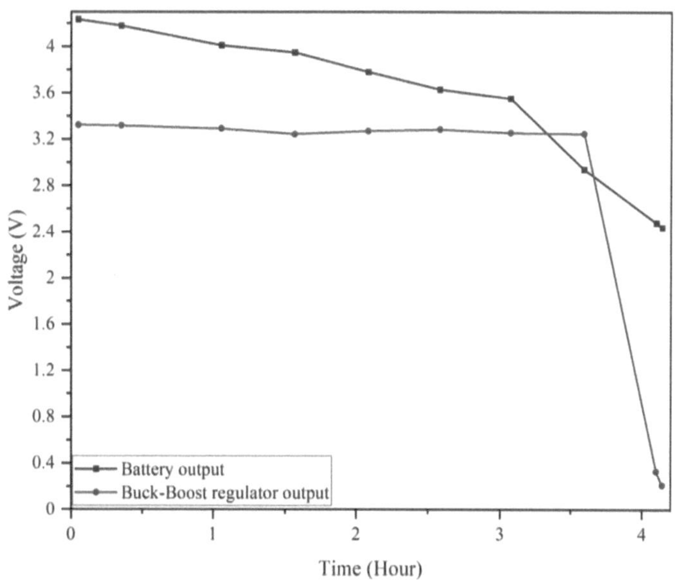

FIGURE 6.10 Output voltage of buck-boost regulator and battery.

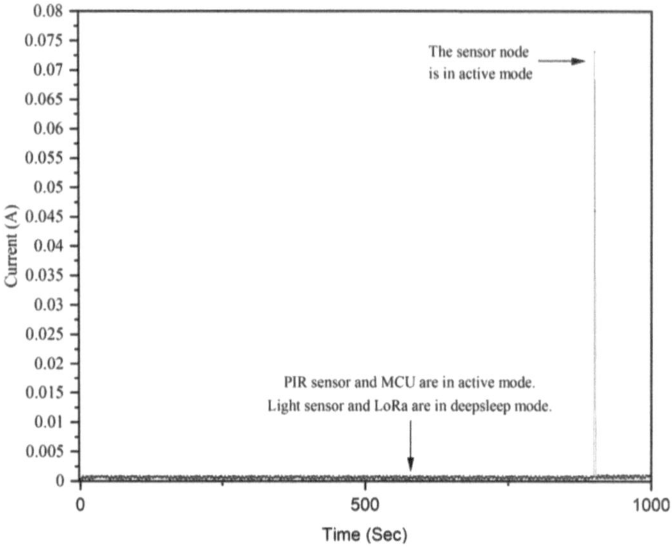

FIGURE 6.11 Measured current consumption of the sensor node during night hours.

has been shown in Table 6.2 using which the average current consumption of the sensor node (I_{SN}) is calculated in one duty cycle using Eq. (6.12).

$$I_{SN} = \frac{1}{T_{DC}}\left(\int_{t=0}^{t=T_{DC}} I_{PIR}dt + \int_{t=0}^{t=T_{DC}} I_{MCU}dt + \int_{t=0}^{t=t_{active}} I_{LS}dt + \int_{t=0}^{t=t_{sleep}} I_{LS}dt + \int_{t=0}^{t=t_{active}} I_{LoRa}dt + \int_{t=0}^{t=t_{sleep}} I_{LoRa}dt \right) \quad (6.12)$$

where I_{PIR}, I_{MCU}, I_{LS}, and I_{LoRa} represent the current consumption of the motion sensor, microcontroller, light intensity sensor, and LoRa, respectively. T_{active} and T_{sleep} denote the duration in active mode and sleep mode, respectively. The duration of one cycle denoted as T_{DC}, is considered to be 900 seconds. The energy consumption of the sensor node is different during day hours and night hours as it executes different sets of tasks following the framework of the system. The average power consumption of the sensor node (P_{SN}) and I_{SN} in a complete day, that is, 24 hours period has been theoretically calculated as 1.648 mW and 499.256 μA.

Subsequently, current consumption of the PMIC and the buck-boost regulator have been measured and the results are shown in Figure 6.12. The average current consumption of both of them is calculated as 478.641 μA and 13.249 μA. Thus, the average power consumption of PMIC (P_{PMIC}) has been calculated as 2.488 mW. It consumes energy from the solar cell and works during the presence of sunlight which is approximately 12 hours during the summer season.

TABLE 6.2
Measurement Results of Current Consumption of Components of Sensor Node

Component	Supply (V)	Operating Mode	Avg. Current Consumption	Duration (Sec)		Avg. Energy Consumption	
				Day	Night	Day	Night
PIR Sensor	3.3	Active	124 μA	0	900	0	368.28 mJ
	3.3	Sleep	3.17 μA	900	0	9.414 mJ	0
MCU	3.3	Active	488 μA	0.1	900	161.04 μJ	1.449 J
	3.3	Sleep	345 μA	899.9	0	1.024 J	0
Light Sensor	3.3	Active	62 μA	0.1	0.1	20.46 μJ	20.46 μJ
	3.3	Deepsleep	1.5 μA	899.9	899.9	4.454 mJ	4.454 mJ
LoRa	3.3	Active	71.67 mA	0	0.23	0	54.397 mJ
	3.3	Sleep	8.5 μA	900	899.77	25.245 mJ	25.238 mJ

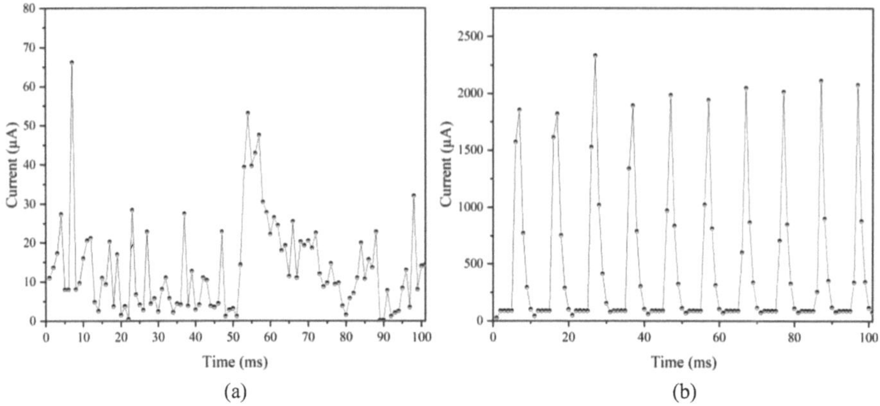

FIGURE 6.12 (a) Measured current consumption of the buck-boost regulator during operation. (b) Measured current consumption of the PMIC during operation.

TABLE 6.3
Summary of Energy Consumption of the System in an Entire Day

Parameter	Energy (J)
E_{PMIC}	107.481
E_{BBReg}	4.807
E_{SN}	142.348
E_{sys}	254.633

The average power consumption of the buck-boost regulator (P_{BBReg}) has been calculated as 55.645 μW. It operates uninterruptedly throughout 24 hours and drags energy from the storage element to power the sensor node. The energy consumption of the system has been summarized in Table 6.3.

6.5.5 Battery Lifetime and Runtime Expectancy

The rated storage capacity of the battery claimed by the manufacturer is 600 mAh. However, the true capacity of the battery never sticks to the rated value due to the difference between tested conditions and real conditions. Temperature works as a key factor as far as the storage capacity of the battery is concerned. To ensure the battery has more than 70% storage capacity of the rated value, the charging temperature of the battery should be between 0°C and 45°C. The discharging temperature should be between −20°C and 60°C. The storage temperature range must be in the range of −20°C to 30°C. The average temperature during the operation is between 20°C and 30°C, where the device has been tested. This satisfies the conditions of the manufacturer to have 70% of the rated storage capacity, that is, 420 mAh. Battery lifetime depends on operating temperature and charge rating (C-rating). The charge cycle of the battery is 500 cycles with a C-rating of 0.5 C. It implies that the battery can undergo 500 full charge cycles with a maximum discharge current of 300 mA. The maximum current the sensor node drags at any point in time is observed as 125 mA, which is much below 300 mA. To calculate the runtime of the battery, the energy consumption of the sensor node and buck-boost regulator should be considered as both of them drags powered from the battery. It can be calculated as 147.15 J which approximately is 2.63% of the total energy capacity of the battery. This can be considered as a macrocycle [32]. The equivalent full cycle can be calculated as 38.017 full cycles. The lifetime of the battery can be calculated as 19008.82 days, which is more than 52 years. The average lifetime of the off-the-shelf components is generally 5 years to 10 years. Thus, it ensures that the battery life is more than the required life of the system, eliminating the need for battery replacement during the entire lifetime of the system.

6.5.6 Comparative Analysis

The comparative analysis of state-of-the-art smart SLMS and LoRaWAN-based solar energy or artificial light energy-powered energy autonomous devices is shown in Tables 6.4 and 6.5, respectively.

- To assess the advancements achieved among the state-of-the-art SLMS, a comparison table has been presented in Table 6.4. The proposed system incorporates state-of-the-art technology to achieve the objective. The proposed SLMS has the necessary features to manage the operation of street lights, ensuring energy efficiency. The novelty lies in introducing energy sustainability and making it affordable, portable, and adaptable as a system to seamlessly integrate into existing LED street light infrastructure, making it easy to retrofit.
- Table 6.5 presents a comparison between solar energy-powered LoRaWAN-based energy-autonomous systems deployed in various real-time applications. The proposed system incorporates relatively smaller solar cells with high output power and maintains a high percentage of duty cycle to ensure high Quality of Service (QoS).

TABLE 6.4
Comparison of State-of-the-Art Smart SLMS

References, Years	Sensing Parameters	Radio Technology	Wireless Range	Average Power Consumption of Sensor Node	Energy Storage	Energy Autonomy	Power Optimization Technique
[24], 2016	Power, Light intensity, Motion	ZigBee	Short	384 mW*	N/A	×	×
[5], 2016	Light intensity, Temperature, Power	ZigBee	Short	414 mW*	N/A	×	×
[14], 2016	Motion	ZigBee	Short	—	N/A	×	×
[6], 2017	Humidity, Power, Particle Concentration	ZigBee	Short	4.13 W*	N/A	×	×
[25], 2018	Temperature, Humidity, Light intensity, and Power	NB-IoT	Long	218 mW*	Battery	×	×
[8], 2018	Motion and Light intensity	N/A	N/A	387 mW*	Battery	×	×
[7], 2021	Temperature, Humidity, Rain, Motion and Light intensity	Wi-Fi	Long	692.4 mW*	N/A	×	×
[9], 2021	Motion and Light intensity	Wi-Fi	Long	525 mW*	N/A	×	×
[10], 2021	Motion, Current, Voltage	LoRaWAN	Long	—	N/A	×	×
[33], 2023	Motion, Light intensity	Wi-Fi	Long	211.37 mW*	N/A	×	×
Proposed Work	Motion, Light intensity	LoRaWAN	Long	**1.648 mW**	Battery	✓	**Duty Cycle**

Note: "—" indicates neither direct nor relevant data for calculation is available in the original manuscript. The notation "N/A" is used to indicate that the specific component being referred to is not available or present in the work being discussed.

* The power consumption of the sensor node has been calculated in this work by analyzing the publicly accessible datasheets of the components for comparison purposes, as it is not reported in the original manuscript.

TABLE 6.5
Comparison of State-of-the-Art LoRaWAN Based Solar Energy or Artificial Light Energy Powered Energy Autonomous Devices

References, Years	Energy Source	Size of Harvester (mm^2)	Maximum Harvester Output	Energy Storage	Application	Current Consumption or Power Consumption of the System	Duty Cycle (%)
[34], 2018	Solar & Artificial light	2826.9	90 mW	Supercapacitor	Environmental Parameter Monitoring	75.57 μA–1.38 mA	15.16
[35], 2019	Solar	—	10 W	Battery	Soil health Monitoring	—	—
[36], 2020	Solar	28900	3.65 W	Battery	Soil health Monitoring	29.33 mW	—
[37], 2020	Solar & Artificial light	23730	3.5 W	Battery	Air Quality Monitoring	25.9 mW	0.16
[38], 2021	Solar	—	3 W	Battery	Air Pollution Monitoring	14.3 mW–14.97 mW	5–6
[19], 2021	Solar	4550	350 mW	Battery	Soil health Monitoring	13 mA	1.65
[39], 2021	Solar	—	6 W	Battery	Ground Water Monitoring	104.081 mW	<1
[40], 2021	Solar	—	330 mW	Battery & Supercapacitor	Environmental Parameter Monitoring and Geolocation Tracking	1.69 mA	2.66
[41], 2021	Solar	—	1 W	Supercapacitor	Environmental Parameter Monitoring	380 mW	—
[20], 2022	Solar	4550	350 mW	Battery	Smart Trashbin	1.5 mA	2.73
Proposed Work	Solar	**1350**	**307 mW**	**Battery**	Smart Street light Management	**2.94 mW**	**50**

Note: The use of the symbol "—" indicates the absence of direct and relevant data for calculation in the original manuscript.

6.6 CONCLUSION

This chapter presents an energy-autonomous SLMS that can energy-efficiently manage the operation of street lights in real time to reduce the electricity budget associated with it. It is powered by solar energy using a small monocrystalline-type solar cell with a surface area of 1350 mm^2. The average power consumption of the system has been calculated as 2.947 mW, and that of the sensor node is 1.648 mW. The system has been deployed in the field and tested in various weather conditions to ensure its feasibility. LoRaWAN has been deployed for wireless data communication, which possesses a long communication range with low power consumption. The proposed system is an IoT-enabled, portable, adaptable, low-power, energy-autonomous solution that can be integrated into any LED-based street light to make it energy-efficient and IoT-enabled. It features remote monitoring which helps the concerned authority to find faulty street lights. In the future, attempts can be made to develop and implement an algorithm to enable multi-hop routing using LoRaWAN. The communication range can be improved using this technique. Attempts can be made to incorporate a task scheduling mechanism incorporating the work done in [44, 45].

REFERENCES

[1] United Nations, "2018 Revision of World Urbanization Prospects," May 16, 2018. [Online]. Available: https://www.un.org/development/desa/publications/2018-revision-of-world-urbanization-prospects.html

[2] S. P. Mohanty, U. Choppali, and E. Kougianos, "Everything You Wanted to Know About Smart Cities: The Internet of Things is the Backbone," *IEEE Consumer Electronics Magazine*, vol. 5, no. 3, pp. 60–70, 2016, doi: 10.1109/MCE.2016.2556879

[3] L. Vailshery, "IoT and Non-IoT Connections Worldwide 2010–2025." [Online]. Available: https://www.statista.com/statistics/1101442/iot-number-of-connected-devices-worldwide/\#statisticContainer [Accessed: March 8, 2021].

[4] "Smart Street Lighting Market Size, Share, Growth | Trends, 2029." [Online]. Available: https://www.fortunebusinessinsights.com/smart-street-lighting-market-106898

[5] G. Shahzad, H. Yang, A. W. Ahmad, and C. Lee, "Energy-Efficient Intelligent Street Lighting System Using Traffic-Adaptive Control," *IEEE Sensors Journal*, vol. 16, no. 13, pp. 5397–5405, 2016, doi: 10.1109/JSEN.2016.2557345

[6] P. T. Daely, H. T. Reda, G. B. Satrya, J. W. Kim, and S. Y. Shin, "Design of Smart LED Streetlight System for Smart City With Web-Based Management System," IEEE *Sensors Journal*, vol. 17, no. 18, pp. 6100–6110, 2017, doi: 10.1109/JSEN.2017.2734101

[7] D. Saha, S. M. Sorif, and P. Dutta, "Weather Adaptive Intelligent Street Lighting System With Automatic Fault Management Using Boltuino Platform," in *Proceedings of the 2021 International Conference on ICT for Smart Society (ICISS)*, Bandung, Indonesia, August 2021, pp. 1–6, doi: 10.1109/ICISS53185.2021.9533234

[8] A. Abdullah, S. H. Yusoff, S. A. Zaini, N. S. Midi, and S. Y. Mohamad, "Smart Street Light Using Intensity Controller," in *Proceedings of the 7th International Conference on Computer and Communication Engineering (ICCCE)*, Kuala Lumpur, September 2018, pp. 1–5, doi: 10.1109/ICCCE.2018.8539321

[9] S. Sorif, D. Saha, and P. Dutta, "Smart Street Light Management System with Automatic Brightness Adjustment Using Bolt IoT Platform," *in Proceedings of the IEEE International IOT, Electronics and Mechatronics Conference (IEMTRONICS)*, Toronto, ON, Canada, April 2021, pp. 1–6, doi: 10.1109/IEMTRONICS52119.2021.9422668

[10] F. Sanchez-Sutil and A. Cano-Ortega, "Smart Regulation and Efficiency Energy System for Street Lighting with LoRa LPWAN," *Sustainable Cities and Society*, vol. 70, pp. 102912–102927, 2021, doi: 10.1016/j.scs.2021.102912

[11] Y. Jiang, Y. Shuai, X. He, X. Wen, and L. Lou, "An Energy-Efficient Street Lighting Approach Based on Traffic Parameters Measured by Wireless Sensing Technology," *IEEE Sensors Journal*, vol. 21, no. 17, pp. 19134–19143, 2021, doi: 10.1109/JSEN.2021.3089208

[12] N. Saokaew, N. Kitsatit, T. Yongkunawut, P. N. Ayudhya, E. Mujjalinvimut, T. Sapaklom, P. Aregarot, and J. Kunthong, "Smart Street Lamp System using LoRaWAN and Artificial Intelligence PART I," in *Proceedings of the 9th International Electrical Engineering Congress (iEECON)*, Pattaya, Thailand, March 2021, pp. 189–192, doi: 10.1109/iEECON51072.2021.9440337

[13] Y.-S. Yang, S.-H. Lee, G.-S. Chen, C.-S. Yang, Y.-M. Huang and T.-W. Hou, "An Implementation of High Efficient Smart Street Light Management System for Smart City," *IEEE Access*, vol. 8, pp. 38568–38585, 2020, doi: 10.1109/ACCESS.2020.2975708

[14] F. Bellido-Outeirino, F. Quiles-Latorre, C. Moreno-Moreno, J. Flores-Arias, I. Moreno-Garcıa, and M. Ortiz-Lopez, "Streetlight Control System Based on Wireless Communication over DALI Protocol," *Sensors*, vol. 16, no. 5, pp. 597–619, 2016, doi: 10.3390/s16050597

[15] F. Leccese, "Remote-Control System of High Efficiency and Intelligent Street Lighting Using a ZigBee Network of Devices and Sensors," *IEEE Transactions on Power Delivery*, vol. 28, no. 1, pp. 21–28, 2013, doi: 10.1109/TPWRD.2012.2212215

[16] F. Leccese, M. Cagnetti, and D. Trinca, "A Smart City Application: A Fully Controlled Street Lighting Isle Based on Raspberry-Pi Card, a ZigBee Sensor Network and WiMAX," *Sensors*, vol. 14, no. 12, pp. 24408–24424, 2014, doi: 10.3390/s141224408

[17] L. Yongsheng, L. Peijie, and C. Shuying, "Remote Monitoring and Control System of Solar Street Lamps Based on ZigBee Wireless Sensor Network and GPRS," in W. Hu (eds.) *Electronics and Signal Processing*, Lecture Notes in Electrical Engineering, Springer, Berlin, Heidelberg, vol. 97, 2011, pp. 959–967.

[18] S. Vishnu, S. R. J. Ramson, S. Senith, T. Anagnostopoulos, A. M. Mahfouz, X. Fan, S. Srinivasan, and A. Kirubaraj, "IoT-Enabled Solid Waste Management in Smart Cities," *Smart Cities*, vol. 4, no. 3, pp. 1004–1017, 2021, doi: 10.3390/smartcities4030053

[19] S. R. J. Ramson, W. D. Leon-Salas, Z. Brecheisen, E. J. Foster, C. T. Johnston, D. G. Schulze, T. Filley, R. Rahimi, M. J. C. V. Soto, J. A. L. Bolivar, and M. P. Malaga, "A Self-Powered, Real-Time, LoRaWAN IoT-Based Soil Health Monitoring System," *IEEE Internet of Things Journal*, vol. 8, no. 11, pp. 9278–9293, 2021, doi: 10.1109/JIOT.2021.3056586

[20] S. R. J. Ramson, S. Vishnu, A. A. Kirubaraj, T. Anagnostopoulos and A. M. Abu-Mahfouz, "A LoRaWAN IoT-Enabled Trash Bin Level Monitoring System," *IEEE Transactions on Industrial Informatics*, vol. 18, no. 2, pp. 786–795, 2022, doi: 10.1109/TII.2021.3078556

[21] S. Bandopadhaya, R. Dey, and A. Suhag, "Integrated Healthcare Monitoring Solutions for Soldier Using the Internet of Things with Distributed Computing," *Sustainable Computing: Informatics and Systems*, vol. 26, pp. 100378–100384, 2020, doi: 10.1016/j.suscom.2020.100378

[22] P. Kumari, R. Mishra, H. P. Gupta, T. Dutta, and S. K. Das, "An Energy Efficient Smart Metering System using Edge Computing in LoRa Network," *IEEE Transactions on Sustainable Computing*, 2021, doi: 10.1109/TSUSC.2021.3049705

[23] W. A. Jabbar, T. Subramaniam, A. E. Ong, M. I. Shu'Ib, W. Wu, and M. A. Oliveira, "LoRaWAN-Based IoT System Implementation for Long-Range Outdoor Air Quality Monitoring," *Internet of Things*, vol. 19, pp. 100540–100564, 2022, doi: 10.1016/j.iot.2022.100540

[24] Z. Kaleem, T. M. Yoon, and C. Lee, "Energy Efficient Outdoor Light Monitoring and Control Architecture Using Embedded System," *IEEE Embedded Systems Letters*, vol. 8, no. 1, pp. 18–21, 2016, doi: 10.1109/LES.2015.2494598

[25] S. Chen, G. Xiong, J. Xu, S. Han, F.-Y. Wang, and K. Wang, "The Smart Street Lighting System Based on NB-IoT," in *Proceedings of the Chinese Automation Congress (CAC)*, Xi'an, China, November 2018, pp. 1196–1200, doi: 10.1109/CAC.2018.8623281

[26] "50 Million Global Street Lights Expected to Be Connected by 2023 – Counterpoint," *Counterpoint Technology Market Research*, November 2, 2023. [Online]. Available: https://www.counterpointresearch.com/insights/50-million-global-street-lights-expected-connected-2023 [Accessed: December 13, 2023].

[27] K. L. Lueth, "Connected Streetlights Market: APAC to Emerge as the Leading Adopter," *IoT Analytics*, April 7, 2022. [Online]. Available: https://iot-analytics.com/connected-streetlights-market-apac-emerges-leading-adopter-2023 [Accessed: December 13, 2023].

[28] MNRE, "Brief on Off-grid Solar PV Programme." [Online]. Available: https://mnre.gov.in/solar-off-grid

[29] European Commission, "Up to 78 Million Batteries Will be Discarded Daily by 2025, Researchers Warn," cordis.europa.eu, July 23, 2021. [Online]. Available: https://cordis.europa.eu/article/id/430457-up-to-78-million-batteries-will-be-discarded-daily-by-2025-researchers-warn [Accessed: December 13, 2023].

[30] "SPV1050 – STMicroelectronics," *STMicroelectronics*. [Online]. Available: https://www.st.com/en/power-management/spv1050.html

[31] ANYSOLAR, "IXOLAR High Efficiency SolarMD," https://ixapps.ixys.com. [Online]. Available: https://ixapps.ixys.com/DataSheet/SM141K10LV.pdf [Accessed: December 9, 2023].

[32] Electropedia, "Battery and Energy Technologies," mpoweruk.com. [Online]. Available: https://www.mpoweruk.com/life.htm#:~:text=This%20is%20because%20battery%20life,100%20cycles%20at%201%25%20DOD [Accessed: December 20, 2021].

[33] N. Valov et al., "Design of a Smart System for Street Light Monitoring and Control," in *Proceedings of the 7th International Symposium on Multidisciplinary Studies and Innovative Technologies (ISMSIT)*, 2023, pp. 1–4, doi: 10.1109/ISMSIT58785.2023.10304998

[34] F. Wu, J. M. Redoute, and M. R. Yuce, "WE-Safe: A Self-Powered Wearable IoT Sensor Network for Safety Applications Based on LoRa," *IEEE Access*, vol. 6, pp. 40846–40853, 2018, doi: 10.1109/ACCESS.2018.2859383

[35] X. Zhang, M. Zhang, F. Meng, Y. Qiao, S. Xu, and S. Hour, "A Low-Power Wide-Area Network Information Monitoring System by Combining NB-IoT and LoRa," *IEEE Internet of Things Journal*, vol. 6, no. 1, pp. 590–598, 2019, doi: 10.1109/JIOT.2018.2847702

[36] S. Sadowski and P. Spachos, "Wireless Technologies for Smart Agricultural Monitoring Using Internet of Things Devices with Energy Harvesting Capabilities," *Computers and Electronics in Agriculture*, vol. 172, pp. 103558–103566, 2020, doi: 10.1016/j.compag.2020.105338

[37] H. Bhusal, P. Khatiwada, A. Jha, J. Soumya, S. Koorapati, and L. R. Cenkeramaddi, "A Self-Powered Long-range Wireless IoT Device based on LoRaWAN," in *Proceedings of the IEEE International Symposium on Smart Electronic Systems (iSES)*, 2020, pp. 242–245, doi: 10.1109/iSES50453.2020.00061

[38] S. Ali, T. Glass, B. Parr, J. Potgieter, and F. Alam, "Low Cost Sensor With IoT LoRaWAN Connectivity and Machine Learning-Based Calibration for Air Pollution Monitoring," *IEEE Transactions on Instrumentation and Measurement*, vol. 70, pp. 1–11, 2021, doi: 10.1109/TIM.2020.3034109

[39] O. H. Kombo, S. Kumaran, and A. Bovim, "Design and Application of a Low-Cost, Low-Power, LoRa-GSM, IoT Enabled System for Monitoring of Groundwater Resources With Energy Harvesting Integration," *IEEE Access*, vol. 9, pp. 128417–128433, 2021, doi: 10.1109/ACCESS.2021.3112519

[40] A. I. Petrariu, A. Lavric, E. Coca, and V. Popa, "Hybrid Power Management System for LoRa Communication Using Renewable Energy," *IEEE Internet of Things Journal*, vol. 8, no. 10, pp. 8423–8436, 2021, doi: 10.1109/JIOT.2020.3046324

[41] M. Yuksel and H. Fidan, "Energy-Aware System Design for Batteryless LPWAN Devices in IoT Applications," *Ad Hoc Networks*, vol. 122, pp. 102625–102645, 2021, doi: 10.1016/j.adhoc.2021.102625

[42] P. Mohanty, U. C. Pati, K. Mahapatra, and S. P. Mohanty, "bSlight: Battery-Less Energy Autonomous Street Light Management System for Smart City," *IEEE Transactions on Sustainable Computing*, doi: 10.1109/TSUSC.2023.3310884

[43] P. Mohanty, U. C. Pati, and K. Mahapatra, "Self-Powered Intelligent Street Light Management System for Smart City," in *Proceedings of the IEEE 18th India Council International Conference (INDICON)*, Guwahati, India, 2021, pp. 1–6, doi: 10.1109/INDICON52576.2021.9691575

[44] C. S. Sandeep, P. Mohanty, and U. C. Pati, "Machine Learning Based Framework for Prediction of Photovoltaic Output Power," in *Proceedings of the IEEE 3rd International Conference on Sustainable Energy and Future Electric Transportation (SEFET)*, August 2023, pp. 1–6, doi: 10.1109/SeFeT57834.2023.10245655

[45] P. Mohanty, U. C. Pati, and K. Mahapatra, "Deep Learning Based Framework for Forecasting Solar Panel Output Power," in *Proceedings of the IFIP Advances in Information and Communication Technology*, October 2023, pp. 1–19, doi: 10.1007/978-3-031-45878-1 16

[46] S. C. Mathi, H. K. Gowra, T. V. Harshith, "IoT Based Smart Street Light Automation using Thermoelectric Transducers," in *Proceedings of the International Conference on Sustainable Communication Networks and Application (ICSCNA)*, Theni, India, 2023, pp. 342–347, doi: 10.1109/ICSCNA58489.2023.10370191

[47] D. Ghai, S. L. Tripathi, S. Saxena, M. Chanda, and M. Alazab, *Machine Learning Algorithms for Signal and Image Processing*, John Wiley & Sons, 2022.

[48] M. S. Priyadarshini, A. Sravani, S. Gochhait, A. Bhatt, M. Bajaj, and M. M. Mahmoud, "IoT Platform-Based Prototype Model of an Adaptive and Intelligent Traffic Lighting System," in *Proceedings of the 4th IEEE Global Conference for Advancement in Technology (GCAT)*, Bangalore, India, 2023, pp. 1–6, doi: 10.1109/GCAT59970.2023.10353407

7 Green Computing in Network Security

N. Sumalatha and K. Baskaran
Alagappa Chettiar Government College of Engineering & Technology (ACGCET), Karaikudi, India

7.1 INTRODUCTION

Green computing seeks to decrease the use of hazardous materials, maximize energy efficiency throughout a product's lifetime, and increase the recycling or biodegradability of obsolete products and factory waste [1]. The computer and IT industries have recently come to understand the value of being green, both in terms of environmental concerns and minimizing costs, which has caused a notable shift in IT sector plans and regulations. The need for corporate computing is constantly expanding, the cost of energy is constantly rising, and people are becoming more aware of the problems with global warming. Energy issues will take on greater importance as carbon emissions, global warming, and climate change heat up. After all, the 21st century belongs to computers, gadgets, and electronic devices. We need to reevaluate our assumptions if we believe that computers are clean and use relatively little energy [2]. Only around 15% of the $250 billion spent annually on powering computers globally is thought to be used for computation; the remaining energy is lost as idle time. According to the Association for Computer Machinery [3], "If climate change is to be slowed in time to avoid catastrophic environmental damage, then the demand for energy and carbon output of computing and the entire ICT sector must be drastically moderated."

The Information, Communications, and Technology (ICT) sector accounts for about 2% of worldwide Co_2 emissions, which is comparable to the sector's contribution from aviation [4]. However, ICT emissions are anticipated to roughly triple by 2030; therefore, without large green investments in the telecom infrastructure that supports ICT services, these services' energy consumption and related CO_2 emissions are anticipated to increase significantly. The primary goals of the United Nations Framework Convention on Climate Change (UNFCC) are to prevent environmental damage while keeping emissions of Greenhouse Gases (GHG) in balance [5]. To meet the needs of future generations, it preserves renewable resources. Companies that focus on Information Technology (IT) use data centers to offer services to customers. Since servers consume more energy, the data center developed green computing life cycle management. Based upon responses to a few questionnaires, the data center takes appropriate action to set the green computing life cycle management into practice [6]. It is used in Malaysia and may eventually be used in

 DOI: 10.1201/9781003546382-7

other nations. Between 1.8% and 3.9% of the world's greenhouse gas emissions are attributable to the ICT industry [7].

The phrase "green computing" refers to a wide range of methods, tools, and approaches that can be used to lessen the effect of computing systems on the environment. These include developing more energy-efficient hardware designs [8], powering computer systems using renewable energy sources [9], and putting more environmentally friendly procedures into data centers and other computing environments [10, 11]. The utilization of natural energy resources for operating computing systems is another topic of study in green computing. This covers the production of power for data centers and other computing centers through the use of the sun, wind, and hydropower. A Natural Resources Defense Council (NRDC) analysis suggests that up to 90% less carbon emissions might be produced by powering data centers with renewable energy.

The significance of green computing and its ability to lessen the IT industry's carbon footprint is covered by the author in [12]. The IT industry's energy usage and related carbon emissions are highlighted in this article, which also gives a general overview of the several strategies and tools that may be used to encourage more environmentally friendly computer activities. These tools include cloud computing and energy-efficient gear. Further hardware and software must be used to make computing more environmentally friendly, which ultimately requires more power [13].

The authors highlight that to encourage the spread of green computing methods and technology, cooperation between various stakeholders—including business, government, and academia—is essential. A meta-heuristic for green computing was provided by [14]. Green computing tools for Erlang were presented in the paper [15], while the author [16] addressed the obstacles and motivations for integrating green computing with sustainable agriculture. In terms of green computing, [17] contrasted Advanced Micro Devices, Inc. (AMD) and Intel processors, and [18] addressed the potential of near-threshold voltage design. An Indonesian green IT policy was proposed by [19, 20], which provided a multi-layer method for creating environmentally friendly digital circuits and many-core architectures, whereas [21] offered a hybrid multicore architecture for green computing. A profile-based building energy-saving service was offered by [22], and multi-label classification techniques for green computing were covered by [23]. To optimize power consumption in Organic Light-Emitting Diode (OLED)-based displays were suggested by GREECOPE [24], a green computing solution utilizing the piezoelectric effect, was described by [25].

Large-scale Internet-based services depend on data centers, which are essential but energy-intensive infrastructures. Moreover, data centers consume 3% of power annually; over 50% has been used in the last ten years. More energy-efficient chips are designed to increase the sustainability of computing. When the energy usage of a single computer chip might appear insignificant, when it is multiplied by millions, it is feasible to achieve significant savings. For example, heterogeneous systems combine frameworks like Central Processing Units (CPUs) and Graphics Processing Units (GPUs) to maximize power and energy efficiency. To promote energy efficiency, the Environmental Protection Agency (EPA) launched the Energy Star

Programme in the US in 1992. The various approaches used for green computing are enlisted as follows:

- Turn off laptops while not in use.
- To save energy, apply sleep or suspended mode.
- Cutting Down on E-Waste.
- Instead of purchasing new printer cartridges, refill existing ones.
- Check out devices with an Energy Star rating.
- Diminishing the brightness of the screen saves electricity.

1. ***Virtualization***: The process of logically combining two or more systems with a single physical hardware architecture is known as virtualization. This method uses less power and less hardware. The concept was executed using x86 processors in the 1990s. New software packages supporting virtualization are being introduced these days. AMD and Intel Corporation implement virtual computing through x86 processor instruction set modifications.
2. ***Servers***: Windows is used on terminal servers that are employed in green computing methods. Users can obtain operating systems through the Mac version of the Aqua Connect Terminal Server. Using this strategy, clients log in to the server. Users communicate with the operating system, and servers handle all computations. Servers and clients are utilized in virtual labs that have been developed. Clients use 12.5 percent of the workstation's energy. Thin client and terminal servers save costs and energy consumption.
3. ***Power Control***: The Advanced Configuration and Power Interface (ACPI), a free industry standard, enables an operating system to directly manage the hardware's power-saving features. After predetermined amounts of inactivity, this enables a system to turn off components like monitors and hard drives. A system may also go into hibernation, where the majority of its components are shut off. Some programs, like undervolting, involve voltage adjustments to the CPU by the user directly, which results in less electricity and heat generation. Depending on the workload, some CPUs can automatically reduce their voltage; this technology is known as "SpeedStep" on Intel processors and Long Run on Transmeta processors.
4. ***Power Source***: Computer power supply units are 70–75% efficient, with the remaining 25–30% being released as heat. The PLUS program recognizes Power Supply Units (PSUs) that have an efficiency of 80% and can be used to replace earlier PSUs that share the same characteristics.
5. ***Storage***: Compact hard disc drives consume less energy than large drives. Solid-state drives require longer times to write data to the drive, consume more power, and store more data. The development of online storage has increased data accessibility and storage capacity.

   The challenge of reducing the electricity consumption of massive storage arrays while maintaining the benefits of online storage remains unexplored.
6. ***Visual Card***: In a computer, the graphics processing unit uses more power. In situations where a GPU is unavailable but a display is required, desktop

sharing and terminal sharing are not feasible. Use a motherboard's low-power video output or an outdated video card for display. Depending on average power usage or performance per watt, a GPU is selected according to the requirement.

7. ***Material Recycling***: With the assistance of various recycling facilities, unwanted computer equipment parts are recycled and donated to charitable organizations. Recycling keeps dangerous materials out of landfills, including lead, mercury, and chromium. Recycling-generated E-waste is shipped to underdeveloped nations, including Europe and North America.

The main contribution of this chapter includes:

1. The security and privacy concerns of the different technologies in terms of energy consumption and emission of gases.
2. The achievement of green computing in different fields of cloud computing, fog computing, Internet of Things (IoT), and Software-Defined Networks (SDNs) are included to reduce the effects of GHG and improve energy efficiency.

The primary contribution made by this chapter comprises:

1. The various technologies' security and privacy issues are examined, along with potential solutions. These issues include assaults, accessibility, secrecy, trust, and identification.
2. The attainment of green computing includes lowering greenhouse gas emissions and enhancing energy efficiency in several domains such as cloud computing, fog computing, the Internet of Things, and Software-Defined Networks (SDNs).

This chapter is organized as follows: Computing, security concerns, and security enhancements are covered in Section 7.2. Fog computing, security concerns, and the implementation of green fog computing are discussed in Section 7.3. IoT technology, security concerns, and privacy issues related to the development of green IoT are covered in Section 7.4. In Section 7.5, the risks associated with Software-Defined Networks (SDNs) at various levels, along with ways to achieve green SDNs, are discussed.

7.2 CLOUD COMPUTING

In actuality, Cloud Computing (CC) and Green Computing (GC) are complementary [26]. Both of these advanced computing gradients are crucial for the development and change of technology. A type of network grid known as cloud computing utilizes network and communication technology to completely virtualize the information technology infrastructure. A key component of green computing is cloud computing and virtualization, which use fewer computers, products, and energy.

When a user submits a request (i.e., query), cloud computing processes that request, computes a response, and then sends that result back to the user over the internet [27]. It does computations of any complexity with the least amount of latency. Data is processed by sophisticated servers in a data center and transferred over the internet for cloud operations. Facebook alone currently requires Petabytes (PB) of storage due to the increase in the number of internet users. Power is needed for data transmission, data processing software and hardware, networking peripherals, and storage. Google uses 1000 servers to process each search engine query, which reduces response time to 0.2 seconds. Figure 7.1 illustrates the energy consumption of one Google search.

In addition to the previously listed, the majority of known attacks include traffic analysis, IP ports, phishing, Internet Protocol (IP) spoofing, message alteration, and so forth. Cloud computing companies accept a wide range of security measures for data protection, all of which offer access control, authorization, and secrecy.

7.2.1 Security in Cloud Computing

Data security, network security, virtualization security, software integrity, and authentication and authorization are just a few of the security concerns surrounding cloud computing that are currently receiving a lot of attention [28]. Data protection is the main objective of security. When data protection is not secure with a cloud service provider, the exchange of information limits the servers. There are several challenging ways to preserve data in cloud computing. The most widely used security methods include intrusion detection systems, multi-tenancy-based access control, Secure Socket Layer (SSL) encryption, and others. The purpose of this study is to review and assess the key security measures for cloud computing data protection. Today, practically all computer systems use cloud computing technology for the exchange of information. It utilizes a network infrastructure that is vulnerable to various

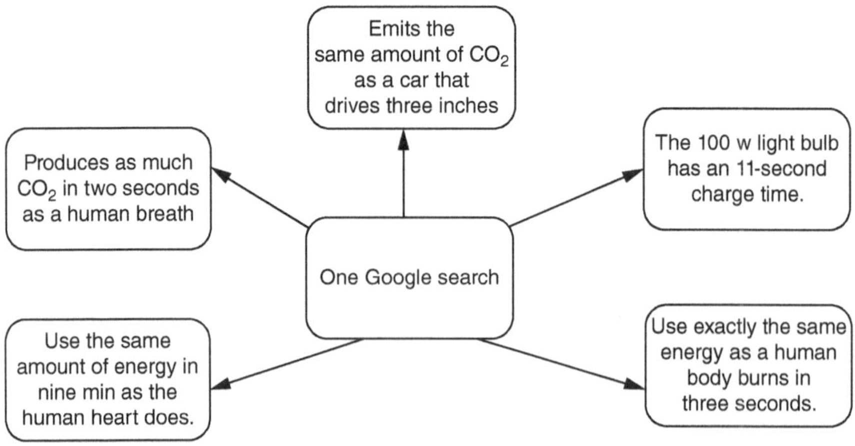

FIGURE 7.1 Energy consumption of one Google search.

attacks [28]. Distributed Denial of Service (DDoS) attacks and man-in-the-middle attacks are the most popular types of attacks. Secure Socket Layer (SSL) is used as a security measure against DDoS attacks. Authenticating clients and servers Client and server authentication are impacted when security mechanisms are not used. To secure the information against man-in-the-middle attacks, authentication is required.

7.2.1.1 Authentication in Cloud Computing

Authentication verifies the user's identity to the service provider and allows them to access cloud-based information. Public and private clouds support different RSA authentication systems, such as knowledge-based and dual-factor authentication.

The Amazon Elastic Compute Cloud (Amazon EC2) provider must use Advanced Encryption Standard (AES) to ensure the most security for user data. The focus of Amazon Web Services (AWS) is on secure data transmission between web servers and browsers, including virtual private clouds [29]. Multi-Factor Authentication (MFA) is the solution among the different authentication schemes as shown in Figure 7.2. To log into cloud instances, users must also submit their username, password, and the dynamically created MFA code [30]. Google has an open-source MFA setup tool called Google Authenticator, which is widely supported across all platforms for MFA or Two-Factor Authentication (TFA), as shown in Figure 7.2.

Additionally, there is an authentication method that enables users to log in to numerous services with just one password [31]. Users of this method are vulnerable to dictionary and honeypot attacks. Google, Microsoft, and Facebook are some of the IT firms that use this type of authentication method. We conclude that AWS uses

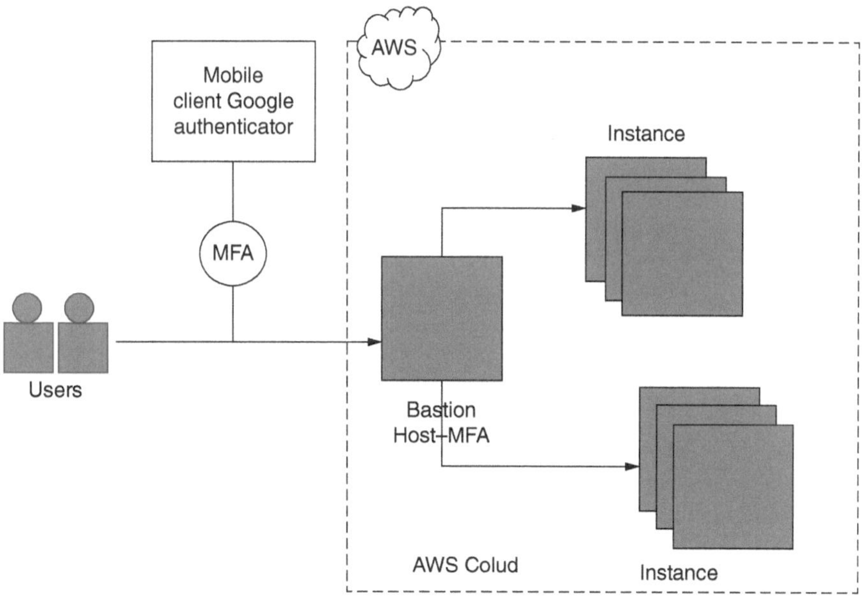

FIGURE 7.2 Google authenticator using MFA in the AWS cloud.

multifactor authentication to protect the data in the cloud. This authentication method has the advantage of making identity and access management possible. Facebook uses single-password authentication to enable cloud data security. This type of authentication mechanism has the advantage of providing security from dictionary and honeypot attacks.

7.2.1.2 Confidentiality in Cloud Computing

Another company that offers encryption for cloud data is Wuala Cloud. Encryption takes place before the data gets uploaded to the cloud, providing good protection by preventing the supplier from accessing the data. The authors of [32] are outlining a hierarchical attribute-based encryption technique for cloud computing. This suggested security method for maintaining secrecy in cloud computing provides excellent access control and fast performance. The authors of [33] suggest an encryption mechanism that would allow owners to govern the cloud-based data they own. The Amazon EC2 provider uses AES to ensure the most security in user data [34].

For the protection of data in the cloud, confidentiality is crucial, and various providers provide a variety of security measures to guarantee it. For instance, DELL provides transparent file encryption in addition to hardware- and software-based encryption. This type of encryption algorithm has the advantages of being simple to use and not requiring human participation. Wuala employs encryption methods on personal computers, and this approach to cloud-based encryption gives users an advantage when accessing the data. Cyber Technology offers Whole Disc Encryption (WDE) or Full Disc Encryption (FDE) to protect the privacy of data stored on cloud servers.

7.2.1.3 Authorization in Cloud Computing

A new client's identity is confirmed upon addition to a cloud service, i.e., authorization is granted upon authentication. Oracle Database Vault is a security feature that shields application data from various customers. An additional authorization technique based on policies secures the privacy of customers and carries out its policies. Organization for the Advancement of Structured Information Standards (OASIS) cloud authorization is based on authorization management, which records user logs that disclose the users' location and the specifics of the devices that they operate.

7.2.1.4 Cloud Computing Access Control

It makes cloud data accessible to approved users. Firewalls, systems to detect intrusions, and responsibility segregation are some of the techniques used in layers and networks for access control. A firewall consists of a set of parameters with user-defined rules and policies. Cloud computing access control is made feasible by the organization McAfee. There are choices for access control, including McAfee Web Gateway, McAfee Single Logon On, and McAfee Single-Use Password. Security techniques improve the prevention of data loss and the management of policies. The McAfee cloud identity manager for cloud computing is shown in Figure 7.3.

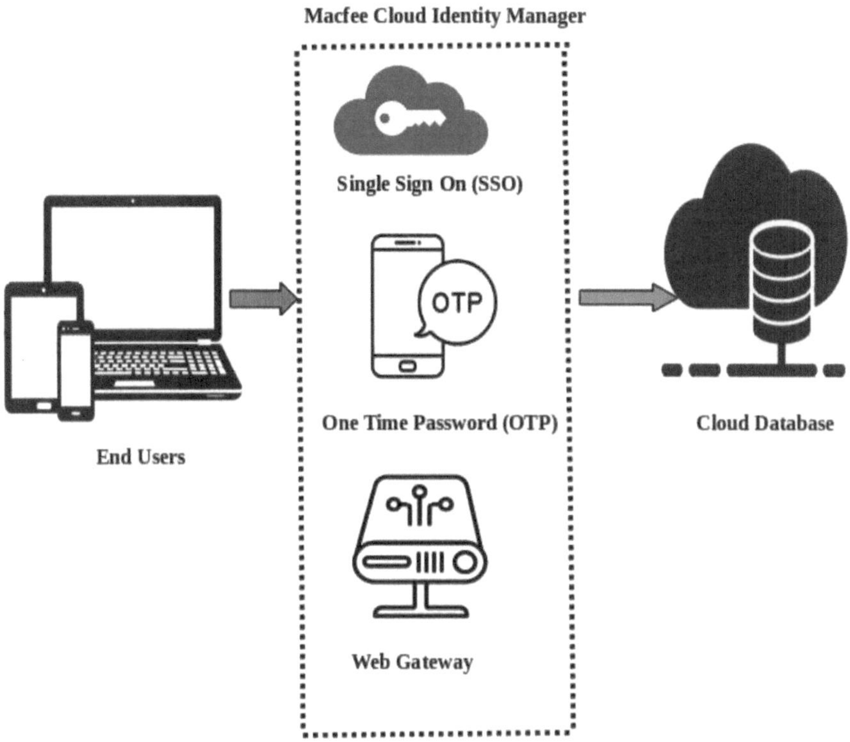

FIGURE 7.3 Cloud identity manager by McAfee.

7.2.2 Improved Security in Cloud Computing

There are various ways to improve security in cloud computing are enlisted as follows:

1. ***Monitoring and Registering***: Threats are identified using the cloud computing monitoring system. Cloud logging captures data from cloud logs. Log data is used to check for discrepancies in the events that are recorded.
2. ***Cloud Visibility and Control***: Cloud visibility means viewing all cloud activities. It aids in discovering potential dangers and areas of insufficient performance in cloud deployment. You can implement regulations to reduce risks after you understand what is causing the process to malfunction. The procedure for cloud visibility and control entails:
   - Address cloud system threats as a preventative measure.
   - Catch an attack in the act before it compromises your data.
   - After an assault has occurred, lessen the impact it has.
3. ***Next Generation Firewall (NGFW)***: In contrast to typical firewalls, this specifies the filtering method with predetermined protocols [35]. Figure 7.4 shows the Next Generation Firewall (NGF). The main features of an NGFW are as follows:
   - Prevent hackers at the network interface.
   - Locating geographically

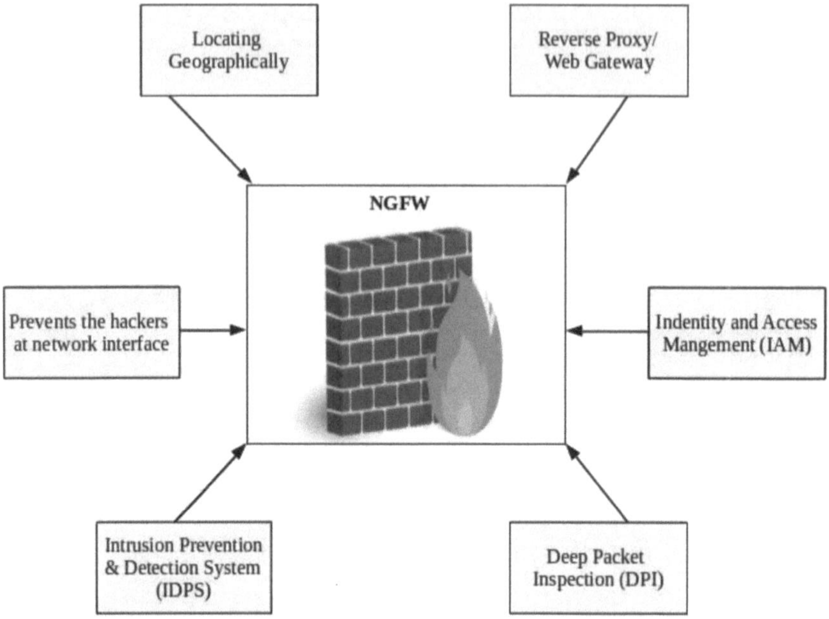

FIGURE 7.4 Next-generation firewall.

- Reverse proxy/web gateway
- Intrusion Detection and Prevention Systems (IDPS)
- Information extraction, or Deep Packet Inspection (DPI)
- Identity and Access Management (IAM)

4. ***Two-Factor Authentication***: Two-factor authentication adds a level of security for users to sign in. It has improvements, including time-dependent codes, strong security, and guaranteed consumer identity.
5. ***Streamline Identity and Access Management***: Identity and Access Management (IAM) is a service on the cloud that permits clients to access cloud tools and regulates them. It enables authorized users to access the system and data. Figure 7.5 shows IAM for cloud service.
   - ***Platform-Specific Accessibility***: restricts the client's ability to approach the particular objective. For example, users can use the operating system, whereas the testing tools are not used.
   - ***Risk-Oriented Access Management***: clients are proved depending on possibility criteria.
   - ***Distributing Rights***: sharing rights are limited to users, preventing them from exchanging information.
6. ***Evaluate Adherence to Data Protection laws***: Cloud storage protects information through a group of instructions known as data protection regulations. Data protection has gotten more difficult as firms transition to hybrid cloud architectures. Gaining user confidence requires General Data Protection Regulation (GDPR) compliance. It helps you avoid hazards and safeguards

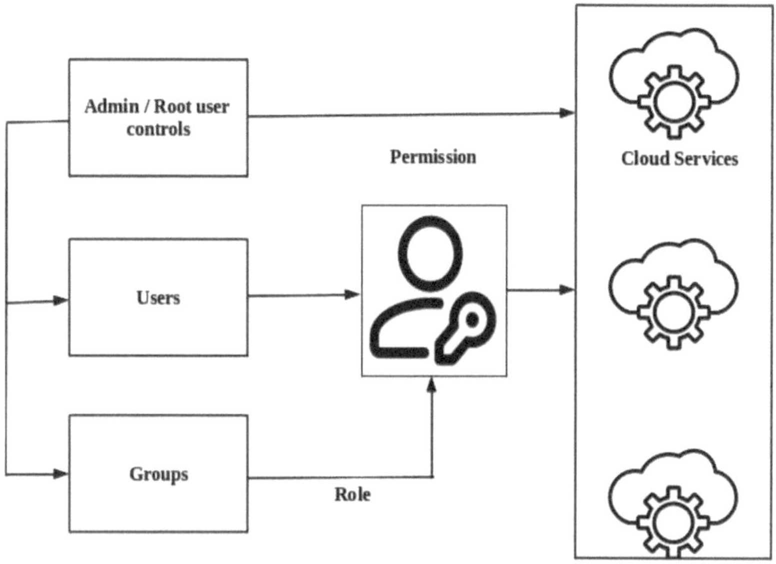

FIGURE 7.5 Identity and access management (IAM) for cloud services.

your private information. Failure to comply could result in financial and reputational losses. Preserving the information involves:

- Hiding the information (ciphering)
- Authentication
- Endpoint security
- Tracking

7. ***Secure Information***: Protecting data centers from denied access includes:
   a. ***Evaluation of Risk***: It includes three steps:
      - Identify the threats.
      - Arranging them according to the degree of severity.
      - Take actions to overcome threats.

   b. ***Data Masking***: A form of security technique known as information masking hides sensitive data by using modified content, such as letters or numerals.

   c. ***Data Protection***: Encrypts the information so that only a valid user can access it with a secure key that is available.

   d. ***Access Controls***: Access management procedures are required by access control policies. It establishes who has access to information and under what conditions.

8. ***Cloud Automation***: Without the need for human involvement, cloud automation may automate system functions. Cloud automation can
   - Strengthen security measures.
   - Avoid setup errors.
   - Maintain compliance at all levels.

Secure deployments during the development phase to reduce the effects of data theft.

7.3 FOG COMPUTING

Cisco claims that Fog Computing (FC) is a cloud extension that goes from the center to the edge to enhance huge data analysis, low latency, and frequent services [36]. To deliver data services and applications, it is a network composed of a large number of geographically dispersed Fog Nodes (FNs) [37]. Each server is a scaled-down version of a cloud server that offers services closer to consumers [38, 39]. FC results in the need for real-time, location-awareness, global distribution, robust mobility, wireless access, real-time transmission, and heterogeneity [40–42]. They can operate together and communicate with one another to create a network that is capable of processing and storing data in real time. Table 7.1 shows the differences between fog computing and cloud computing [43].

The fog computing services are situated near the endpoints [44]. The computer paradigm's intimate relationship to end devices gives it a significant advantage over other traditional computing approaches. Figure 7.6 shows some significant characteristics of fog computing with cloud computing and IoT.

7.3.1 Security Issues in Fog Computing

Similar to cloud computing, fog computing provides end users with storage and data processing capabilities. The reviewed literature highlighted many security vulnerabilities related to fog computing, including authentication, privacy, data security,

TABLE 7.1
Comparison Between Cloud Computing and Fog Computing

Sr. No.	Cloud Computing	Fog Computing
1.	High lag	Low lag
2.	A reduction in data is not possible.	Reducing the amount of data is possible.
3.	The speed of response is low.	The speed of response is high.
4.	reduces the certainty	improves the certainty
5.	Access time is high, which depends on the VM connectivity.	Accessing time is more expensive compared to cloud computing.
6.	Integration of several information sources is possible.	Integration of several information sources and components is possible.
7.	Portability is limited.	Portability is supported.
8.	Location-based computing is supported in cloud computing.	Location-based computing is supported in fog computing.
9.	The limited number of host nodes.	The large number of host nodes.
10.	Centralized coverage	Decentralized coverage.
11.	Services are provided via the Internet.	Services are provided at the edge of the local network.
12.	The mode of communication is an IP network.	Modes of communication include wireless communication (WLAN, WiFi, 3G, 4G, ZigBee, etc.) or wired

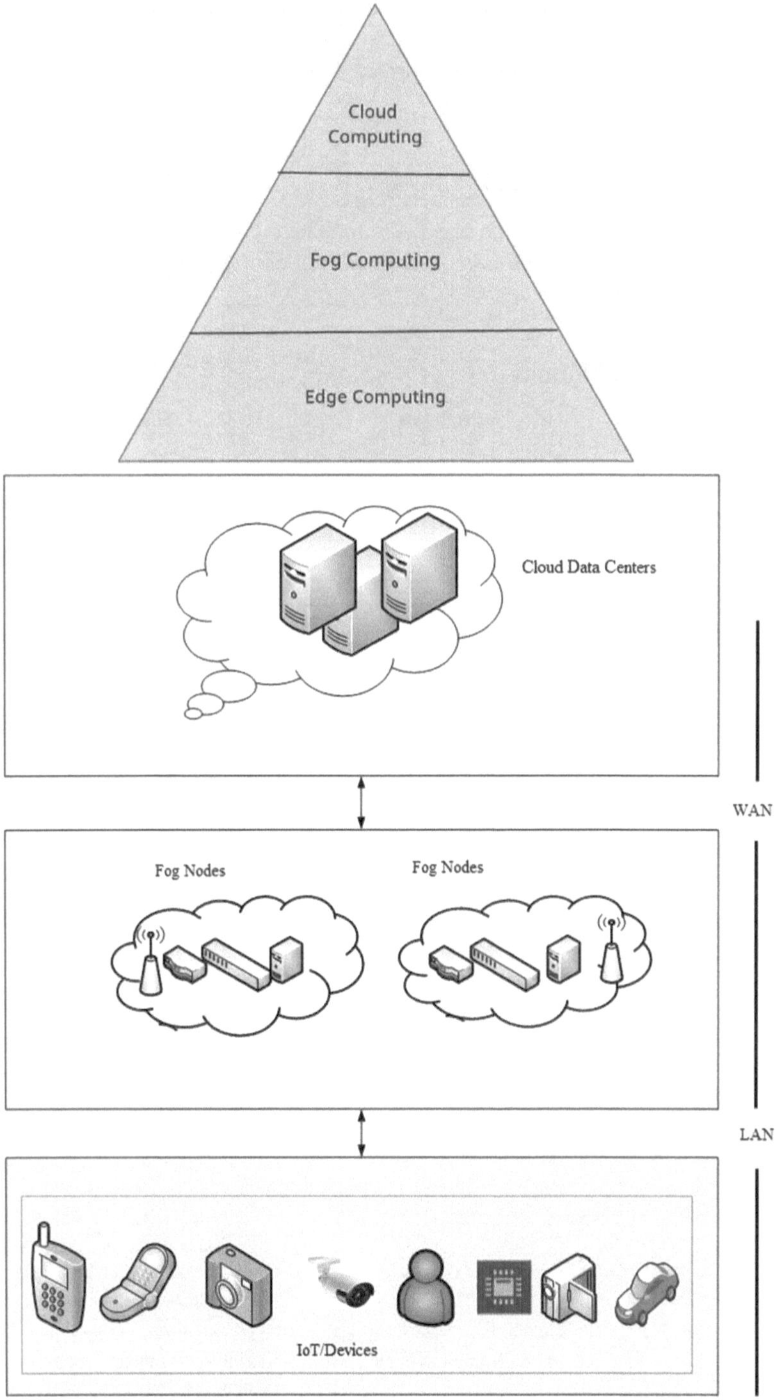

FIGURE 7.6 Fog computing with cloud computing and IoT.

and other harmful assaults. The researchers are particularly interested in the developing field of fog computing. In-depth studies are being conducted to determine the model's benefits [45]. This computer approach has certain obstacles and unresolved security issues [46], as shown in Table 7.2.

7.3.1.1 Authentication

The primary security concern across several gateway tiers is authentication, as fog computing has enabled numerous end users to access extensive services through a single fog node. Authentication is required for both entities and communications in

TABLE 7.2
Security Issues and Solutions in Fog Computing

Sr. No.	Challenges	Problems	Solutions
1.	Authentication	Middle-man attacks occur without authentication.	1. Public key cryptography [RSA and ECC] [47] 2. Biometric authentication in mobile computing 3. Fingerprint authentication in cloud computing
2.	Malicious attacks	DoS, internal attacks, flooding attacks, port scanning, and attacks on the virtual machine and hypervisor	By observing, closely examining, and poking a lot of comprehensive inquiries about access control procedures, log files, and customer login information, an intrusion detection system can be delivered to the fog node's system side to identify sniffing activities.
3.	Data Protection	The integrity of data must be guaranteed during the processing of distributed data.	1. Techniques for masking and minimal encryption are required [48]. 2. Two approaches are presented in [49]: behavior profiles and the decoy system. a. Unusual activity, including gaining more access to different records at odd times, will cause the scheme to report the entry as suspicious and restrict the associated user. b. A decoy system comprises fictitious data, including honeypots, honey files, and other things that can be used to locate, confuse, and determine potential insider threats.
4.	Privacy	Right to keep their location secret from other nodes.	Preserving useful information during communication can be achieved with fuzzing, segregation, encoding, decoding, arranging, and rearranging steps [50].

fog computing [51]. The possibility of a Man-In-The-Middle (MITM) attack exists in the absence of sufficient authentication. The issue of MITM in a fog computing environment is yet unresolved. Since fog devices are typically not under monitoring, attackers can readily respond to communications. Because encryption and decryption methods use a lot of battery life, especially on 3G mobile phones, they are not appropriate for HTTPS MITM assaults [52]. Even though an earlier study indicated that it uses little network resources, they used deception techniques and public-key cryptography to enable authentication. To determine which algorithm would use more resources, public key cryptography was implemented using traditional cryptosystems such as Rivest Shamir Adleman (RSA) and Elliptic Curve Cryptography (ECC). When they finally examined the outcomes of the RSA and ECC algorithms, they found that, in resource-constrained fog devices, ECC produced the best results when compared to RSA [47]. Biometric authentication—such as fingerprint, face, and touch-based authentication—plays a significant role in cloud computing and mobile computing. Fog computing, which was examined in [48], will benefit more from the deployment of various authentication methods. Since AES encryption requires less computer power and is widely used [53], it is a viable option for fog computing. Nevertheless, no existing encryption method is contrasted with AES in this experiment.

7.3.1.2 Malicious Attacks

Fog computing uses a variety of edge devices to process collected data with latency awareness. Fog computing is vulnerable to several malicious assaults, which can seriously impair system performance if they are not prevented. Denial of Service (DoS) assaults are one type of malicious attack that has been launched. A particular kind of network assault called Distributed Denial-of-Service (DDoS) prevents authorized users from accessing cloud or fog resources. The standard, recommended approach to fixing the issue is intrusion detection. Unfortunately, as of right now, there isn't a solution that can properly tackle DDoS difficulties in a fog environment [54]. This kind of attack occurs when an attacker requests limitless processing and storage services from several connected devices in an Internet of Things context [48, 55].

By spoofing the IP addresses of many devices and sending a fake request to access processing and storage services, the intruders stop a recognized user from using the intended computer. Attacks of this kind can happen at several system levels. When multiple nodes launch this attack at the same time, its severity increases. Because fog computing networks are open, existing preventive measures designed for other types of networks are not appropriate for fog computing. The Man-in-the-Middle assault is another malevolent cyberattack. In this way, the fog node gateway can be compromised or swapped out for a fake one.

7.3.1.3 Data Protection

In IoT, as the number of devices rises, the information generated increases exponentially. These data also need to be processed at the processing level and saved at the communication level. Handling the data on IoT devices is very challenging due to resource limitations [56]. Data is sent to a nearby fog node by the Internet of Things device when it detects data. Dealing with a lot of data on Internet-of-Things devices is challenging.

As a result, the data is split up and sent to different fog nodes for processing. At this point, it is necessary to analyze the material without disparaging it. When processing dispersed data, data integrity must be ensured. Due to the scarcity of resources, the encryption and decryption procedures are exceedingly challenging in this case. Thus, masking and lightweight encryption approaches are required [57]. The authors of [48] provide a means to secure data from fraudulent users for cloud and fog computing elements. Table 7.2 shows the security issues and solutions in fog computing.

Behavior profiles and the decoy system were the two methods they offered. These methods' primary goal is to lessen security breaches. If any reports indicate abnormal behavior, such as growing access to different data at odd times, the network will flag an entry as suspicious and ban the associated user. Behavior profiling methods are frequently used in a conventional client-server architecture with unrestricted access to computational resources. By thoroughly evaluating and choosing workable machine learning strategies and the training data needed for behavior profiling, the method can be further enhanced. The fact that there are many users and files makes this more important. Other works employ similar behavior profiling and decoy approaches to identify and stop malevolent insider threats [47, 58]. The behavioral profiling, evaluation, and client verification methods will prevent genuine information piracy and strain resources in the cloud without disclosing any critical data. A decoy system comprises fictitious data, including honeypots, honey files, and other records that can be used to locate, confuse, and identify potential insider threats. They demonstrated that, on average, the suggested technique may detect anomalous behavior with better than 90% accuracy.

7.3.1.4 Privacy in Fog Computing

Compared to cloud computing, maintaining privacy in fog computing is challenging since fog servers are closer to clients and can collect more relevant content. End users must be granted privacy through security measures. Privacy of location, privacy of services, and privacy of data are critical in fog computing. In fog computing, each node communicates with other nodes and can transmit confidential information at any given moment. They are entitled to keep their whereabouts a secret from other nodes. Thus, fog computing needs to guarantee all these rights to provide dependable communication [56]. The following summarize protecting the privacy and safeguarding the data for end-user devices and Fog networks [50]:

- Collecting sensor information and extracting its characteristics.
- Data fuzzing involves adding Gaussian noise to data at a specific variance level to reduce the likelihood of sniffing and eavesdropping.
- Data segregation involves dividing data into blocks and rearranging them to prevent Man-In-The-Middle (MITM) attacks.
- Public key infrastructure is implemented to encrypt each data block.
- Data packets are decrypted and rearranged at the fog node.

Additionally, the system minimizes communication with fog nodes using a feature reduction capability, which lowers risk because it concentrated on protecting sensitive and private data while it was being transmitted. By choosing an algorithm for regulating keys and encoding that prioritizes protecting data privacy, the suggested method can be strengthened. Furthermore, the necessary processing overheads for carrying out considerable data manipulation (fuzzing, segregation, encryption, decryption, and ordering and reordering) both before and after the communication are not well discussed. Because creating a fog network may not be possible due to the necessary computing overheads.

7.3.1.5 Access Control

When equipment or a consumer can access the sources, this is known as access control. like writing or reading data, running programs, and managing actuators. In the fog paradigm, an access control system permits authorization to be obtained from a different node [59]. Fog computing authorization is a critical component. Verifying the identities of the various systems is required to grant their requests to carry out specific tasks. Anyone can access the system and misuse the resources if the fog node lacks an authorization mechanism [60]. In a similar vein, controls should be put in place to govern data and services if users of the fog or cloud desire to employ computing services. As a result, the fog system must require the implementation of an authorization system and an access control mechanism.

7.3.1.6 Intrusion Detection System

The purpose of an intrusion detection system is to stop attackers from gaining unauthorized access and determine whether warnings are appropriate to stop incursions or lessen their effects. Attacks on cloud systems can take many forms, including port scanning, internal flooding, and attacks on virtual machines and hypervisors. To prevent these kinds of attacks, intrusion detection mechanisms are typically implemented in cloud systems. To find intrusions, this system examines and keeps an eye on the log file, the access control policy, and user registration data. On the network side, it must operate to recognize fraudulent activity such as DoS attempts and port scanning [49, 57, 60]. In fog computing, sniffing activities can be identified by sending an intrusion detection system to the fog node's system side. It does this by observing, examining, and probing a great deal about log files, client login information, and access control procedures. To differentiate dangerous attacks, they can also be relayed to the fog network side. For instance, denial-of-service attacks, port scanning, etc. Fog computing opens up new possibilities for investigating how fog computing can assist with client-side and cloud-side siding and binding in the event of an intrusion [61].

7.3.1.7 Policy-Driven Secure Management of Resources

An essential policy management architecture for Fog computing resources is suggested to enhance safe exchange and interoperability among user-requested services [61]. Five main modules comprise the system shown in Table 7.3.

- Application Administrator (AA) is responsible for managing multiple users;
- Policy Resolver (PR) manages authentication depending on factors;
- Policy Repository (PRep): regulations and policies are stored;
- The Policy Decision Engine (PDE) makes decisions based on specified policy guidelines in advance;
- Policy Enforcer (PE) looks for inconsistencies in policy implementation.

TABLE 7.3
Policy Management Framework

AA	While considering various tenants, apps, data exchange, and communication services, policies and regulations are specified (stored in PRep).
PR	It uses a particular set of characteristics and access rights about the requested resource to identify the user. A database contains the user attributes and the corresponding permissions for each user.
PDE	Data from PR is gathered, and rules from PRep are studied and applied through PE. The eXtensible Access Control Markup Language (XACML) is used to design the rules.
PE	The Policy Enforcer module can be found in a physical device like a mobile device, GPS, or linked car, or it can be found in a virtual instance like an FN, FI, or cloud computing data center.
PRep	After the Policy Resolver matches user attributes, the Policy Decision Engine consults the policy rules to ascertain (i) the user's access to the requested applications and (ii) the necessary constraints to be imposed based on the user's access privileges.

7.3.2 Green Fog Computing

Reducing energy usage in fog computing without sacrificing functionality is the aim of the Green-Demand-Aware Fog Computing (GDAFC) method [62]. To determine which fog nodes are operational, backup, and idle, this technique applies a prediction algorithm. When processing power is out, fog nodes transition to active nodes. It also determines the proper sleep interval for the fog nodes, accounting for the applications' latency requirements. This strategy can save up to 65% of energy without sacrificing the required latency, according to the mathematical formulation.

Fog computing architecture's theoretical modeling [63] and performance compared with the conventional cloud computing approach Fog computing was found to have a far lower service latency than cloud computing on a system that included many IoT apps operating in real-time and with low latency. Furthermore, real-time, low-latency services are required by IoT applications by 25%, and fog computing uses 40.48% less energy on average than traditional cloud computing.

Green fog computing in the agriculture sector [64] uses onboard computers as low-power fog nodes to gather data from sensors. The minimal energy requirements can be easily met by adding renewable energy supplies, which will increase its sustainability. For the smart agriculture sector as well as other application areas, the recommended green fog-based architecture would positively impact the creation of a green environment.

7.4 INTERNET OF THINGS

The Internet of Things (IoT) enables connections and communications between machines and objects [65]. This new technology's primary goals are to automate tasks and connect consumers' everyday devices to the Internet. Although the Internet of Things offers numerous advantages, it also has significant drawbacks, including poor administration, improper energy use, identity management, security concerns, and privacy concerns [66]. The most important problems affecting the development of IoT are security and privacy. In the Internet of Things, all gadgets have access to the Internet since they cannot function without it. There are numerous ways to access sensitive data on objects over the internet. Attackers can illegally use information

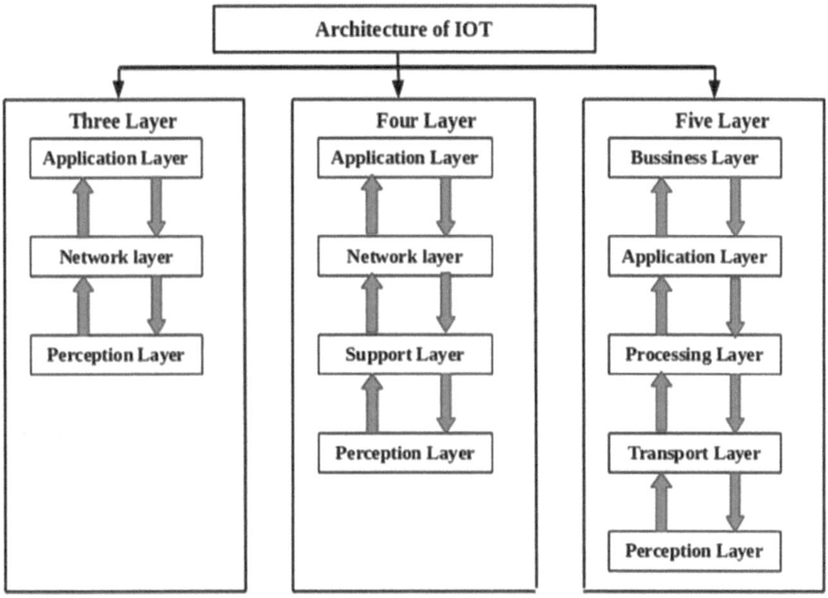

FIGURE 7.7 The layered architectures of IoT (three, four, or five layers).

for their purposes, which can cause significant losses for users [67]. IoT security and privacy have also become problems. Figure 7.7 depicts the layer design of the Internet of Things (IoT), each of which has three, four, and five layers to represent the hierarchy of all suggested layered architectures.

1. ***Perception Layer (Sensor Layer)***: Its primary purpose is to locate objects and get data from them. It includes technologies like WSN, RFID, and NFC that are connected to objects to collect information. The encryption technique preserves the integrity and confidentiality of the information. Attackers who want to use resources to swap out the sensors with their own are mostly after them [68]. As a result, sensors may be vulnerable to the majority of threats.
2. ***Network Layer (Transmission Layer)***: It serves as a bridge between the application layer and the perception layer. Through sensors, it sends the data gathered from the physical things. Data can be transmitted wirelessly or over wires as the medium. It also assumes responsibility for interconnecting networks, network devices, and smart things. The transport layer of IoT has DoS/DDoS assaults, forgery/middle attacks, heterogeneous network attacks, the application risk of IPv6, and WLAN application conflicts. In terms of security concerns, such as the authenticity and integrity of data being transmitted over a network.
3. ***Application Layer***: It describes all IoT-related applications and environments. Smart cities, smart homes, smart health, animal tracking, etc. are a few examples of IoT applications. The primary duty is to offer service to the applicants. Because services rely on the data gathered by sensors, each application contains a unique service. Issues with application

security include information access, privacy, user authentication, data stream destruction and tracking, stability of the IoT platform, security of the middleware, governance platform, and others. The key challenge for an Internet of Things (IoT)-based smart house is implementing robust security. The ZigBee-based components used in IoT-based smart homes utilize poor computing capacity and little storage [69].

4. ***Support Layer***: The security in the IoT architecture is the primary reason for adding a fourth layer because a three-layer architecture sends data straight to the network layer. Threats are more likely to arise because the information is routed straight to the network layer. A new layer is suggested because the three-layer architecture has several faults. However, in a four-layer architecture, data gathered from a perception layer is transmitted to a support layer. It is accountable for two things. It first verifies that information is safe from threats and sent by legitimate users. The users and the information can both be verified in a variety of ways. The authentication method is the most popular. Passwords, keys, and pre-shared secrets are used to implement it. The second task is to communicate with the network layer. Both wireless and wired methods of information transmission between the support layer and network layer are possible. This layer may be subject to some threats, including DoS attacks, malicious insider assaults, unauthorized access, etc.
5. ***Processing Layer (Middleware Layer)***: It gathers the necessary data from the transport layer by discarding additional data that is not relevant and processing valid data. It also solves the IoT's large data issue. Because big data generates a lot of information, IoT performance may be impacted [70, 71]. Current IoT security concerns and suggested solutions to all IoT layers [72] should be taken into account while implementing IoT security mitigation, as shown in Figure 7.7. An Internet of Things (IoT) network is thought to include technologies like Radio Frequency Identification (RFID) and Wireless Sensor Networks (WSNs). Consequently, Table 7.4 lists potential attacks on these two systems, that is, RFID and WSN, and Table 7.5 lists the challenges and mitigations of IoT layers.

TABLE 7.4
Possible Threats to WSN and RFID

Layers	Threats of RFID	Threats of WSN
Physical/Link	Impairment of RFID readers, relay attacks, Sybil attacks, selective forwarding, and synchronization attacks	Passive interference, active jamming or temporarily disabling the device, Sybil, destruction of RFID readers, replay attacks
Network/Transport layer	The sinkhole, unfairness, false routing, hello and session flooding, eavesdropping	Tag attacks: cloning, spoofing Reader attacks: impersonation, eavesdropping network protocol attacks
Application layer	Injection, buffer overflows	Injection, buffer overflows, unauthorized tag reading, and tag modification
Multi-layer attacks	Side channel attacks, replay attacks, traffic analysis, and crypto attacks	Side channel attacks, replay attacks, traffic analysis, and crypto attacks

TABLE 7.5
Security Challenges and Mitigation of IOT Layers

Sr. No.	Layers	Security Challenges	Mitigation
1.	Perception layer	Recognition of the odd sensor node	Algorithm for fault detection, decentralized intrusion prevention system
		The preferred cryptography methods and key management system	A large-scale network demands public-key encryption
		Device vulnerabilities	Procedure for slot reservations Access control and attack mitigation for resource depletion
2.	Network layer	IPSec communication with IPv6 nodes enabled.	Examining whether IPv6 and IPSec are appropriate for secure communication
3.	Application layer	Configurable embedded computer systems.	Implementing secure coding principles
4.	Support layer	DoS attacks, malicious insider assaults, unauthorized access	Lightweight authentication and encryption
5.	Processing layer	Protecting storage data from malware	Confidentiality

7.4.1 IoT Technologies

IoT's main technologies are radio frequency identification, wireless sensor networks, and near-field communication [73].

1. ***Radio Frequency Identification (RFID)***: IoT includes radio frequency identification as a basic technology, which is described in [74] and [75]. RFID parts are discussed in [76], classified as active RFID and passive RFID. All IoT things have IDs and smart tags, making it possible for computers to manage them. The extremely lightweight method of authentication for RFID has been discussed in [77], along with the existing attacks, levels of security, and design flaws.
2. ***Wireless Sensor Network (WSN)***: Wireless Sensor Network (WSN) is frequently used for information collection and remote sensing applications. Sensor nodes are distributed geographically. These networks are power-efficient, economical, and cost-effective [78]. RFID and WSN both have common characteristics. However, WSN has the advantage because of their intelligence and processing abilities. Paper [79] mentions difficulties that need to be overcome to assess WSN strength. Additionally, [80] proposes a deterministic algorithm that can be utilized to address the issue of coverage for well-known regions using WSNs.
3. ***Near-Field Communication (NFC)***: Near-Field Communication (NFC) is essential for the Internet of Things and is used for short-range, low-power,

and low-data-rate communication links whenever required. Such technology enables a wide range of services, including smart cards, transportation, access control, etc., particularly in the context of the IoT [81].

7.4.2 Security Issues

IoT architecture ensures the confidentiality and protection of clients. Protecting the client's information from third parties is termed secrecy. The IoT's functionality also depends on the interoperability of items. A specific endpoint's data transmission tends not to raise any privacy concerns on its own [82]. However, even fragmented data from several endpoints that have been put together, sorted, and analyzed might produce sensitive data. A person or entity has the right to confirm how much information they are willing to share with other parties. A person's data set can be created without their authorization. Paper [83] discusses upcoming possibilities, trends, and suggestions about privacy for IoT-based apps and services. Collection, sharing and management, and security concerns are the three primary axes of research activity in data privacy that are covered in [84, 85]. The safety hazards in IoT technologies have been discussed in [86]. Following are some of the defense and secrecy requirements of IoT to be fulfilled, as shown in Figure 7.8:

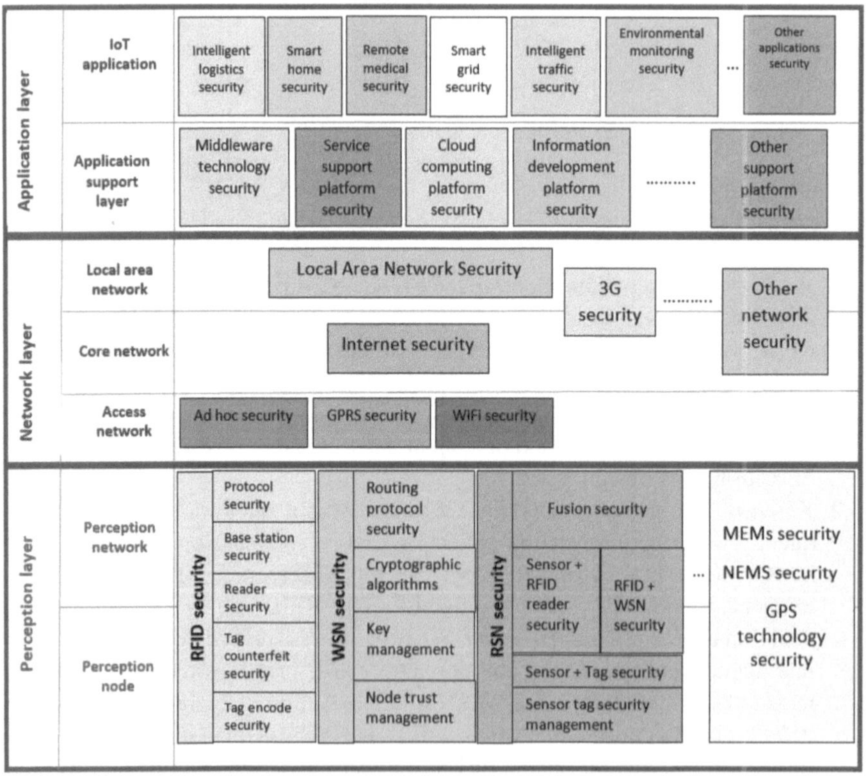

FIGURE 7.8 Typical IoT security architecture.

1. ***User Privacy***: Enhancing user protection and confidentiality at all stages is now a top priority. Tag strategy is recommended for Internet of Things privacy management in [86], and [87] illustrates the privacy model known as the k-anonymity model to protect important data. Paper [86] provides an examination of the privacy issue that arises when an IoT node is given a fixed domain name.
2. ***Access Control (Authorization)***: Informatics providers need to apply access control measures to safeguard data from perversion caused by third parties to users' private information. Only those who own the data should have access to it [88]. Two words are used to define access control in [89]. These terms are data holder and data collector, respectively. You can see issues with the authentication for an external data stream in [90]. Access control is described for the situation of streaming data in [88].
3. ***Confidentiality***: In the Internet of Things, data confidentiality [82] is a key restriction that ensures access and modification to certified entities through a system of access control and object authentication with an associated identity supervision system [91, 92]. Two key ideas in confidentiality are the definition of a system for access control and an object authentication technique. [93] explains a suitable query language for enabling applications to enhance the needed information recognized using confidentiality in an IoT environment. [94] proposes a security architecture that considers user privacy, security concerns, and confidentiality. The author addresses the challenges of IoT scalability, availability, and security with a higher priority. Authenticating and protecting the devices and ensuring the confidentiality and integrity of data [88]
4. ***Integrity***: The term "integrity" in the context of the Internet of Things (IoT) refers to the necessity to verify that data coming from platforms, devices, or other things has not been altered in any way before being used. IoT devices cannot function accurately, become exploited, or serve as starting points for other assaults if sufficient integrity measures are not followed. Integrity is the assurance that the information received has not been changed while in transit [95]. When data is protected from outside physical interference or cybercriminals during transmission using several common tracking techniques, the information can't be changed without the system being made aware of the dangers [96].
5. ***Availability***: Data accessibility guarantees that authorized parties have quick access to their information resources. Many IoT devices have full or incomplete connectivity to the Internet. Reliability and recoverability are related to availability. IoT availability includes providing programming and hardware at any time and location for supporters. Existing technology is accessible and compatible with IoT capabilities and protocols because of its hardware availability. [97, 98] present IoT difficulties in addition to security challenges at several tiers based on the security concepts of data confidentiality, integrity, and availability. [99] mentions various IoT levels with security issues. The IoT vulnerabilities that enable the assaults should be considered to maintain information security.

6. ***Trust***: Trust depends on the quality of the data, which is one of the basic requirements for IoT. Trust for devices, entities, and data are the three parts of trust [68]. We cannot utilize full security suites on IoT devices due to their limited resource availability. We must either create a unique security framework or select an option from the available ones. To keep IoT secure, we must go towards minimal security measures since otherwise, device resources will be burdened. IoT trust management seeks to provide safe access control while spotting and removing rogue nodes [72]. There is a crucial requirement for an automated, transparent, and simple access control administration to grant different access levels to different nodes or users due to scalability and the enormous number of smart things that carry sensitive data [100]. According to [101], although Trust-Based Access Control (TBAC) is still fairly new, it has been effectively used in commercial applications for access control in an IoT network.
7. ***Ability to Resist Attacks***: In an IoT environment, attackers will identify and exploit the weaknesses in the system. Any defense mechanism for the system must prevent such assaults. In the event of a node failure, it must adjust and be protected against single points of failure. It should be able to defend itself from a variety of assaults.
8. ***Mobile Security***: Mobile nodes are constantly switching between clusters in the Internet of Things. A protocol based on cryptography is widely used for this purpose to allow protection for identification, privacy, and authentication. An ad-hoc protocol has been described in [102] for the case where mobile nodes reconfigure with new clusters. This protocol prevents attacks like replay attacks, eavesdropping, tracking, and location privacy attacks [103].
9. ***Secure Middleware***: In the IoT, there are different types of devices interacting with each other, which results in several types of middleware layers that will affect the security and integrity of data and devices used within the same network. In the IoT, data is gathered from machine-to-machine and machine-to-user interactions. To enable the program to be distributed on various platforms or operating systems, middleware [67] in IoT is designed using specific core technologies, such as conventional middleware servers, as a communication component. However, because IoT data is so large and constantly changing, middleware for the IoT must have a large storage capacity and be able to grow linearly to accommodate it [104].

7.4.3 Privacy-Enhancing Technologies

In the open IoT era, user data privacy is a serious concern that must be protected under all circumstances. There are a few technologies that can be utilized to improve the privacy of user personal data, as discussed in [103]. Here are a few of them:

1. ***Transport Layer Security***: Transport Layer Security (TLS) enhances the security and integrity of data. TLS [72] is a commonly used protocol for

communication encryption and authentication. TLS offers two authentication methods for limited devices: Transport Layer Security Pre-Shared Key (TLS-PSK) cipher suites, which uses pre-shared keys, and Transport Layer Security-Diffie–Hellman key Exchange-Rivest–Shamir–Adleman (TLS-DHE-RSA), which employs the public key and cryptographic algorithms Rivest–Shamir–Adleman (RSA) and Diffie-Hellman (DH) key exchange. The drawback of transport layer security is that it requires its connection, lags in finding information, and adds more overhead.

2. ***Encryption***: Encryption is used to achieve data integrity for battery-operated IoT devices with low power consumption [72]. Only application-specific ICs can be embedded in devices with limited resources [105]. Therefore, because of their low processing power, short battery life, compact size, little memory, and restricted power supply, conventional cryptographic primitives are not appropriate for low-resource smart devices. Therefore, lightweight cryptography is used for such devices. The goal of research in [106, 107] and [108] has been to implement lightweight, low-cost encryption in both the physical world and the network. On the other hand, [107] suggests an attribute-based decryption method to support user revocation.
3. ***Virtual Private Network***: A close group of partners can create Virtual Private Networks (VPNs), which can be accessed from the outside. Groups of partners have access to the system and hide personal information to preserve data integrity [73]. Virtual private networks are confined to small areas and do not allow for dynamic global information sharing; improving privacy is not achieved. The majority of these studies [109] have concentrated on the creation of simple VPN security methods for smart IoT objects. Others [110] concentrated on enhancing the features and removing the flaws in the current light VPN security methods. Although they may not be directly related to this study, other studies [111] have many additional VPN security difficulties in common, including the kind of smart IoT gadgets they dealt with, the similarity of the VPN security challenges, and the solutions employed.

7.4.4 Major Security Issues and Solutions

The computer-based Internet gave way to the Internet of Things (IoT), which includes Machine-to-Machine (M2M) communication capabilities. It is crucial to lower the cost of IoT and expand the number of devices it supports to enable broader adoption. Before attaining the objective of broader use of IoT, several technical and security concerns must be resolved.

Energy consumption, wireless communication, scalability, security, and other technical concerns are associated with IoT [73]. The topic of discussion here is IoT security-related topics shown in Table 7.6. Among the principal security concerns are:

TABLE 7.6
Core Security Threats in IoT Technologies

Sr. No.	Security Issues	Problems	Solutions
1.	Identification	Identify the device, whether it is an original or malicious node.	1. Bar codes and visual-based identification 2. Technologies such as RFID and NFC have been utilized for scanning.
2.	Authentication	Authenticating every device is not an easy job to accomplish.	1. RFID can also be used for integrated data encryption, anti-counterfeiting, and to protect data on documents, certifications, and other domains [112]. 2. The authentication procedure uses symmetric key encryption, which is appropriate for limited devices like sensors [113]. 3. In an Internet of Things system, mutual authentication is essential for verifying the legitimacy of the server and the device. The era of mutual authentication [114–116], and [117]. 4. In [118], [119], [116], [120], [121], [122], [115], [123], and [124], the goal is to offer secure communication and lightweight authentication for access control. 5. Other approaches to achieving authentication in the IoT are multi-factor authentication, which uses bio-hashing and provides confidentiality, as proposed by [114, 117, 125, 126]. 6. Device-level authentication involves a unique fingerprint that identifies the location and status of the device [127]. All devices employ the Infinite Gaussian Mixture Model (IGMM) to create their fingerprints. 7. Use Pervasive Authentication Protocol (PAuthKey), an authentication protocol with a key-established method for distributed IoT [128]. The key is divided into two phases. The first is the registration phase, which uses key registration to start cryptography between the user and the Internet of Things device. 8. SDN with software-defined networking [129]. Every device is supposed to be linked to a gateway that has access to central data. Three nodes—the device, gateway, and controller—will receive the message.

3.	Data Management	• Utilizing IPv6 to handle devices and their respective IP addresses • Pre-loaded data management • Regularly validating alterations	1. Bar codes: The method of bar code identification is precise and quick. It produces results quickly and with a low error rate. When a bar code scanner scans a bar code, data that computers can recognize is sent from the bar code's information. 2. Vision-based identification is another practical option. It matches the features that are chosen to identify the items. Both local and global approaches are available. Local methods look for prominent areas like entropy or corners. A global approach takes an image's entirety into account [130]. 3. Structured Query Language (SQL) Lite
4.	Device heterogeneity	Various devices demand distinct security measures and management techniques. It is difficult to apply one solution to all the objects because each one demands a different strategy.	1. Physical and hardware addresses can be used for device identification, or IPv6 can be deployed. 2. The Information-Driven Architecture (IDRA) [73], which was created specifically to combine all of the devices, must be employed. IDRA doesn't require a gateway to connect items directly. 3. The Intelligent Transport System (ITS) uses risk analysis, another security technique. In this manner, certificates are given to the authorities using a key (public key) infrastructure to guarantee that data won't be interrupted. 4. The Key Performance Indicator (KPI)-like protocol from [101] is used for the Internet of Things. The routers are encrypted [for source and destination data flow] using this protocol. The key is used to perform the decryption process.

TABLE 7.7
Objectives and Methods to Implement Green Technologies

Objectives for Green Technology	Methods to Implement Green Technologies in IoT
Reduction of energy consumption	The design should be sustainable.
Recycle batteries	Utilization of renewable energy
Renew the harvesting of energy	Reduce the amount of data and transfer data if required.
Limit energy waste and consumption	Decentralized should be moved.
Reduction of power wastage	Communication constraints should be defined.

7.4.5 Green IoT

The Internet of Things (IoT) rapid growth in technology has drastically changed the way of life. It's important to keep in mind that the Internet of Things uses energy in addition to its many advantages. It produces electronic garbage and pollutes the environment. These two put additional pressure on the smart world and the environment. We can boost IoT's benefits while lowering its drawbacks, thanks to the growing demand for green IoT. The idea of the "Green IoT (GIoT)" refers to an environmentally friendly Internet of Things, which requires several steps to be taken to lower carbon emissions, conserve resources, and promote energy-efficient behaviors [131]. Table 7.7 lists the objectives and methods for green IoT [132].

7.4.5.1 Green IoT Technologies

Green IoT technologies are enlisted as follows:

7.4.5.1.1 Green RFID Tags

RFID is regarded as one of the greatest wireless technologies for IoT. RFID can be used to transport real-world data into the visual world without requiring loss. It can hold data about the items. This approach has two kinds of indications: negative and active signs [133]. Numerous studies have been conducted on green RFID, and it has been determined that for green RFID, various technologies are required:

1. Limiting the size of RFID since recycling the tags is a difficult and involved process.
2. Utilization of energy-conserving equipment and procedures to dynamically modify the amount of energy transmitted, prevent signs from colliding, and prevent overheating.

Many applications, including transport, control, shipping, receiving, and organization retrieval management, are tailored to the green RFID. Standard features and scalable options are also included [134].

7.4.5.1.2 Green WSN Technology

WSN is used for IoT communication. A wireless sensor network (WSN) is made up of numerous base station nodes and sensors. WSNs can be used for a wide range of purposes, including industrial procedure monitoring, defense limitations, item tracking, identification of fire, environment control and monitoring machine health, and more [135]. To conserve power, WSN technology needs to be able to transmit a signal effectively and support sleep mode. Additionally, sensor microprocessors must have intelligent waking and sleeping mechanisms. Consequently, lower energy consumption and quicker processors are the prevailing trends in microprocessors for WSNs. The novel idea of "green WSN" seeks to reduce Co_2 emissions while increasing lifespan and throughput. Green WSN technology can employ the following tactics:

1. Take advantage of renewable energy sources to offset the energy used, such as the sun, vibrational energy, kinetic energy, and temperature.
2. Sensor nodes should be kept in sleep mode for the majority of their lifespan and only used when necessary to conserve energy.
3. Use of energy-efficient technology in antennas with directional and energy-efficient radio, such as energy transmission and reception, cooperative communication, and energy efficiency.
4. To lower multiple kinetic energy consumption, efficient-energy steering approaches like multipath steering are used to convey nodes of the steering energy.
5. Reduce the amount of data by using methods like network computing, contraction, adaptive sampling, and aggregation; to reduce the amount of storage, employ data awareness algorithms.

7.4.5.1.3 Green Cloud Computing (GCC)

Virtualization via the internet is known as Cloud Computing (CC). It provides infinite computing, storage, and internet-based service delivery. IoT is commonplace, but cloud-based computing technology is pervasive. The combination of CC and IoT offers enormous research potential. GCC's primary objective is to increase the use of reusable, easily recyclable, and ecologically friendly products. The energy efficiency of Data Centers (DC) is becoming more and more crucial [136].

The smart world uses a vast amount of data that is growing through a variety of devices, sensors, wireless networks, and mobile phones. This makes it more important than ever to develop solutions that will increase energy efficiency for DC and address various issues.

1. The renewable green energy sources include wind, solar, water, and heat.
2. Constant support for computing and communication technology, along with advancements in circumstances like optical communication and other things.
3. Creation of multiple energy-saving gadgets that utilize Variable On/Variable Off (VOVO) and Dynamic Voltage and Frequency Scaling (DVFS) technology.

4. Implement energy-saving techniques, such as nano data centers.
5. Making use of numerous dynamic energy management technologies.

A framework built on Intrusion Detection and Prevention (IDPS) [137] has been developed; it detects harmful behavior, logs information about it, tries to halt it, and reports back to the security administrator. It manages green cloud computing in addition to network security. The hybrid IDPS, which combines anomaly- and signature-based techniques, provides real-time protection, active reaction time, and monitoring. Green cloud computing uses virtualization [138]. By replacing the physical switch with a virtual one, an energy-efficient environment with very little power consumption has been achieved.

7.4.5.1.4 Machine-to-Machine (M2M)

Wireless machine-to-machine (M2M) communications have emerged as the most promising solution for revolutionizing future "intelligent" pervasive applications due to the exponential growth of wireless communication devices and the ubiquitous nature of wireless communication networks. The main benefit of M2M communications is that a large number of intelligent wireless devices can function as "servers," working together to gather and provide users with real-time monitoring data. M2M communications are quickly evolving into a game-changing force for the next generation of intelligent real-time networked applications since it doesn't require direct human participation. The Green, Reliability, and Security (GRS) requirements [139], as indicated in Figure 7.9, must be met to implement M2M communications systems for next-generation real-time monitoring applications, and challenges of GRS are given in Table 7.8.

Both public and private clouds' energy usage for switching, data processing, transmission, and storage was investigated. A significant amount of the energy used in cloud computing can be attributed to circuit switching and transportation.

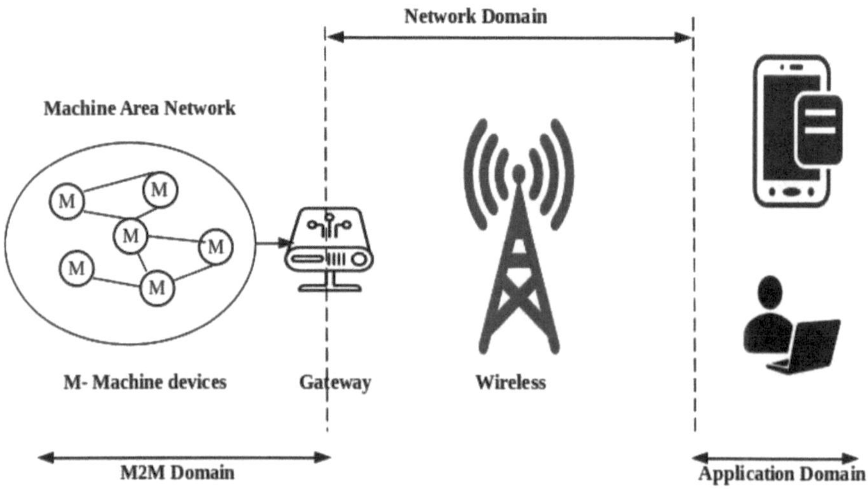

FIGURE 7.9 GRS requirement for M2M architecture.

TABLE 7.8
Challenges of GRS

Challenges	Requirements
Green	1. Optimizing M2M nodes to prolong the M2M communication. 2. To achieve green, environmentally friendly M2M communications, efforts also need to be made on the Base Station (BS) (it consumes more power).
Reliability	M2M communications are expanding quickly, which makes high reliability necessary.
Security	1. Through M2M applications, an attacker can more easily compromise M2M nodes by launching physical attacks. 2. M2M nodes may choose to go into sleep mode to save energy, making these attacks even more undetectable.

The following are the findings, regardless of the substantial research on green cloud computing that has been done and the potential solutions that have been offered:

1. Lower energy consumption by utilizing hardware and software.
2. Power-saving virtual machine strategies. For instance, Virtual Machine (VM) placement, migration, consolidation, and distribution.
3. Multiple approaches for allocating energy-efficient resources, along with associated tasks.
4. Effective strategies to save energy.

7.4.5.1.5 Green Data Centre (GDC)

A novel technology for data management, storage, and distribution is called Green Data Centre (GDC). Data Centers (DCs), which handle various types of data and applications, have large energy consumption, expensive operating expenses, and noticeable carbon dioxide footprints. Furthermore, a variety of commonplace items like mobile phones, sensors, etc. are contributing to the rise in big [140] data generation. The need for DC energy efficiency is growing as we move towards a smarter world [138]. Several methods are used for efficient energy consumption, and data centers are monitored by [141]. Apart from the research conducted by authors [140–142], they also introduced an optimization technique for DC energy efficiency that supports quality of service. Moreover, GDCs are supplying data services for 5G Mobile Ad Hoc Networks (MANETs), or cloud-assisted mobile ad hoc networks [143, 144]. To green the Internet of Things, the study in [141] offers a practical way to lower power usage without sacrificing DC cooling efficiency. Reducing routing and searching transactions is one of the cloud data servers' energy-saving mechanisms. To control next-generation DCs, Peoples et al. investigated the strategies that integrated effectiveness into the energy-efficient context-aware broker (e-CAB) framework. Several approaches are given in [138, 140, 141] to enhance the energy efficiency of GDC. The following techniques are used to

1. Make use of effective dynamic power management technology.
2. Create hardware with more energy-efficient design principles.
3. Create innovative, energy-efficient data center architectures to save power.
4. Create precise and effective data center power models.
5. Utilize computing and communication methods to assist.

7.5 SOFTWARE-DEFINED NETWORKING (SDN)

The use of cloud computing, big data, virtualization technology, and other factors is driving the emergence of new network architectures and applications, along with the advancement of information and communications technology. Software-Defined Networking (SDN) is a revolutionary network architecture that achieves control plane and data plane separation. The software platform controls the hardware called the central controller [145]. SDN gives managers the ability to swiftly establish network resources and dynamically modify network-wide traffic flow in response to shifting demands [146]. But as it develops quickly, difficulties arise when putting a full-scale carrier SDN into practice. SDN security is among the biggest obstacles.

Both industry and academia have expressed a significant amount of interest in the SDN idea. A diverse range of establishments and associations collaborate to investigate standards and technologies relevant to SDN. Among them, the Open Networking Foundation (ONF) presents a unique initiative that defines the interaction between the control plane and the data plane. The open flow protocol was developed by the Open Networking Foundation [147, 148], implemented in network hardware, and maintained by the SDN communication interface. Figure 7.10 illustrates that SDN architecture comprises three layers: resource, control, and application.

SDN architecture comprises three layers: resource, control, and application.

1. ***Application Layer***: SDN applications define a programmatic service-aware behavior of network resources, thereby specifying network services or business applications. Through application-control interfaces, applications communicate with the SDN control layer to automatically alter the characteristics and behavior of network resources [149].
2. ***Control Layer***: This layer regulates the dynamic behavior of network resources in the application layer. Using application-control interfaces, SDN apps govern the network and resources. Control signals are sent to the network resources via the resource control interface [149].
3. ***Resource Layer***: The network elements carry and deal with packets of data at the resource layer according to choices made by the SDN control layer.

There are two interface controls in SDN are enlisted as follows:

1. ***Application-Control Interface***: The application-control interface facilitates communication between the control and application layers.
2. ***Interface for Resource Control***: The resource control interface and the control layer.

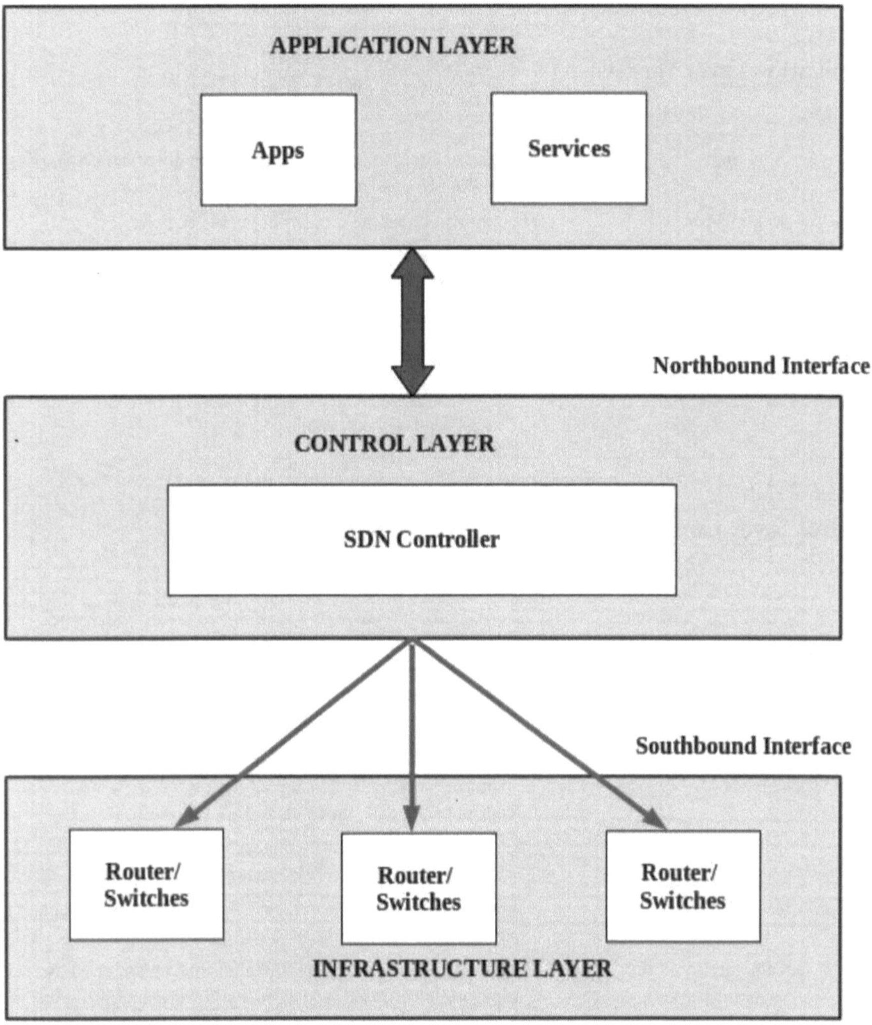

FIGURE 7.10 Layers of SDN.

7.5.1 Threats to the Application Layer

The attacker modifies the application and implements a malicious network policy, which affects the SDN application layer, as shown in Table 7.9.

7.5.2 Threats to the Control Layer

The SDN controller is the hub of the entire network and should maintain a high level of security. Any threat at this layer would affect the whole system. Table 7.10 is a list of the threats at the control layer.

TABLE 7.9
Application Layer Threats

Sr. No.	Threats	Description
1.	Spoofing	An attacker could access user information or services by posing as an SDN controller and using it for other attacks.
2.	Repudiation	The user can reject the threatening network policy.
3.	Disclosure of information	An invader could pretend to be an authorized user and introduce counterfeit flows onto the network by using SDN apps.
4.	Application vulnerability	SDN application flaws, including insecure or defective code, can be used by an attacker to get unauthorized access to resources.

TABLE 7.10
Control Layer Threats

Sr. No.	Threats	Description
1.	Conflict of flow rules	Secure detection prevents unauthorized flows, which goes against the security policy and harms the SDN controller.
2.	Fake flow rule addition	An attacker may use an SDN application to deliver some fictitious flow rules.
3.	Spoofing	An attacker acts as the head of an SDN application and performs some measures, like altering information, capturing routing, and using network topology to access the control of the SDN controller.
4.	DoS attack	An invader could use fake congestion to launch denial-of-service assaults on the SDN controller.
5.	Repudiation	When the user enters the wrong flow rules in the flow table, an admin or SDN application will reject it.
6.	Vulnerability in the operating system	Operating Systems (OS) are the platforms on which SDN controllers are based, and as such, the vulnerabilities present in the OS also present themselves to the SDN controller. Attackers could take advantage of operating system flaws like backdoor accounts and default passwords, which would have a major negative effect on the SDN controller.

7.5.3 Threats to Resource Layers

The threats at the resource layer are listed in Table 7.11.

SDN's security defense capabilities are essential to combating various SDN security threats. Currently, there are two methods for resolving the problem: evolution, which develops security modules and improves the controller architecture to achieve the required security mitigation capabilities [150]. Another method is revolution, which modifies the current controller into a new SDN controller with additional security functions [151, 152]. Based on the previously examined SDN certainty, the

TABLE 7.11
Resource Layer Threats

Sr. No.	Threats	Description
1.	Spoofing	An intruder behaves as a network head or SDN regulator alters information from SDN switches, and modifies entire flow tables.
2.	Eavesdropping	An attacker can intercept communications between SDN switches and learn details about relevant traffic, devices, and flows.
3.	Flow table overflow	A flow table overflow is caused when the flow table capacity reaches a bottleneck.
4.	Repudiation	A network head or SDN regulator refuses to accept the improper configuration.

protection of the SDN layers is determined. The SDN security architecture is suggested in Figure 7.11.

There are two types of security capacity within SDN: general capacities and specialized skills. Traditional networking and other targets share security objectives such as authorization, authentication, integrity protection, and confidentiality protection.

- ***Authentication***: Three layers must validate one another to ensure the identity's validity.
- ***Authorization***: Approves access to system data or network policy management by users, applications, and controllers.
- ***Protection of Confidentiality***: Information transferred via a communication interface or stored in a controller should be handled with care.
- ***Integrity Protection***: Integrity protection should be applied to data that is sent via a communication interface or stored in a controller.

As stated in Table 7.12, the framework claims that numerous new functional things, standards, and interfaces have led to advanced security issues.

The security requirements of the following reference papers are given in Table 7.13.

7.5.4 Green SDN

In SDN architecture, provide a green scheme (called GreSDN) where a controller periodically checks the status of the links. GreSDN promotes reducing the energy utilization of the network without altering the traffic flow's transmission channels until it is complete. Then, to determine the paths with the lowest energy consumption for the traffic demands, two heuristic routing methods that can be employed in GreSDN are proposed [166]. Finally, through simulation, the effectiveness of the routing algorithms is assessed in terms of their capacity to save energy as well as their influence on the network's quality of service. Using the constant original parameters of the links, the Constant Weight Greedy Algorithm (CWGA) determines

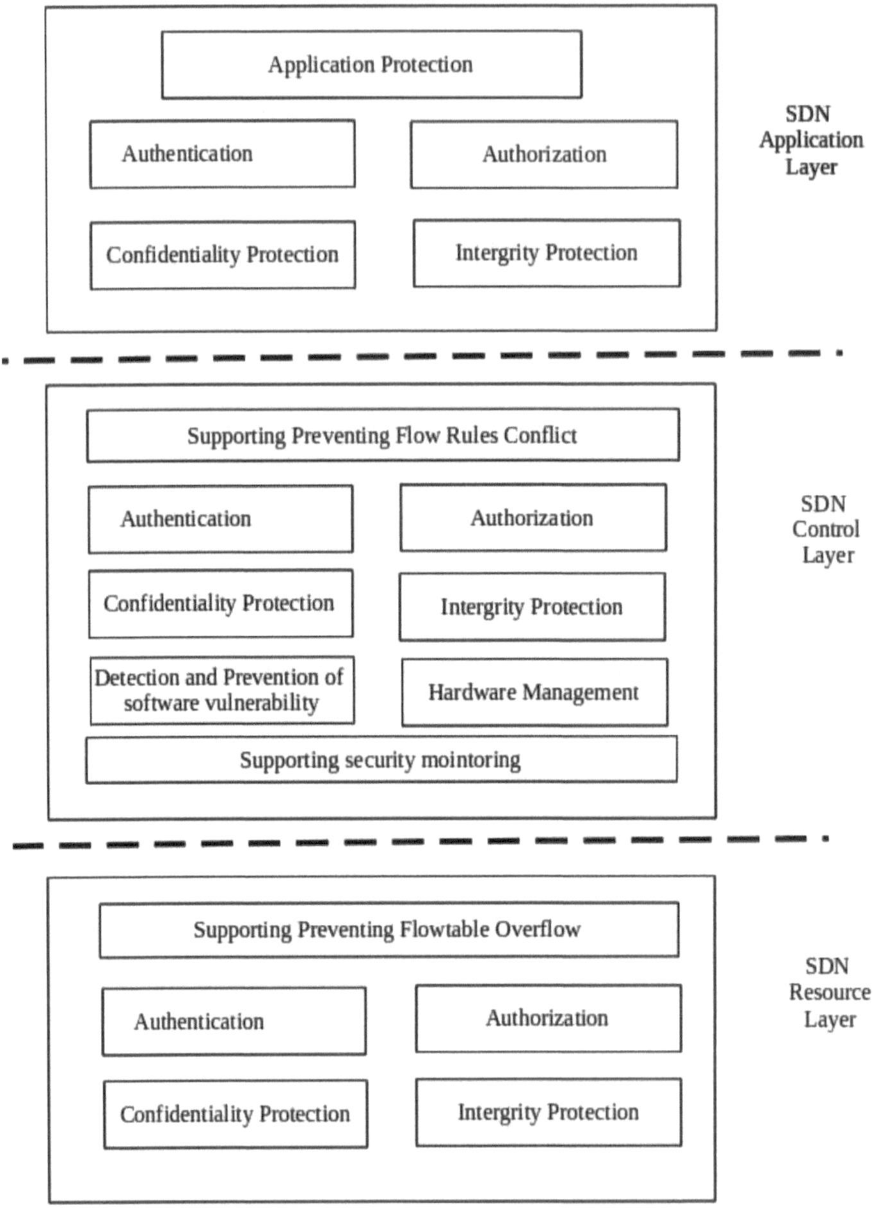

FIGURE 7.11 SDN architecture.

constant pathways for the traffic. By dynamically distributing the connection weights according to their current state, the Dynamic Weight Greedy Algorithm (DWGA) finds the paths with the least amount of energy consumption.

In ICT, network device control becomes essential, and SDN makes this possible. When compared to traditional networks, networks with SDN controllers use 50% of the energy in a network. Divide the energy-saving strategies into the

TABLE 7.12
Security Vulnerabilities in Layers

Sr. No.	Layers	Security Abilities
1.	Application layer	The application layer protects against vulnerabilities caused by apps.
2.	Control layer	To prevent the circumvention of obligatory network regulations, the control layer must follow: a. Prevention of flow rules from conflicting; b. Detection and prevention of software vulnerabilities. c. Anti-DoS protection is implemented by the control layer. d. The control layer supports hardware management to identify hardware failures.
3.	Resource layer	The resource layer prevents flow table overflow.

TABLE 7.13
Security Requirements Used in Different Research Papers

Reference Papers	Security Requirement	Proposed Method
[153]	Unauthorized devices linked to a network that gives one or more customers unauthorized wireless access are known as rogue access points or RAPs. Insiders and hackers use these devices to conceal harmful information.	Web Real-Time Communication (WebRTC) uses SDN and a Trusted Agent (TA) to identify and prevent Rogue Access Points (RAPs) from accessing networks using both standard and unique techniques, with the least amount of performance effect.
[154]	Attacks via packet injection impact the control plane's networking applications and services, and they mostly use data plane resources.	Packet Checker is a lightweight extension module on SDN controllers that can identify and mitigate the flooding of bogus packets in an efficient manner as a defense against the packet injection attack.
[155]	A security architecture that is efficient and based on policies.	Four policy functions are taken into account in the proposed scheme: separating, chaining, merging, and reordering. Only a part of the requirement documents is submitted to the SDN policy-based architecture through the Network Function Virtualization (NFV) system.
[156]	Techniques for security and dependability, like multi-path or access control.	The creation of a stable and secure SDN control platform is a practical application of the idea put forth here.
[157]	A policy-based strategy is used to coordinate various security processes and identify a variety of security threats in the SDN.	The strength of the suggested design is its capacity to handle both dynamic shifts in security assaults and the trust that the infrastructure's network devices enjoy. A dynamic policy framework provides dynamic changes to several security methods and components via feedback.

(Continued)

TABLE 7.13 (Continued)

Reference Papers	Security Requirement	Proposed Method
[158]	Software-Defined Networking (SDN) controllers.	SDN environments now include security solutions for identifying and preventing clients from breaking network policies.
[159]	Device communication and control plane relationships.	To reduce the cost of security, we measure how secure primitives affect the scalability and performance of the control plane. the performance of various TCP versus TLS implementations and delving deeper into the hashing and Message Authentication Code (MAC) primitives that underlie them.
[160]	Northbound interface that the SDN controller provides, such as a Representational State Transfer Application Program Interface (REST API). Malicious apps exploit APIs to launch hostile attacks, posing a major risk to network security.	SEAPP is a secure application management platform that uses access control via a REST API. To prevent malicious attacks, our primary strategy is to encrypt REST API calls and restrict application permissions at a granular level.
[161]	Attack surface area grows as new devices and procedures are put into place.	Device fingerprinting-based authentication to improve security in situations where cryptographic methods aren't available.
[162]	The controller serves as the network's brain, managing several functions like load balancing, routing, and delivering the necessary Quality of Service (QoS). However, the network becomes less secure due to the centralized controller.	SDN Secure COntroller (SECO) is a new and easy-to-use defense and detection algorithm that runs in the controller and enhances SDN security features against DoS assaults.
[163]	To stop DDoS attacks, use the network's controller or several hosts.	The security plane functions in tandem with the data plane, which handles packet forwarding between SDN switches, and in addition to the control plane, which manages rule and data communication between SDN controllers and switches.
[164]	SDN controller	Four open-source SDN controllers—OpenDaylight, ONOS, Floodlight, and Ryu—as well as the app-to-control risks and the four permission categories—READ, ADD, UPDATE, and REMOVE—are presented. To safeguard SDN controllers against API misuse, we thus introduce the SDN Controller Dynamic Access Control (DAC) system, a controller-independent dynamic access control system.

(*Continued*)

TABLE 7.13 (Continued)

Reference Papers	Security Requirement	Proposed Method
[165]	SDN controllers are hacked, and network elements like end hosts and soft switches breach network topology and data plane forwarding.	SPHINX to identify attacks on network topology and data plane forwarding that originate within an SDN, both known and may be undiscovered. SPHINX allows for the incremental validation of all network changes and constraints by utilizing the innovative abstraction of flow graphs, which closely resemble the actual network activities. SPHINX dynamically picks up new network behavior and sounds an alarm if it notices questionable alterations to the way the network control layer behaves.

following groups [167–169]. Based on controlling the behavior of switches, dynamic resource allocation, power management, and traffic engineering, although it is a relatively simple technique, turning on and off-network devices depending on utilization becomes more complex when deploying an SDN that has been partially deployed. This is because we have to make compromises to increase device and throughput performance, making it a Non-Deterministic Polynomial-time (NP)-hard problem. While turning off idle network devices might help save energy, unexpected spikes in traffic and device outages can cause packet loss and congestion. As a result, any downed network equipment should be restored to service as soon as possible.

The other technique of queue management is employed to reduce congestion and packet loss. Analyzing the trade-off between queue management and network device uptime is necessary, though. One significant problem with SDN is that the location of the controller inside the network directly affects energy conservation; this can be resolved by conjuring appropriate topologies. The SDN levels are referred to as the Green Application Layer, the Green Control Layer, and the Green Infrastructure Layer. Additionally, the need for "green hosts" is covered. Green SDN controllers are discussed in [167–172].

7.6 CONCLUSION

Green computing boosts the utilization of renewable resources, improves network performance, and decreases E-waste from hardware devices. Green computing is used to enhance various technologies, resulting in a reduction of hazardous gases and a greener environment. Green data centers, green IoT, green cloud computing, and green SDN with AI and machine learning algorithms can all be developed with more research in this area. Future advancements in green technology development must address the concerns of security and privacy. Artificial Intelligence (AI) and Machine

Learning (ML) techniques are being used in many cities to create "smart cities," which could eventually be paired with green computing to produce even more effective results. Green computing and smart technologies would be paired to increase the network's energy efficiency.

REFERENCES

[1] K. Sourabh, S. M. Aqib, and A. Elahi, "Sustainable Green Computing: Objectives and Approaches," *International Conference on Recent Innovations in Science, Agriculture, Engineering, and Management*, 2017, pp. 452–461.

[2] G. S. G. Singh, "Green Computing Initiatives for Environmental Issues," *Proceedings of the International Academic Conferences*, Harvard, USA, pp. 87–90, 2015.

[3] E. S. Development, "Learn How Green Computing Reduces Energy Consumption and Lowers Carbon Emissions from the Design, Use, and Disposal of Technology Products. What Organizations Can Do What You Can Do," https://www.ibm.com/blog/greencomputing/

[4] C. A. Chan, A. F. Gygax, E. Wong, C. A. Leckie, A. Nirmalathas, and D. C. Kilper, "Methodologies for Assessing the Use-Phase Power Consumption and Greenhouse Gas Emissions of Telecommunications Network Services," *Environ. Sci. Technol.*, vol. 47, no. 1, pp. 485–492, 2013.

[5] B. Saha, "Green Computing Current Research Trends," *Int. J. Comput. Sci. Eng.*, vol. 6, no. 3, pp. 467–469, 2018, doi: 10.26438/ijcse/v6i3.467469

[6] B. Anthony, M. Abdul Majid, and A. Romli, "A Descriptive Study towards Green Computing Practice Application for Data Centers in IT Based Industries," *MATEC Web Conf.*, vol. 150, pp. 1–8, 2018, doi: 10.1051/matecconf/201815005048

[7] T. Nazare, J. Gadelha, E. Nepomuceno, and R. Lozi, "Green Computing for Energy Transition: A Survey," *IEEE Lat. Am. Trans.*, vol. 21, no. 9, pp. 937–948, 2023, doi: 10.1109/TLA.2023.10251799

[8] H. A. Alharbi, T. E. H. Elgorashi, and J. M. H. Elmirghani, "Energy Efficient Virtual Machines Placement over Cloud-Fog Network Architecture," *IEEE Access*, vol. 8, pp. 94697–94718, 2020, doi: 10.1109/ACCESS.2020.2995393

[9] X. Deng, D. Wu, J. Shen, and J. He, "Eco-Aware Online Power Management and Load Scheduling for Green Cloud Datacenters," *IEEE Syst. J.*, vol. 10, no. 1, pp. 78–87, 2016, doi: 10.1109/JSYST.2014.2344028

[10] F. Shakeel and S. Sharma, "Green Cloud Computing: A Review on Efficiency of Data Centres and Virtualization of Servers," *Proc. IEEE Int. Conf. Comput. Commun. Autom. ICCCA 2017*, vol. 2017-Janua, pp. 1264–1267, 2017, doi: 10.1109/CCAA.2017.8230012

[11] D. Saxena, A. K. Singh, C. N. Lee, and R. Buyya, "A Sustainable and Secure Load Management Model for Green Cloud Data Centres," *Sci. Rep.*, vol. 13, no. 1, pp. 1–23, 2023, doi: 10.1038/s41598-023-27703-3

[12] S. P. Raja, "Green Computing and Carbon Footprint Management in the IT Sectors," *IEEE Trans. Comput. Soc. Syst.*, vol. 8, no. 5, pp. 1172–1177, 2021, doi: 10.1109/TCSS.2021.3076461

[13] K. W. Cameron, "Energy Oddities, Part 2: Why Green Computing is Odd," *Computer (Long. Beach. Calif).*, vol. 46, no. 3, pp. 90–93, 2013, doi: 10.1109/MC.2013.94

[14] U. U. Tariq, H. Ali, L. Liu, and X. Zhai, "A Novel Meta-Heuristic for Green Computing on VFI-NoC-HMPSoCs," *Proc. 2019 IEEE Smart World, Ubiquitous Intell. Comput. Adv. Trust. Comput. Scalable Comput. Commun. Internet People Smart City Innov. Smart World/UIC/ATC/SCALCOM/IOP/SCI 2019*, pp. 1545–1552, 2019, doi: 10.1109/SmartWorld-UIC-ATC-SCALCOM-IOP-SCI.2019.00278

[15] G. Nagy, Á. A. Mészáros, I. Bozó, and M. Tóth, "Tools Supporting Green Computing in Erlang," *Erlang 2019- Proc. 18th ACM SIGPLAN Int. Work. Erlang, co-located with ICFP 2019*, pp. 30–35, 2019, doi: 10.1145/3331542.3342570
[16] A. Al-Zamil and A. K. J. Saudagar, "Drivers and Challenges of Applying Green Computing for Sustainable Agriculture: A Case Study," *Sustain. Comput. Informatics Syst.*, vol. 28, 2020, doi: 10.1016/j.suscom.2018.07.008
[17] B. Krithika and N. Keerthana, "Comparison of Intel Processor with AMD Processor with Green Computing," *Proc. 2013 Int. Conf. Green Comput. Commun. Conserv. Energy, ICGCE 2013*, pp. 737–742, 2013, doi: 10.1109/ICGCE.2013.6823531
[18] S. Khare and S. Jain, "Prospects of Near-Threshold Voltage Design for Green Computing," *Proc. IEEE Int. Conf. VLSI Des.*, pp. 120–124, 2013, doi: 10.1109/VLSID.2013.174
[19] H. Sukarman, and N. K. S. Putri, "Green Information Technology Policy in Indonesia. In *2018 IEEE International Conference on Information Management and Technology (ICIMTech)*, September 2018, pp. 309–314.
[20] A. Joshi, C. Chen, Z. Takhirov, and B. Nazer, "A Multi-Layer Approach to Green Computing: Designing Energy-Efficient Digital Circuits and Manycore Architectures," *2012 Int. Green Comput. Conf. IGCC 2012*, no. June, pp. 6–9, 2012, doi: 10.1109/IGCC.2012.6322276
[21] H. Mogale, M. Esiefarienrhe, N. Gasela, and L. Letlonkane, "Introducing DOMINO: An Eco-Friendly Asynchronous Hybrid Multicore Architecture for Green Computing," *2018 Int. Conf. Adv. Big Data, Comput. Data Commun. Syst. icABCD 2018*, pp. 1–7, 2018, doi: 10.1109/ICABCD.2018.8465463
[22] H. Lee, J. Han, Y. K. Jeong, and I. W. Lee, "Profile-Based Building Energy Saving Service in Green Computing Environment," *2011 Int. Conf. ICT Converg. ICTC 2011*, pp. 768–769, 2011, doi: 10.1109/ICTC.2011.6082530
[23] L. Guo, B. Jin, R. Yu, C. Yao, C. Sun, and D. Huang, "Multi-Label Classification Methods for Green Computing and Application for Mobile Medical Recommendations," *IEEE Access*, vol. 4, no. January, pp. 3201–3209, 2016, doi: 10.1109/ACCESS.2016.2578638
[24] S. Asnani, M. G. Canu, and B. Montrucchio, "Producing Green Computing Images to Optimize Power Consumption in OLED-Based Displays," *Proc.- Int. Comput. Softw. Appl. Conf.*, vol. 1, pp. 529–534, 2019, doi: 10.1109/COMPSAC.2019.00081
[25] M. Kshirsagar, R. Lahoti, T. More, and C. Ryan, "GREECOPE: Green Computing with Piezoelectric Effect," *Int. Conf. Smart Cities Green ICT Syst. (SMARTGREENS)-Proc.*, vol. 2021-April, no. January, pp. 164–171, 2021, doi: 10.5220/0010445801640171
[26] R. Sharma, P. Mane, N. Sharma, S. S. Nikam, and A. A. Manjrekar, "Green Cloud Computing: Challenges and Solutions," *Eur. Chem. Bull.*, vol. 12, no. 5, pp. 6828–6831, doi: 10.48047/ecb/2023.12.si5a.0616
[27] A. Jain, M. Mishra, S. K. Peddoju, and N. Jain, "Energy Efficient Computing- Green Cloud Computing," In *2013 International Conference on Energy Efficient Technologies for Sustainability*, Nagercoil, India, pp. 978–982, 2013.
[28] K. Jakimoski, "Security Techniques for Data Protection in Cloud Computing," *Int. J. Grid Distrib. Comput.*, vol. 9, pp. 49–56, 2016, doi: 10.14257/ijgdc.2016.9.1.05
[29 U. Khalid, A. Ghafoor, M. Irum, and M. A. Shibli, "Cloud Based Secure and Privacy Enhanced Authentication & Authorization Protocol," *Procedia Comput. Sci.*, vol. 22, pp. 680–688, 2013, doi: 10.1016/j.procs.2013.09.149
[30] P. Internet, "How to Protect Your Server with Multi-Factor Authentication on AWS," pp. 2–5, https://cloudacademy.com/blog/how-to-protect-your-server-with-multi-factor-authentication-on-aws/
[31] T. Acar, M. Belenkiy, and A. Küpçü, "Single Password Authentication," *Comput. Networks*, vol. 57, no. 13, pp. 2597–2614, 2013, doi: 10.1016/j.comnet.2013.05.007

[32] G. Wang, Q. Liu, J. Wu, and M. Guo, "Hierarchical Attribute-Based Encryption and Scalable User Revocation for Sharing Data in Cloud Servers," *Futur. Gener. Comput. Syst.*, vol. 30, no. 5, pp. 1716–1724, 2013, doi: 10.1016/j.future.2012.05.005
[33] C. I. Fan and S. Y. Huang, "Controllable Privacy Preserving Search Based on Symmetric Predicate Encryption in Cloud Storage," *Futur. Gener. Comput. Syst.*, vol. 29, no. 7, pp. 1716–1724, 2013, doi: 10.1016/j.future.2012.05.005
[34] E. M. Mohamed, H. S. Abdelkader, and S. El-Etriby, "Enhanced Data Security Model for Cloud Computing," In *2012 8th International Conference on Informatics and Systems (INFOS)*, Giza, Egypt, pp. 12–17, 2012.
[35] S. Deepak, "10 Tips to Improve Security in Cloud Computing," https://www.cloudpanel.io/blog/how-to-improve-security-in-cloud-computing/
[36] A. B. Manju and S. Sumathy, "Efficient Load Balancing Algorithm for Task Preprocessing in Fog Computing Environment," In *Smart Intelligent Computing and Applications*, Satapathy, S. C., Bhateja, V., and Das, S., Eds., Springer: Singapore, 2019; pp. 291–298, doi: 10.1007/978-981-13-1927-3_31
[37] M. Díaz, C. Martín, and B. Rubio, "State-of-the-Art, Challenges, and Open Issues in the Integration of Internet of Things and Cloud Computing," *J. Netw. Comput. Appl.*, vol. 67, pp. 99–117, 2016, doi: 10.1016/j.jnca.2016.01.010
[38] Z. Shu, J. Wan, D. Zhang, and D. Li, "Cloud-Integrated Cyber-Physical Systems for Complex Industrial Applications," *Mob. Networks Appl.*, vol. 21, no. 5, pp. 865–878, 2016, doi: 10.1007/s11036-015-0664-6
[39] Y. Chen, E. Sun, and Y. Zhang, "Joint Optimization of Transmission and Processing Delay in Fog Computing Access Networks," *2017 9th International Conference on Advanced Infocomm Technology (ICAIT)*, 2017, pp. 155–158, 2018, doi: 10.1109/ICAIT.2017.8388906
[40] S. Sarkar and S. Misra, "Theoretical Modelling of Fog Computing: A Green Computing Paradigm to Support IoT Applications," *IET Netw.*, vol. 5, pp. 23–29, doi: 10.1049/iet-net.2015.0034
[41] Z. Mahmood, *Fog Computing: Concepts, Frameworks and Technologies*, Springer International Publishing, 2018. doi: 10.1007/978-3-319-94890-4
[42] A. Khakimov, A. Muthanna, and M. S. A. Muthanna, "Study of Fog Computing Structure," *Proceedings of the 2018 IEEE Conference of Russian Young Researchers in Electrical and Electronic Engineering (ElConRus)*, vol. 2018, pp. 51–54, 2018, doi: 10.1109/EIConRus.2018.8317028
[43] J. Pan and J. Mcelhannon, "Future Edge Cloud and Edge Computing for Internet of Things Applications," *IEEE Internet Things J.*, vol. 5, pp. 439–449, 2017, doi: 10.1109/JIOT.2017.2767608
[44] I. Bouzarkouna, M. Sahnoun, N. Sghaier, D. Baudry, and C. Gout, "Challenges Facing the Industrial Implementation of Fog Computing," *Proceedings of the 2018 IEEE 6th International Conference on Future Internet of Things and Cloud (FiCloud)*, pp. 341–348, 2018, doi: 10.1109/FiCloud.2018.00056
[45] Y. Guan, J. Shao, G. Wei, and M. Xie, "Data Security and Privacy in Fog Computing," *IEEE Netw.*, vol. 32, pp. 106–111, 2018, doi: 10.1109/MNET.2018.1700250
[46] S. Khan, S. Parkinson, and Y. Qin, "Fog Computing Security: A Review of Current Applications and Security Solutions," *J. Cloud Comput.*, vol. 6, pp. 1–22, 2017, doi: 10.1186/s13677-017-0090-3
[47] M. T. Dong and X. Zhou, "Fog Computing: Comprehensive Approach for Security Data Theft Attack Using Elliptic Curve Cryptography and Decoy Technology," *Open Access Library J.*, vol. 3, pp. 1–14, 2016, doi: 10.4236/oalib.1102802
[48] S. J. Stolfo, M. Ben Salem, and A. D. Keromytis, "Fog Computing: Mitigating Insider Data Theft Attacks in the Cloud," *Proc. IEEE CS Secur. Priv. Work. SPW 2012*, vol. 8, no. 2, pp. 125–128, 2012, doi: 10.1109/SPW.2012.19

[49] H. J. Nam, H. Y. Choi, H. J. Shin, H. S. Kwon, J. M. Jeong, C. H. Hahn, and J. B. Hur, "Security and Privacy Issues of Fog Computing," *J. Korean Inst. Commun. Inf. Sci.*, vol. 42, pp. 257–267, 2017, doi: 10.7840/kics.2017.42.1.257

[50] S. Kulkarni, S. Saha, and R. Hockenbury, "Preserving Privacy in Sensor-Fog Networks," In *9th International Conference for Internet Technology and Secured Transactions (ICITST)*, pp. 96–99, 2014.

[51] M. H. Ibrahim, "Octopus: An Edge-Fog Mutual Authentication Scheme," *Int. J. Netw. Secur.*, vol. 18, no. 6, pp. 1089–1101, 2016.

[52] H. Atabo Christopher, J. Yakubu, S. Muhammad Abdulhamid, and A. D. Mohammed, "An Architectural Framework for Ant Lion Optimization-Based Feature Selection Technique for Cloud Intrusion Detection System Using Bayesian Classifier," *I-Manager's J. Cloud Comput.*, vol. 5, pp. 36–44, 2018, doi: 10.26634/jcc.5.2.15691

[53] R. I. Emori, "Scale Models of Automobile Collisions with Breakaway Obstacles-Investigation Indicates that Scale Models can be Used to Show the Motion of Breakaway Signposts and Lightposts After Being Struck by Automobiles," *Exp. Mech.*, vol. 13, pp. 64–69, 1973, doi: 10.1007/BF02322384

[54] J. Yakubu, M. Abdulhamid, H. A. Christopher, H. Chiroma, and M. Abdullahi, "Security Challenges in Fog-Computing Environment: A Systematic Appraisal of Current Developments," *J. Reliab. Intell. Environ.*, vol. 5, pp. 209–233, 2019, doi: 10.1007/s40860-019-00081-2

[55] R. Rios, R. Roman, J. A. Onieva, and J. Lopez, "From SMOG to Fog: A Security Perspective," *2017 2nd International Conference on Fog and Mobile Edge Computing (FMEC)*, pp. 56–61, 2017, doi: 10.1109/FMEC.2017.7946408

[56] A. Alrawais, A. Alhothaily, C. Hu, and X. Cheng, "Fog Computing for the Internet of Things: Security and Privacy Issues," *IEEE Internet Comput.*, vol. 21, pp. 34–42, 2017, doi: 10.1109/MIC.2017.37

[57] K. Lee, D. Kim, D. Ha, U. Rajput, and H. Oh, "On Security and Privacy Issues of Fog Computing Supported Internet of Things Environment," *2015 6th International Conference on Network of the Future (NOF)*, pp. 1–3, 2015, doi: 10.1109/NOF.2015.7333287

[58] I. Sudha, A. Kannaki, and S. Jeevidha, "Alleviating Internal Data Theft Attacks by Decoy Technology in Cloud," *Int. J. Comput. Sci. Mobile Comput.*, vol. 3, pp. 217–222, 2014.

[59] R. Roman, J. Lopez, and M. Mambo, "Mobile Edge Computing, Fog et al.: A Survey and Analysis of Security Threats and Challenges," *Futur. Gener. Comput. Syst.*, vol. 78, pp. 680–698, 2018, doi: 10.1016/j.future.2016.11.009

[60] C. Modi, D. Patel, B. Borisaniya, H. Patel, A. Patel, and M. Rajarajan, "A Survey of Intrusion Detection Techniques in Cloud," *J. Netw. Comput. Appl.*, vol. 36, pp. 42–57, 2013, doi: 10.1016/j.jnca.2012.05.003

[61] K. A. Fakeeh, "Privacy and Security Problems in Fog Computing," *Commun. Appl. Electron.*, vol. 4, pp. 1–7, 2016, doi: 10.5120/cae2016652088

[62] D. S. N. K. P. Ali Kumar, S. H. S. Newaz, F. H. Rahman, G. M. Lee, G. Karmakar, and T. W. Au, "Green Demand Aware Fog Computing: A Prediction-Based Dynamic Resource Provisioning Approach," *Electronics*, vol. 11, pp. 1–23, 2022, doi: 10.3390/electronics11040608

[63] S. Sarkar and S. Misra, "Theoretical Modelling of Fog Computing: A Green Computing Paradigm to Support IoT Applications," *IET Netw.*, vol. 5, pp. 23–29, 2016, doi: 10.1049/iet-net.2015.0034

[64] R. Qureshi, S. H. Mehboob, and M. Aamir, "Sustainable Green Fog Computing for Smart Agriculture," *Wirel. Pers. Commun.*, vol. 121, pp. 1379–1390, 2021, doi: 10.1007/s11277-021-09059-x

[65] M. Burhan, R. A. Rehman, B. Khan, B. S. Kim, "IoT Elements, Layered Architectures and Security Issues: A Comprehensive Survey," *Sensors*, vol. 18, no. 9, 2018, pp. 2796–2833.

[66] I. Yaqoob, E. Ahmed, I. A. T. Hashem, A. I. A. Ahmed, A. Gani, M. Imran, and M. Guizani, "Internet of Things Architecture: Recent Advances, Taxonomy, Requirements, and Open Challenges," *IEEE Wirel. Commun.*, vol. 24, pp. 10–16, 2017, doi: 10.1109/MWC.2017.1600421

[67] Q. Jing, A. V. Vasilakos, J. Wan, J. Lu, and D. Qiu, "Security of the Internet of Things: Perspectives and Challenges," *Wirel. Networks*, vol. 20, pp. 2481–2501, 2014, doi: 10.1007/s11276-014-0761-7

[68] S. Sicari, A. Rizzardi, L. A. Grieco, and A. Coen-Porisini, "Security, Privacy and Trust in Internet of Things: The Road Ahead," *Comput. Networks*, vol. 76, pp. 146–164, 2015, doi: 10.1016/j.comnet.2014.11.008

[69] N. Koshizuka and K. Sakamura, "Ubiquitous ID: Standards for Ubiquitous Computing and the Internet of Things," *IEEE Pervasive Comput.*, vol. 9, pp. 98–101, 2010, doi: 10.1109/MPRV.2010.87

[70] Z. Bi, Y. Liu, J. Krider, J. Buckland, A. Whiteman, D. Beachy, and J. Smith, "Real-Time Force Monitoring of Smart Grippers for Internet of Things (IoT) Applications," *J. Ind. Inf. Integr.*, vol. 11, pp. 19–28, 2018, doi: 10.1016/j.jii.2018.02.004

[71] R. Want, "An Introduction to RFID Technology," *IEEE Pervasive Comput.*, vol. 5, pp. 25–33, 2006, doi: 10.1109/MPRV.2006.2

[72] M. Noor and W. H. Hassan, "Current Research on Internet of Things (IoT) Security: A Survey," *Comput. Networks*, vol. 148, pp. 283–294. doi: 10.1016/j.comnet.2018.11.025

[73] A. U. Rehman, S. U. Rehman, I. U. Khan, M. Moiz, and S. Hasan, "Security and Privacy Issues in IoT," *Int. J. Commun. Netw. Inf. Secur.*, vol. 8, 2022, doi: 10.17762/ijcnis.v8i3.2074

[74] E. Welbourne, L. Battle, G. Cole, K. Gould, K. Rector, S. Raymer, M. Balazinska, and G. Borriello, "Building the Internet of Things Using RFID: The RFID Ecosystem Experience," *IEEE Internet Comput.*, vol. 13, pp. 48–55, 2009, doi: 10.1109/MIC.2009.52

[75] A. Juels, "RFID Security and Privacy: A Research Survey," *IEEE J. Sel. Areas Commun.*, vol. 24, no. 2, pp. 381–394, 2006, doi: 10.1109/JSAC.2005.861395

[76] G. Shen and B. Liu, "The Visions, Technologies, Applications and Security Issues of Internet of Things," In *2011 International Conference on E-Business and E-Government (ICEE)*, Shanghai, China, pp. 1–4, 2011, doi: 10.1109/ICEBEG.2011.5881892

[77] G. Avoine, X. Carpent, and J. Hernandez-Castro, "Pitfalls in Ultralightweight Authentication Protocol Designs," *IEEE Trans. Mob. Comput.*, vol. 15, pp. 2317–2332, 2016, doi: 10.1109/TMC.2015.2492553

[78] J. Yick, B. Mukherjee, and D. Ghosal, "Wireless Sensor Network Survey," *Comput. Netw.*, vol. 52, no. 12, pp. 2292–2330, 2008, doi: 10.1016/j.comnet.2008.04.002

[79] V. Potdar, A. Sharif, and E. Chang, "Wireless Sensor Networks: A Survey," In *2009 International Conference on Advanced Information Networking and Applications Workshops*, Bradford, UK, pp. 636–641, 2009, doi: 10.1109/WAINA.2009.192

[80] F. Frattolillo, "A Deterministic Algorithm for the Deployment of Wireless Sensor Networks," *Int. J. Commun. Networks Inf. Secur.*, vol. 8, pp. 1–10, 2016, doi: 10.17762/ijcnis.v8i1.1476

[81] P. Urien, "LLCPS: A New Security Framework Based on TLS for NFC P2P Applications in the Internet of Thing," In *2013 IEEE 10th Consumer Communications and Networking Conference (CCNC)*, Las Vegas, NV, pp. 845–846, 2013, doi: 10.1109/CCNC.2013.6488560

[82] P. M. Chanal and M. S. Kakkasageri, "Security and Privacy in IoT: A Survey," *Wirel. Pers. Commun.*, vol. 115, pp. 1667–1693, 2020, doi: 10.1007/s11277-020-07649-9
[83] A. A. Abi Sen, F. A. Eassa, K. Jambi, and M. Yamin, "Preserving Privacy in Internet of Things: A Survey," *Int. J. Inf. Technol.*, vol. 10, pp. 189–200, 2018, doi: 10.1007/s41870-018-0113-4
[84] N. Miloslavskaya and A. Tolstoy, "Internet of Things: Information Security Challenges and Solutions," *Cluster Comput.*, vol. 22, pp. 103–119, 2019, doi: 10.1007/s10586-018-2823-6
[85 P. Seneviratne, "Beginning LoRa Radio Networks with Arduino: Build Long Range, Low Power Wireless IoT Networks," *Begin. LoRa Radio Networks with Arduino Build Long Range, Low Power Wirel. IoT Networks*, pp. 1–309, 2019, doi: 10.1007/978-1-4842-4357-2
[86] D. Evans and D. M. Eyers, "Efficient Data Tagging for Managing Privacy in the Internet of Things," In *2012 IEEE International Conference on Green Computing and Communications*, Besancon, France, pp. 244–248, 2012, doi: 10.1109/GreenCom.2012.45
[87] J. Cao, B. Carminati, E. Ferrari, and K. L. Tan, "CASTLE: Continuously Anonymizing Data Streams," *IEEE Trans. Dependable Secur. Comput.*, vol. 8, pp. 337–352, 2011, doi: 10.1109/TDSC.2009.47
[88] S. Babar, P. Mahalle, A. Stango, N. Prasad, and R. Prasad, "Proposed Security Model and Threat Taxonomy for the Internet of Things (IoT)," *Commun. Comput. Inf. Sci.*, vol. 89, pp. 420–429, 2010, doi: 10.1007/978-3-642-14478-3_42
[89] A. Alcaide, E. Palomar, J. Montero-Castillo, and A. Ribagorda, "Anonymous Authentication for Privacy-Preserving IoT Target-Driven Applications," *Comput. Secur.*, vol. 37, pp. 111–123, 2013, doi: 10.1016/j.cose.2013.05.007
[90] Y. Wang and Q. Wen, "A Privacy Enhanced DNS Scheme for the Internet of Things," In *IET International Conference on Communication Technology and Application (ICCTA)*, Beijing, pp. 699–702, 2011, doi: 10.1049/cp.2011.0758
[91 S. Papadopoulos, Y. Yang, and D. Papadias, "CADS: Continuous Authentication on Data Streams," *33rd Int. Conf. Very Large Data Bases (VLDB)-Conf. Proc.*, September 2007, pp. 135–146, 2007.
[92] J. Cao, B. Carminati, E. Ferrari, and K. L. Tan, "ACStream: Enforcing Access Control Over Data Streams," *Proc. Int. Conf. Data Eng.*, pp. 1495–1498, 2009, doi: 10.1109/ICDE.2009.25
[93] R. Mehta, J. Sahni, and K. Khanna, "Internet of Things: Vision, Applications and Challenges," *Procedia Comput. Sci.*, vol. 132, pp. 1263–1269, 2018, doi: 10.1016/j.procs.2018.05.042
[94] M. Usman, I. Ahmed, M. I. Aslam, S. Khan, and U. A. Shah, "SIT: A Lightweight Encryption Algorithm for Secure Internet of Things," *Int. J. Adv. Comput. Sci. Appl.*, vol. 8, pp. 402–411, 2017, doi: 10.14569/IJACSA.2017.080151
[95] S. Li, L. Da Xu, and S. Zhao, "The Internet of Things: A Survey," *Inf. Syst. Front.*, vol. 17, pp. 243–259, 2015, doi: 10.1007/s10796-014-9492-7
[96] S. Bhattacharjee, M. Salimitari, M. Chatterjee, K. Kwiat, and C. Kamhoua, "Preserving Data Integrity in IoT Networks Under Opportunistic Data Manipulation," In *2017 IEEE 15th Intl Conf on Dependable, Autonomic and Secure Computing, 15th Intl Conf on Pervasive Intelligence and Computing, 3rd Intl Conf on Big Data Intelligence and Computing and Cyber Science and Technology Congress (DASC/PiCom/DataCom/CyberSciTech)*, Orlando, FL, USA, pp. 446–453, 2017, doi: 10.1109/DASC-PICom-DataCom-CyberSciTec.2017.87
[97] H. Geng, "Internet of Things and Data Analytics Handbook," *Internet Things Data Anal. Handb.*, pp. 1–776, 2017, doi: 10.1002/9781119173601

[98] S. Pokorni, "Reliability and Availability of the Internet of Things," *Vojnoteh. Glas.*, vol. 67, pp. 588–600, 2019, doi: 10.5937/vojtehg67-21363
[99] M. Kolisnyk and V. Kharchenko, "A Markov Model of IoT System Availability Considering DDoS Attacks, Patching and Energy Modes," *Stud. Syst. Decis. Contr.*, vol. 171, pp. 185–207, 2019, doi: 10.1007/978-3-030-00253-4_9
[100] M. Eisenhauer, P. Rosengren, and P. Antolin, "HYDRA: A Development Platform for Integrating Wireless Devices and Sensors into Ambient Intelligence Systems," In *The Internet of Things*, Giusto, D., Iera, A., Morabito, G., and Atzori, L., Eds., Springer: New York, doi: 10.1007/978-1-4419-1674-7_36
[101 Z. Li, X. Yin, Z. Geng, H. Zhang, P. Li, Y. Sun, H. Zhang, and L. Li, "Research on PKI-Like Protocol for the Internet of Things," In *2013 5th International Conference on Measuring Technology and Mechatronics Automation*, Hong Kong, China, pp. 915–918, 2013, doi: 10.1109/ICMTMA.2013.227
[102] J. Miao and L. Wang, "Rapid Identification Authentication Protocol for Mobile Nodes in Internet of Things with Privacy Protection," *J. Networks*, vol. 7, pp. 1099–1105, 2012, doi: 10.4304/jnw.7.7.1099-1105
[103] A. Hameed and A. Alomary, "Security Issues in IoT: A Survey," In *2019 International Conference on Innovation and Intelligence for Informatics, Computing, and Technologies (3ICT)*, Sakhier, Bahrain, pp. 1–5, 2019, doi: 10.1109/3ICT.2019.8910320
[104] D. Mendez Mena, I. Papapanagiotou, and B. Yang, "Internet of Things: Survey on Security," *Inf. Secur. J.*, vol. 27, pp. 162–182, 2018, doi: 10.1080/19393555.2018.1458258
[105] V. A. Thakor, M. A. Razzaque, and M. R. A. Khandaker, "Lightweight Cryptography for IoT: A State-of-the-Art," *Cryptogr. Secur.*, pp. 1–19, arXiv:2006.13813.
[106] A. K. Nain, J. Bandaru, M. A. Zubair, and R. Pachamuthu, "A Secure Phase-Encrypted IEEE 802.15.4 Transceiver Design," *IEEE Trans. Comput.*, vol. 66, pp. 1421–1427, 2017, doi: 10.1109/TC.2017.2672752
[107] M. Mangia, F. Pareschi, R. Rovatti, and G. Setti, "Low-Cost Security of IoT Sensor Nodes with Rakeness-Based Compressed Sensing: Statistical and Known-Plaintext Attacks," *IEEE Trans. Inf. Forensics Secur.*, vol. 13, pp. 327–340, 2018, doi: 10.1109/TIFS.2017.2749982
108] Z. Mahmood, H. Ning, and A. U. Ghafoor, "A Polynomial Subset-Based Efficient Multi-Party Key Management System for Lightweight Device Networks," *Sensors (Switzerland)*, vol. 17, p. 670, 2017, doi: 10.3390/s17040670
[109] R. Roman, J. Zhou, and J. Lopez, "On the Features and Challenges of Security and Privacy in Distributed Internet of Things," *Comput. Networks*, vol. 57, pp. 2266–2279, 2013, doi: 10.1016/j.comnet.2012.12.018
[110] J. King and A. I. Awad, "A Distributed Security Mechanism for Resource-Constrained IoT Devices," *Informatica*, vol. 40, pp. 133–143, 2016.
[111] T. Heer, O. Garcia-Morchon, R. Hummen, S. L. Keoh, S. S. Kumar, and K. Wehrle, "Security Challenges in the IP-Based Internet of Things," *Wirel. Pers. Commun.*, vol. 61, pp. 527–542, 2011, doi: 10.1007/s11277-011-0385-5
[112] T. Shinzaki, I. Morikawa, Y. Yamaoka, and Y. Sakemi, "IoT Security for Utilization of Big Data: Mutual Authentication Technology and Anonymization Technology for Positional Data," *Fujitsu Sci. Tech. J.*, vol. 52, pp. 52–60, 2016.
[113] R. Amin, S. H. Islam, G. P. Biswas, M. K. Khan, L. Leng, and N. Kumar, "Design of an Anonymity-Preserving Three-Factor Authenticated Key Exchange Protocol for Wireless Sensor Networks," *Comput. Networks*, vol. 101, pp. 42–62, 2016, doi: 10.1016/j.comnet.2016.01.006
[114] X. Li, J. Peng, J. Niu, F. Wu, J. Liao, and K. K. R. Choo, "A Robust and Energy Efficient Authentication Protocol for Industrial Internet of Things," *IEEE Internet Things J.*, vol. 5, pp. 1606–1615, 2018, doi: 10.1109/JIOT.2017.2787800

[115] O. Salman, S. Abdallah, I. H. Elhajj, A. Chehab, and A. Kayssi, "Identity-Based Authentication Scheme for the Internet of Things," In *2016 IEEE Symposium on Computers and Communication (ISCC)*, Messina, Italy, pp. 1109–1111, 2016, doi: 10.1109/ISCC.2016.7543884

[116] M. Safkhani and N. Bagheri, "Passive Secret Disclosure Attack on an Ultralightweight Authentication Protocol for Internet of Things," *J. Supercomput.*, vol. 73, pp. 3579–3585, 2017, doi: 10.1007/s11227-017-1959-0

[117] R. Giuliano, F. Mazzenga, A. Neri, and A. M. Vegni, "Security Access Protocols in IoT Capillary Networks," *IEEE Internet Things J.*, vol. 4, pp. 645–657, 2017, doi: 10.1109/JIOT.2016.2624824

[118] B. C. Chifor, I. Bica, V. V. Patriciu, and F. Pop, "A Security Authorization Scheme for Smart Home Internet of Things Devices," *Futur. Gener. Comput. Syst.*, vol. 86, pp. 740–749, 2018, doi: 10.1016/j.future.2017.05.048

[119] P. K. Dhillon and S. Kalra, "A Lightweight Biometrics Based Remote User Authentication Scheme for IoT Services," *J. Inf. Secur. Appl.*, vol. 34, pp. 255–270, 2017, doi: 10.1016/j.jisa.2017.01.003

[120] W. Feng, Y. Qin, S. Zhao, and D. Feng, "AAoT: Lightweight Attestation and Authentication of Low-Resource Things in IoT and CPS," *Comput. Networks*, vol. 134, pp. 167–182, 2018, doi: 10.1016/j.comnet.2018.01.039

[121] M. Yun and B. Yuxin, "Research on the Architecture and Key Technology of Internet of Things (IoT) Applied on Smart Grid," In *2010 International Conference on Advances in Energy Engineering*, Beijing, China, 2010, pp. 69–72, doi: 10.1109/ICAEE.2010.5557611

[122] F. Wu, X. Li, L. Xu, S. Kumari, M. Karuppiah, and J. Shen, "A Lightweight and Privacy Preserving Mutual Authentication Scheme for Wearable Devices Assisted by Cloud Server," *Comput. Electr. Eng.*, vol. 63, pp. 168–181, 2017, doi: 10.1016/j.compeleceng.2017.04.012

[123] J. Srinivas, S. Mukhopadhyay, and D. Mishra, "Secure and Efficient User Authentication Scheme for Multi-Gateway Wireless Sensor Networks," *Ad Hoc Networks*, vol. 54, pp. 147–169, 2017, doi: 10.1016/j.adhoc.2016.11.002

[124 G. Glissa and A. Meddeb, "6LowPSec: An End-to-End Security Protocol for 6LoWPAN," *Ad Hoc Networks*, vol. 82, pp. 100–112, 2019, doi: 10.1016/j.adhoc.2018.01.013

[125] M. Lavanya and V. Natarajan, "Lightweight Key Agreement Protocol for IoT Based on IKEv2," *Comput. Electr. Eng.*, vol. 64, pp. 580–594, 2017, doi: 10.1016/j.compeleceng.2017.06.032

[126] S. Shin and T. Kwon, "Two-Factor Authenticated Key Agreement Supporting Unlinkability in 5G-Integrated Wireless Sensor Networks," *IEEE Access*, vol. 6, pp. 11229–11241, 2018, doi: 10.1109/ACCESS.2018.2796539

[127] Y. Qiu and M. Ma, "A Mutual Authentication and Key Establishment Scheme for M2M Communication in 6LoWPAN Networks," *IEEE Trans. Ind. Inf.*, vol. 12, pp. 2074–2085, 2016, doi: 10.1109/TII.2016.2604681

[128] P. Porambage, C. Schmitt, P. Kumar, A. Gurtov, and M. Ylianttila, "PAuthKey: A Pervasive Authentication Protocol and Key Establishment Scheme for Wireless Sensor Networks in Distributed IoT Applications," *Int. J. Distrib. Sens. Networks*, vol. 10, 2014, doi: 10.1155/2014/357430

[129] Y. Sharaf-Dabbagh and W. Saad, "On the Authentication of Devices in the Internet of Things," In *2016 IEEE 17th International Symposium on a World of Wireless, Mobile and Multimedia Networks (WoWMoM)*, Coimbra, Portugal, pp. 1–3, 2016, doi: 10.1109/WoWMoM.2016.7523532

[130] L. H. Lauerman, "Advances in PCR Technology," *Anim. Heal. Res. Rev.*, vol. 5, pp. 247–248, 2004, doi: 10.1079/ahrr200477

[131] I. Avci and Y. H. Dakhil, "Survey About Green IoT: Applications, Technologies, Challenges, and Future Directions," *In 2022 International Congress on Human-Computer Interaction, Optimization and Robotic Applications (HORA)*, Ankara, Turkey, pp. 1–7, 2022, doi: 10.1109/HORA55278.2022.9800104
[132] M. Maksimovic and E. O. Miklicanin, "Green Internet of Things and Green Nanotechnology Role in Realizing Smart and Sustainable Agriculture," In *8th International Scientific Agriculture Symposium (AGROSYM)*, Jahorina, Bosnia and Herzegovina, October 2017.
[133] E. Manavalan and K. Jayakrishna, "A Review of Internet of Things (IoT) Embedded Sustainable Supply Chain for Industry 4.0 Requirements," *Comput. Ind. Eng.*, vol. 127, pp. 925–953, 2019, doi: 10.1016/j.cie.2018.11.030
[134] F. K. Shaikh, S. Zeadally, S. Member, and E. Exposito, "Enabling Technologies for Green Internet of Things," *IEEE Syst. J.*, vol. 11, pp. 983–994, 2017.
[135] C. S. Nandyala and H. K. Kim, "Green IoT Agriculture and Healthcare Application (GAHA)," *Int. J. Smart Home*, vol. 10, pp. 289–300, 2016, doi: 10.14257/ijsh.2016.10.4.26
[136] M. A. Hoque, M. Siekkinen, and J. K. Nurminen, "Energy Efficient Multimedia Streaming to Mobile Devices – A Survey," *IEEE Commun. Surv. Tutorials*, vol. 16, pp. 579–597, 2014.
[137] J. Kizza and F. Migga Kizza, "Intrusion Detection and Prevention Systems," In *Securing the Information Infrastructure*, IGI Global, pp. 239–258, 2011, doi: 10.4018/978-1-59904-379-1.ch012
[138] M. M. K. M. S. Akshaya and M. M. N. Priya, "Green Internet of Things for Smart World Green Internet of Things for Smart World," *Int. J. Sci. Res. Dev.*, vol. 6, pp. 1024–1027, 2018.
[139] R. Lu, X. Li, X. Liang, X. Shen, and X. Lin, "GRS: The Green, Reliability, and Security of Emerging Machine to Machine Communications," *IEEE Commun. Mag.*, vol. 49, pp. 28–35, 2011, doi: 10.1109/MCOM.2011.5741143
[140] J. Shuja, K. Bilal, S. A. Madani, M. Othman, R. Ranjan, P. Balaji, and S. U. Khan, "Survey of Techniques and Architectures for Designing Energy-Efficient Data Centers," *IEEE Syst. J.*, vol. 10, pp. 507–519, 2016, doi: 10.1109/JSYST.2014.2315823
[141] M. Dayarathna, Y. Wen, and R. Fan, "Data Center Energy Consumption Modeling: A Survey," *IEEE Commun. Surv. Tutorials*, vol. 18, pp. 732–794, 2016, doi: 10.1109/COMST.2015.2481183
[142] N. Cordeschi, M. Shojafar, D. Amendola, and E. Baccarelli, "Energy-Efficient Adaptive Networked Datacenters for the QoS Support of Real-Time Applications," *J. Supercomput.*, vol. 71, pp. 448–478, 2015, doi: 10.1007/s11227-014-1305-8
[143] N. D. Han, Y. Chung, and M. Jo, "Green Data Centers for Cloud-Assisted Mobile Ad-Hoc Networks in 5G," *IEEE Network*, vol. 29, pp. 70–76, 2015.
[144] A. Roy, "Energy-Efficient Data Centers and Smart Temperature Control System with IoT Sensing," In *2016 IEEE 7th Annual Information Technology, Electronics and Mobile Communication Conference (IEMCON)*, pp. 1–4, 2016, doi: 10.1109/IEMCON.2016.7746251
[145] Y. Shi, F. Dai, and Z. Ye, "An Enhanced Security Framework of Software Defined Network Based on Attribute-based Encryption," In *2017 4th International Conference on Systems and Informatics (ICSAI)*, pp. 965–969, 2017.
146 M. A. B. Pérez, N. Y. S. Losada, E. R. Sánchez, and G. M. Gaona, "State of the Art in Software Defined Networking (SDN)," *Visión electrónica*, vol. 13, pp. 178–194, 2019.
[147] K. Kaushal and V. Sahni, "Early Detection of DDoS Attack in WSN," *Int. J. Comput. Appl.*, vol. 134, pp. 14–18, 2016, doi: 10.5120/ijca2016908117

[148] Open Networking Foundation, "Software-Defined Networking: The New Norm for Networks," ONF White Paper, pp. 1–12, 2012, https://opennetworking.org/sdn-resources/whitepapers/software-defined-networking-the-new-norm-for-networks/
[149] S. Sector and O. F. International Telecommunication Union, "ITU-T Telecommunication Standardization Sector of ITU," X.1038, 2016, https://www.itu.int/rec/T-REC-X.1038-201610-I/en
[150] P. Shuping, G. Bingli, S. Yi, G. Zervas, R. Nejabati, and D. Simeonidou, "Software Defined Optical Data Centre Networks," *China Commun.*, vol. 12, pp. 1–9, 2015, doi: 10.1109/CC.2015.7224692
[151] D. Jin and D. M. Nicol, "Parallel Simulation of Software Defined Networks," In *Proceedings of 1st ACM SIGSIM Conference on Principles of Advanced Discrete Simulation (SIGSIM PADS)*, pp. 91–102, 2013, doi: 10.1145/2486092.2486104
[152] L. Liu, R. Muñoz, R. Casellas, T. Tsuritani, R. Martínez, and I. Morita, "OpenSlice: An OpenFlow-Based Control Plane for Spectrum Sliced Elastic Optical Path Networks," In *2012 38th European Conference and Exhibition on Optical Communications*, Amsterdam, Netherlands, 2012, pp. 1–3, doi: 10.1364/ECEOC.2012.Mo.2.D.3
[153] J. H. Cox, R. Clark, and H. Owen, "Leveraging SDN and WebRTC for Rogue Access Point Security," *IEEE Trans. Network Serv. Manag.*, vol. 14, pp. 756–770, 2017, doi: 10.1109/TNSM.2017.2710623
[154] S. Deng, X. Gao, Z. Lu, and X. Gao, "Packet Injection Attack and Its Defense in Software-Defined Networks," *IEEE Trans. Inf. Forensics and Secur.*, vol. 13, pp. 695–705, 2018.
[155] W. Lee and N. Kim, "Security Policy Scheme for an Efficient Security Architecture in Software-Defined Networking," *Information*, vol. 8, p. 65, 2017, doi: 10.3390/info8020065
[156] D. Kreutz, F. M. V. Ramos, and P. Verissimo, "Towards Secure and Dependable Software-Defined Networks," In *Proceedings of 2nd ACM SIGCOMM Workshop on Hot Topics in Software Defined Networking*, pp. 55–60, 2013, doi: 10.1145/2491185.2491199
[157] A. Abubakar and B. Pranggono, "Machine Learning Based Intrusion Detection System for Software Defined Networks," In *2017 17th International Conference on Emerging Security Technologies (EST)*, pp. 138–143, 2017.
[158] J. H. Cox, R. J. Clark, and H. L. Owen, "Security Policy Transition Framework for Software Defined Networks," In *Guide to Security in SDN and NFV: Challenges, Opportunities, and Applications*, pp. 149–169, 2017.
[159] D. Kreutz, J. Yu, P. E. Verissimo, C. Magalhaes, and F. M. Ramos, "The Kiss Principle in Software-Defined Networking: A Framework for Secure Communications," *IEEE Secur. Priv.*, vol. 16, pp. 60–70, 2018, doi: 10.1109/MSP.2018.3761717
[160] T. Hu, Z. Zhen, Y. Peng, L. Dong, L. Ziyong, R. Quan, H. Yuxiang, and L. Julong, "SEAPP: A Secure Application Management Framework Based on REST API Access Control in SDN-Enabled Cloud Environment," *J. Parallel Distrib. Comput.*, vol. 147, pp. 108–123, 2021, doi: 10.1016/j.jpdc.2020.09.006
[161] N. Gray, T. Zinner, and P. Tran-Gia, "Enhancing SDN Security by Device Fingerprinting," In *2017 IFIP/IEEE Symposium on Integrated Network and Service Management (IM)*, pp. 879–880, 2017.
[162] S. Wang, K. G. Chavez, and S. Kandeepan, "SECO: SDN sEcure COntroller Algorithm for Detecting and Defending Denial of Service Attacks," In *2017 5th International Conference on Information and Communication Technology (ICoIC7)*, pp. 1–6, 2017.
[163] A. Hussein, I. H. Elhajj, A. Chehab, and A. Kayssi, "SDN Security Plane: An Architecture for Resilient Security Services," In *2016 IEEE International Conference on Cloud Engineering Workshop (IC2EW)*, pp. 54–59, 2016.

[164] Y. Tseng, M. Pattaranantakul, R. He, Z. Zhang, and F. Na, "Controller DAC: Securing SDN Controller with Dynamic Access Control," In *2017 IEEE International Conference on Communications (ICC)*, pp. 1–6, 2017, doi: 10.1109/ICC.2017.7997249

[165] M. Dhawan, R. Poddar, K. Mahajan, and V. Mann, "SPHINX: Detecting Security Attacks in Software-Defined Networks," *NDSS*, vol. 15, pp. 8–11, 2015.

[166] Y. Hu, T. Luo, W. Wang, and C. Deng, "GreSDN: Toward a Green Software Defined Network," In *18th Asia-Pacific Network Operations and Management Symposium (APNOMS)*, pp. 1–6, 2016, doi: 10.1109/APNOMS.2016.7737209

[167] A. Jeyasekar, S. Nanda, and A. Uthra, "Green SDN: Trends of Energy Conservation in Software Defined Network," *Int. J. Eng. Technol.*, vol. 7, pp. 9–13, 2018, doi: 10.14419/ijet.v7i3.12.15853

[168] "Next-Generation Firewall Technology: Protecting Networks from Advanced Threats," https://edfuturetech.com/product/next-generation-firewall-technology-protecting-networks-from-advanced-threats/

[169] "What to Expect: Future Trends in Identity and Access Management," https://www.veritis.com/blog/what-to-expect-future-trends-in-identity-and-access-management/

[170] D. Ghai, S. L. Tripathi, S. Saxena, M. Chanda, and M. Alazab, *Machine Learning Algorithms for Signal and Image Processing*, John Wiley & Sons, 2022.

[171] B. A. N. Raju, D. Ghai, and K. Rawal, "Design of Futuristic Trolley System with Comparative Analysis of Previous Models," In *Big Data Analytics and Intelligent Techniques for Smart Cities*, CRC Press, pp. 223–247, 2021.

[172] D. Ghai, H. K. Gianey, A. Jain, and R. S. Uppal, "Quantum and Dual-Tree Complex Wavelet Transform-Based Image Watermarking," *Int. J. Mod. Phys. B*, vol. 34, 2050009, 2020.

8 Key Concepts in AI Models for Remote Sensing Applications

Jami Venkata Suman
GMR Institute of Technology, Rajam, India

Mamidipaka Hema
JNTUGVCEV, Vizianagaram, India

Babji Prasad Chapa
GMR Institute of Technology, Rajam, India

Jhansi Bharathi Madavarapu
University of Cumberlands, Williamsburg, United States

8.1 INTRODUCTION

The techniques of remote sensing are also used for different types of applications like the range of classifications of Hyperspectral Imaging (HSI), mangroves detection, environmental level of pollution, and other objects to target, rainfall estimation, and disaster prevention [1]. The methods of deep learning have also been applied in the studies on the technologies of remote sensing of their ideal performance in the particular extraction and the data interpretation and classification. Developing the ideal level of DL for a particular range of applications needs a considerable level of relevant data [2], because the majority of the applications of remote sensing technologies include the assessment of big data. The methods of the DL are specifically very useful in the techniques of remote sensing. The researchers have made good progress in the process of applying the learning methods of machine learning to the aspect of remote sensing. However, these techniques and methods have several kinds of drawbacks. First majority of the conventional techniques are ideally based on parameter-tuning and heuristics, which also rely on the personal experience and the knowledge of the domain of the person specifically developing the particular level of model [3]. However, the factor of personal experience and knowledge of the domain might also be very helpful in particular types of tasks and cases, this ideal dependence also limits the concept of generalizability of the

DOI: 10.1201/9781003546382-8

models of Machine Learning (ML) and also makes them quite unsuitable for usage in the combination with the systems of the remote sensing. Second, the ML models of conventional techniques also extract only the range of shallow features [4]. These types of shallow features are extracted from simple and statistical nonlinear levels of correlations. Models that particularly rely on such type of features have limited type of performance for recognizing the tasks, like the classification HIS and nonprecipitating-precipitation level of classification, or could also be taken in the usage in the procedures (preprocessing) like the reduction in the dimension [5]. The goal of this chapter is to demonstrate, via particular examples, mostly from remote sensing that AI has enormous potential for usage in various applications and for altering the utilization of environmental data in the future. Artificial Intelligence will profoundly alter how people do business across various activities, including research, operations, and user interactions. In a multitude of areas such as Autonomous cars, music production, financial market predictions, voice recognition, smart assistance, quantum physics, medical diagnostics, and other applications, AI has already shown to be a revolutionary and value-enhancing, disruptive technology.

8.2 PROBLEM STATEMENT

With the factor of increment in the volume and quality of data from the platforms of remote sensing, there is a specific requirement from the range of platforms (computational) and the efficient range of tools to extract and handle the ideal information from the datasets of the remote sensing [6]. The AI tools could proceed to assist in the factor to manage the large volumes of the different forecasting, analysis, modeling, and environmental levels of observations [7].

8.3 MULTIPLAYER PERCEPTRON

A Multilayer Perceptron (MLP) contains input and output layers, as well as one or more hidden layers made up of numerous neurons, layered on top of each other. While neurons in a Perceptron must employ an activation function that enforces a threshold, such as ReLU or sigmoid, neurons in a Multilayer Perceptron can utilize any arbitrary activation function. Summer will collect all the weights and send them to the activation function. The entire scenario is depicted in Figure 8.1.

The DL is a specific field of the concept of machine learning that has specifically developed all out of the particular type of research on MLPs [8]. However, the convention and ideal multiplayer perceptron that also contain only one particular layer (hidden), the architectures of the deep learning that have numerous levels of layers, therefore the process of enabling the usage of the labeled data or raw data sets in the fact of model training. As the labeled or raw data are the major type of input into the model of deep learning and are also ideally processed in every type of layer (hidden), the model particularly proceeds to learn quite increasingly the features of high and deep levels. Ultimately, the labeled or raw data are specifically encoded as the vector of the high dimensional level of discriminants aspect [9].

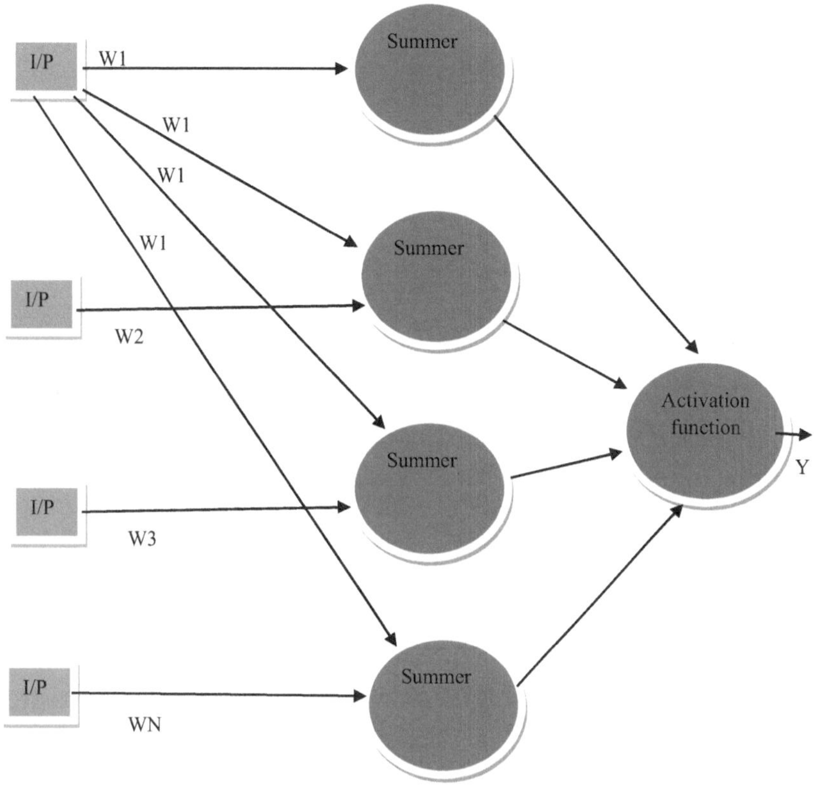

FIGURE 8.1 Stages of multilevel perceptron model.

However, the numerous architectures of deep learning have also been ideally proposed, majorly the share normal components like the SoftMax, connected, pooling, and convolutional layers [10]. The models of deep learning also expand upon the normal architecture of the MLP by the process of incorporating the numerous levels of layers that are hidden to learn the regressions (complicated) and to map the raw data for the outputs. Because of their capabilities of regression, the models of deep learning also contain different types of parameters that should also be ideally tuned [11]. Hence, the factor of constructing the models of deep learning also needs considerable resources and effort, involving the training and time sets of data, specifically, most models of deep learning are also trained via the supervised level of learning [12]. The process of developing the models of deep learning in the early days of deep learning was also quite complex. However, two major levels of solutions have also provided a big help that provided the researchers to overcome the obstacles (aforementioned) [13]. Firstly, because of the recent level of advancements in the software and hardware (computational), the entity of the researchers could also efficiently and conveniently execute the models of deep learning [14]. The deep learning range of platforms involving the processing of tensors with the units,

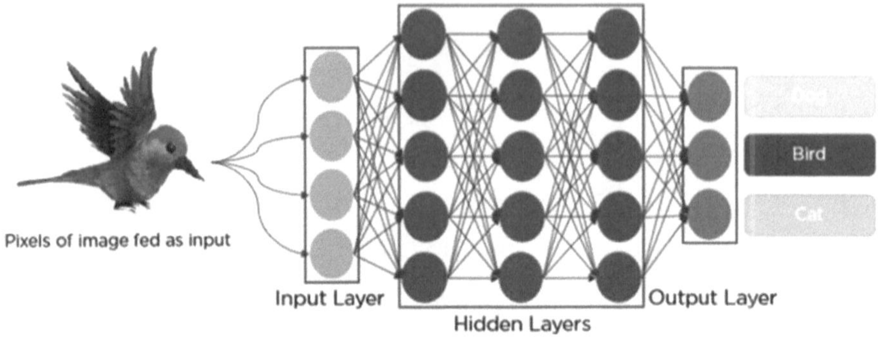

FIGURE 8.2 Convolutional neural networks architecture.

Graphics Procedure Units (GPUs), and CPUs each have distinct levels of advantages for certain levels of models in deep learning. Secondly, as discussed above, the majority of the applications of remote sensing include the assessment of the data and the large scale that ideally annotates the concept of the remote sensing sets of data that could easily be used for training the methods of deep learning [15].

8.4 CONVOLUTIONAL NEURAL NETWORK

Convolutional Neural Network (CNN) architecture is specifically the most representative and typical architecture of the deep learning concept since it has ideally been applied in the process (image) and is also being considered in the vision of the computer [16]. The architecture of the convolutional neural network is structured and specifically very suitable to process the layers of data in multiple levels of arrays. Figure 8.2 is responsible for illustrating the basic architecture of the CNN, which also contains the pooling, convolutional, and ideally connected form of layers and also the layer of the SoftMax [17].

The convolutional specified layers are taken into use for enhancing and extracting the range of spatial features in the form of input data. The entity of the pooling layers that are also responsible for reducing the dimensions (spatial) of the input form of data, therefore the process to reduce the trainable range of parameters in the different layers that are designed subsequently and eventually proceeding to enable them to ideally concentrate on the major patterns which are ultimately input [18]. As this input is ideally trying to proceed in the deep layers, the majority of features are also extracted at the high levels. Ultimately, SoftMax layers and fully connected aspects are taken into use for the classification of the data [19].

8.5 FUNDAMENTAL PRINCIPLES OF REMOTE SENSING

To understand the key principles of the remote sensing technique, it is really important to comprehend its different types of diversified applications and techniques and also to integrate them with all the techniques of artificial intelligence [20–22]. The systems of remote sensing are ideally built to take the benefit of the different

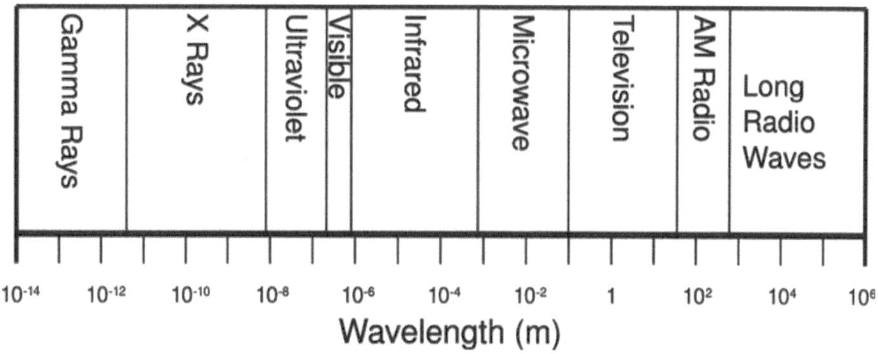

FIGURE 8.3 Ideal representation of electromagnetic specified spectrum [22].

modules of the spectrum of electromagnetism, as per Figure 8.3 and it also includes the description of the windows (atmospheric) to observe different types or targets. The sensors (passive) work to detect the natural form of energy being reflected or emitted by the surroundings of the earth like the optical range of sensors that are responsible for capturing the reflection of the sunlight [23].

On the other hand, the active forms of sensors emit energy and also measure the backscattered or reflected signals. This particular wider range of active sensors which are responsible for enabling the remote sensor data to be ideally acquired via different types of satellites for international coverage, and also aircraft for the major resolution (spatial), and drones for data collection (small-scale) [24]. Once the procedure of remote sensing is ideally acquired, the factor to interpret the images and the digital range of data also becomes very important in the process of extracting the meaningful form of information [25]. The processing of digital images and its key techniques involve the process of enabling the extraction, algorithms-based classification, feature-based extraction, fusion of images, and filtering of valuable forms of insights. The process of the following paragraphs proceeds to describe the major techniques of remote sensing, while the methods of artificial intelligence that proceed to assist with the processing of data [26] are presented in Figure 8.2.

8.5.1 Optimal Remote Sensing

This ideal technique is responsible for focusing on interpreting and gathering the range of optical data, specifically within the near-infrared and visible form of sections of the electromagnetism-based spectrum. The interaction of sunlight with the surface of the earth and specific materials of the particular surface is responsible for absorbing and also reflecting the light wavelengths [27, 28]. This ideal level of interaction is responsible for creating the signatures of the unique spectral aspect that is the range of characteristics of major features of the surface. These particular sensors which are available in the airborne, handheld, detectors and models of spaceborne are responsible for containing the key detectors that ideally play the record of the intensity of light all across the several kinds of wavelength [29]. The recorded form of data is transmitted to the ground level of stations or to the centers to process, where they are ideally transformed and processed into the spectral or image form of data [30, 31].

Considering the Remote sensing Image (RI) and its object of detection, the primary level objective is to specifically stay certain whether a preferred satellite or aerial form of images and also to contain the range of objects (pertinent) and determine (precisely) their level of locations [32–34]. To ensure the quality of the images, several levels of processing and similar kinds of steps are being undertaken [35]. The factor of the preprocessing includes the contrast enhancement and noise level of removal to improve the interpretability and clarity, followed by the level of feature-specified extraction, where the different types of characteristics are also extracted and identified from the different types of images for further assessment [36]. Eventually, the objective is to proceed with classifying the objects within the assessment and images of the particular accuracy of the different types of results. The procedure of classification also proceeds to allow for efficient execution and interpretation and the procedure to understand the information of the image [37]. An accurate form of assessment is also ideally performed for trying to verify the precision and reliability of the outcomes.

8.5.2 Radar-Based Remote Sensing

This particular technique is responsible for operating in the region (microwave) of the spectrum based on electromagnetism, including the reception and the key transmission of the different types of microwave-based waves [38, 39]. The antenna (radar) proceeds to emit the different types of pulses of the radiation-based microwave all toward space or earth, to capture the echoes specified reflection by the factor of targets and also to contain the form of data regarding the characteristics of the targets involving the dielectric based properties, roughness, size, shape, direction and distance [40]. By the procedure to analyze the intensity and time of the range of echo-based signals, radar-based sensing can also generate maps or images of the different types of targets with different types of perspectives and varying ranges of resolutions [41]. It is specifically been used in the process of mapping the surfaces of land, and also the process to monitor the patterns of weather, studying the currents of the ocean, and also the procedure to detect objects like vehicles and buildings [42, 43].

The synthetic-based aperture form of radar also produces surface (high resolution) images and is specifically quite a valuable form of the forest (large level of scale) that covers the factor of mapping since it can be very responsible for penetrating the clouds and also the foliage, alongside the enable the mapping (accurate) even in the factor of challenging the range of weather or the limited form of visibility and its key conditions [44]. The technology of dual-polarization is employed by the factor of synthetic aperture-based radar allows for the factor of differentiation between the types of the forest canopy and the vegetation of underlying. When the radar-based signal also encounters the canopy of the forest, it also scatters, with the signal range of the portion proceeding to return to the instrument of the radar [45]. This form of return signal is responsible for carrying an important range of information about the structure of the forest and the ideal aspect of the biomass [46]. By the process of incorporating the radar (dual-polarization) the comprehensiveness and accuracy of the mapping of the forest which is also enhanced, by the factor providing a detailed form of insights into the underlying form of vegetation and the structure of the forest [47]. The SAR-based ability to efficiently distinguish between the vegetation beneath and the forest range of canopy types is an important benefit. This particular capability enables the SAR to generate a higher level of resolution and data that could also detect the different types of changes in the forest covering an exceptional form of precision [48, 49].

8.5.3 LiDAR

The LiDAR is responsible for operating by the factor to emit the pulsed range of lasers that also the particular form of target, and the particular time that takes form the reflected form of the light in order return to the range of the sensor is ideally measured to calculate the particular form of distance between the object and the key sensor [50]. For the aspect of the surveys (airborne), the distance being traveled is then ideally converted to the form of elevation, and the different return allows the forming of the forests (mapping) and the heights of the trees.

8.5.4 Microwave-Based Remote Sensing

Microwave remote sensing is the process of examining the data gathered by sensors that operate in the microwave region of the electromagnetic spectrum. The wavelengths in the microwave portion of the spectrum fall roughly between 1 mm and 1 m. In the visible and infrared regions of Electromagnetic Radiation (EMR), we frequently experience atmospheric effects. However, these longer waves can pass through the clouds. Microwave sensors are time-independent because their active mode of microwave reflection (backscattering) and passive mode of emissions from the earth's surface are not confined by the time of data acquisition. Furthermore, there is no correlation between these emissions and reflections and their counterparts in the thermal, infrared, or visible regions of the spectrum.

However, the type and quantity of backscattered electromagnetic radiation can reveal details about the dimensions, structure, electrical characteristics, and other characteristics of the exposed surfaces and objects. These answers provide us with a very different perspective on the surroundings. Although the most basic systems only record the amplitude, it is possible to measure the return signal's polarization, phase, and amplitude. Owing to the aforementioned distinct reactions, microwave remote sensing offers the following benefits over other EMR regions:

- Independent of time
- Independent of weather
- Sensitive to soil, plant, and snow moisture
- Improvement of relief and surface roughness
- Soil and vegetation cover penetration
- The capacity to gather information from a distance off the flight path

Due to these benefits, they are useful for timely monitoring of the following: ocean wind vector, wave spectra, wave height, and atmospheric parameters; soil moisture; crop/vegetation; snow cover; geological features; coastal zone; urban extent; and man-made targets. The two main categories of microwave sensors are passive and active. Radiometers are examples of passive sensors. This includes atmospheric sounders, multifrequency scanning and imaging radiometers, etc.

Radar stands for Radar Ranging and Detection. An active microwave remote sensing system is called Active. Imaging radar is described by several systems, including Active Microwave Imager (AMI), Synthetic Aperture Radar (SAR), and Side Looking Radar (SLAR), also known as Real Aperture Radar (RAR). Active microwave sensors also include rain mapping radar, scatterometers, and altimeters.

8.6 METHODOLOGY

The secondary research methodology will be used in this research article. The methodology of the secondary research aspect is ideally suitable for exploring the range of artificial intelligence in the aspect of remote sensing because of the amount of current data and literature on this particular topic [51]. The concept of remote sensing is an ideal domain with the current form of extensive research, making it the process conducive to secondary-based research. The aspect of access to the datasets, reports, and studies allows the entity of the researchers to analyze the patterns, advancements, and trends in the applications of artificial intelligence efficiently [52]. Furthermore, the entity of the secondary research enables the ideal review of the past form of work, proceeding to facilitate the ideal understanding of the particular form of subject, without the requirement for the time-consuming and costly collection of primary data in remote or geographically based locations [53].

8.7 RESULT AND DISCUSSION

Considering the above discussion, multiple levels of sensor which is specifically combined to gain the ideal understanding of the structure investigated [54, 55]. Table 8.1 ideally provides a particular overview of the cons and pros of each technique of remote sensing, with its applications, limitations, and advantages [56–60].

TABLE 8.1
Summary of Different Remote Sensing Techniques

Techniques	Advantages	Limitations	Sample Range of Applications
Optimal range of remote sensing	Capturing the reflected radiation of solar and emitted form of thermal radiation for the particular assessment [61].	Impacting accuracy of data.	Land usage mapping.
Radar form of remote sensing	For operating in the region of microwave that provides distance and valuable data [62, 63].	Data proceedings could be very complex.	To map land surfaces.
LiDAR	For providing the elevation measurements and précised distance.	Atmospheric-based conditions [64].	Creating detailed 3D maps.

8.8 CONCLUSION AND FUTURE SCOPE

The execution of the techniques of artificial intelligence in the aspect of remote sensing has also emerged as the ideal form of paradigm with practical application considering the tremendous potential aspect. This particular convergence creates opportunities for advancing the understanding of the dynamics of the earth, supporting the procedure of decision-making, and fostering sustainability and its development. This article provides an ideal review of the present state of AI-based techniques in remote sensing tools, considering emphasizing their impact and significance. In the future, remote sensing can ideally hold the major potential. The key advancement in the AI-based algorithm, specifically coupled with the increment availability of satellite imagery (high resolution) and the factor of censored data, will also enable real-time and accurate assessment of the earth's changes and features.

REFERENCES

[1] D. Hong et al., "Interpretable hyperspectral artificial intelligence: When nonconvex modelling meets hyper spectral remote sensing," *IEEE Geoscience and Remote Sensing Magazine*, vol. 9, no. 2, pp. 52–87, 2021.

[2] Mellit and S. Kalogirou, "Artificial intelligence and internet of things to improve efficacy of diagnosis and remote sensing of solar photovoltaic systems: Challenges, recommendations and future directions," *Renewable and Sustainable Energy Reviews*, vol. 143, p. 110889, 2021.

[3] X. Liu et al., "A remote sensing and artificial neural network-based integrated agricultural drought index: Index development and applications," *Catena*, vol. 186, p. 104394, 2020.

[4] J. Jung et al., "The potential of remote sensing and artificial intelligence as tools to improve the resilience of agriculture production systems," *Current Opinion in Biotechnology*, vol. 70, pp. 15–22, 2021.

[5] S. A. Boukabara et al., "Leveraging modern artificial intelligence for remote sensing and NWP: Benefits and challenges," *Bulletin of the American Meteorological Society*, vol. 100, no. 12, pp. ES473–ES491, 2019.

[6] S. S. Virnodkar et al., "Remote sensing and machine learning for crop water stress determination in various crops: A critical review," *Precision Agriculture*, vol. 21, no. 5, pp. 1121–1155, 2020.

[7] G. Veselov et al., "Applications of artificial intelligence in evolution of smart cities and societies," *Informatica*, vol. 45, no. 5, pp. 603–604, 2021.

[8] Y. Afaq and A. Manocha, "Analysis on change detection techniques for remote sensing applications: A review," *Ecological Informatics*, vol. 63, p. 101310, 2021.

[9] R. P. Sishodia, R. L. Ray, and S. K. Singh, "Applications of remote sensing in precision agriculture: A review," *Remote Sensing*, vol. 12, no. 19, p. 3136, 2020.

[10] M. Mohajane et al., "Application of remote sensing and machine learning algorithms for forest fire mapping in a Mediterranean area," *Ecological Indicators*, vol. 129, p. 107869, 2021.

[11] W. Shi et al., "Change detection based on artificial intelligence: State-of-the-art and challenges," *Remote Sensing*, vol. 12, no. 10, p. 1688, 2020.

[12] A. Mohan et al., "Review on remote sensing methods for landslide detection using machine and deep learning," *Transactions on Emerging Telecommunications Technologies*, vol. 32, no. 7, p. e3998, 2021.

[13] M. Gonzalez-Rivero et al., "Monitoring of coral reefs using artificial intelligence: A feasible and cost-effective approach," *Remote Sensing*, vol. 12, no. 3, p. 489, 2020.
[14] G. Furano et al., "Towards the use of artificial intelligence on the edge in space systems: Challenges and opportunities," *IEEE Aerospace and Electronic Systems Magazine*, vol. 35, no. 12, pp. 44–56, 2020.
[15] H. Shirmard et al., "A review of machine learning in processing remote sensing data for mineral exploration," *Remote Sensing of Environment*, vol. 268, p. 112750, 2022.
[16] R. Dash, M. McMurtrey, C. Rebman, and U. K. Kar, "Application of artificial intelligence in automation of supply chain management," *Journal of Strategic Innovation and Sustainability*, vol. 14, no. 3, pp. 43–53, 2019.
[17] N. C. Eli-Chukwu, "Applications of artificial intelligence in agriculture: A review," *Engineering, Technology & Applied Science Research*, vol. 9, no. 4, pp. 4377–4383, 2019.
[18] W. Wu et al., "Application of local fully Convolutional Neural Network combined with YOLO v5 algorithm in small target detection of remote sensing image," *PloS one*, vol. 16, no. 10, p. e0259283, 2021.
[19] S. Bera and V. K. Shrivastava, "Analysis of various optimizers on deep convolutional neural network model in the application of hyperspectral remote sensing image classification," *International Journal of Remote Sensing*, vol. 41, no. 7, pp. 2664–2683, 2019.
[20] Z. Chang et al., "Landslide susceptibility prediction based on remote sensing images and GIS: Comparisons of supervised and unsupervised machine learning models," *Remote Sensing*, vol. 12, no. 3, p. 502, 2020.
[21] Q. Guo et al., "Applications of artificial intelligence in the field of air pollution: A bibliometric analysis," *Frontiers in Public Health*, vol. 10, p. 933665, 2022.
[22] H. Loisel et al., "Remote sensing," *Surface Ocean–Lower Atmosphere Processes Geophysical Research Series*, vol. 187, pp. 27–301, 2009.
[23] Wikimedia, "Remote sensing illustration.jpg," 20 November published, Accessed on 8 November, 2023.
[24] X. Li et al., "Retrieval of crop biophysical parameters from Sentinel-2 remote sensing imagery," *International Journal of Applied Earth Observation and Geoinformation*, vol. 80, pp. 187–195, 2019.
[25] Q. Yuan et al., "Deep learning in environmental remote sensing: Achievements and challenges," *Remote Sensing of Environment*, vol. 241, p. 111716, 2020.
[26] H. Zha et al., "Improving unmanned aerial vehicle remote sensing-based rice nitrogen nutrition index prediction with machine learning," *Remote Sensing*, vol. 12, no. 2, p. 215, 2020.
[27] X. Li et al., "Deep-learning-based information mining from ocean remote-sensing imagery," *National Science Review*, vol. 7, no. 10, pp. 1584–1605, 2020.
[28] M. Sheykhmousa et al., "Support vector machine versus random forest for remote sensing image classification: A meta-analysis and systematic review," *IEEE Journal of Selected Topics in Applied Earth Observations and Remote Sensing*, vol. 13, pp. 6308–6325, 2020.
[29] R. Pires de Lima and K. Marfurt, "Convolutional neural network for remote-sensing scene classification: Transfer learning analysis," *Remote Sensing*, vol. 12, no. 1, p. 86, 2019.
[30] L. P. Osco et al., "A review on deep learning in UAV remote sensing," *International Journal of Applied Earth Observation and Geoinformation*, vol. 102, p. 102456, 2020.
[31] A. Barela et al., "Applications of proximal remote sensing in agriculture: A review," *The Pharma Innovation Journal*, vol. 12, no. 2, pp. 1124–1130, 2021.

[32] I. Indirabai et al., "Optical remote sensing for biophysical characterisation in forests: A review," *International Journal of Applied Engineering Research*, vol. 14, no. 2, pp. 344–354, 2019.
[33] N. Gnann et al., "Close-range remote sensing-based detection and identification of macroplastics on water assisted by artificial intelligence: A review," *Water Research*, vol. 222, p. 118902, 2022.
[34] L. Ma et al., "Deep learning in remote sensing applications: A meta-analysis and review," *ISPRS Journal of Photogrammetry and Remote Sensing*, vol. 152, pp. 166–177, 2019.
[35] A. Asokan and J. Anitha, "Change detection techniques for remote sensing applications: A survey," *Earth Science Informatics*, vol. 12, pp. 143–160, 2019.
[36] H. Shahabi et al., "Flood detection and susceptibility mapping using sentinel-1 remote sensing data and a machine learning approach: Hybrid intelligence of bagging ensemble based on k-nearest neighbour classifier," *Remote Sensing*, vol. 12, no. 2, p. 266, 2020.
[37] S. N. Topp et al., "Research trends in the use of remote sensing for inland water quality science: Moving towards multidisciplinary applications," *Water*, vol. 12, no. 1, p. 169, 2020.
[38] R. Costache et al., "Flash-flood susceptibility assessment using multi-criteria decision making and machine learning supported by remote sensing and GIS techniques," *Remote Sensing*, vol. 12, no. 1, p. 106, 2019.
[39] M. Amani et al., "Google earth engine cloud computing platform for remote sensing big data applications: A comprehensive review," *IEEE Journal of Selected Topics in Applied Earth Observations and Remote Sensing*, vol. 13, pp. 5326–5350, 2020.
[40] A. Arabameri et al., "Assessment of landslide susceptibility using statistical-and artificial intelligence-based FR–RF integrated model and multiresolution DEMs," *Remote Sensing*, vol. 11, no. 9, p. 999, 2019.
[41] Benami et al., "The rise of artificial intelligence in healthcare applications," In *Artificial Intelligence in Healthcare*, Academic Press, 2020, pp. 25–60.
[42] Z. Ullah et al., "Applications of artificial intelligence and machine learning in smart cities," *Computer Communications*, vol. 154, pp. 313–323, 2020.
[43] J. Li, X. Huang, and J. Gong, "Deep neural network for remote-sensing image interpretation: Status and perspectives," *National Science Review*, vol. 6, no. 6, pp. 1082–1086, 2019.
[44] W. Wu, D. Hong, and J. Chanussot, "Convolutional neural networks for multimodal remote sensing data classification," *IEEE Transactions on Geoscience and Remote Sensing*, vol. 60, pp. 1–10, 2021.
[45] E. Ben Ayed and M. R. Carter, "Uniting remote sensing, crop modelling and economics for agricultural risk management," *Nature Reviews Earth & Environment*, vol. 2, no. 2, pp. 140–159, 2021.
[46] L. Tan et al., "Can we detect trends in natural disaster management with artificial intelligence? A review of modelling practices," *Natural Hazards*, vol. 107, pp. 2389–2417, 2021.
[47] N. C. Nhu et al., "Landslide susceptibility mapping using machine learning algorithms and remote sensing data in a tropical environment," *International Journal of Environmental Research and Public Health*, vol. 17, no. 14, p. 4933, 2020.
[48] T. Kattenborn et al., "Review on Convolutional Neural Networks (CNN) in vegetation remote sensing," *ISPRS Journal of Photogrammetry and Remote Sensing*, vol. 173, pp. 24–49, 2021.
[49] Y. Li, J. Ma, and Y. Zhang, "Image retrieval from remote sensing big data: A survey," *Information Fusion*, vol. 67, pp. 94–115, 2021.

[50] S. Durrieu, "Design of a European space borne LiDAR system for vegetation mapping-LEAF: LiDAR for earth and forests," *Conference on Silvilaser*, Freiburg, Germany, 14–17 September 2010.

[51] M. Newman and D. Gough, "Systematic reviews in educational research: Methodology, perspectives and application," in: Zawacki-Richter, O., Kerres, M., Bedenlier, S., Bond, M., and Buntins, K. (eds.), *Systematic Reviews in Educational Research*. Springer VS: Wiesbaden, pp. 3–22, 2020.

[52] K. J. Sileyew, "Research design and methodology," *Cyberspace*, pp. 1–12, 2019.

[53] V. Bairagi and M. V. Munot, *Research Methodology: A Practical and Scientific Approach*, CRC Press, 2019.

[54] E. Maxwell, T. A. Warner, and L. A. Guillén, "Accuracy assessment in convolutional neural network-based deep learning remote sensing studies-Part 1: Literature review," *Remote Sensing*, vol. 13, no. 13, p. 2450, 2021.

[55] H. Jiang et al., "Quantitative assessment of soil salinity using multi-source remote sensing data based on the support vector machine and artificial neural network," *International Journal of Remote Sensing*, vol. 40, no. 1, pp. 284–306, 2019.

[56] C. Sun et al., "Using of multi-source and multi-temporal remote sensing data improves crop-type mapping in the subtropical agriculture region," *Sensors*, vol. 19, no. 10, p. 2401, 2019.

[57] D. Ghai, S. L. Tripathi, S. Saxena, M. Chanda, and M. Alazab, *Machine Learning Algorithms for Signal and Image Processing*, John Wiley & Sons, 2022.

[58] V. K. A. Somayajula, D. Ghai, and S. Kumar, "Land use/land cover change analysis using NDVI, PCA," In *2021 5th IEEE International Conference on Computing Methodologies and Communication*, pp. 849–855, 2021.

[59] V. K. A. Somayajula, D. Ghai, S. Kumar, S. L. Tripathi, C. Verma, C. O. Safirescu, and T. C. Mihaltan, "Classification and validation of spatio-temporal changes in land use/ land cover and land surface temperature of multitemporal images," *Sustainability*, vol. 14, no. 23, pp. 15677, 2022.

[60] V. K.A. Somayajula, D. Ghai, and S. Kumar, "Land cover classification using landsat images, normalized difference vegetation index in Vijayawada, AP," *International Journal of Early Childhood Special Education*, vol. 14, no. 3, pp. 1159–1171, 2022.

[61] J. Yu et al., "Application of a convolutional neural network to land use classification based on GF-2 remote sensing imagery," *Arabian Journal of Geosciences*, vol. 14, pp. 1–14, 2021.

[62] Y. A. Khan and M. Shrivastava, "Artificial intelligence to improve the food and agriculture sector," *Journal of Food Quality*, vol. 2021, pp. 1–7.

[63] A. Abdollahi et al., "Deep learning approaches applied to remote sensing datasets for road extraction: A state-of-the-art review," *Remote Sensing*, vol. 12, no. 9, p. 1444, 2020.

[64] M. Weiss, F. Jacob, and G. Duveiller, "Remote sensing for agricultural applications: A meta-review," *Remote Sensing of Environment*, vol. 236, p. 111402, 2020.

9 Artificial Intelligence Models for Remote Sensing Applications

Divya Shivani Thangi
Department of Genetics and Plant Breeding, Angrau, Bapatla, India

9.1 INTRODUCTION

The success of sustainable development in any region depends upon what is known regarding resource management and hazards in the area. While there are many ways to keep an eye on natural resources and potential threats, Remote Sensing (RS) technology has gained a lot of traction since the 1970s due to its low acquisition costs and great usefulness for gathering, analyzing, and managing data. RS tools and approaches have been used for a variety of applications in different timespans over the last few decades. RS offers near-real-time and archival data on Earth systems. RS is used in several Earth system scientific domains to get spatial data. One reason why RS is a good choice for solving global environmental, ecological, and socioeconomic concerns is its capacity to monitor Earth systems at different geographical and temporal scales. RS may offer a global, regional, and local synoptic view of spatial data, enabling quick decision-making and action [1].

RS is the primary surveying method used to gather data in distant and inaccessible areas because it provides immediate access to information. Numerous benchmark studies on the application of RS in sustainable development have been conducted; these studies address a range of subtopics in the domains of socioeconomic development, natural hazards, and environmental evaluation. among others [2, 3]. Franklin [4] reported the use of RS in sustainable forest management. Huete et al. [5] reported the development of a global vegetation index that is used to monitor the behavior of growth of plants. Wilson et al. [6] reported the influence of zoning on vegetation indices and temperature in urban ecosystems using RS, and Dudhani et al. [3] mapped water resources in plain, hilly, and mountain regions with the use of RS data sources. Van Westen [7] reported natural disaster management as though there is no satellite specifically designed for use in disaster mitigation but through the orbital satellites, they provided useful information that helped in the prevention of the disaster, its preparedness, and also helped to relief its efforts.

Over the past three decades, RS has been used more often to evaluate initiatives for sustainable development. Data analysis has greatly improved as a result of

DOI: 10.1201/9781003546382-9

advances in RS technology and the availability of enormous amounts of data, particularly when paired with Machine Learning (ML) and Geographic Information System (GIS) algorithms. Since the early 1990s, RS data has been analyzed using Machine Learning (ML) techniques such as convolutional neural networks, random forests, and support vector machines for environmental evaluations and socioeconomic development monitoring [8–10]. These algorithms will probably be essential for optimizing the advantages of geographical data. When employed to monitor sustainable development initiatives, these approaches were not always accurate and efficient due to the lack of pictures with fine spatial and temporal resolution. But over the past ten years, there has been a significant improvement in the mapping and tracking of sustainable development activities thanks to the development of new platforms and interfaces like graphics processing units, cloud platforms (like Google Earth Engine), open data sources (like USGS Earth Explorer, Copernicus Data Hub, Bhuvan, and Open Topography), and graphics processing units. An additional factor contributing to the ten-year increase in the use of RS to evaluate sustainable development is the expansion of worldwide partnerships amongst RS community members, partly enabled by conversations on various social media platforms like Stack Exchange, GitHub, Quora, Facebook, and LinkedIn. The expanding use of RS to collect data for environmental and natural resource monitoring has also been facilitated by the proliferation of open-source RS software and several advanced analytical tools (e.g., SAGA, QGIS, SNAP, SeaDAS, LAS).

Almost all areas of Earth and environmental research now use RS, which is regarded as a scientific instrument. This assessment attempts to evaluate how developments in RS technology have impacted three key areas of sustainability, taking into account the significance of sustainable development in the 21st century. To start, we go over how RS is used for natural resource development, monitoring, and management. We go into how RS is used for hazard monitoring and environmental evaluations in our second section. Third, we evaluate the usefulness of RS for enhancing quality of life, population estimates, and transportation planning. We tried to give a general overview of the idea of sustainable development in this study, as well as the functions that RS and GIS play in attaining sustainability in the face of expanding human activity and climate change.

Despite these obstacles, artificial intelligence has become a technical marvel with great potential for environmental preservation. With AI's capacity to analyze massive volumes of data, spot patterns, and make deft judgments instantly, we have an unmatched chance to completely transform how we approach sustainable growth and environmental preservation. RS is used in many different contexts for the development and management of natural resources. The applications of RS technology for natural resource management and development, especially in the context of sustainable development, are briefly presented in the sub-sections below.

9.2 BIODIVERSITY

Life on Earth depends on ecosystem services and biodiversity because they enable the supply of cultural, regulatory, supporting, and provisioning functions. For the sake of present and future generations, biodiversity monitoring and conservation are therefore crucial. Numerous field-tested strategies and tactics have been created to aid in the preservation of biodiversity. Nonetheless, their efficacy and scope are typically restricted. For example, traditional maps of Land Use and Land Cover (LULC) derived from field surveys have not been able to fully identify and track biodiversity and ecosystems, particularly those located in remote and wider geographic areas. Considering these constraints, it is imperative to devise efficacious methods for gathering data in less-than-ideal circumstances. RS approaches reliably provide baseline data across large regions are more effective in observing and tracking changes in the environment and produce precise and accurate data [11].

RS is frequently used to investigate a variety of ecological roles as well as anthropogenic and natural sources of landscape changes. For example, RS may be used not just to determine regional variation in species richness but also to detect the biophysical features of species habitats, distributions, and locations. To address new difficulties, RS has been progressively developed and refined during the last few years. RS can be used directly to monitor biodiversity, for example, by gathering data on species assemblages in biological groups or individual animals using satellite and aircraft sensors. Moreover, RS may be implemented indirectly by obtaining environmental factors and using them as standings [11, 12].

9.3 CLIMATE

The utilization of remote sensing techniques to gather climate data might be beneficial in comprehending the spatial patterns of microclimatic behavior and its connections to biodiversity. A multitude of parameters, such as temperature, relative humidity, and soil moisture, influence the survival and production of several species [12]. In recent years, many satellites from which climate parameters can be derived have been launched. United States launched the TERRA and AQUA satellites in the years 1999 and 2002. TERRA is equipped with five onboard sensors to track climate change and Earth's surroundings. (i) the Advanced Spaceborne Thermal Emission and Reflection Radiometer (ASTER), (ii) Clouds and the Earth's Radiant Energy System (CERES), (iii) Multi-angle Imaging Spectroradiometer (MISR), (iv) MODIS, and (v) Measurements of Pollution in the Troposphere (MOPITT) another model AQUA has six onboard sensors for water studies: (i) the Advanced Microwave Scanning Radiometer for the Earth Observing System (AMSR-E), (ii) MODIS, (iii) Advanced Microwave Sounding Unit (AMSU-A), (iv) Atmospheric Infrared Sounder (AIRS), (v) Humidity Sounder for Brazil (HSB), and (vi) CERES [13]. These sensors gather data about the water cycle on Earth, including cloud cover, precipitation, soil moisture, sea ice, land ice, and snow cover on both land and ocean surfaces. Measurements are also made of aerosols, water temperature, phytoplankton, plant cover, and radiating energy fluxes. These variables aid in our comprehension of the connection between biodiversity and climate data.

9.4 FOREST FIRES

Among the many environmental dangers that face forest ecosystems is fire, which has the potential to be quite dangerous. Depending on its location, timing, and cause, fire can either be a necessary component of the forest ecosystem's cycle or it can just be a destructive, unnatural threat to the existence of related plants and animals.

Indonesia, Brazil, Mexico, Canada, USA, France, Turkey, Greece, India, and Italy are all severely impacted by wildfires. Fire lookout towers, which are positioned at high locations inside a forest, have historically been used to detect forest fires. A person whose job it is to search for fires with binoculars or other advanced tools like an Osborne fire locator is housed in a fire lookout tower.

Weather factors including clouds, light reflection, and smoke from industry have a big impact on how accurate these systems are. Satellite imaging serves as the basis for more sophisticated forest fire detection systems. The Indian Remote Sensing Satellite-Advanced Wide Field Sensor (IRS AWiFS), the Moderate Resolution Imaging Spectroradiometer (MODIS), and the Advanced Very High-Resolution Radiometer (AVHRR) are utilized to identify active forest fires. Data from this equipment is used for forest fire monitoring by the current satellite-based forest fire detection systems. Weather has a major influence on satellite-based systems' accuracy and dependability, unlike ground-based monitoring. Rain and clouds both absorb portions of the frequency spectrum, lowering the spectral resolution of satellite imaging and thus affecting the accuracy of detection. Despite their ability to monitor a vast region, satellite-based systems have very low resolution a fire can be detected only after it has grown large.

9.5 OCEAN STUDIES

Systems for remote sensing offer useful data for charting and tracking many oceanic characteristics. Because of their distance and wide coverage, seas provide good targets for Remote Sensing (RS). Systems such as Altimeter, Synthetic Aperture Radar (SAR), Scatterometer, Microwave radiometer, Thermal Infrared radiometer (TIR), Glonass, Global Positioning System (GPS), Optical System, Synthetic Aperture Radar (SAR), Light Detection and Ranging (LiDAR), and High Frequency (HF) radars are examples of non-spaceborne radar systems.

9.5.1 Optical System

The optical range or horizontal visibility may be determined with the use of optical diffusion meters. They are made up of a receiver and a light source, which is often a laser. Aiming at a shared region, both are positioned at a 35° angle downward. An attenuation coefficient is used to quantify the amount of lateral scattering caused by air along a light beam. The visibility is inversely proportional to any deviation from the clear air extinction coefficient (such as in fog), with the larger the loss, the poorer the visibility. These sensors can be found in automatic weather stations to monitor general visibility, ocean currents, runway visual range, and road conditions. Their primary flaw is that the measurement is made over a small amount of air between the transmitter and the receiver.

9.5.2 Synthetic Aperture Radar (SAR)

An imaging radar installed on a moving platform is called a Synthetic Aperture Radar (SAR). The system circuitry successively transmits electromagnetic waves, gathers echoes, digitizes the data, and stores it for further processing. Transmission and reception map to distinct tiny places because they happen at separate times. The virtual aperture created by the well-organized combination of the received signals is substantially longer than the actual antenna width. Its origins give rise to the phrase "synthetic aperture," which confers on it the capability of imaging radar. Because it aligns with the position of the object within the antenna's field of vision, the azimuth direction—also referred to as the along-track direction—and the flight track are both perpendicular to the range direction.

There are two steps to the 3D processing. After focusing on the azimuth and range directions to create 2D (Azimuth-range) high-resolution pictures, phase differences between complex images are measured using a Digital Elevation Model (DEM), which is derived from various look angles to recover height information. The elevation is the third dimension, which is obtained by combining the azimuth-range coordinates obtained from 2-D SAR focusing with the height data. Standard processing algorithms are all that are needed for the first step; extra pre-processing, including phase calibration and picture co-registration, is employed for the second.

9.5.3 Scatterometer

A microwave energy pulse is sent toward the Earth's surface to operate a radar scatterometer, and the reflected energy is then measured. To calculate the backscatter signal power, a second measurement of the noise-only power is produced and subtracted from the signal+noise measurement. Through the use of the distributed target radar equation, sigma-0 (σ^0) is calculated from the signal power measurement. To get accurate backscatter readings, scatterometer devices must be calibrated with extreme precision. Measurements of near-surface winds over the ocean have been the main use of spaceborne scatterometry. Wind scatterometers are the name given to these devices. A Geophysical Model Function (GMF) that links wind and backscatter may be used to predict the near-surface wind vector over the ocean's surface by integrating sigma-0 observations from various azimuth angles. Radar backscatter over the water is caused by capillary-gravity waves that are scattered by wind and are usually in balance with the near-surface wind. Bragg scattering is the name given to the scattering process that results from waves that resonate with microwaves.

The wind's direction and speed determine how much electricity is backscattered. The backscatter from these waves changes when seen from various azimuth angles. The speed and direction of the sea surface wind may be estimated by taking advantage of these fluctuations. "Wind retrieval" or "model function inversion" are other names for this estimation procedure. This non-linear inversion process links the scatterometer backscatter and the vector wind and is predicated on precise knowledge of the Global Mapping Function (GMF) (in an empirical or semi-empirical form). An angular diversity scatterometer measurement with the GMF is necessary for retrieval. This measurement is given by the scatterometer taking several backscatter measurements of the same location on the ocean's surface from various azimuth angles. Wind readings from scatterometers are utilized in climate studies, air-sea interaction research, and hurricane monitoring. Backscatter data from scatterometers are used to track Antarctic icebergs, research polar ice, analyze vegetation, and investigate world change. Winds over sand and snow dunes have been measured from space using scatterometer observations.

9.5.4 Altimeter

An instrument used to measure an object's height above a given level is called an altimeter or altitude meter. The term altimetry, which refers to the measuring of height, is connected to bathymetry, which is the measurement of depth beneath water. The basis of radio altimeters is the idea that electromagnetic wave pulses are reflected off the sea or earth's surface. The radio spectrum includes these wavelengths. Since electromagnetic waves move at the speed of light, the distance may be calculated very instantly. While surface flaws might cause variations in the radio signal, radio altimeters offer a dependable and precise way to measure height. Altimeters are also used by mountaineers and skydivers to determine their exact location in the sky or on the ground. Barometric altimeters are the most popular kind. By monitoring air pressure, they can calculate altitude. Air pressure drops with increasing height. This is because air at high altitudes has a lower density, or is thinner. Less pressure is applied to the Earth below it. Because air pressure drops during storms, weather may also affect altitude readings. A spring, a sealed metal chamber, and a pointer that displays altitude in feet or meters make up a basic barometric altimeter. Bending the spring and moving the pointer, the chamber expands with decreasing air pressure and shrinks with increasing air pressure. An altimeter can be worn on the wrist or positioned on the instrument panel of an aircraft.

9.5.5 HF Radar

A distant sensing device called High-Frequency (HF) radar utilizes radio waves to determine sea surface height, waves, and ocean currents. It's an economical, non-intrusive way to learn about the water. Antennas for HF radar systems are positioned at the water's edge. High-frequency radio wave pulses are emitted by the antennas, and these pulses reflect off the water's surface and return to the antenna. Depending on the radar frequency, HF radar systems can monitor surface currents up to 200 km distant with resolutions of 500 m to 6 km. Ocean surface currents may be measured in almost real-time by HF radar systems, both in terms of direction and speed. Ocean wave spectra and surface current fields have been measured using High-Frequency (HF) radars.

The backscattering from a moving, rough sea surface is the basis of the physics underlying HF radar. By using ground wave propagation, the radar sends out electromagnetic waves with a wavelength of 50–10 m (between 6 and 30 MHz). These waves travel over the sea surface beyond the horizon before being scattered back by waves in the water that have half the electromagnetic wavelength (Bragg scattering). The Doppler spectrum, which is produced by moving waves and the speed at which surface currents convey ocean waves, is measured by the dispersed signals. Measurements beyond the horizon are possible by guided propagation along the conductive sea surface (ground wave).

Second-order sea echoes of the Doppler spectrum may also be used to deduce the wave directional spectrum and the height of the ocean waves. The radial current speed concerning the radar site is determined using the Doppler shift of the backscattered signal. The two horizontal components of the surface velocity may be computed if the two radar stations measure the radial velocity of a patch of water from two distinct angles. The surface current was measured as a horizontal mean across a few kilometers in both azimuth and range, during about 10 minutes, and over the upper 0.5–1.0 m of the ocean (the penetration depth of scattering ocean waves). These radar locations offer data on waves and surface currents in the coastal and ocean waters up to 300 km offshore.

9.5.6 Thermal Infrared Radiometer (TIR)

Through clouds, Thermal Infrared Radiometer (TIR) radiation cannot pass through. Because of haze and particles, the atmosphere's scattering and absorption can have a detrimental impact on TIR radiation even when there are no clouds present. The wavelength and atmospheric gas absorptions determine the clear-sky atmosphere's transmissivity in the TIR region of the electromagnetic spectrum. As a result, the atmospheric window—where the atmosphere is more transparent—should be carefully considered while determining the TIR wavelength intervals in an RS system. Within two atmospheric windows, the TIR radiometers detect Sea-Surface Temperature (SST). One of the biggest obstacles to detecting SST using Equation is the presence of clouds, which necessitates the development of a precise plan for eliminating pixels tainted by weather and clouds. Finding the clear sky pixels is a crucial first step in obtaining a precise time-series SST estimation.

Numerous techniques, such as BT minima, binary tests in a decision tree based on BT uniformity, and comparisons with lower-resolution gap-free reference fields, have been proposed in this respect for cloud screening in TIR measurements. These techniques, however, are dependent on the threshold values used, which might lead to inaccuracies in SST estimates at high latitudes and close to ocean thermal fronts at clouds that are semi-transparent. To overcome these constraints, a Bayesian probabilistic method was presented for cloud screening of TIR imagery. This method was extensively employed for operational SST estimation in several satellite missions, including the Japanese geostationary meteorological Himawari-8 satellite, the Advanced Along-Track Scanning Radiometer (AATSR), and the Geostationary Operational Environmental Satellite (GOES). Additionally, it was shown that alternating decision-tree methods enhance the effectiveness of decision-tree approaches in cloud screening. In these approaches, ML algorithms are used to establish threshold values and their weights rather than trial-and-error techniques. Figure 9.1 shows Remote Sensing (RS) applications in ocean studies.

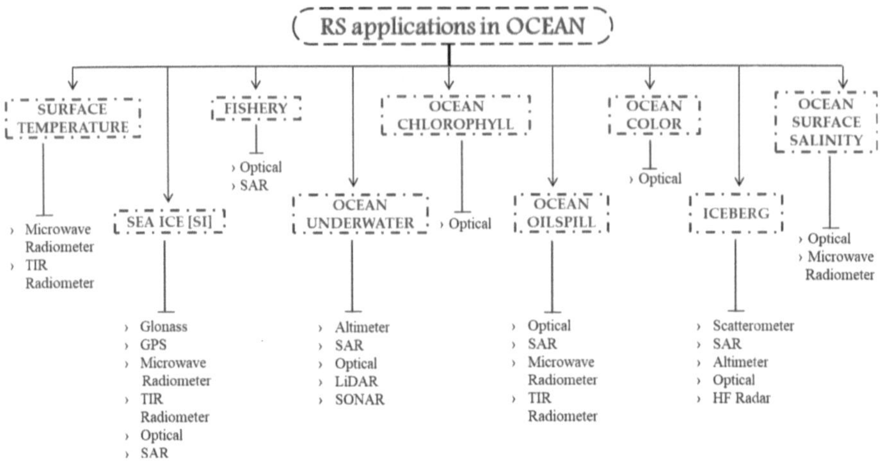

FIGURE 9.1 Remote sensing (RS) applications in ocean studies.

9.6 ARCHAEOLOGICAL RESEARCH

Experts worldwide are increasingly favoring the non-destructive method of remote sensing for the protection of Archaeological and Cultural Heritage (ACH). This is because remote sensing enables quick searches and mapping at various scales, quick analysis of data sets from multiple sources, and dynamic monitoring of ACH sites and their surroundings. Archaeological research and cultural heritage have become more and more reliant on the use of remote sensing data and its products in recent years. To differentiate between archaeological remains and identify changes in the environment over time, several spatial and spectral analytic datasets have been used. In the past 10 years, archaeologists have also embraced more comprehensive automated object recognition techniques for possible sites. These methods included, among other things, active methods (Synthetic Aperture Radar (SAR) and Light Detection and Ranging Radar (LiDAR)), multispectral and hyperspectral images, Airborne and Spaceborne Remote Sensing (ASRS), Convolutional Neural Networks (CNN) and Deep Learning (DL) models using aerial and satellite images, and multispectral and hyperspectral images. Scholars also discuss how archaeologists may investigate these AI methods in different contexts, such as recognizing and categorizing archaeological elements.

9.7 HABITAT STRUCTURE

It is possible to get insights into the patterns and distributions of species by comprehending their habitat architecture. RS technologies have shown to be beneficial in this regard. The topography, canopy height, and vertical distribution of canopy elements—the latter of which serves as a proxy for the diversity of bird species in trees—were all determined using LiDAR data. There was a correlation between the vertical distribution analysis results and the bird survey data. To estimate forest structural factors such as canopy height and biomass, data from LiDAR, Landsat-7,

QuickBird, and Synthetic Aperture Radar/Interferometric Synthetic Aperture Radar (SAR/InSAR) were combined and compared.

9.7.1 Earth Observation

An unparalleled perspective of the Earth's surface is provided by satellite imaging, which also provides vital information for environmental monitoring. To find relevant trends, though, the sheer amount of data created demands advanced processing skills. With the use of Artificial Intelligence (AI) technologies, such as Convolutional Neural Networks (CNNs), it is possible to detect deforestation, habitat loss, and land degradation with previously unheard-of precision from satellite photos. Critical environmental indicators may be monitored almost instantly with the use of AI-powered remote sensing instruments. Artificial Intelligence (AI)-driven systems can quickly identify illicit logging, encroachments, and unsustainable farming practices by continually analyzing changes in plant cover, forest density, and land use. This early warning system encourages a proactive approach to environmental preservation by enabling politicians and environmentalists to react quickly to new dangers.

9.7.2 Wildlife Protection

To keep endangered species from going extinct, extensive monitoring is required. Conventional approaches to tracking animals can be costly, time-consuming, and have a narrow focus. However, the use of AI in GPS tracking, acoustic monitoring, and camera trap picture processing has completely changed the field of animal protection. Artificial Intelligence (AI) supports conservation efforts by offering priceless insights into species behavior and habitat utilization through the identification of individual animals, estimation of population levels, and tracking of movement patterns. Endangered animals and their habitats are seriously threatened by poaching and the illicit wildlife trade. Artificial Intelligence (AI) tools like machine vision and natural language processing can scan through enormous volumes of web information to find and disrupt networks involved in the illicit wildlife trade. Moreover, artificial intelligence-powered surveillance systems with face recognition capabilities can help law enforcement catch poachers and traffickers, acting as a deterrent to illicit activities.

9.7.3 Rainfall Prediction

Predicting the amount of rain is a significant meteorological issue that has a big impact on humankind in areas like agriculture productivity, drought, flooding, and sustainable water resource management. It is hard for standard methodologies to produce rainfall forecasts with a sufficient level of accuracy due to the dynamic and non-linear character of the meteorological circumstances. The intricacy of the meteorological processes that led to rainfall makes it exceedingly difficult to forecast rainfall using quantitative methods. The study suggested four non-linear methods for predicting rainfall, including Artificial Neural Networks (ANN). ANNs can map a variety of input and output patterns. Rainfall was predicted using the Elman Neural Network (ENN), Recurrent Neural Network (RNN), Cascade Forward Neural Network (CFNN), and Feed Forward Neural Network (FFNN). The meteorological variables for the years 2015–2019, including temperature, wind speed, humidity, rainfall, visibility, and others, are included in the dataset utilized for this work. According to simulation data, the Elman NN model outperformed all other suggested Neural Network (NN) models in terms of performance. Additionally, we discovered that Elman NN performed the best in 2018 with the lowest Root Mean Square Error (RMSE), MSE, and Mean Absolute Error (MAE) are 6.460, 40.45, and 0.54, respectively. According to the findings, NN algorithms are trustworthy, strong algorithms that can be used to predict rainfall on a daily, monthly, or annual basis.

9.8 AI-ENABLED SUSTAINABLE DEVELOPMENT

9.8.1 Smart Cities and Urban Planning

With more people living in cities throughout the globe, the idea of smart cities is becoming more and more popular. Artificial Intelligence (AI) is revolutionizing urban living by streamlining traffic, public transit, and energy use. AI-enabled smart grids facilitate real-time energy distribution monitoring and management, lowering waste and encouraging the incorporation of renewable energy sources. The spread of AI-powered waste management systems helps to reduce the negative environmental effects of cities. By streamlining garbage collection routes and sorting procedures, AI-powered waste collection and recycling algorithms increase efficiency and lower costs. AI-driven urban planning models also make it possible to construct resilient and sustainable cities by taking into account elements like public facilities, green areas, and optimized infrastructure.

9.8.2 Renewable Energy and Resource Management

Shifting to renewable energy is essential to reducing greenhouse gas emissions and halting global warming. Improved solar, wind, and energy storage technologies have been made possible by AI's capacity to evaluate intricate energy data and optimize renewable energy systems. The global switch to clean energy is accelerated by these developments, which increase the economic viability and accessibility of renewable energy. Degradation of the environment is mostly caused by ineffective resource management. Organizations may optimize resource allocation and minimize waste by utilizing AI algorithms to analyze data on resource utilization, supplier networks, and consumption trends. This optimization promotes sustainability and ecological balance in several industries, including manufacturing, water management, agriculture, and recycling.

9.8.3 Precision Agriculture and Sustainable Food Production

It is a difficult task to feed the world's expanding population while reducing agriculture's environmental impact. A solution is provided by AI-driven precision agriculture, which combines information from sensors, satellites, and drones to produce a detailed picture of crop health, soil conditions, and water use. Precision nutrient delivery, intelligent irrigation, and pest management are made easier by AI-powered insights, which support productive and sustainable farming methods. Food waste has a significant negative impact on both the environment and world food security. Because of AI's predictive powers, supply chains can be monitored in real time, allowing for prompt actions to stop food loss and spoiling. Moreover, AI systems can reduce food waste at the retail and consumer levels by analyzing trends in customer behavior and optimizing inventory management.

9.9 DIGITAL AGRICULTURE

Digital agriculture is the fourth revolution of agriculture, wherein sensors, computation, and Artificial Intelligence (AI) are used to improve crop management leading to an increase in yield. The model PROLOG uses weather data, machinery capacities, labor availability, and information on permissible and prioritized operators, tractors, and implements for evaluating the operational behavior of a farm system. Demeter is a computer-controlled speed-rowing machine, equipped with a pair of video cameras and a global positioning sensor for navigation. Models like Artificial neural networks use one or more layers of functions for example DefoNet, a neural network designed to recognize defoliation by giving input in the form of images with good pixels. Decision trees are another model that gives information about the canopy coverage in the forests [14]. For weed management, models like Unmanned Aerial Vehicle (UAV)-imagery to divide images, compute and convert to binary the vegetation indexes, detect crop rows, optimize parameters, and learn a classification model [15].

Crop simulation models have become important tools to integrate physiology, genetics, and phenomics. They use input factors including weather, soil data, and crop management information to estimate crop yield. Because large data is becoming more freely available via the usage of Unmanned Aircraft Systems (UAS), Artificial Intelligence (AI) is garnering major interest within agriculture disciplines. Awika et al. [16] reported that genetic analysis and UAS-based agricultural characteristics, including excess green index (ExG), canopy cover, and canopy volume in spinach. Using genotypic and phenotypic data, Deep Convolution Neural Network (DCNN) approach is used for high throughput phenotyping of crops such as soybeans and wheat. Using images from UAS, partial least square regression, Artificial Neural Network (ANN), and Random Forest (RF) are utilized in wheat and maize for predicting yield. Using UAS images of rice, beans, and spinach, weed detection can be completed using Fully Convolutional Network (FCN) and Convolutional Neural Network (CNN) models. Using UAS and field images, disease detection in wheat, bananas, and maize was identified using CNN, RF, and DCNN. Barley biomass was identified by RF analysis of the UAS images [17].

9.10 REMOTE SENSING APPLICATIONS IN PRODUCTION AGRICULTURE

9.10.1 Mapping of Topography

Topographic characteristics (such as a field's slope, aspect, and elevation) frequently influence preseason management decisions, including when to conduct field operations, what kind of crop to plant, and how much seed to use. Hydrological balance, which affects soil properties (such as temperature and moisture content), is influenced by topography. Digital Elevation Models (DEMs) created by survey-grade GPS equipment, GPS devices installed on agricultural equipment, or remote sensing photos can be used to determine field topography. Although more accurate, survey-grade GPS technology is costly and labor-intensive to install. At the moment, field equipment-mounted pseudo-range GPS devices are frequently utilized to deliver elevation data while on the go. Because of their lower accuracy, topographic mapping seldom makes use of this data [1–5].

RS data gathered from satellites and aircraft may greatly minimize the cost, time, and accuracy related to topographic mapping. The most popular methods for producing DEMs are GPS, photogrammetry, and laser surveying. In the United States, the most widely utilized DEM data at the moment are those produced from satellite images. Even though these data are freely available, PA finds little use for them because of their poor vertical precision, which makes it difficult to discern in-field elevation variations (RMSE was found to be 4.01 m). Satellite data is not as good as DEM data generated from airborne light detection and Ranging (LiDAR) found relatively minor variations when comparing field survey elevation points with a high-resolution (1 m) LiDAR DEM [18].

9.10.2 Mapping of Subsurface

A thorough grasp of how tile drainage systems are distributed spatially in farming areas may help with better water management, which raises crop yields while lowering nitrogen losses to streams. The positions, breadth, and density of the existing tile drains, some of which were built more than 50 years ago, are now poorly understood (the phrases "tile drains," "drain lines," and "tile lines" are used interchangeably). Most of the time, data on former tile lines is either nonexistent or has been lost. Traditionally, large-scale mapping has included the laborious, time-consuming, and wasteful use of handheld tile probes and heavy trenching equipment to detect drain lines. RS technology has the potential to be an accurate, scalable, and affordable method for detecting and mapping drain lines [19].

Currently, tile drains are a large blind spot in our understanding of water routing and nutrient exports to water resources. While hydrologic and nutrient models such as SPAtially Referenced Regressions On Watershed attributes (SPARROW) [20] and Soil Water Assessment Tool (SWAT) [21] have been widely used to assess nutrient exports, these models depend on an accurate understanding of river hydrography from datasets such as NHDPlus, which entirely neglect the dense networks of unmapped tile drains that supply water and nutrients to agricultural streams. These tile drain networks have potentially large implications for storm hydrology and nutrient fates at the watershed scale.

9.10.3 Mapping of Soil Moisture and Temperature

To make management decisions about irrigation, fertilizer application, and planting, a field's temperature, and moisture state are crucial. Cool planting circumstances during planting place major strains on the emergence of warm-season crops like maize and soybeans because soil moisture affects soil temperature. The ideal soil temperature range for maize germination and emergence is between 30 and 32°C.

Signals in the microwave range are less likely to be impacted by atmospheric and cloud conditions than RS data obtained in the visible, near-infrared, and short-wave infrared bands. As a result, they have a higher potential to yield precise soil moisture estimations. Currently, several satellites, including Sentinel-1 and Soil Moisture Active Passive (SMAP) satellites [22, 23] are equipped with active and passive microwave sensors for monitoring soil moisture. To downscale SMAP data, several studies have combined optical RS data and Synthetic Aperture Radar (SAR) from Sentinel 1 with machine learning algorithms. The spatial-temporal resolution of downscaled soil moisture data lacks sufficient spatial precision for PA, even with advancements in downscaling methods.

9.10.4 For Assessing the Soil Compaction

Reduced agricultural output is the outcome of soil compaction's detrimental effects on soil health, which include decreased porosity, soil hydraulic conductivity, and nutrient availability. Gaining a better knowledge of the temporal and spatial extents of soil compaction in a field can assist farmers in mitigating crop production losses associated with in-field compaction. Cone penetrometers are often used to measure soil compaction as a function of penetration resistance per unit area. However, because the data gathered is discontinuous, this approach is time-consuming, difficult, and incomplete. Only a small number of studies have employed RS technologies to measure and identify soil compaction so far. Changes in the Green Normalised Difference Vegetation measure (GNDVI), a measure created from the green and near-infrared spectral bands of spectral bands of imagery. However, the relationship between the cone penetrometer and NIR data was found to be too weak to identify compacted soil areas [24].

9.10.5 Crop Emergence and Density Detection

Grain and biomass yields, as well as the logistics of harvesting, can be significantly impacted by the geographical and temporal variabilities of crop populations and their densities within a field. When such information is timely made available, it can impact mid-season choices about pesticide, fertilizer, and herbicide applications, as well as replanting. High spatial resolution photos are used to quantify crop attributes, such as individual crop stands, sizes, and forms (e.g., area, diameter, main axis length, minor axis length), utilizing powerful computer vision algorithms and analytics that have recently been created.

These algorithms have demonstrated that crop development phases and picture spatial resolution affect how well such information may be extracted. For example, it has been discovered that photos taken during the early phases of development, with a resolution ranging from 3.88 μm to 2.4 mm, are beneficial for crop counting. Few, if any, research have examined the quantification of agricultural growth phases, despite current efforts being concentrated on the detection and counting of crop seedlings as well as the estimation of plant spacing. Accurate supply forecasting for crop sectors may be developed by integrating crop development phases with weather forecasts [25–29].

9.10.6 Yield Prediction

To get data on yield during harvest, some farmers use yield-monitoring devices installed on combines. When harvesting crops, a yield monitor usually combines yield data from several crop rows (for example, a contemporary corn combine usually utilizes a 6-, 8-, 12-, or 16-row head). As a result, crop yield per row detection becomes more difficult and yield maps might have extremely coarse resolutions. Studies have shown how RS imagery can be used to create high-resolution yield maps that evaluate within-field yield variability at both the field and landscape scales. By doing so, researchers can gain a better understanding of the total production potential of agricultural fields. These studies have used empirical approaches.

These studies predict crop yields with an R^2 range from 0.57 to 0.94 by using VIs obtained from RS imagery and fitting the data into machine learning algorithms. These experiments show that even using visible photography, crop production may be forecast with excellent accuracy. It has been demonstrated, however, that crop growth phases affect the accuracy of yield forecast models. For example, it has been discovered that yield prediction models are more accurate when they are based on footage obtained in the middle of the growing season as opposed to early development phases. However, minimizing possible agricultural production losses frequently depends on the capacity to anticipate crop output early in the growing season [30–35].

9.10.7 Assessing the Grain Quality

Because grain quality affects both the nutritional content and the production system's profitability, it is just as significant as grain quantity. Improved knowledge of grain quality before harvest is crucial to assist logistics and handling choices linked to feedstock. There aren't many studies out there right now that concentrate on evaluating grain quality using RS. According to Jensen et al. [36], there has been modest success (R^2 in the 0.64–0.85) in predicting grain protein using RS imaging. They have also emphasized the significance of spectral resolution and the development stage for a precise evaluation of grain protein. Given that genotype has a significant influence on yield quality, more research should be done on the application of RS for mapping crop genotypes, and the function of genotypes in grain quality assessment is thus warranted [37–39].

9.10.8 Assessing the Crop Residue

Agricultural production and soil quality can only be increased by wise agricultural residue management, which also reduces operational difficulties and harmful environmental effects associated with excessive residue. Using multispectral satellite imagery from Landsat ETM+ and Landsat OLI, Sharma et al. [40] found that hyperspectral TIR imagery from NASA's Airborne Terrestrial Application Sensor (ATLAS) was able to distinguish between varying heat capacities between soil and residues in different residue management systems more effectively than VIS and NIR imagery. The spectral indices derived from VIS and NIR bands, such as the Normalized Difference Tillage Index (NDTI), could be useful in differentiating the extent of residue cover related to different tillage practices for maize and soybean fields in South Central Nebraska. These studies stayed mostly at a landscape size and paid little attention to within-field variations in residue management because of the limited spatial resolution of satellite photography. The fact that relatively few studies have examined site-specific tillage techniques for residue management suggests that there may be opportunities to monitor residue using UAS-based technologies, which will aid in our understanding of how residue management affects the dynamics of soil, water, and nutrients.

9.11 CONCLUSION

Artificial Intelligence is rapidly expanding its potential in all areas and demonstrating its potential impact on environmental sustainability. With its diverse range of applications, AI can help create a more sustainable future for humanity by predicting environmental trends, designing resilient infrastructure, and optimizing resource usage. We can create a sustainable future that balances human growth with the preservation of the rich biodiversity and natural resources of our world by incorporating AI technology into the ecosystem.

REFERENCES

[1] Jensen, J.R. and Cowen, D.C., 1999. Remote sensing of urban/suburban infrastructure and socio-economic attributes. *Photogrammetric Engineering and Remote Sensing*, 65, pp. 611–622.
[2] Avtar, R., Kumar, P., Singh, C.K., Sahu, N., Verma, R.L., Thakur, J.K. and Mukherjee, S., 2013. Hydrogeochemical assessment of groundwater quality of Bundelkhand, India using statistical approach. *Water Quality, Exposure and Health*, 5, pp. 105–115.
[3] Dudhani, S., Sinha, A.K. and Inamdar, S.S., 2006. Assessment of small hydropower potential using remote sensing data for sustainable development in India. *Energy Policy*, 34(17), pp. 3195–3205.
[4] Franklin, S.E., 2001. *Remote Sensing for Sustainable Forest Management*. CRC Press.
[5] Huete, A.R., Liu, H.Q., Batchily, K.V. and Van Leeuwen, W.J.D.A., 1997. A comparison of vegetation indices over a global set of TM images for EOS-MODIS. *Remote Sensing of Environment*, 59(3), pp. 440–451.
[6] Wilson, J.S., Clay, M., Martin, E., Stuckey, D. and Vedder-Risch, K., 2003. Evaluating environmental influences of zoning in urban ecosystems with remote sensing. *Remote Sensing of Environment*, 86(3), pp. 303–321.
[7] Van Westen, C.J., 2000. The modeling of landslide hazards using GIS. *Surveys in Geophysics*, 21(2–3), pp. 241–255.
[8] Lary, D.J., Alavi, A.H., Gandomi, A.H. and Walker, A.L., 2016. Machine learning in geosciences and remote sensing. *Geoscience Frontiers*, 7(1), pp. 3–10.
[9] Singh, T., Sharma, S. and Nagesh, S., 2017. Socio-economic status scales updated for 2017. *International Journal of Research in Medical Sciences*, 5(7), pp. 3264–3267.

[10] Merghadi, A., Yunus, A.P., Dou, J., Whiteley, J., ThaiPham, B., Bui, D.T., Avtar, R. and Abderrahmane, B., 2020. Machine learning methods for landslide susceptibility studies: A comparative overview of algorithm performance. *Earth-Science Reviews*, 207, 103225.

[11 Duro, D.C., Coops, N.C., Wulder, M.A. and Han, T., 2007. Development of a large area biodiversity monitoring system driven by remote sensing. *Progress in Physical Geography*, 31(3), pp. 235–260.

[12] Turner, B.L., Kasperson, R.E., Matson, P.A., McCarthy, J.J., Corell, R.W., Christensen, L., Eckley, N., Kasperson, J.X., Luers, A., Martello, M.L. and Polsky, C., 2003. A framework for vulnerability analysis in sustainability science. *Proceedings of the National Academy of Sciences*, 100(14), pp. 8074–8079.

[13] King, M.D., Platnick, S., Menzel, W.P., Ackerman, S.A. and Hubanks, P.A., 2013. Spatial and temporal distribution of clouds observed by MODIS onboard the Terra and Aqua satellites. *IEEE Transactions on Geoscience and Remote Sensing*, 51(7), pp. 3826–3852.

[14] Romero-Gainza, E. and Stewart, C., 2023. AI-driven validation of digital agriculture models. *Sensors*, 23(3), p. 1187.

[15] Eli-Chukwu, N.C., 2019. Applications of artificial intelligence in agriculture: A review. *Engineering, Technology & Applied Science Research*, 9(4), pp. 4377–4383.

[16] Awika, H.O., Bedre, R., Yeom, J., Marconi, T.G., Enciso, J., Mandadi, K.K., Jung, J. and Avila, C.A., 2019. Developing growth-associated molecular markers via high-throughput phenotyping in spinach. *Plant Genome*, 12, pp. 1–19.

[17] Jung, J., Maeda, M., Chang, A., Bhandari, M., Ashapure, A. and Landivar-Bowles, J., 2021. The potential of remote sensing and artificial intelligence as tools to improve the resilience of agriculture production systems. *Current Opinion in Biotechnology*, 70, pp. 15–22.

[18] Vaze, J., Teng, J. and Spencer, G., 2010. Impact of DEM accuracy and resolution on topographic indices. *Environmental Modelling & Software*, 25, pp. 1086–1098.

[19] Allred, B., Eash, N., Freeland, R., Martinez, L. and Wishart, D.B., 2018. Effective and efficient agricultural drainage pipe mapping with UAS thermal infrared imagery: A case study. *Agricultural Water Management*, 197, pp. 132–137.

[20] Schwarz, G.E., Hoos, A.B., Alexander, R.B. and Smith, R.A., 2006. The SPARROW surface water-quality model: Theory, application and user documentation. *US Geological Survey Techniques and Methods Report B*, 6, p. 248.

[21] Koch, S., Bauwe, A. and Lennartz, B., 2013. Application of the SWAT model for a tile-drained lowland catchment in North-Eastern Germany on subbasin scale. *Water Resources Management*, 27, pp. 791–805.

[22] Babaeian, E., Sadeghi, M., Franz, T.E., Jones, S. and Tuller, M., 2018. Mapping soil moisture with the OPtical TRApezoid Model (OPTRAM) based on long-term MODIS observations. *Remote Sensing of Environment*, 211, pp. 425–440.

[23] Verstraeten, W.W., Veroustraete, F. and Feyen, J., 2008. Assessment of evapotranspiration and soil moisture content across different scales of observation. *Sensors*, 8, pp. 70–117.

[24] Wells, L.G., Stombaugh, T.S. and Shearer, S.A., 2013. *Application and Assessment of Precision Deep Tillage*; American Society of Agricultural and Biological Engineers: St. Joseph, MI, Volume 1.

[25] Jin, X., Liu, S., Baret, F., Hemerlé, M. and Comar, A., 2017. Estimates of plant density of wheat crops at emergence from very low altitude UAV imagery. *Remote Sensing of Environment*, 198, pp. 105–114.

[26] Fleming, J. and Robertson, R.G., 2003. Fire management tech tips: The Osborne fire finder, Tech. Rep. 0351 1311-SDTDC, USDA Forest Service, October.

[27] Jones, M., Smith, P. and Patel, R., 2021. The role of artificial intelligence in environmental conservation. *Nature Sustainability*, 4(7), pp. 546–558.

[28] Kaur, A., Chen, Y. and Gupta, A., 2022. AI and biodiversity monitoring: A comparative study of camera traps and acoustic monitoring. *Biodiversity and Conservation*, 31(2), pp. 527–543.

[29] Li, Y., Wang, C. and Chen, J. 2022. AI applications in climate change mitigation and adaptation: A review. *Journal of Environmental Management*, 303, 114151.

[30] Doraiswamy, P.C., Sinclair, T.R., Hollinger, S., Akhmedov, B., Stern, A. and Prueger, J., 2005. Application of MODIS derived parameters for regional crop yield assessment. *Remote Sensing of Environment*, 97, pp. 192–202.

[31] Marconi, R., Brown, T. and Martinez, G., 2021. AI-powered smart cities: Advancements and opportunities for sustainable urban planning. *Sustainability*, 13(5), 2556.

[32] Miller, B., Turner, W. and Comber, A., 2023. Challenges and opportunities for data collaboration in AI-driven conservation projects. *Environmental Research Letters*, 18(3), 035009.

[33] Ng, L., Park, J. and Johnson, R., 2023. Ethical considerations in AI applications for conservation: Lessons from anti-poaching efforts in Kenya. *Conservation Ethics*, 9(1), pp. 34–48.

[34] Rayhan, A., 2023. AI and the environment: Toward sustainable development and conservation. Research Gate, July 10.

[35] Rayhan, A., 2023. The role of artificial intelligence in climate change mitigation and adaptation. *Artificial Intelligence*. doi: 10.13140/RG.2.2.10346.70087

[36] Jensen, J., 2007. Remote sensing of soils, minerals, and geomorphology. In *Remote Sensing of the Environment*; Pearson Education: London, pp. 457–524.

[37] Robinson, K., Garcia, S. and Lee, D., 2020. AI for wildlife conservation: Current applications and future directions. *Conservation Letters*, 13(2), e12696.

[38] Santos, M., Zhang, L. and Chaves, A., 2022. AI-based early warning systems for extreme weather events: A case study in Bangladesh. *Environmental Science & Policy*, 125, pp. 39–47.

[39] Williams, A., Jackson, L. and Adams, S., 2021. AI-driven precision agriculture for sustainable food production: A case study from California. *Frontiers in Sustainable Food Systems*, 5, 614216.

[40] Sharma, V., Irmak, S., Kilic, A., Sharma, V., Gilley, J.E., Meyer, G.E., Knezevic, S.Z. and Marx, D., 2016. Quantification and mapping of surface residue cover for maize and soybean fields in South Central Nebraska. *Transactions of the ASABE*, 59, pp. 925–939.

10 Artificial Intelligence for Energy Storage System

Manoj Singh Adhikari, Yogesh Kumar Verma, Manoj Sindhwani, and Shippu Sachdeva
School of Electronics and Electrical Engineering, Lovely Professional University, Phagwara, India

Manoj Kumar Shukla
Department of Robotics and Automation, Symbiosis Institute of Technology, Pune, India

10.1 INTRODUCTION

Energy Storage Systems (ESS) play an important role in stabilizing and modernizing energy infrastructures in the entire world. As the demand is increasing for efficient energy, reliable, and sustainable solutions, the importance of ESS cannot be overstated [1–4]. Energy Storage Systems consist of technologies and solutions designed to capture and store energy for subsequent use. Fundamentally it acts as a buffer between energy production and consumption. In this situation, ESS plays a significant role in balancing demand and supply in power grids [4–8].

As the increasing global energy demands and the imperative to minimize reliance on fossil fuels, ESS has emerged as a cornerstone in the transition for a more sustainable and resilient energy ecosystem. For efficient energy capture and distribution from recurrent renewable sources (i.e., solar and wind), ESS reports the characteristic variability of these resources, guaranteeing a reliable and steady power supply [9–14]. ESS plays an important role in modernizing the electrical grid for the integration of renewable energy sources. It serves as a bridge between intermittent energy generation (e.g., solar and wind) and the constant power demand. Artificial Intelligence (AI) has emerged as a powerful tool to optimize the efficiency, performance, and reliability of these energy storage systems [15–19].

AI for energy storage refers to the application of Data-Driven (DD) techniques and Machine Learning (ML) algorithms to improve the control and management of energy storage technologies. The convergence of AI and energy storage grips the probability of reforming the way we store and use electrical energy, facing challenges, that is, cost optimization, grid stability, and energy supply-demand balancing [20–24]. AI is composed to revolutionize the energy storage industry by revealing new levels of flexibility, reliability, and efficiency. With the help of data and advanced

DOI: 10.1201/9781003546382-10

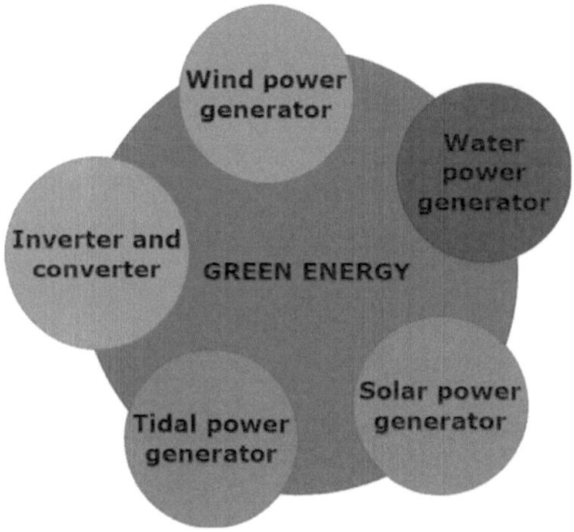

FIGURE 10.1 Foundation of green energy.

algorithms, AI-empowered energy storage systems have the potential to speed the transition to a more sustainable energy future [25–31]. However, it is important to discuss challenges associated with data, interoperability, and regulations, and appreciate the profits of this transformative technology. Figure 10.1 shows the foundation of green energy.

In this chapter types of energy storage technologies, an overview of AI, improved grid stability and reliability, data acquisition and sensors, types of data required in AI-based energy storage systems, predictive modeling for energy demand, machine learning algorithms for ESS, communication protocols for energy storage system, and current challenges in AI for energy storage are discussed as given below.

10.2 TYPES OF ENERGY STORAGE TECHNOLOGIES

Energy storage systems include a wide range of technologies, individually with unique applications, advantages, and characteristics. These technologies consist of:

1. ***Pumped Hydro Storage***: Relies on gravitational potential energy with the help of pumping water to a higher elevation for later release through turbines to produce power.
2. ***Battery Storage***: Uses chemical reactions to store and release electrical energy. Variants contain lead-acid, lithium-ion, and flow batteries.
3. ***Flywheel Energy Storage***: Uses the kinetic energy of a spinning mass to store and release energy.
4. ***Thermal Storage***: Stores energy in the form of heat, further can be used for power production, Cooling, or heating.
5. ***Increased Renewable Energy Capacity***: Many nations have continued to invest in and expand their renewable energy capacity. Solar and wind power installations have seen substantial growth globally. The rate of renewable

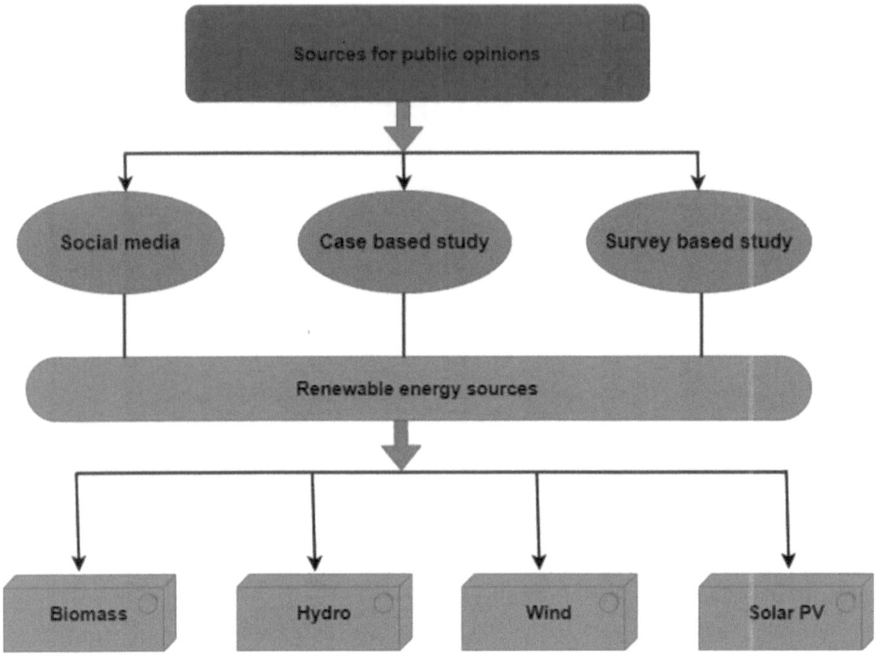

FIGURE 10.2 Renewable energy sources and public opinions.

energy technologies has also been reduced, making them more competitive with traditional fossil fuel-based sources. Figure 10.2 shows the renewable energy sources and public opinions.

6. ***Supercapacitors***: Store and release energy electrostatically. It offers fast charging and discharging capability. Hydrogen Storage: Converts electrical energy into hydrogen gas through electrolysis. Further, it can be used for several applications.
7. ***Compressed Air Energy Storage***: The energy is stored in compressed air within underground reservoirs. The compressed air is released when it is desirable to drive turbines.

To decouple energy production from consumption, all the above technologies contribute to a more resilient and adaptive energy grid. Energy storage systems are instrumental in confirming a sustainable, efficient, and reliable energy supply. Through various innovative technologies, ESS reports the challenges modeled by recurrent renewable sources and supports the global transition concerning a cleaner and additional secure energy future. This guide will investigate greater into the intricacies of ESS, discovering the applications, benefits, and advancements that are determining the landscape of energy storage. Figure 10.3 shows the solar tower system.

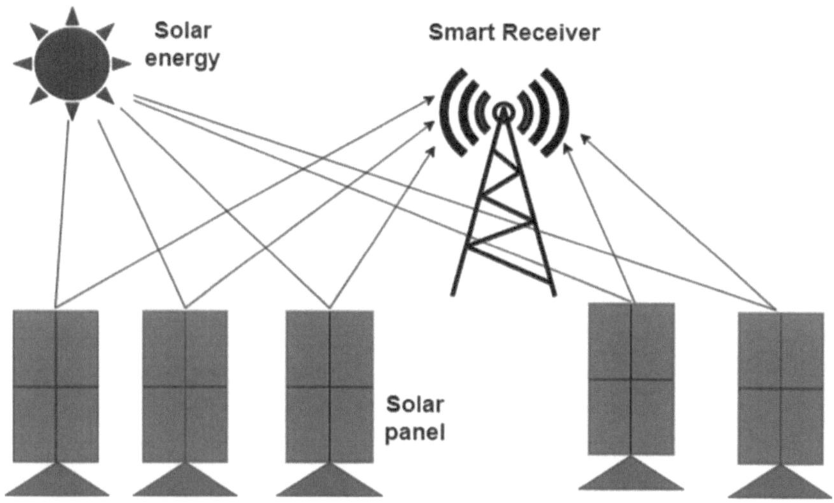

FIGURE 10.3 Solar tower system.

10.3 OVERVIEW OF ARTIFICIAL INTELLIGENCE

Artificial Intelligence (AI) signifies a transformative technology that simulates human intelligence, allowing machines to execute tasks that involve human cognition. The AI-based applications across a wide range of industries, decision-making, revolutionizing processes, and efficiency. AI denotes the simulation of human intelligence in machines, permitting them to problem-solve, learn, and make conclusions autonomously. It includes several subfields, that is, machine learning, natural language processing, and computer vision.

1. ***Computer Vision***: It is required for the enabling machines to interpret and investigate visual data, enabling tasks such as facial recognition, object recognition, and image analysis.
2. ***Machine Learning***: Machine Learning (ML) is a subset of AI that permits machines to learn patterns and perform predictions from data, without being programmed. Figure 10.4 shows the schematic of machine learning models.
3. ***Natural Language Processing***: Natural Language Processing (NLP) is helpful to provide empowerment to machines for interpreting, understanding, and generating human language, aiding tasks such as sentiment analysis, translation, and chatbots.
4. ***Deep Learning***: Deep Learning (DL) is a specific form of ML that includes neural networks with multiple layers, permitting complex pattern acknowledgment.

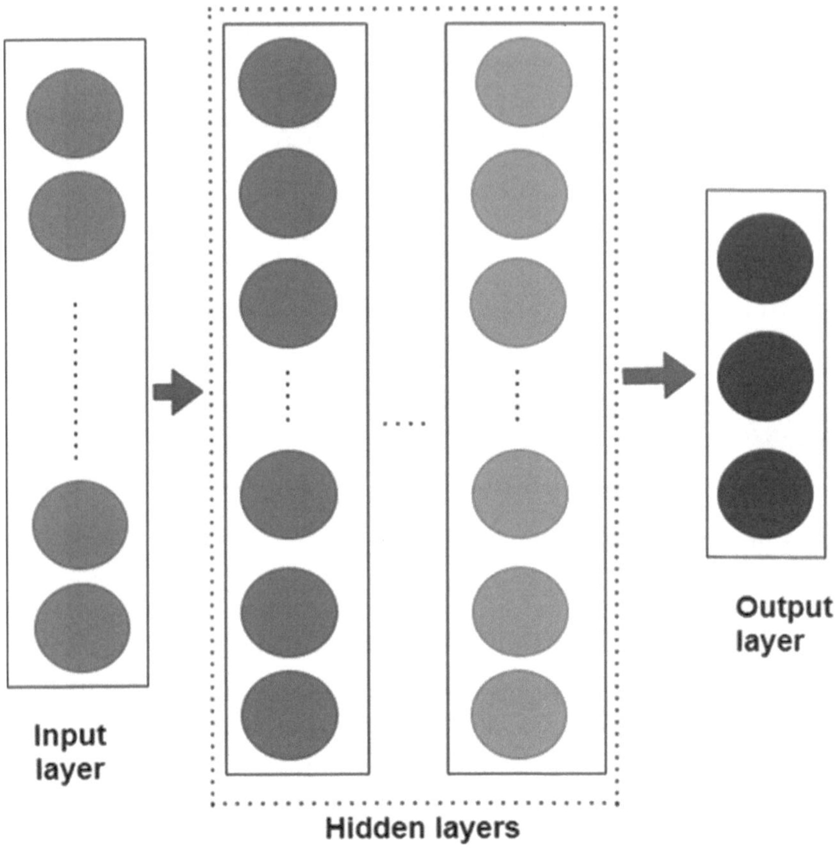

FIGURE 10.4 A schematic machine learning models.

10.4 IMPROVED GRID STABILITY AND RELIABILITY

Grid stability and reliability are dominant in confirming a consistent and secure energy supply to customers. The major role of AI in the integration of energy systems has suggestively contributed to enhancing both grid stability and reliability. Figure 10.5 shows the grid-connected photovoltaic (PV) and energy storage charging station. There are numerous ways in which AI attains all these objectives.

1. ***Predictive Maintenance and Fault Detection***: AI-powered systems investigate information from many sensors to predict equipment failures before they occur. By detecting irregularities in real time, maintenance can be planned proactively, diminishing the risk of unexpected outages and disturbances.
2. ***Load Forecasting and Demand Response***: AI-based algorithms examine historic consumption patterns, weather forecasts, and additional pertinent data to predict accurately future energy demand. This data enables values

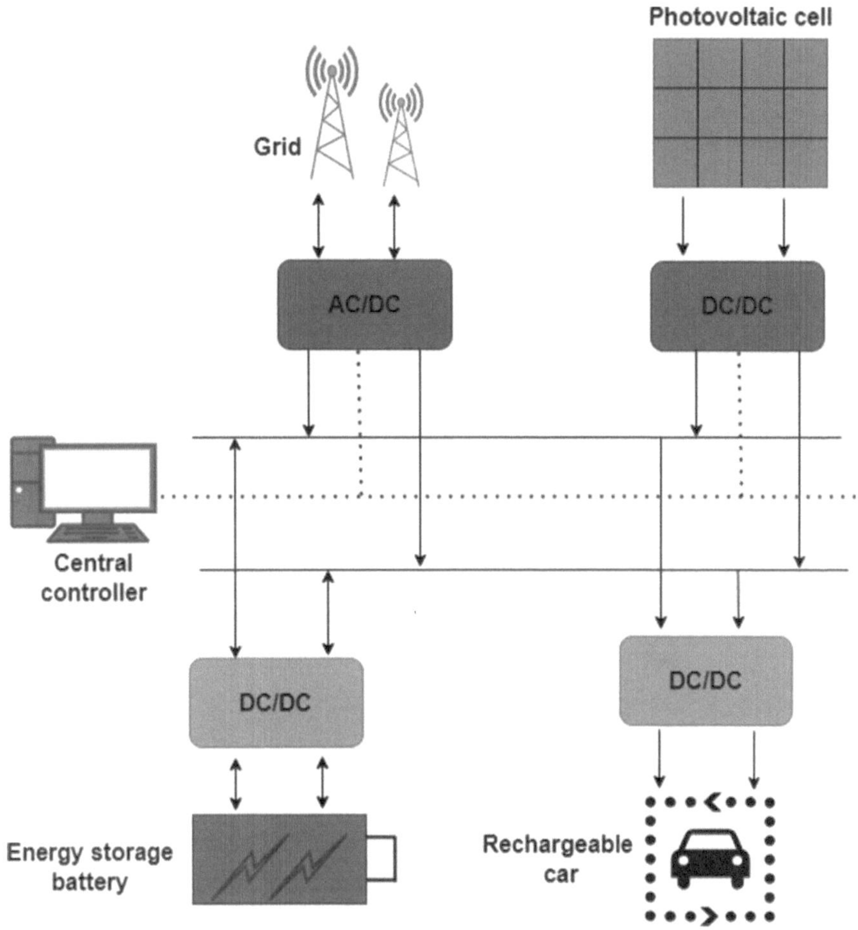

FIGURE 10.5 Grid-connected PV and energy storage charging station.

to regulate their generation and distribution plans, guaranteeing that supply matches demand, thus preventing overloads.

3. ***Voltage and Frequency Regulation***: AI-based control systems monitor voltage and frequency levels continuously in the grid. It can make quick modifications to stabilize these parameters, confirming that electrical machinery receives a consistent and reliable power supply.
4. ***Integration of Renewable Energy Sources***: Renewable energy sources (e.g. solar and wind) can be variable and intermittent. With the support of AI integrate these sources seamlessly into the grid by forecasting their output and managing with conventional power sources to sustain stability even with fluctuations in production of renewable energy.
5. ***Grid Balancing and Frequency Control***: AI-based algorithms quickly answer to changes in load or generation. It automatically regulates the output of power plants or storage arrangements to maintain the grid's frequency within suitable limits.

6. ***Cybersecurity and Threat Detection***: AI-based schemes are perfectly working to monitor network traffic and recognize suspicious activities suggestive of cybersecurity threats. By quickly detection and replying to probable attacks, the grid's reliability and integrity are protected.
7. ***Weather Forecast Integration***: AI-based programs can integrate weather forecasts into grid operation approaches. This allows services to prepare for risky weather conditions, change the generation strategies, and implement load-shedding plans when essential to maintain stability.
8. ***Hydrogen Energy***: Hydrogen is emerging as a potential green energy carrier. Hydrogen is produced through electrolysis powered by renewable energy. Its use in industry, transportation, and energy storage, contributes to a cleaner sustainable energy system. The block diagram of hydrogen production from seawater is shown in Figure 10.6.

Hence, the integration of AI in energy grids signifies an enormous step toward achieving improved stability and reliability. With autonomous decision-making,

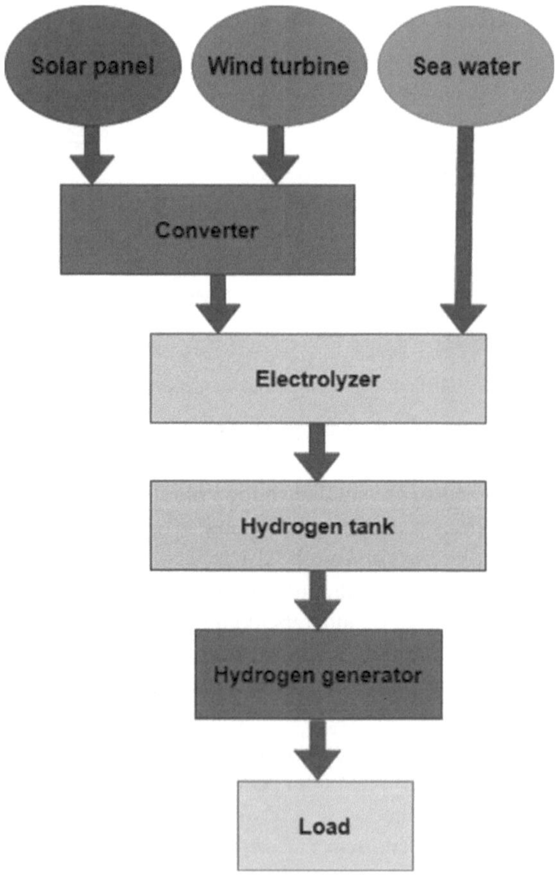

FIGURE 10.6 Hydrogen energy production from seawater.

AI technologies allow energy systems to familiarize themselves and respond to changing conditions in real time. This leads to a more robust and reliable energy infrastructure. It can provide better assistance to customers, even in the appearance of unexpected challenges.

10.5 DATA ACQUISITION AND SENSORS

Data acquisition and sensors serve as the basis for AI-oriented energy storage systems. It empowers the gathering of important information related to the performance, state, and environmental conditions of the system. There is a lot of importance in data acquisition and the role of sensors in optimizing energy storage operations.

10.5.1 Role of Data Acquisition

Data acquisition consists of gathering and recording several types of data from sensors. In ESS, data acquisition plays a key role in providing the information required for informed decision-making and performance analysis.

10.5.2 Types of Sensors in ESS

There are various types of sensors in ESS:

1. ***State-of-Charge (SOC) Sensors***: For the measurement of the current charge level of a battery or ESS. This data is important to consider the existing energy capacity and confirm optimal usage.
2. ***State-of-Health (SOH) Sensors***: To monitor the complete health and state of the energy storage system, delivering perceptions into factors such as cycle life, battery degradation, and performance over time.
3. ***Temperature Sensors***: These sensors are used for monitoring the temperature of various components in the energy storage system. This is useful for avoiding overheating, so that not reduce the efficiency, and also important concerning safety hazards.
4. ***Voltage and Current Sensors***: Voltage and current sensors are used to gather data in real time related to electrical parameters, permitting precise monitoring of charging and discharging progressions.
5. ***Flow Sensors***: It is used to measure the flow of fluids in a system, confirming that cooling and operative processes are working optimally.
6. ***Data Accuracy and Precision***: The accuracy and precision of sensor data are very important so for the measurement of data it must be ensured. dominant. Regular maintenance and calibration of sensors are essential to assurance consistent measurements. In addition, data validation techniques are used to classify and rectify any erroneous readings.
7. ***Data Communication and Integration***: The sensors are used for the data collection and the data is efficiently transmitted to a central monitoring and control system. It consists of communication protocols such as Modbus, CANbus, IoT protocols MQTT for real-time data transfer.

8. ***Data Logging and Storage***: The useful stored data is logged and stored for trend identification, historical analysis, and compliance reporting. Scalable and secure data storage solutions are crucial to achieving the large volumes of data produced by sensors.

Hence, for the AI-enhanced energy storage system the data acquisition and sensors are the foundation elements. It provides the vital information desirable to optimize operations, informed decisions, and confirm the performance and reliability of the system. With accurate and reliable sensor data, AI models efficiently improve the effectiveness and efficiency of energy storage solutions, contributing towards further sustainable and resilient energy infrastructure.

10.6 TYPES OF DATA REQUIRED IN AI-BASED ENERGY STORAGE SYSTEMS

For the implementation of AI successfully in an ESS, a diverse range of data is required. This data includes real-time, historical, and external factors that collectively inform decision-making and optimize operations. There are different types of data required which are explained as follows:

10.6.1 Historical Data

Historical data delivers perceptions of past patterns, performance, and trends. It creates the basis for training machine learning models and finding baseline expectations. For ESS, the key historical data includes:

1. ***Load Profiles***: It provides information about records of historical energy consumption patterns at different time intervals (i. e. seasonal, hourly, daily).
2. ***Environmental Conditions***: There are various factors for historical records as air quality temperature, and humidity in the vicinity of the energy storage system.
3. ***Grid Data***: The information related to grid conditions, that is, frequency, voltage levels, and stability metrics over time.
4. ***Charge and Discharge Cycles***: It gives information on how the energy storage system has been used earlier, comprising the frequency and charge-discharge cycles.

10.6.2 Real-Time Data

Real-time data is key for instant decision-making. It confirms the ESS responds dynamically to current conditions. It contains:

1. ***Current State Parameters***: Instantaneous readings of voltage, current, state of charge, state of health, and temperature. Load and Demand Data: Current energy consumption patterns, which help in load forecasting and demand response.

2. ***Grid Conditions***: Real-time information on grid voltage, frequency, and other parameters necessary for grid integration and stability.

10.6.3 Weather Data

Weather data is particularly important for ESS integrated with renewable energy sources. It helps in anticipating and responding to variations in renewable energy generation. Relevant weather data includes:

1. ***Solar Radiation***: The intensity and duration of sunlight, are crucial for systems integrated with solar energy.
2. ***Wind Speed and Direction***: For systems integrated with wind energy, this data informs about potential fluctuations in generation.
3. ***Temperature and Humidity***: These factors affect the efficiency and performance of energy storage systems and associated components.

10.6.4 Market and Price Data

For ESS integrated into grid systems with market participation, market and price data is essential. This includes:

1. ***Energy Prices***: Information about current and forecasted energy prices, helping in optimizing charge and discharge cycles.
2. ***Grid Frequency and Ancillary Services Markets***: Data relevant to grid balancing and frequency regulation services.

10.6.5 Operational Data

Data related to the actual operations and maintenance of the ESS is crucial for performance monitoring and maintenance planning. This includes:

1. ***Cycle Count and Depth***: Information on the number and depth of charge-discharge cycles the energy storage system has undergone. Hence, the main key factor for the successful implementation of AI in energy storage systems is the accessibility and quality of diverse data types. By considering real-time, historical, and operational data, AI models are capable of informed decisions, contributing to more reliable, optimized energy storage operations, and efficient energy infrastructure.

10.7 PREDICTIVE MODELING FOR ENERGY DEMAND

One of the critical applications of AI in energy storage systems is predictive modeling for energy demand. It includes historical and real-time data to estimate future energy consumption outlines. The process, benefits, and key considerations of predictive modeling for energy demand as

10.7.1 Process of Predictive Modeling

1. ***Data Collection and Preparation***: Collection of historical energy consumption data, with pertinent landscapes as time of day, day of the week, and temperature.
2. ***Model Selection***: To select an appropriate predictive modeling technique. The basic approaches include time series analysis, regression models, and machine learning algorithms (such as Gradient Boosting, Neural Networks, and Random Forest).
3. ***Training and Validation***: Use historical data to train the predictive model. Prove the model's performance using an individual dataset to confirm it generalizes well to new data.
4. ***Prediction and Evaluation***: Apply the trained model to real-time or future data to generate energy demand forecasts. Evaluate the model's accuracy and adjust as needed.

10.7.2 Benefits of Predictive Modeling for Energy Demand

1. ***Improved Grid Planning***: Accurate demand forecasts enable utilities and grid operators to plan for infrastructure upgrades and expansions to meet future energy needs.
2. ***Optimized Resource Allocation***: Predictive modeling helps allocate resources efficiently, such as scheduling maintenance during periods of lower demand.
3. ***Integration of Renewable Energy***: Forecasting energy demand aids in effectively integrating flexible renewable energy sources like solar and wind into the grid.
4. ***Demand Response Programs***: Enables benefits to realize demand reaction initiatives, incentivizing consumers to modify their energy consumption through peak periods.

Hence, predictive modeling for energy demand is a powerful tool that permits effectiveness and grid operators to propose, optimize operations, and integrate renewable energy sources effectively. By leveraging AI-driven forecasting techniques, energy storage systems can contribute to a more reliable, sustainable, and efficient energy infrastructure.

10.8 MACHINE LEARNING ALGORITHMS FOR ESS

Machine learning algorithms play a crucial role in optimizing the performance and operation of ESS. These algorithms leverage data from various sensors, historical patterns, and real-time information to make intelligent decisions about how to charge, discharge, and manage energy within the system. Here are some key machine-learning algorithms commonly used for ESS:

1. ***Regression Analysis***: Linear Regression is used to model the connection between dependent and independent variables. In ESS, it can be employed for tasks like expecting the State of Charge (SOC) or State of Health (SOH) of batteries based on historical data.
2. ***Time Series Analysis***: Autoregressive Integrated Moving Average (ARIMA) is particularly useful for forecasting energy demand and generation patterns over time. It can assist in optimizing the charging and discharging schedules of ESS.
3. ***Classification Algorithms***: Support Vector Machines (SVM), Random Forests, and Neural Networks (NN) come under this category. All these algorithms are used to classify events in an ESS (i.e., fault detection or decisive the optimal operational mode) based on current conditions.
4. ***Clustering Algorithms***: K-Means clustering is used for grouping analogous operating conditions, which supports recognizing optimal charging and discharging strategies for diverse clusters of situations.
5. ***Reinforcement Learning***: Deep Q-Networks (DQN) reinforcement learning is used for the optimization of control policies for ESS. DQN learns the best action to take in different states to maximize rewards, that is, increase energy efficiency and reduce the cost.
6. ***Neural Networks***: Neural networks use deep learning models. It is used for complex tasks such as anomaly detection, predicting battery degradation, and state estimation.

Hence, the selection of the appropriate algorithm depends on the desired outcome, available data, and application. Often, a combination of all algorithms is used in a hybrid method to address various characteristics of energy storage system optimization. Real-time data processing and model arrangement are key factors for practical implementation. Figure 10.7 illustrates the opportunities for renewable energy sources.

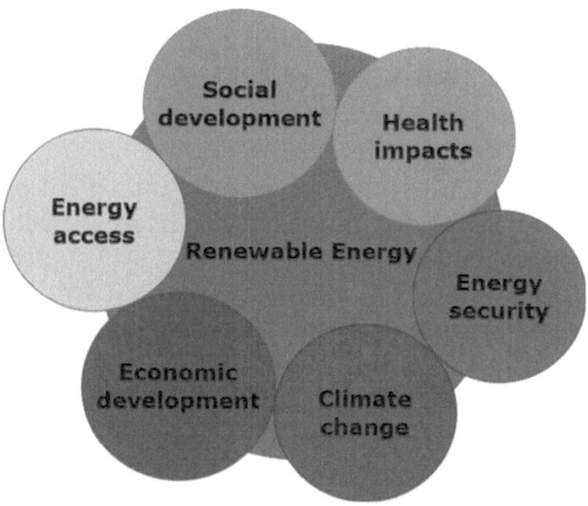

FIGURE 10.7 Opportunities of renewable energy sources.

10.9 COMMUNICATION PROTOCOLS FOR ENERGY STORAGE SYSTEM

For the energy-efficient exchange of information or data between various components in an energy storage system, the choice of appropriate communication protocols is very critical. The selection of appropriate protocols guarantees the seamless coordination, control, and monitoring of the process. Communication protocols which are mostly used in ESS are given as follows:

10.9.1 Supervisory Control and Data Acquisition

Supervisory Control and Data Acquisition (SCADA) is the most widely used control system architecture which aids in remote monitoring and control of industrial processes. The operator can have accessibility to real-time data which further allows him/her to interact with the ESS and monitor it by making appropriate decisions.

10.9.2 Distributed Network Protocol 3

Distributed Network Protocol 3 (DNP3) protocol is generally used for electric utility automation systems. Point-to-point as well as multipoint configurations are feasible in this case. It is robust and reliable.

10.9.3 Message Queuing Telemetry Transport

Message Queuing Telemetry Transport (MQTT) which is a lightweight, publish-subscribe messaging protocol is compatible with environments where the bandwidth is restricted, and the networks are unreliable. Efficient and reliable communication between devices is possible.

10.9.4 Modbus

Modbus is an industrial networking protocol and is widely accepted for its simplicity and versatility, which makes it suitable for various types of devices and equipment.

The reliable and effective operation of an energy storage system depends on choosing the right communication protocol. System architecture, scalability, security requirements, and compatibility with existing infrastructure are just a few examples of the variables that affect protocol choice. Each of the protocols listed here has unique advantages and applications, and it's crucial to take these things into account while developing and putting an ESS into use.

10.10 CURRENT CHALLENGES IN AI FOR ENERGY STORAGE

The field of AI for energy storage faces several challenges. These challenges arise from the complex nature of energy systems and the integration of AI technologies. The key challenges are listed below:

1. ***Data Availability and Quality***: Poor data might make it difficult for AI models to be trained and perform well. It can also be difficult to gather reliable data from a variety of sources.

2. ***Interpretability and Explainability***: A lot of AI models, in actual deep learning models, are repeatedly regarded as "black boxes," making it challenging to understand how they come to their conclusions or suggestions.
3. ***Scalability and Generalizability***: Ensuring that AI models created for a particular energy storage system can be expanded upon, extended, and used with bigger systems.
4. ***Model Complexity and Training Time***: Complex AI models may need a lot of processing power and training time, which might be a barrier in real-world scenarios.
5. AI applications with real-time processing and response times.
6. ***Integration with Existing Infrastructure***: It can be difficult, especially in brownfield projects, to ensure seamless integration of AI-enhanced energy storage systems with current technologies and infrastructure.

Researchers, business leaders, lawmakers, and regulators must work cooperatively to address these issues. To improve the capabilities and lessen the constraints of AI in the field of energy storage, ongoing research, and development are essential.

10.11 CONCLUSION

The development of an energy infrastructure that is robust and sustainable will be significantly aided by the incorporation of Artificial Intelligence (AI) methods into Energy Storage Systems (ESS). This chapter gave a thorough review of AI's use in ESS, emphasizing its potential to solve some of the major problems that traditional energy storage systems face. With the use of machine learning algorithms, ESS can now anticipate trends in energy consumption, adjust to changing inputs from renewable energy sources, and improve charge-discharge cycles. ESS can make dynamic decisions in real time using reinforcement learning techniques, resulting in optimal energy use. The dependability and performance of energy storage systems are further enhanced using neural networks, which improve pattern identification and defect detection. It's crucial to recognize the difficulties that come with this paradigm change, though. To guarantee the secure functioning of AI-powered ESS, effective data collecting, privacy protection, and cybersecurity measures must be put in place. Additionally, continual research and development activities are necessary due to the cost and scalability issues associated with using AI technology in energy storage systems. Even further breakthroughs in energy storage are possible in the future. We foresee additional development and innovation in the field of energy storage as AI technologies advance. In addition to making the electricity system more dependable and sustainable, this will be essential to meeting the world's renewable energy ambitions.

REFERENCES

[1] A. Entezari, A. Aslani, R. Zahedi, Y. Noorollahi, "Artificial intelligence and machine learning in energy systems: A bibliographic perspective," *Energy Strategy Reviews*, vol. 45, pp. 101017, 2023.

[2] A. Legala, X. Li, "Hybrid data-based modeling for the prediction and diagnostics of Li-ion battery thermal behaviors," *Energy and AI*, vol. 10, pp. 100194, 2022.

[3] R. Machlev, L. Heistrene, M. Perl, K. Y. Levy, J. Belikov, S. Mannor, Y. Levron, "Explainable Artificial Intelligence (XAI) techniques for energy and power systems: Review, challenges and opportunities," *Energy and AI*, vol. 9, pp. 100169, 2022.
[4] N. Kharlamova, S. Hashemi, C. Træholt, "Data-driven approaches for cyber defence of battery energy storage systems," *Energy and AI*, vol. 5, pp. 100095, 2021.
[5] D. Liu, Y. Chen, K. K. Chai, T. Zhang, M. Elkashlan, "Two-dimensional optimization on user association and green energy allocation for HetNets with hybrid energy sources," *IEEE Transactions on Communications*, vol. 63, no. 11, pp. 4111–4124, 2015.
[6] C. C. Lin, D. J. Deng, C. C. Kuo, Y. L. Liang, "Optimal charging control of energy storage and electric vehicle of an individual on the internet of energy with energy trading," *IEEE Transactions on Industrial Informatics*, vol. 14, no. 6, pp. 2570–2578, 2018.
[7] A. Tahsin, P. Roy, Md. A. Razzaque, Md. M. Rashid, M. Siraj, S. A. AlQahtani, Md. R. Hassan, M. M. Hassan, "Energy cooperation among sustainable base stations in multi-operator cellular networks," *IEEE Access*, vol. 11, pp. 19405–19417, 2023.
[8] A. Jahid, M. S. Hossain, M. K. H. Monju, M. F. Rahman, M. F. Hossain, "Techno-economic and energy efficiency analysis of optimal power supply solutions for green cellular base stations," *IEEE Access*, vol. 8, pp. 43776–43795, 2020.
[9] M. Sadiq, S. W. Ali, Y. Terriche, M. U. Mutarraf, M. A. Hassan, K. Hamid, Z. Ali, J. Y. Sze, C. L. Su, J. M. Guerrero, "Future greener seaports: A review of new infrastructure, challenges, and energy efficiency measures," *IEEE Access*, vol. 9, pp. 75568–75587, 2021.
[10] C. Chen, B. He, X. Tang, "Green-aware workload scheduling in geographically distributed data centers," *IEEE International Conference on Cloud Computing Technology and Science Proceedings*, pp. 82–89, 2012.
[11] S. Homsi, S. Liu, G. A. Chaparro-Baquero, O. Bai, S. Ren, G. Quan, "Workload consolidation for cloud data centers with guaranteed qos using request reneging," *IEEE Transactions on Parallel and Distributed Systems*, vol. 28, no. 7, pp. 2103–2116, 2016.
[12] Y. Jin, Y. Wen, Q. Chen, "Energy efficiency and server virtualization in data centers: An empirical investigation," *Proceedings IEEE INFOCOM Workshops*, pp. 133–138, 2012.
[13] J. Sekhar, G. Jeba, S. Durga, "A survey on energy efficient server consolidation through vm live migration," *International Journal of Advances in Engineering & Technology*, vol. 5, no. 1, pp. 515, 2012.
[14] Q. Fan, N. Ansari, X. Sun, "Energy driven avatar migration in green cloudlet networks," *IEEE Communications Letters*, vol. 21, no. 7, pp. 1601–1604, 2017.
[15] M. Dayarathna, Y. Wen, R. Fan, "Data center energy consumption modeling: A survey," *IEEE Communications Surveys Tutorials*, vol. 18, no. 1, pp. 732–794, 2016.
[16] S. M. B. Billah, K. M. Kabir, M. O. Islam, S. Barua, M. S. Mahmud, M. S. Hossain, "Hydrogen energy storage based green power plant in seashore of Bangladesh: Design and optimal cost analysis," *International Conference on Innovations in Green Energy and Healthcare Technologies (IGEHT)*, Coimbatore, India, pp. 1–5, 2017.
[17] Y. Goyal, M. S. Arya, S. Nagpal, "Energy efficient hybrid policy in green cloud computing," *International Conference on Green Computing and Internet of Things (ICGCIoT)*, Greater Noida, India, pp. 1065–1069, 2015.
[18] T. Bhattacharya, X. Qin, "Modeling energy efficiency of future green data centers," *International Green and Sustainable Computing Workshops (IGSC)*, Pullman, WA, pp. 1–3, 2020.
[19] B. Delinchant, F. Wurtz, S. Ploix, J. L. Schanen, Y. Marechal, "GreEn-ER living lab: A green building with energy aware occupants," *International Conference on Smart Cities and Green ICT Systems (SMARTGREENS)*, Rome, Italy, pp. 1–8, 2016.
[20] T. N. F. Dos Reis, M. M. Teixeira, C. D. Salles Soares Neto, "Relation of energy consumption in green cloud computing with big data," *IEEE Green Technologies Conference*, Denver, CO, USA, pp. 280–284, 2023.

[21] N. Kumar, "A study on green energy powered cognitive radio network for communication network architecture of smart grid," *International Innovative Applications of Computational Intelligence on Power, Energy and Controls with their Impact on Humanity (CIPECH)*, Ghaziabad, India, pp. 3–7, 2018.
[22] M. Sithan, L. L. Lai, "Application of green technologies in developing countries-reduced carbon emission and conservation of energy," *IEEE Power and Energy Society General Meeting*, Detroit, MI, USA, pp. 1–7, 2011.
[23] N. Yarlagadda, Y. K. Verma, M. S. Adhikari, V. Mishra, "Opto-VLSI devices and circuits for biomedical and healthcare applications," *A Review of Multi-material, Multi-gate MOSFET Structures*, pp. 29–40, CRC Press, 2023.
[24] X. Ma, S. Huang, Z. Li, Z. Yang, F. Li, L. Chen, "Quantitative evaluation method of green power development level," *International Conference on Power and Energy Systems (ICPES)*, Chengdu, China, pp. 420–425, 2020.
[25] N. Goyal, S. Sharma, A. Kumar Rana, S. L. Tripathi, *Internet of Things: Robotic and Drone Technology*, CRC Press, pp. 1–288, 2022.
[26] K. Zhang, J. Zhang, P. D. Xu, T. Gao, D. W. Gao, "Explainable AI in deep reinforcement learning models for power system emergency control," *IEEE Transactions on Computational Social Systems*, pp. 1–9, 2021.
[27] D. Ghai, S. L. Tripathi, S. Saxena, M. Chanda, M. Alazab, *Machine Learning Algorithms for Signal and Image Processing*, John Wiley & Sons, 2022.
[28] S. L. Tripathi, M. K. Dubey, V. Rishiwal, S. Padmanabhan, *Introduction to AI techniques for Renewable Energy System*, Taylor & Francis, Boca Raton, FL, 2021.
[29] S. L. Tripathi, S. Ganguli, A. Kumar, T. Magradze, *Intelligent Green Technologies for Sustainable Smart Cities*, Wiley, 2022.
[30] P. Umapathy, J. Hemanth, S. Khera, A. Inbamani, S. L. Tripathi, *Machine Learning and the Internet of Things in Solar Power Generation*, CRC Press, Boca Raton, FL, 2023.
[31] S. L. Tripathi, M. Mahmud, *Explainable Machine Learning Models and Architecture*, Wiley & Scrivener Publishing LLC, USA, 2023.

11 Revolutionizing Energy Storage in Electric and Hybrid Vehicles

Empowering the Future with Artificial Intelligence

Ayush Behera, Madhurima Sit, and Manjushree Nayak
NIST Institute of Science and Technology (Autonomous), Berhampur, India

11.1 INTRODUCTION TO ENERGY STORAGE SYSTEM

The idea behind energy storage is the preservation of generated energy in one state so that it can be used in a different one at a later date. An accumulator is a device that stores chemical energy. Energy naturally exists in a variety of phases and forms, each of which must be transformed into a different form to facilitate easier storage. Some of the favored forms of energy storage technology are batteries and dams. Glycogen and starch are two forms of energy storage found in living things. Camels can survive in endless deserts thanks to their high water storage capacity. Intermittent clean energy sources like the sun, wind, and water require energy storage devices to preserve excess energy during times of abundant supply and low consumption and release it during times of scarce supply and high consumption. To control the varying solar and wind energies, energy storage technologies are also vital [1]. In Karachi, coastal winds slow down during scorching temperatures, as well as solar output, begins to change when cloud patches are moving across the sky. Rainfall in the mountains affects the movement of water in streams. Energy storage devices, both mechanical and chemical, are essential components of renewable energy systems. Some examples of electrical energy storage devices include Plug-in Electric Vehicles (PEVs), supercapacitors, extended-life batteries, etc. The most significant and effective method for electrical network stabilization is battery-based energy storage [2]. Energy transmission and storage are essential components for ensuring consumers have stable access to energy. Globally, the production of electricity has

 DOI: 10.1201/9781003546382-11

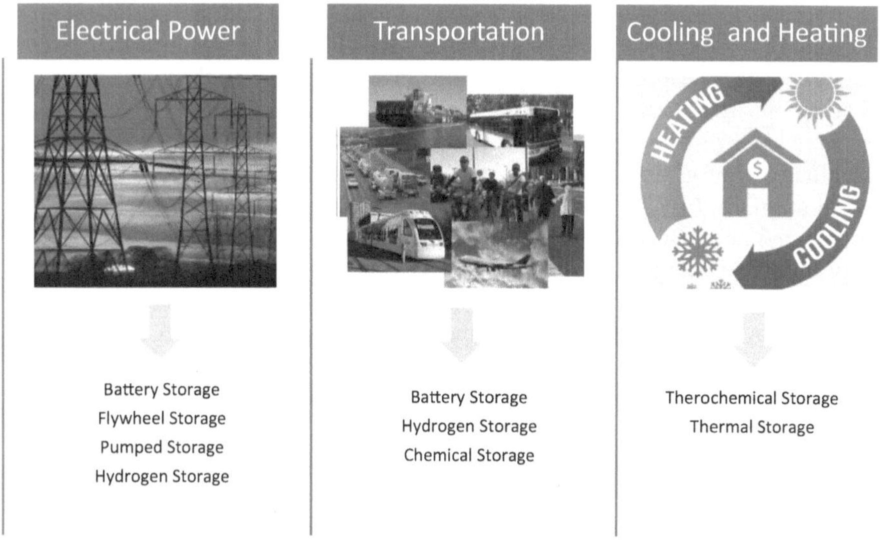

FIGURE 11.1 Diverse energy storage solutions for a sustainable future.

shifted dramatically due to Greenhouse Gases (GHGs) originating from fossil fuels [3]. In addition to being a clean and renewable energy source, photocatalytic H2 production using readily available cocatalysts to aid in water splitting is a breakthrough in the field of renewable energy [4]. Mechanical energy storage devices include compressed air reservoirs, hydrogen storage, flywheels, pumped storage hydropower, and other systems. Figure 11.1 illustrates a spectrum of diverse energy storage solutions, showcasing a roadmap toward a sustainable future. Compared to mechanical energy storage systems, chemical energy storage solutions perform faster. The rates of deep charging and deep discharge influence the choice of electrical energy storage systems. There is a large variety of DC batteries available, and each usage requires a different choice. Hydrogen storage as an engine fuel is slow since it requires a long time to ignite.

Engines and turbines are not as rapid in charging and discharging as common lead-acid, sodium sulfur, nickel hydride, nickel cadmium, and lithium-ion battery cells. Flow-type cells can store energy from external reservoirs to boost their capacity. Since batteries deteriorate and eventually die, there are life issues with all kinds of battery energy storage systems. The efficiency coefficient of systems that use both heat and power is higher than that of systems that simply use heat or electricity. The primary uses of electricity are in motor driving, lighting, heating, and cooling. Systems for storing heat can significantly improve the efficiency of power usage. Water can be directly heated by solar collectors, and hot plant water can also be stored. Although heat energy can be stored in solids and gases, water is frequently chosen because, at 70°C, its high specific heat capacity is 290 MJ/m^3. High latent heat capacity materials are used in latent heat thermal energy storage systems. Thermal energy storage systems utilize Phase Change Materials (PCM).

As water has a large specific heat capacity, it is used in steam heat accumulators. Sensible heat storage makes use of a material's sensible heat to store energy. Systems designed to store heat or cold for the summer or winter can store the warmth of summer or winter cold and disperse it in the appropriate season. Thermoelectric generators are a good way to convert the darkness of the night to light, just like solar cells. The efficiency of generation is increased in biomass facilities and solar thermal by storing steam [5, 6]. Considering the temperature threshold, a comparison between sensible and latent heat storage systems reveals that the latent system has a higher temperature and energy efficiency than the sensible system [7–10].

Power density and energy density serve as essential characteristics of energy storage technologies. Fuel Cells (FCs) and batteries are examples of energy storage system technologies with limited power concentration but substantial energy concentration [11–20]. These technologies present power regulation issues as a result of their delayed unpredictable reaction. On the other hand, excessive power demands from technologies like flywheels and supercapacitors (SCs) can shorten the storage system's lifespan [21]. Presently available storage technologies are unable to simultaneously meet energy density and power requirements. Owing to advancements in storage technology, it is often necessary to enhance the dynamic and stasis state performance of Hybrid Energy Storage Systems (HESS) [22, 23]. The HESS has been presented with several review papers. The majority of review publications concentrate on HESSs in electrical vehicles, while some [24–26] concentrate on HESSs in renewable energy. Achieving decarbonization requires the production and preservation of renewable energy. Hydrogen fuel cells and storage batteries have exceptional energy conversion efficiency as energy from green sources. Due to its compact size and great versatility, this application is frequently taken into consideration for transportation and the mobility of remote towns [27]. Renewable energy sources are predicted to surpass other energy sources as the main energy source in the long run, even though efforts to enhance energy efficacy and progressively include them seem the most rational in the near future [28]. This demands that electrochemical technologies like fuel cells, electrolyzers, and batteries be widely used in addition to the substantial usage of hydrogen as a form of fuel or energy source [29]. By 2040, renewable energy is predicted to provide about 40% of the world's electricity.

The ability to convert excess green power into hydrogen is undoubtedly a breakthrough. In addition, algorithms working with sensors and the interconnected network of devices can stabilize main grids and optimize the efficiency of dispatch [30]. Many factors, including shifting supply, growing demand, inefficiencies, and inadequate analytics for optimal management, are contributing to the energy sector's current problems. Several issues, such as the necessity for decentralization in power generation, the demand for increased operational efficiency, and the growth of energy efficiency, may be related to the economic sustainability and growth of Artificial Intelligence (AI) within the energy sector [31]. Artificial intelligence is used in renewable energy technology to forecast energy together with its efficacy and attainability [32]. AI methods can be used to address a variety of issues, such as the best customer choice and its attributes and inclinations. It's widely accepted that the goal of artificial intelligence is to create intelligent programs and robots with a higher degree of automation and intelligence to carry out particular tasks or address particular issues [33]. Numerous important industries, including the food industry, business, education, agriculture, safety and security, health and welfare, and the arts, have used artificial intelligence. In a similar vein, AI is crucial to the development of the renewable energy industry [34]. Artificial intelligence (AI) holds the promise to completely transform the energy industry in the future years by helping to overcome energy's inherently uncertain and unpredictable nature and fostering the use of renewable energy sources. In the field of renewable energy, artificial intelligence is becoming more and more significant, especially in the areas of hydrogen and battery technology [35].

11.2 CONVENTIONAL TECHNIQUES FOR OPTIMIZING HYBRID ENERGY

New energy sources are always being developed as a result of the pollution that fossil fuels cause [8, 9]. These days, the primary component of embedded energy storage systems present in contemporary electric vehicles is Li-ion batteries, which have a high energy density and can provide long-distance endurance. Li-ion batteries have a slower response time than supercapacitors when compared to one another [10, 11]. To match the performance of fuel vehicles, electric vehicles use a Hybrid Energy Storage System (HESS) comprising Li-ion batteries and supercapacitors. This makes it possible for quick transient acceleration, a plentiful supply of energy, and long-range endurance [12]. Improving the energy storage gadget is essential to the development of electric cars. It becomes necessary to think about increasing the battery's capacity and simultaneously decreasing its size and weight to increase the charging pace [13]. Figure 11.1 shows diverse energy storage solutions for a sustainable future.

Selecting a suitable plan for energy management is essential when using hybrid energy storage systems. Numerous energy management strategies have been documented in the literature in recent years. These methods include battery power limiting, state machine control, Dynamic Programming (DP), Deep Neural Networks (DNN), fuzzy algorithms, frequency decoupling as well as on/off-line optimal methods [14]. The main goal of the best management strategies is to minimize a cost function to guarantee a continuous supply. Offline global optimization and online local optimization are two categories into which these tactics can be separated. To achieve off-line global optimization, the optimal power distribution between various sources must be obtained. Accurate driving condition prediction is also required for online local optimization.

11.2.1 Energy Storage Systems Tailored for Electric and Hybrid Vehicles

In Plug-in Hybrid Electric Vehicles (PHEVs), Electric Vehicles (EVs), and Hybrid Electric Vehicles (HEVs), the strategy for energy management and Energy Storage System (ESS) component sizing has a substantial influence on performance and fuel economy. Long cycle life is a requirement shared by all of the aforementioned vehicle applications for batteries. Additionally, because EVs use a significant portion of the battery's energy (80% for EVs, 50% for PHEVs, and 10% for HEVs), they put more strain on the battery than HEV and PHEV applications do [15]. Furthermore, the frequent charging and discharging that EV batteries must endure hurts their lifespan.

Three main categories can be used to classify HESS topologies: completely active, semi-active, and passive. The supercapacitor's potential is limited by passive HESSs, despite being the least expensive topology due to their lack of a DC/DC converter. Fully active HESSs use two DC/DC converters plus an additional control circuit for optimal control effect because of their flexibility. However, there are trade-offs between cost, weight volume, simplicity, and efficiency with this design. With just one DC/DC converter, the semi-active HESS offers a well-balanced combination of system cost and performance. Accordingly, a widely studied semi-active HESS is commonly used in this work.

According to earlier research, optimizing the HESS is essential for achieving high overall efficiency, cutting costs, saving energy, and improving system dynamics. To achieve optimal energy management, a variety of online strategies have been developed and discussed for Hybrid Energy Storage Systems (HESS) in recent literature. These strategies include the "all or nothing" control strategy, fuzzy logic control strategy, filtration-based strategy, model predictive control strategy, and rule-based control strategy. These control algorithms are empirically designed and try to reduce the current's peak and Root Mean Square (RMS) values to prolong the battery's life. These online techniques, however, are unable to locate the global optimization solution. Additionally, these studies ignore the effects of various environments.

When compared to online strategies, Pontryagin's Minimum Principle (PMP) and Dynamic Programming (DP) can identify the actual best solution. These techniques, however, are limited to situations in which the driving cycle is known ahead of time. Furthermore, the computational cost of these methods is very high, making their practical application difficult. Due to the absence of a dynamic degradation model for the LiFePO4 battery, most of the referred research was unable to provide an accurate assessment of the capacity loss. Moreover, it was viewed that the HESS setup and the energy management system design were two different issues.

11.3 ROLE OF ARTIFICIAL INTELLIGENCE IN ENERGY STORAGE

For the integration of renewable energy and Energy Storage Systems (ESSs), academics have created an immense number of algorithms and approaches for state estimations, optimization modeling, and behavior expressions. Three factors can be used to summarize these:

i. ***Improving the Configuration of the System:*** By analyzing the link between the energy management algorithm and power matching during device operation and simultaneously optimizing both power matching and energy management algorithms, this type of work seeks to identify the ideal battery and ultra-capacitor configurations. Numerous techniques are used in optimization, including the hybrid optimization approach, the Particle Swarm Optimization (PSO) algorithm, the harmony search algorithm, and artificial bee colony optimization.

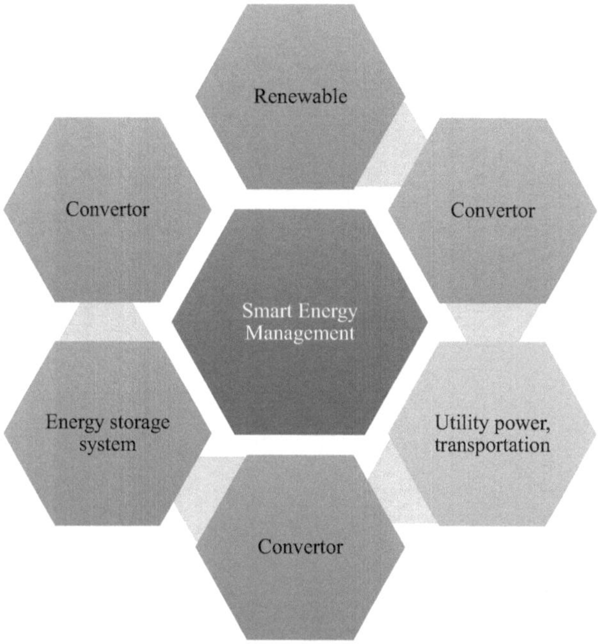

FIGURE 11.2 Smart energy management.

ii. ***Energy Management Strategy:*** The goal of this type of work is to create smart and efficient management mechanisms that will improve the ESS's resilience and dependability as well as the control system's flexibility in the face of changing operating circumstances. Figure 11.2 shows smart energy management. Increasing energy efficiency and resource utilization requires the use of a HESS control technique. Since Renewable Energy (RE) sources are sporadic and have to accomplish several objectives, the monitoring method is usually intricate and requires continuous operation. Techniques including predictive control, neuro-fuzzy inference systems control, variable control, and dynamic programming are commonly used. Certain studies on energy storage systems driven by artificial intelligence are shown in Table 11.1.

iii. ***Estimating Parameter States:*** The goal of this kind of research is to create highly accurate, adaptable, and dependable methods for system identification and status assessments. By examining how stress factors impact electrode materials and electrolytes from an electrochemical or material science perspective, as well as how power supply aging laws are established using signal analysis and features of thermal and electrical behaviors, it is also used to explore the connections between stress factors and aging mechanisms. Neural networks and Bayesian filters are the most popular techniques.

TABLE 11.1
Prior Studies on Artificial Intelligence-Driven Energy Storage Systems

Smart Algorithms	Types of Energy Storage	Green Energy	Aspects	Discovery
Agglomerative hierarchical clustering Algorithm (AHC)	Cell	Solar-powered, wind-driven	Duration	This approach shows optimization of solar/wind and battery integration: agglomerative hierarchical clustering. The results show that 5–15 days' worth of time series data is sufficient to improve system performance by five percent. The precession of temporal chronology, which is essential for applications involving energy storage, gives AHC an edge over other clustering algorithms.
Non-dominated Genetic Sorting Algorithm	Pumped hydropower, Storage cell	Solar-powered, wind-driven	Price and emissions	The incorporation of solar, wind, and pumped storage is optimized by the GA algorithm for both economic and environmental system optimization.
Particle Swarm Optimization (PSO) Algorithm	Electric cells and hydrogen	Photovoltaic cells, wind energy	Expenses, Effectiveness, and longevity	The energy management system uses the PSO algorithm to reduce overhead expenses (29.36%), increase productivity (27.21%), and lengthen device lifetimes (43.43%).
Hybrid Particle Swarm Optimization and Teaching-Learning-based Optimization (HPSO-TLBO)	Cell	Wind Power	Exhalation, Interval, Overhead	Numerical findings show that, when wind turbine instability is considered, a versatile multi-target dispatch model meets the requirements of solutions. Meanwhile, similar results show that the PSO-TLBO approach effectively resolves the proposed shipping issues.

11.3.1 Artificial Intelligence in Different Sustainable Energy Storage Systems

Artificial Intelligence is becoming more and more influential in all areas of engineering, but especially in sustainable energy systems. Numerous applications of artificial intelligence have been implemented, including novel solar technologies [36], improving the electrical stability of Unified Power Flow Controllers (UPFCs) and wind [37], solar, load [38], gas [39], and electricity price forecasting; additionally, occupant satisfaction and smart buildings [40–42]; IoT security and safety system in smart cities [43]; demand forecast and demand-side management [44]; predictive maintenance [45]; renewable energy generation forecast [46, 47]; photovoltaic generation maximal power point monitoring on a fuzzy logic basis [48, 49], etc. Table 11.2 shows the various stages of development of AI in the energy sector. This section covers the application of AI in seven domains: (i) energy applications; (ii) power delivery; (iii) electric distribution networks; (iv) energy storage; (v) energy applications; (vi) energy efficiency and nanotechnology in energy systems; and (vii) energy policy and economics.

11.3.2 Artificial Intelligence Usage in the Generation of Energy

The global energy exchange is confronted with increasing growth, productivity, shifting trends in supply and demand, and inadequate technology to manage it all. These difficulties are particularly severe in developing nations. Efficiency problems are especially problematic when many informal power grid connections lead to a considerable quantity of power not being counted or measured. Because consumers lack incentives to use energy efficiently, this results in losses and higher CO_2 emissions. Industrialized nations' power corporations have already started integrating AI and associated technologies to enable communication between smart meters, smart grids, and the industrial Internet of Things. These systems can continue to expand renewable energy sources while improving power management, efficiency, and transparency. Smart meters are a choice made by consumers based on their preferences. Consumers have the option to modify their consumption patterns or to turn their electricity "ON" or "OFF" during peak hours.

TABLE 11.2
AI's Role in the Energy Sector and Its Many Stages of Development [18]

Sr. No.	Safeguarding and Management	Decision Formulation	Consumer Engagement and Logistics
1.	Pillaging, deconstructing, servicing	Efficiency maximization	Invoice delivery and management
2.	Proactive maintenance	Prediction	Customer involvement and ease of use of the system
3.	Safety Procedures	Making strategic business decisions and optimizing inventory	Branding strategies and product adaptation for various types

Fair access to inexpensive, safe, and sustainable clean electricity is one of the Sustainable Development Goals (SDGs). However, this will only ever be a goal if innovative thinking and creative technologies can solve the many energy-related issues that the markets are currently facing, such as insufficient power generation, deficient transmission and dissemination infrastructure, sustainability issues, and ecological problems. It also presents a variety of issues for the generation, storage, distribution, and use of power among nations, in addition to new and developing technological developments and changes in consumer demand. AI has the potential to lower energy costs and consumption while accelerating the use of green, safe energy sources by global grids. The incorporation of AI in the power sector is being driven by emerging economies.

A smart grid that uses artificial intelligence (AI) can adapt to changes in the amount and load of renewable resources that are flowing amidst the current framework. AI will make it easier to formulate decisions for dispersed power generation.

11.3.3 Usage of Artificial Intelligence in Energy Storage

Artificial intelligence (AI) can help assess the safety of equipment for small new customers, such as buildings, by predicting the service life of storage facilities and their integration with power sources [16]. Renewable Energy Sources Map (REmap) analysis predicts that global energy storage will increase from an estimated 4.67 TWh in 2017 to 6.62 TWh in 2030, a 42% increase to 68% in 2017. If the world's energy system doubles in size by 2014 (REmap doubles), storage capacity could rise to 11.89 TWh in 2030 and 15.27 TWh in 2030; this is an increase of 155% compared to 227% in 2030. Pumped hydro storage space has long been utilized to lower production costs by shifting energy sources from periods of low demand to high demand. Determining the cost-effectiveness of grid infrastructure for batteries and other mechanical and thermal energy storage devices remains a difficult task. The economies of today are very market-specific due to generally high costs and occasionally inexpensive flexibility replacements. Nevertheless, a range of services are currently offered by battery-electric storage systems, and this list will only grow as costs come down and efficiency rises. Utility-scale competitive undertakings are becoming more prevalent. The possible applications for energy storage are illustrated. The increasing need for novel battery technologies for energy production, distribution, and thermal storage in the residential and commercial domains can be attributed to a variety of storage locations.

11.4 AI TECHNOLOGY FOR ELECTRIC VEHICLES

The widespread adoption of Electric Vehicles (EVs) depends on their economic viability, safety, and dependability—qualities that AI can greatly enhance. AI applications for EVs have been extensively studied and can be broadly categorized into multiple areas, such as EV battery architecture, production, and control, range optimization, and design and optimization of EV control systems. Figure 11.3 covers EVCSs, the linking of EVs with smart grid systems, and EVs themselves are some of the application areas for AI. The system for battery management in electric vehicles

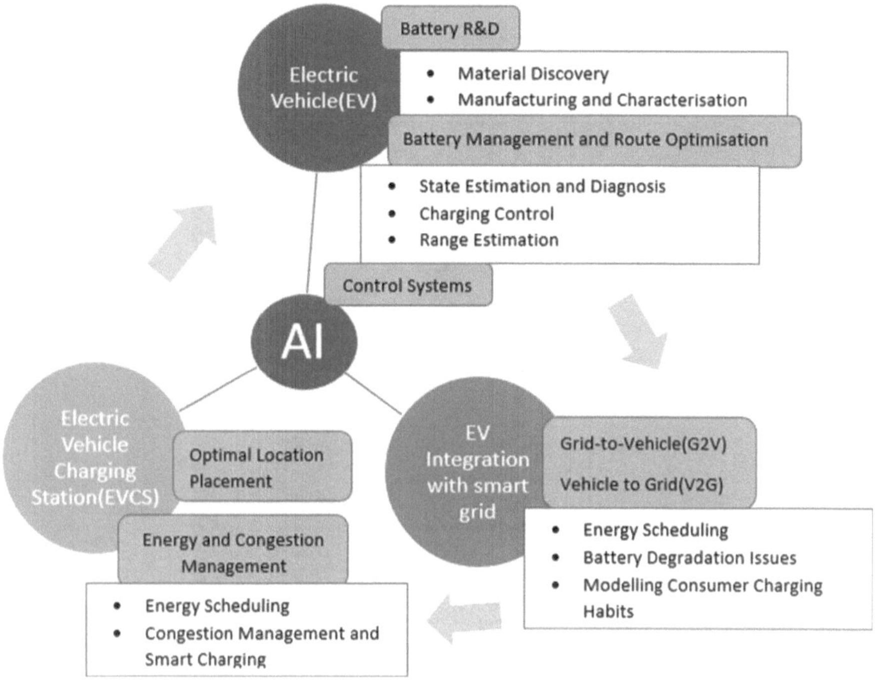

FIGURE 11.3 Overview of EVCS, integration of EV with smart grid, and AI's role in EV.

is essential for battery state assessment, battery pack sensing, etc. Figure 11.4 depicts how Machine learning can be implemented in Battery Management [17].

11.4.1 Information Gathering by AI

By using sophisticated data processing methods, Artificial Intelligence (AI) is essential for obtaining information from the environment and identifying patterns. In the field of transportation, AI gathers data in real-time from a variety of sensors, cameras, and data sources about the surrounding environment and the actions of moving vehicles. This data is analyzed by machine learning algorithms, which then use the results to comprehend traffic patterns, spot possible dangers, and optimize routes for effective navigation.

AI also makes a substantial contribution to efficient energy storage management. AI systems can evaluate energy consumption patterns, pinpoint peak usage periods, and maximize energy storage system charging and discharging cycles by utilizing predictive analytics and pattern recognition.

11.4.2 Usage of Optimization Algorithms

The demand for more sustainable and efficient energy solutions has caused a major shift in the energy storage system market in recent years. The use of optimization

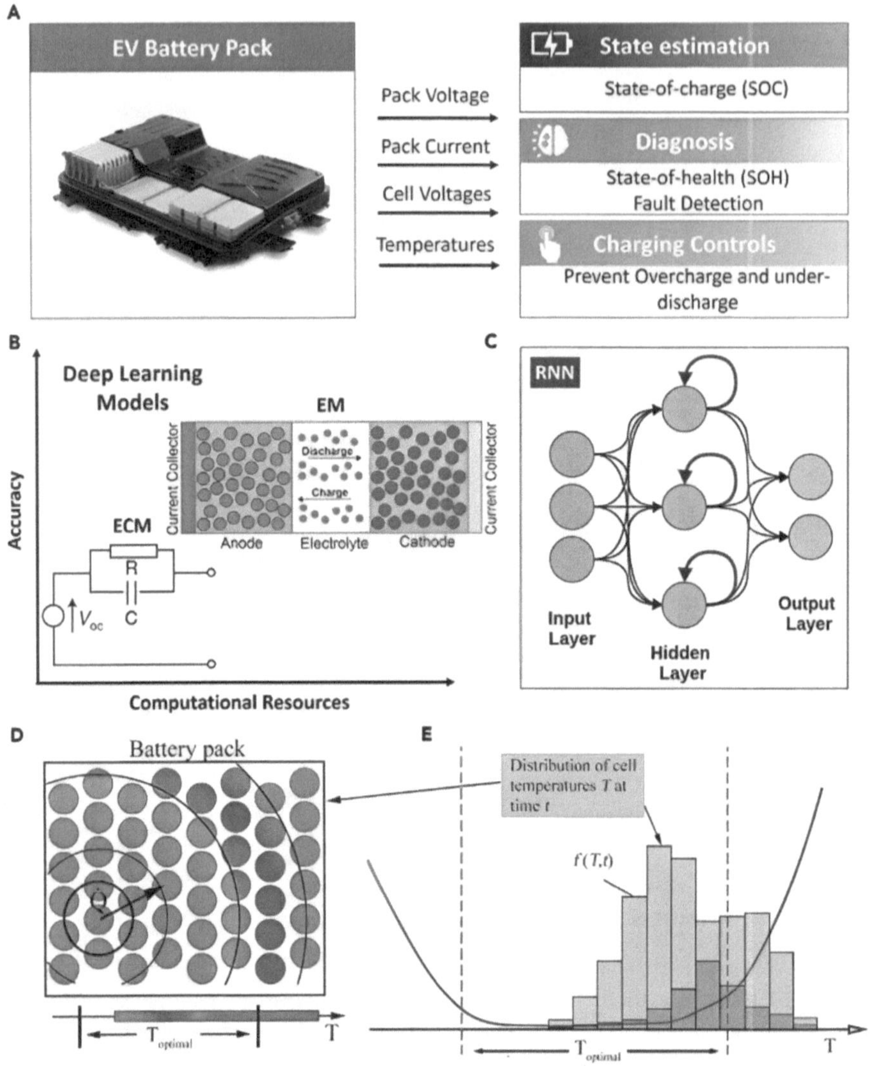

FIGURE 11.4 Use of machine learning in battery management [20]: (a) The battery-management system receives information from the battery-pack sensor. Periodically, the temperature probes' readings, pack voltage, pack current, individual cell voltages, and pack temperatures are gathered by the battery management system; (b) Accuracy versus the amount of computing power needed to estimate State of Charge (SOC) and State of Health (SOH). Once Deep learning algorithms-powered data-driven models that measure SOC and SOH demonstrate higher accuracy when compared to Equivalent Circuit Models (ECMs) and significantly less computational power when compared to physical models, including models with a single particle; (c) Recurrent Neural Network (RNN) schematic diagram; (d) The battery pack's battery cells' temperature profile. Used with permission under the Creative Common License from Karlsen; (e) A histogram can be used to display the temperature profile of the batteries.

algorithms is a significant factor in this transition. These algorithms are essential for improving energy storage systems' efficiency, especially when it comes to hybrid systems. We will delve into the nuances of optimization algorithms in this talk, and we will look at some examples that show how they affect energy storage efficiency.

Algorithms for optimization are computer techniques created to identify the optimal answer to a particular issue. These algorithms seek to optimize resource utilization, minimize losses, and maximize efficiency in the context of energy storage systems. Numerous optimization methods, including particle swarm optimization, genetic algorithms, and linear programming, have been applied to energy storage to tackle challenging problems.

An effective mathematical method for allocating resources is called linear programming. When it comes to energy storage, linear programming is useful in figuring out how best to distribute energy among many elements, including cost, storage capacity, and demand. For example, linear programming can be used to optimize battery charging and discharging cycles in a grid-connected energy storage system, guaranteeing a balance between energy supply and demand.

Natural selection serves as the inspiration for genetic algorithms, which are used in energy storage to maximize system sizing. The algorithm selects the best-performing solutions and combines them to create better configurations by iteratively evolving alternative solutions. This method is very useful for figuring out how big energy storage systems should be, considering things like load requirements, the patterns of renewable energy generation, and total system cost.

A heuristic optimization method called Particle Swarm Optimization (PSO) mimics how people interact with one another in a group. PSO is used for dynamic energy management in applications involving energy storage. For instance, PSO can dynamically modify the distribution of energy storage resources in a microgrid that combines renewable and non-renewable energy sources to adapt to shifting patterns of energy generation and demand.

11.4.2.1 Case Studies of Optimization Algorithms on Energy Storage Systems

Some case studies of optimization algorithms on energy storage systems are explained as follows:

a. ***Integrated Renewable Energy:*** The integration of renewable energy sources into the power grid is made possible in large part by optimization algorithms. Optimization algorithms can be used in a hybrid energy storage system that combines wind and solar electricity to manage the transition between different energy sources, predict weather patterns, and modify energy storage parameters. As a result, there is less reliance on conventional energy sources and a seamless integration of renewable energy into the grid.
b. ***Optimization of Electric Vehicle Charging:*** When it comes to Electric Vehicles (EVs), optimization algorithms play a crucial role in controlling battery charging and discharging. Using evolutionary algorithms to improve the scheduling of electric vehicle charging stations while accounting for grid demand, electricity pricing, and customer preferences is one example.

Preventing peak loads, not only improves the efficiency of the infrastructure for charging but also adds to grid stability.

c. ***Grid Stability by Control of Frequency:*** Energy storage devices that offer frequency regulation services can help maintain grid stability. Energy storage devices' output can be continually adjusted using optimization methods, like model predictive control, in response to variations in the frequency of the grid. This dynamic regulation contributes to grid stabilization and consistent power delivery.

Energy storage systems can be made more efficient with the use of optimization algorithms, but there are some issues and problems that must be taken into account. One difficulty is that some algorithms are computationally complex and may need a lot of computing power. Achieving ideal solutions is further complicated by the precise modeling of system parameters and the unpredictable nature of some elements, such as weather in renewable energy systems.

11.4.3 Current State-of-Art for Hybrid Energy Storage

The use of Artificial Intelligence (AI) in hybrid energy storage systems is a significant move in the current energy storage landscape [19]. The increasing demand for effective, adaptable, and sustainable energy solutions is the reason for this integration. We examine the state-of-the-art artificial intelligence (AI) applications for hybrid energy storage in this thorough assessment, looking at success stories and addressing the difficulties encountered when applying AI to practical situations.

a. ***Algorithms for Optimization to Increase Efficiency:*** Among the fundamental building blocks of AI applications for hybrid energy storage are optimization algorithms. These algorithms, which include machine learning-based methods, genetic algorithms, and particle swarm optimization, are essential for upgrading the functionality and efficiency of hybridized energy storage systems. These algorithms maximize total system efficiency by dynamically adjusting parameters to ensure optimal energy storage, distribution, and usage through continuous data analysis.
b. ***Predictive Analytics in the Integration of Renewable Energy:*** Predictive analytics powered by AI is essential for smoothly integrating renewable energy sources into hybrid storage systems. To forecast future energy generation [20] and demand, machine learning models can examine historical data, weather patterns, and trends in energy usage. This insight allows for wise choices to be made when distributing and storing energy from renewable sources, guaranteeing a steady and dependable supply of electricity.
c. ***Battery Management Systems using Machine Learning:*** Energy storage systems depend heavily on Battery Management Systems (BMS) to be functional and healthy. In BMS, Artificial Intelligence (AI), especially machine learning, is being used more and more for state-of-health monitoring, predictive maintenance, and real-time battery charging and discharging cycle optimization. By using this application, batteries last longer and hybrid energy storage systems continue to operate efficiently.

11.4.3.1 Case Studies of AI Integration into Energy Storage

Some case studies of AI integration into energy storage are explained as follows:

a. ***The Powerwall and Powerpack from Tesla:*** The Powerpack and Powerwall from Tesla are prime examples of how AI has been successfully incorporated into energy storage. AI algorithms are used by these systems, which are intended for both commercial and domestic use, to optimize patterns of energy consumption. To find the most effective times to charge and discharge the batteries, Tesla's AI systems examine sensor data, weather predictions, and past usage trends. By carefully controlling energy demands, this helps maintain grid stability and saves users' costs.
b. ***Australia's Hybrid Microgrid:*** One example of how AI has been successful in optimizing energy storage in a complicated system is the installation of a hybrid microgrid in South Australia. To balance energy supply and demand, artificial intelligence (AI) algorithms examine data from solar panels, wind turbines, and conventional energy sources. This improves the microgrid's dependability and helps the area reach its objective of having a large share of renewable energy in its total energy mix.
c. ***Singapore's Smart Grids:*** Building smart grids in Singapore is an example of how AI can be used effectively for both energy distribution and storage. These smart networks can forecast energy use, control variations in renewable energy production, and maximize the use of energy storage devices by integrating AI algorithms. As a result, the energy infrastructure is more adaptive and resilient and can react quickly to changing circumstances.

11.4.3.2 Difficulties in Using AI in Practical Situations

Some difficulties of using AI in practical situations are explained as follows:

a. ***Data Accessibility and Quality:*** Data availability and quality are major obstacles to AI integration in hybrid energy storage systems. For training and making decisions, Artificial Intelligence (AI) algorithms mostly depend on precise and thorough data. Achieving high-quality data in real-world scenarios can be difficult because of sensor constraints, privacy issues with data, and the requirement for big datasets to train complex machine-learning models.
b. ***Complexity of Computation:*** One major obstacle is the computational complexity of some AI algorithms, which is particularly problematic for real-time applications. Rapid decision-making is necessary because hybrid energy storage systems frequently operate in dynamic and uncertain contexts. Putting computationally complex algorithms into practice could impose a strain on the system's processing power, causing reaction times to lag and possibly even inefficiency.
c. ***Policy and Regulatory Obstacles:*** There are regional differences in the legislative and policy obstacles that AI integration in energy storage systems must overcome. Different regulations apply to cybersecurity, data protection, and the use of AI technology, which affects how widely these systems

are adopted. It is difficult for developers and other stakeholders in the energy sector to navigate various regulatory environments.

11.4.3.3 Prospective Routes and Oncoming Patterns

Some prospective routes and oncoming patterns are explained as follows:

a. ***Real-time Processing with Edge Computing*:** Integrating edge computing is one new approach in AI for hybrid energy storage. Edge computing improves real-time decision-making by processing and analyzing data closer to the point of data generation. This lowers latency. This is especially important for energy storage systems that have to react quickly to changing circumstances.
b. ***AI Explainable for Openness*:** Explainable AI (XAI) is becoming more and more in demand as AI systems become more complex. Establishing confidence among stakeholders, regulators, and users in the energy storage space requires transparent and comprehensible AI models. Effective collaboration and well-informed decision-making are made possible by explainable AI, which guarantees that decision-making processes are comprehensible.
c. ***AI Hybrid Models*:** Hybrid artificial intelligence models, which integrate various AI methods like rule-based systems, machine learning, and optimization algorithms, are showing promise. By combining the advantages of each method, these models address certain energy storage problems and offer a more reliable and flexible solution.

The state-of-the-art in artificial intelligence for hybrid energy storage offers a constantly changing set of opportunities and difficulties. The Powerpack from Tesla, microgrids in South Australia, and smart grids in Singapore are just a few examples of the success stories that highlight how AI is revolutionizing energy storage efficiency. To fully utilize AI in practical situations, however, some obstacles including those about data quality, computational complexity, interoperability, and regulatory concerns need to be overcome. Emerging innovations in the sector, such as explainable AI, edge computing, and hybrid AI models, have the potential to overcome these obstacles and influence the development of intelligent and sustainable energy storage systems in the future. To create resilient, flexible, and environmentally sustainable energy infrastructures for the future, AI integration in hybrid energy storage is still an important step forward.

11.5 CONCLUSION

Artificial Intelligence (AI) and energy storage together in electric and hybrid cars is a game-changer for a more empowered and sustainable future. The combination of energy storage and AI offers previously unheard-of possibilities to completely change the automotive industry in the never-ending quest for greener and more effective modes of transportation. The wide range of AI applications in vehicle energy storage has been covered in this thorough investigation, from predictive analytics for ideal charging to intelligent battery management systems. The transformational potential of this synergy is demonstrated by the success stories of trailblazers such as Tesla, which demonstrate the superiority of AI-driven power storage in electric vehicles. As we read on to the end, it becomes clear that the usage of AI in-vehicle energy storage is not just a technological advance but also a catalyst for a fundamental change in the way that people view and engage with cars. The achievements discussed in this discussion, especially Tesla's Powerpack and Powerwall, serve as prime examples of the revolutionary effects artificial intelligence (AI) can have on energy storage in the automotive industry. Tesla's AI algorithms are an example of a model of efficiency and intelligence that goes beyond conventional vehicle paradigms. They are continuously monitoring and reacting to user behavior, weather patterns, and grid circumstances.

But this trip through the fusion of artificial intelligence and energy storage in electric and hybrid cars also highlights a variety of difficulties. The challenges of applying AI solutions in the actual automotive industry are highlighted by the availability and quality of data, computational complexity, and interoperability requirements. The emergence of explainable AI has brought attention to the need for transparency in AI decision-making, which is critical to gaining the trust of users and authorities. To build a peaceful ecology that supports the widespread use of AI-powered energy storage, researchers, engineers, legislators, and industry stakeholders must work together to overcome these obstacles.

Future directions for resolving these issues and expanding the potential of energy storage in cars include edge computing, explainable AI, and hybrid AI models. With the emergence of edge computing, the problem of computational complexity and latency in dynamic vehicular contexts is addressed by bringing real-time processing closer to the source of data generation. Explainable AI promotes trust and makes it easier for the car industry and regulators to work together effectively by guaranteeing transparency in decision-making processes.

Furthermore, the integration of machine learning, optimization algorithms, and rule-based systems through the hybridization of AI models presents a comprehensive strategy to address the various facets involved in energy storage within automobiles. Hybrid models offer resilient, flexible, and intelligent systems that can handle the complexities of various driving situations, user behaviors, and changing energy landscapes by utilizing the advantages of various AI techniques.

Beyond individual cars, AI-driven energy storage is empowering the future by influencing the dynamics of resilient grids, smart cities, and sustainable energy infrastructures. The achievements and obstacles discussed in this talk point to the future and encourage all parties involved to work together, be creative, and take advantage of artificial intelligence's capacity to revolutionize the automobile industry. The future is full of promise for cleaner, smarter, and more sustainable transportation as energy storage and artificial intelligence (AI) collide in the crucible of this technological revolution. The combination of artificial intelligence and energy storage in electric and hybrid cars is a monument to human creativity and a lighthouse pointing the way toward a more intelligent, connected, and environmentally friendly automotive future as we forge ahead through this new territory.

REFERENCES

[1] T. Funabashi, *Integration of distributed energy resources in power systems: implementation, operation and control*. Academic Press, 2016.

[2] G. J. May, A. Davidson, and B. Monahov, "Lead batteries for utility energy storage: A review," *Journal of Energy Storage*, vol. 15, pp. 145–157, 2018.

[3] N. Khan, S. Dilshad, R. Khalid, A. R. Kalair, and N. Abas, "Review of energy storage and transportation of energy," *Energy Storage*, vol. 1, pp. 49, 2019.

[4] M. B. Tahir, M. Sagir, and N. Abas, "Enhanced photocatalytic performance of CdO-WO3 composite for hydrogen production," *International Journal of Hydrogen Energy*, vol. 44, no. 45, pp. 24690–24697, 2019.

[5] M. R. Kargar, E. Baniasadi, and M. Mosharaf-Dehkordi, "Numerical analysis of a new thermal energy storage system using phase change materials for direct steam parabolic trough solar power plants," *Solar Energy*, vol. 170, pp. 594–605, 2018.

[6] R. M. Greenough, M. Stark, F. Conti, S. Abdessamad, and W. Zörner, "Steam storage systems for flexible biomass CHP plants-Evaluation and initial model-based calculation," 2019.

[7] J. Guo, X. Huai, and K. Cheng, "The comparative analysis on thermal storage systems for solar power with direct steam generation," *Renewable Energy*, vol. 115, pp. 217–225, 2018.

[8] Z. Shuai, C. Shen, X. Yin, X. Liu, and Z. J. Shen, "Fault analysis of inverter-interfaced distributed generators with different control schemes," *IEEE Transactions on Power Delivery*, vol. 33, no. 3, pp. 1223–1235, 2017.

[9] Z. Shuai et al.,"Microgrid stability: Classification and a review," *Renewable and Sustainable Energy Reviews*, vol. 58, pp. 167–179, 2016.

[10] N. R. Tummuru, M. K. Mishra, and S. Srinivas, "Dynamic energy management of renewable grid integrated hybrid energy storage system," *IEEE Transactions on Industrial Electronics*, vol. 62, no. 12, pp. 7728–7737, 2015.

[11] T. Mesbahi, N. Rizoug, F. Khenfri, P. Bartholomeüs, and P. Le Moigne, "Dynamical modeling and emulation of Li-ion batteries–supercapacitors hybrid power supply for electric vehicle applications," *IET Electrical Systems in Transportation*, vol. 7, no. 2, pp. 161–169, 2017.

[12] A. Santucci, A. Sorniotti, and C. Lekakou, "Power split strategies for hybrid energy storage systems for vehicular applications," *Journal of Power Sources*, vol. 258, pp. 395–407, 2014.

[13] J. Shen, S. Dusmez, and A. Khaligh, "Optimization of sizing and battery cycle life in battery/ultracapacitor hybrid energy storage systems for electric vehicle applications," *IEEE Transactions on Industrial Informatics*, vol. 10, no. 4, pp. 2112–2121, 2014.

[14] M.-E. Choi, S.-W. Kim, and S.-W. Seo, "Energy management optimization in a battery/supercapacitor hybrid energy storage system," *IEEE Transactions on Smart Grid*, vol. 3, no. 1, pp. 463–472, 2011.

[15] J. R. Belt, "Battery test manual for plug-in hybrid electric vehicles," Idaho National Lab. (INL), Idaho Falls, ID (United States), 2010.

[16] N. Silaparasetty and N. Silaparasetty, "An Overview of Machine Learning," Mach. Learn. Concepts with Python Jupyter Noteb. Environ. Using Tensorflow 2.0, pp. 21–39, 2020.

[17] C. Chen, Y. Zuo, W. Ye, X. Li, Z. Deng, and S. P. Ong, "A critical review of machine learning of energy materials," *Advanced Energy Materials*, vol. 10, no. 8, p. 1903242, 2020.

[18] T. Ahmad et al., "Energetics Systems and Artificial Intelligence: Applications of Industry 4.0," *Energy Reports*, vol. 8, pp. 334–361, 2022.

[19] T. Ahmad et al., "Artificial intelligence in the sustainable energy industry: Status Quo, challenges, and opportunities," *Journal of Cleaner Production*, vol. 289, p. 125834, 2021.
[20] A. N. Abdalla et al.,"Integration of energy storage system and renewable energy sources based on artificial intelligence: An overview," *Journal of Energy Storage*, vol. 40, p. 102811, 2021.
[21] Etxeberria, A. et al. (2010) "Hybrid Energy Storage Systems for renewable energy sources integration in microgrids: A Review," In *2010 Conference Proceedings IPEC*, 2010, doi:10.1109/ipecon.2010.5697053
[22] R. Hemmati, H. Saboori, "Emergence of hybrid energy storage systems in renewable energy and transport applications – A review," *Renewable and Sustainable Energy Reviews*, vol. 65, pp. 11–23, 2016, doi: 10.1016/j.rser.2016.06.029
[23] T. Zimmermann, P. Keil, M. Hofmann, M. F. Horsche, S. Pichlmaier, A. Jossen, "Review of system topologies for hybrid electrical energy storage systems," *Journal of Energy Storage*, vol. 8, pp. 78–90, 2016, doi: 10.1016/j.est.2016.09.006
[24] L. W. Chong, Y. W. Wong, R. K. Rajkumar, R. K. Rajkumar, D. Isa, "Hybrid energy storage systems and control strategies for stand-alone renewable energy power systems," *Renewable and Sustainable Energy Reviews*, vol. 66, pp. 174–189, 2016, doi: 10.1016/j.rser.2016.07.059
[25] T. Bocklisch, "Hybrid energy storage approach for renewable energy applications," *Journal of Energy Storage*, vol. 8, pp. 311–319, 2016, doi: 10.1016/j.est.2016.01.004
[26] S. Ahmad Hamidi, D. M. Ionel, A. Nasiri, "Modeling and management of batteries and ultracapacitors for renewable energy support in Electric Power Systems–an overview," *Electric Power Components and Systems*, vol. 43, pp. 1434–1452, 2015, doi:10.1080/15325008.2015.1038757
[27] M. A. Hannan et al. "Impact of renewable energy utilization and artificial intelligence in Achieving Sustainable Development Goals," *Energy Reports*, vol. 7, pp. 5359–5373, 2021, doi: 10.1016/j.egyr.2021.08.172
[28] P. Moriarty, D. Honnery, "What is the global potential for renewable energy?" *Renewable and Sustainable Energy Reviews*, vol. 16, pp. 244–252, 2012, doi: 10.1016/j.rser.2011.07.151
[29] S. A. Kalogirou, (2001) "Artificial neural networks in Renewable Energy Systems Applications: A Review," *Renewable and Sustainable Energy Reviews*, vol. 5, pp. 373–401, 2001, doi: 10.1016/s1364-0321(01)00006-5
[30] Q. He, et al. "Artificial intelligence application in a renewable energy-driven desalination system: A critical review," *Energy and AI*, vol. 7, pp. 100123, 2022, doi: 10.1016/j.egyai.2021.100123
[31] C. Chen, et al. "Artificial Intelligence on economic evaluation of energy efficiency and Renewable Energy Technologies," *Sustainable Energy Technologies and Assessments*, vol. 47, pp. 101358, 2021, doi: 10.1016/j.seta.2021.101358
[32] A. N. Abdalla, et al. "Integration of energy storage system and renewable energy sources based on Artificial Intelligence: An overview," *Journal of Energy Storage*, vol. 40, pp. 102811, 2021. doi: 10.1016/j.est.2021.102811
[33] T. Ahmad, et al. "Artificial Intelligence in sustainable energy industry: Status quo, challenges and opportunities," *Journal of Cleaner Production*, vol. 289, pp. 125834, 2021. doi: 10.1016/j.jclepro.2021.125834
[34] E. Elahi, C. Weijun, S. K. Jha, and H. Zhang, "Estimation of realistic renewable and non-renewable energy use targets for livestock production systems utilising an artificial neural network method: A step towards livestock sustainability," *Energy*, vol. 183, pp. 191–204, 2019, doi: 10.1016/j.energy.2019.06.084

[35] J. Yuan, C. Farnham, C. Azuma, and K. Emura, "Predictive artificial neural network models to forecast the seasonal hourly electricity consumption for a University Campus," *Sustainable Cities and Society*, vol. 42, pp. 82–92, 2018, doi: 10.1016/j.scs.2018.06.019
[36] A. Badiei, Y.G. Akhlaghi, X. Zhao, S. Shittu, X. Xiao, J. Li, … G. Li, "A chronological review of advances in solar assisted heat pump technology in 21st century," *Renewable and Sustainable Energy Reviews*, vol. 132, 110132, 2020.
[37] A. Alhejji, M.E. Hussein, S. Kamel, S. Alyami, "Optimal power flow solution with an embedded center-node unified power flow controller using an adaptive grasshopper optimization algorithm," *IEEE Access*, vol. 8, pp. 119020–119037, 2020.
[38] S. Wang, L. Jing, Y. Zhao, H.R. Wickramasinghe, X. Wu, G. Konstantinou, "Operation of unified power flow controller as virtual synchronous generator," *IEEE Access*, vol. 8, pp. 162569–162580, 2020.
[39] N. Wei, C. Li, X. Peng, F. Zeng, X. Lu, "Conventional models and artificial intelligence-based models for energy consumption forecasting: A review," *Journal of Petroleum Science and Engineering*, vol. 181, 106187, 2019.
[40] T. Ouahiba, B. Fatima, H. Thafath, "Smart Buildings and Occupants Satisfaction: The Case of Cyber Park of Sidi Abdallâh and Some Residential Buildings in Algeria", In *Artificial Intelligence in Renewable Energetic Systems: Smart Sustainable Energy Systems* (pp. 3–14). Springer International Publishing, 2018.
[41] B.A.N. Raju, D. Ghai, K. Rawal, "Design of Futuristic Trolley System with Comparative Analysis of Previous Models," In *Big Data Analytics and Intelligent Techniques for Smart Cities*, pp. 223–247, CRC Press, 2021.
[42] D. Ghai, S.L. Tripathi, S. Saxena, M. Chanda, M. Alazab, *Machine Learning Algorithms for Signal and Image Processing*, John Wiley & Sons, 2022.
[43] H. Zahmatkesh, F. Al-Turjman, "Fog computing for sustainable smart cities in the IoT era: Caching techniques and enabling technologies-an overview," *Sustainable Cities and Society*, vol. 59, 102139, 2020.
[44] I. Antonopoulos, V. Robu, B. Couraud, D. Kirli, S. Norbu, A. Kiprakis, S. Wattam, "Artificial intelligence and machine learning approaches to energy demand-side response: A systematic review," *Renewable and Sustainable Energy Reviews*, vol. 130, 109899, 2020.
[45] R. Foresti, S. Rossi, M. Magnani, C.G.L. Bianco, N. Delmonte, N. (2020). "Smart society and artificial intelligence: big data scheduling and the global standard method applied to smart maintenance," *Engineering*, vol. 6, pp. 835–846, 2020.
[46] O. Ruhnau, P. Hennig, R. Madlener, "Economic implications of forecasting electricity generation from variable renewable energy sources," *Renewable Energy*, vol. 161, pp. 1318–1327, 2020.
[47] T. Ahmad, H. Zhang, B. Yan, "A review on renewable energy and electricity requirement forecasting models for smart grid and buildings," *Sustainable Cities and Society*, vol. 55, 102052, 2020.
[48] O. Erixno, N. Abd Rahim, F. Ramadhani, N.N. Adzman, (2022). "Energy management of renewable energy-based combined heat and power systems: A review," *Sustainable Energy Technologies and Assessments*, vol. 51, 101944, 2022.
[49] M. Kermadi, E. M. Berkouk, "Artificial intelligence-based maximum power point tracking controllers for Photovoltaic systems: Comparative study," *Renewable and Sustainable Energy Reviews*, vol. 69, pp. 369–386, 2017.

12 Revolutionizing Storage *The Artificial Intelligence Era in Energy Management*

Senthil Kumar Ramu
Vellore Institute of Technology, Chennai, India

Saravanan Subramani
Amrita School of Engineering, Coimbatore,
Amrita Vishwa Vidyapeetham, India

Balakumar Palaniyappan
Vellore Institute of Technology, Chennai, India

Pandiyan Pitchai
KPR Institute of Engineering and Technology,
Coimbatore, India

12.1 INTRODUCTION

Since climate change is affecting many countries, sustainable development is becoming more and more crucial to global commercial operations [1]. Sustainability is an established term that emphasizes generational fairness and is commonly understood to have three dimensions: economic, social, and environmental. Degrading the environment and thriving economies are incompatible because attaining environmental sustainability involves risks to corporate operations and aspirations in a highly competitive market [2]. It would be assumed that scientific organizations would endorse the work done by policymakers. The Carbon Management Plan: PAS 2060 Qualified Explanatory Declaration [3] outlines the agreement to attain and confirm carbon neutrality and the steps industries or nations undertake to do so. This study aims to illustrate the efforts that businesses from all over the globe have taken to bargain for agreements that will increase energy efficiency and lower emissions of Greenhouse Gases (GHG) [4]. Many industries, including mining, building, and transportation, need non-renewable resources. These industries harm the natural world and provide severe problems for nations, such as social unrest and financial difficulties [5].

DOI: 10.1201/9781003546382-12

Recent years have seen a significant increase in the development of ESS, which uses sustainable energy to satisfy emission reduction and energy-saving objectives. Voltage and frequency variations will occur because ESSs, whether operated on an island or in a grid, have some unpredictability and intermittency difficulties [6]. In keeping with their global environmental goals, Renewable Energy Sources (RES) can offer a substitute for reliance on fossil fuels by developing green energy solutions that lower peak demand and emissions of greenhouse gases. The utilization of RE and frequency and peak management of the power grid are facing increasing difficulties due to emerging technologies, and the power grid's function has grown more complex. EST offers an efficient way to address the issues above by applying different storage mechanisms to the power system and promptly and flexibly adjusting the system power [7]. The total installed capacity of stored energy worldwide is expected to rise by 42%–68% by 2030, according to the International Renewable Energy Agency. Australia and Japan will hold the highest percentages of energy storage deployments by 2025, while India and China will have the most significant number of energy storage deployments [8]. Utilizing EST may aid in the distribution of energy peaks, frequency modulation, smoothing of fluctuations, and the production of excellent electrical energy. Furthermore, EST offers significant financial advantages and a temporary energy source that can be smoothly turned off the grid.

Utilizing Smart Grid (SG) technology to integrate RES can be advantageous for electricity systems in the future. The principle behind SG is to convert the present electrical grid from an electromechanically managed network to a digitally managed network. The report on the SG system was released by the US Department of Energy [9]. Digitally based sensors and field equipment make up SG systems, which are designed to manage various electrical operations, handling of information, communication methods, and control methods. As the SG idea has advanced, traditional grid planning and operating issues have changed into three major tasks. The information generated by digital technologies during the grid is processed and analyzed, and operators receive assistance finding and integrating the details. Devices and systems can share data. Real-time process monitoring, data transmission back to operating centers, and a regular automatic reaction when methods require to be modified are all possible. Power stability on the grid, intelligent grid protection, demand forecasting, and fault detection are among the issues with SG [10]. These crucial components allow the collection of enormous amounts of multi-type and high-dimensional data about how the electric power system operates. However, when handling extensive information, traditional models, control schemes, and optimization have several limitations. Consequently, AI techniques in the SG are getting into greater focus.

Large amounts of data are used in AI techniques to build intelligent computers that can carry out tasks that generally need human intellect. AI can be separated into Machine Learning (ML). In specific contexts, the phrases AI and ML are employed identically. On the other hand, machine learning is but one approach to attaining AI. More all-encompassing methods for creating AI systems include automation, Expert Systems (ES), Fuzzy Logic (FL), Neural Networks (NNs), and drones. AI generally speeds up and increases the precision of making decisions. AI in SG applications is best described as computers that mimic grid operators' thought processes to develop healing capabilities. In some situations, AI might be unable to take the grid operator role. Even while AI systems have the potential to be more accurate, dependable, and unlimited, there are still a lot of issues with incorporating AI techniques into SG technology. Physical AI and virtual AI are the two different types of AI systems that the smart grid enables. Self-aware AI platforms that can manage and enhance certain grid operations with or without human assistance are examples of physical AI systems. Virtual AI solutions include computing as an element that can help utility grid technicians with their tasks [9]. The two categories of AI systems found in the SG are Narrow Intelligence (NI) and General Intelligence (GI). A GI is created to learn and develop independently, just like humans. However, an NI is a type of AI system that is specifically created for a given task, with its own set of parameters and restrictions, such as an AI system that employs many datasets to anticipate load. The advancement of GI systems might eventually aid in the creation of entirely intelligent grid structures.

Developing sustainable and dependable energy systems appears possible by incorporating RES into SG [11]. The Internet of Things (IoT) has been instrumental in the growth of the installation of SGs, which has gained significant traction in recent years. To optimize the generation, transportation, and utilization of electricity in an SG, real-time information from various sources can now be collected and analyzed thanks to IoT devices and technology. IoT devices can monitor vital data in real time, including electrical reliability and energy consumption. This data is necessary to promptly identify and address problems, maintaining the grid's stability. IoT devices could be used for network infrastructure maintenance planning, which enables utilities to find and fix faults before they result in disruptions or other concerns. Demand response programs are made possible by IoT devices and systems, which encourage users to use less energy during peak hours. This lowers peak demand, maximizes the use of RES, and improves the grid's overall effectiveness [12].

Incorporating AI into initiatives for sustainable development enables stakeholders to make data-driven decisions, comprehend intricate systems, forecast results, and carry out focused interventions [9]. Furthermore, the uses of AI go well beyond increasing productivity; they are essential in transforming sectors, empowering local communities, and creating a more just and inclusive global community. A few key areas are focused in this chapter where AI is significantly advancing sustainable development. The next sections will delve into the many applications of AI in a variety of disciplines, ranging from the optimization of RES to the improvement of SGs, and ESS, monitoring the environment. The integration of AI with cutting-edge technologies and IoT is also covered in this chapter to provide an overview of the linked future of ESS.

12.2 AI-ENABLED RENEWABLE ENERGY INTEGRATION AND MANAGEMENT

AI plays a crucial role in the energy sector due to its ability to handle vast amounts of data and navigate increasingly intricate systems. AI can revitalize the Renewable Energy (RE) industry through improved monitoring, operation, maintenance, and storage of RE. Additionally, it ensures the timely operation and control of systems in the sector. Several important uses of AI are involved in the integration of RE into power systems [13], including:

- Controlling the production of renewable energy by tackling supply volatility and renewable source unpredictability.
- Ensuring safe operations, dependability, and stability of the grid.
- Providing precise weather and demand forecasts.
- Putting into practice effective demand-side management.
- Improving energy storage system performance.
- Supporting the planning and execution of markets.
- Improving communication between microgrids and grid components.

12.2.1 Predictive Analytics

Predictive analytics involves employing advanced Artificial Intelligence algorithms with an impressive ability to analyze extensive historical data, weather patterns, and real-time energy consumption. Through harnessing these cutting-edge technologies, we can make precise predictions about future energy demand. This capability is particularly valuable for utility companies and grid operators, providing a myriad of benefits and advantages. By using accurate energy demand projections, we can optimize the generation and distribution of sustainable energy sources, thereby reducing both wastage and expenses effectively [13].

12.2.2 Smart Grids

Smart grids constitute a vital element in fostering a sustainable energy future. By incorporating advanced technologies and communication systems into our electrical infrastructure, these grids facilitate more effective and reliable energy distribution. AI-enabled smart grids play a pivotal role in the establishment and sustenance of sustainable energy systems. The deployment of sophisticated sensor technologies, resilient communication networks, and state-of-the-art AI algorithms allows for seamless real-time monitoring and efficient control of energy distribution across the grids. It is imperative to implement measures that prevent power outages, reduce transmission losses, and bolster the overall resilience of the grid. The adoption of sustainable energy policies becomes crucial in addressing these challenges and ensuring the reliability and robustness of our energy infrastructure [14].

12.2.3 Intelligent Storage

Renewable energy systems face potential unreliability without adequate storage capacity, especially considering future shifts in market complexity, demand fluctuations, and the emergence of virtual customers. In the absence of substantial long-term meteorological data, recent trends indicate that AI can still optimize these systems [15]. Intelligent storage enhances flexibility in managing variable renewable inputs and fluctuating demand due to changing climate conditions. Moreover, it maximizes the return on investment when incorporated into renewable energy projects. A crucial element in the development of intelligent renewable energy systems is intelligent storage, essential for unlocking the full potential of renewable energy. This outcome benefits both energy system producers and consumers by providing access to low-cost energy.

Incorporating renewable energy sources into the power grid provides a significant advantage in the improvement of storage and transmission network quality [13, 16]. The ability to seamlessly transition between power sources becomes a valuable adjustment tool. Storage systems address the cyclical evolution of demand and the unpredictability of renewable sources, particularly wind and solar. This capability enables the generation of excess energy during periods of low demand.

12.2.4 Centralized Control System

Incorporating AI into centralized control systems is essential for proactively avoiding energy production shortages through early problem identification and reducing repair time. To effectively address these challenges, the AI system should include statistically based alerts, reporting tools, security keys enabling user authentication from multiple locations, an intuitive web interface, and a backup server for unforeseen recovery situations.

The necessity of using AI in RE becomes apparent due to the growing interconnections between grids, driven by the substantial volume of information and data. In this scenario, centralized intelligent control platforms are crucial for supervising designated sites. AI plays a vital role in handling exponentially growing data by offering strategies to manage variations in RE through predictions and real-world knowledge. This approach, by enhancing the integration of RE into the energy network, allows for a more effective utilization of the potential of these sources, even in the face of their inherent unpredictability [13].

To sustain efficiency, it is essential to interconnect and standardize various assets given their diverse capacities, ages, and technologies. In response to changing market conditions, this efficiency needs validation, necessitating a centralized intelligent unit capable of adapting to and addressing new challenges.

12.2.5 Maintenance and Diagnostics

The potential of Artificial Intelligence (AI) to transform the realm of sustainable energy lies in its ability to facilitate predictive maintenance within power plants and distribution systems. Through the utilization of sophisticated algorithms and the analysis of sensor data, AI can accurately predict equipment failures, enabling proactive interventions and minimizing downtime. This not only improves the reliability and efficiency of energy infrastructure but also diminishes the necessity for reactive repairs, thereby fostering a more sustainable and resilient energy sector. The adoption of predictive maintenance strategies stands as a critical measure toward achieving heightened reliability in energy systems while concurrently lowering downtime and maintenance costs [17].

a. ***Emission Reduction:*** By strategically employing artificial intelligence (AI), we possess the capacity to substantially reduce carbon emissions by optimizing both energy generation and consumption. This revolutionary technology stands as a vital tool in our continuous efforts to combat climate change.

b. ***Fault and Islanding Detection:*** Islanding is the process wherein Distributed Generation (DG) from renewable sources continues to power the load after the grid is disconnected, posing a risk to site workers and associated equipment. In such instances, maintenance personnel may not be aware that they are being powered and connected by DG [17]. Common causes of unintentional islanding encompass events like electrical grid failures, intentional breaker disconnection for maintenance, and other incidents leading to breakers being opened towards the grid. Considering situations involving imbalance, non-detection zones, and fault misoperation, Artificial Neural Networks (ANN) demonstrate effectiveness in diagnosing islanding detection.

   In [18] utilized Multi-Layer Perceptual Neural Networks (MLPNNs) and artificial neural network methodologies that incorporated decision-making tree characteristics. Backpropagation was employed to train MLPNNs for diagnosing defects, resulting in an impressive 99.1% fault diagnosis accuracy. In comparison, experiments with existing Decision Tree Algorithms (DTA), Bagging, Support Vector Machine (SVM), Random Forest (RF), and accuracy ranges of 83.33%, 98.9%, 98.9%, and 97.8%, were observed. Consequently, the proposed approach in this study demonstrated increased accuracy, signifying better diagnostic quality compared to previous methods.

c. ***Demand Side:*** Demand-side management strategies that target boosting the share of RE use, controlling peak loads, or cutting electricity costs can be built upon the predictive results for energy suppliers and consumers. Similar strategies have already been widely used for load demand forecasting, much like the extensive deployment of AI algorithms in RE prediction. Shah and Ansari [19] have demonstrated that the integration of RE sources with an intelligent energy management system in a DC microgrid can reduce the amount of energy drawn from the AC grid. This is accomplished by planning crucial energy load events and obtaining energy from effective RE sources. Intelligent electronic devices that possess the ability to transmit power and exchange information carry out the system's functionalities.

12.2.6 Hybrid Control Method

The integration of AI techniques with optimization algorithms proves to be pivotal in overseeing load balancing, demand response, and forecasting RE in Hybrid Renewable Energy Systems (HRES) within a smart grid environment [20].

a. ***Load Balancing:*** One of the most important AI techniques for optimizing load balancing in HRES is reinforcement learning. Strategies to balance energy loads among several sources are established by closely examining patterns of energy production and use. These strategies are then improved over time by using metaheuristic optimization algorithms, which adjust to shifting patterns of energy production and consumption.

b. ***Demand Response:*** Long Short-Term Memory and Reinforcement Learning (LSTM-RL) is a novel technique that is proposed to predict patterns of energy demand and find opportunities for demand response. By analyzing data that includes patterns of energy consumption, weather, and other variables, these techniques determine when demand is likely to increase or decrease. Optimization algorithms are then used to create strategies for managing demand response, like ranking it according to the availability of renewable energy or different energy.

c. ***Renewable Energy Forecasting:*** Forecasting the generation of RE is made easier by the use of AI techniques such as decision trees and neural networks. By utilizing meteorological data, past energy output, and additional factors, these methods forecast the quantity of energy that will be produced from renewable sources.

12.3 AI-ENABLED SMART GRIDS AND OPTIMAL ENERGY DISTRIBUTION

Electrical energy is essential to society because it provides a high standard of living and sustained economic growth. Electric energy consumption has gradually increased in recent years, and this need will continue to rise. Nowadays, non-renewable and ecologically hazardous energy sources, including fossil fuels, natural gas, and oil, account for a large share of the world's electrical energy production. A heavy reliance on fossil fuels might cause an energy catastrophe down the road, raising gasoline costs gradually worldwide. Emerging environmental and energy issues throughout the world are expected to be addressed by distributed RES. There is a worldwide initiative toward utilizing RES for electricity generation. RES looked to be a feasible alternative to hazardous energy sources. Due to the inexpensive cost and unlimited Photovoltaic (PV) power accessibility, PV energy is one of the most popular sustainable energy sources. By adding PV panels, this final use consumption of energy becomes a generator in the residence. As a result, an apartment building's user power turns a prosumer. RES provides highly unreliable electricity, relies on environmental circumstances, and cannot be immediately integrated into present electrical grids. In this regard, to maximize the amount of renewable energy produced without discarding any, the Distributed Energy Sharing Program (DESP) has been recommended [21]. The smart grid's topology is seen in Figure 12.1.

An increased Distributed Renewable Energy (DRE) in the future will require sophisticated planning tools and models and planning approaches that integrate decisions across the transmission, distribution, and customer domains. Existing resources, infrastructure planning tools, and techniques are not designed for a complex grid, in this proposed work DREs can deliver power back to the grid and significantly reduce or shift load. The generation of power from solar PV plants is changeable due to solar irradiation and temperature. Remote monitoring is

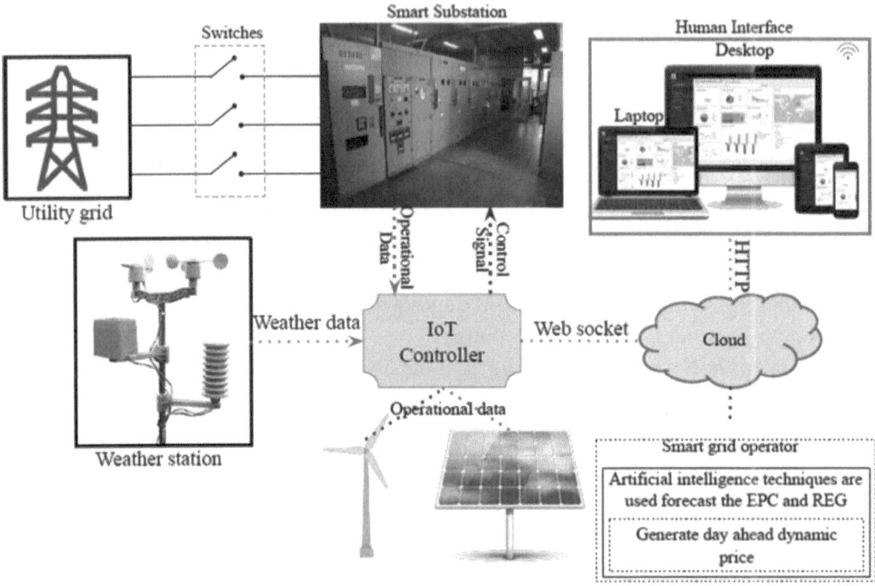

FIGURE 12.1 AI-based smart grid system.

required to manage power generation and operate efficiently. An IoT strategy to construct a remote monitoring system for a hybrid power plant and home appliances. Remote monitoring eliminates the risks involved with traditional wire systems, making data acquisition and monitoring considerably more accessible and less expensive.

However, renewable energy sources cannot provide constant power generation during the day, and hence, Artificial Intelligence (AI) techniques are used to manage the distributed energy sources effectively. Figure 12.2 shows the flowchart of the basic model regression model. Several Machine Learning (ML) algorithms have been designed to deliver an accurate PV power prediction for the next few minutes to years. Usually, such forecast schemes can be divided into physical forecast models, analytical forecast models, and ML forecast models based on historical data. The modern big data scenario uses a large volume of data to get new insights and acquire knowledge that helps the daily deciding process. One major source of these data is IoT systems that collect and transfer a large amount of sensor data. Figure 12.3 shows the flowchart of the IoT Controller. The power system's main challenge is providing a secure and reliable power supply for the end users. Therefore, Demand Side Management (DSM) is important to the smart grid system. The DRE's prediction has a significant effect on the DSM system. Accurate load forecasting is substantial for energy efficiency, minimizing power generation costs, and improving financial and social benefits. As the percentage of PV systems increases, the irregular and fluctuating nature of the generated power—which is contingent upon meteorological conditions—threatens the

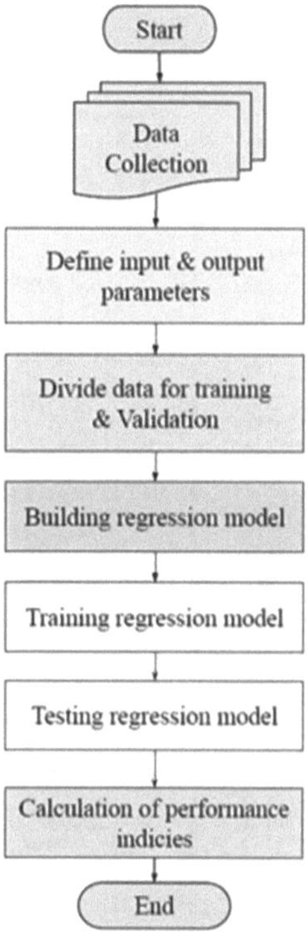

FIGURE 12.2 Flowchart of basic regression model.

electrical grid's stability. PV power forecasting is a significant energy management aspect for end-use prosumers and utility grid operators that could alleviate unfavorable PQ disturbances posed through higher shares of PV systems. Figure 12.4 shows the forecasting horizons with the applications.

DSM is essential to the performance of following SG systems because of the rising energy demand. An intelligent approach for end users to use or preserve electric energy is provided by an Internet of Things (IoT) based Load Scheduling Program (LSP) [22]. Customers can choose from a variety of pricing schemes, including period-of-use [23], dynamic rates [24], critical prices, peak and off-season time prices, and incentives through the Demand Response (DR) program. Customers that utilize the DR program that is based on incentives have advantages over the electric grid. By adjusting their power utilization over peak times in anticipation of time-based price or other monetary incentives, consumers can participate significantly in the grid's functioning through Demand Response (DR). DR programs are a resource alternative that some electrical system designers and operators utilize to balance demand and supply [25]. These initiatives can reduce retail rates by lowering the price of power in wholesale markets. One option to include consumers in DR services is to provide time-based costs, such as immediate

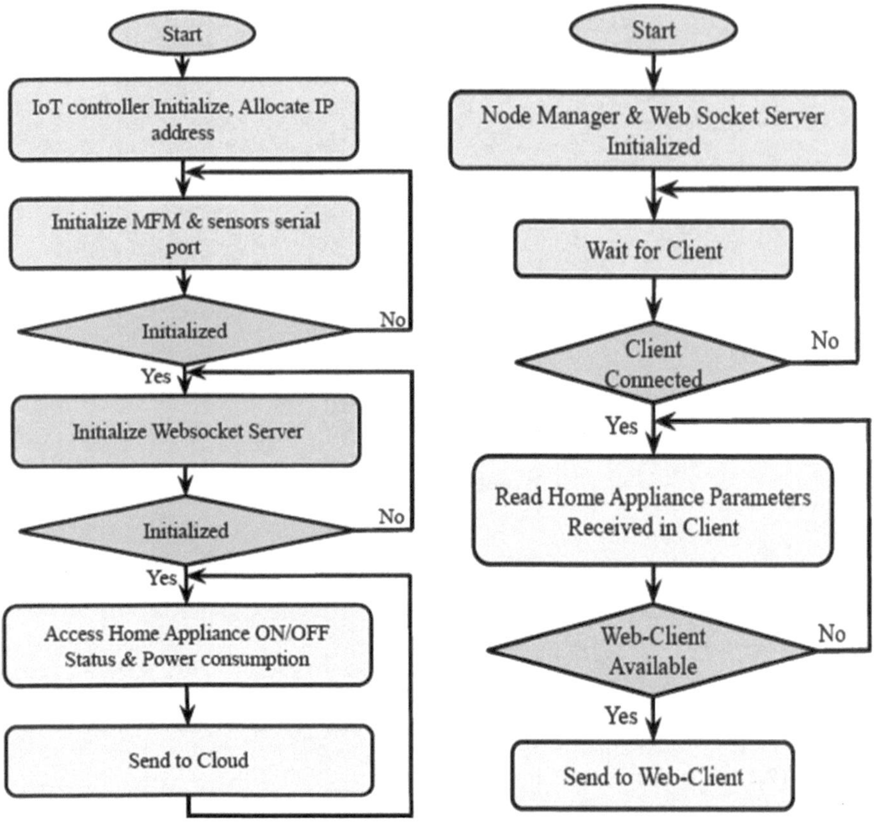

FIGURE 12.3 Flowchart of the IoT controller.

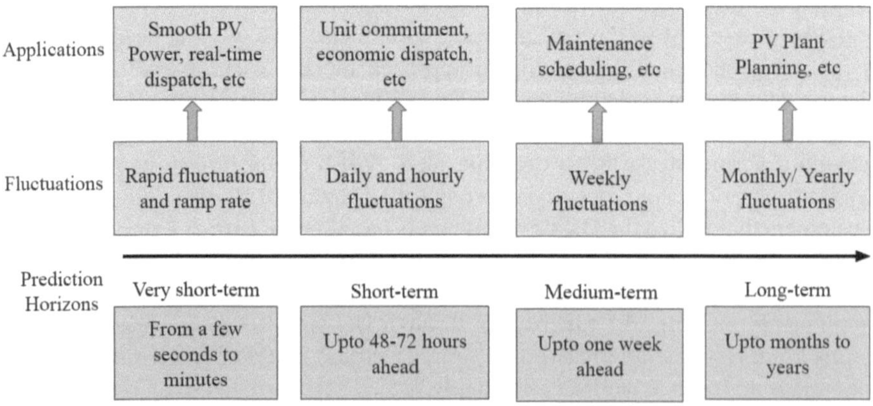

FIGURE 12.4 Forecasting horizons.

pricing, time-of-use costs, crucial peak prices, configurable peak costs, and crucial peak discount rates. Since modernizing the grid enhances DR programs' capabilities and potential rewards, the electric power industry views them as a more critical resource alternative.

With the help of the binary firefly algorithm, a DSM scheme is proposed that minimizes the electricity tariff and utility grid Peak to Average Ratio (PAR). By adjusting their power utilization over peak times in anticipation of time-based price or other monetary incentives, consumers can contribute significantly to the grid's functioning through DR. The DR programs are a resource alternative that some electrical system designers and operators utilize to balance demand and supply [25]. These initiatives can reduce retail rates by lowering the price of power in wholesale markets. One option to include consumers in DR services is to provide time-based costs, such as instantaneous time-of-use costs, crucial peak prices, configurable peak costs, and crucial peak discount rates. Since modernizing the grid enhances DR programs' capabilities and potential rewards, the electric power industry views them as a more critical resource alternative [26].

Numerous studies on price-based DR have been conducted, with an emphasis on appliance management immediately to optimize the societal implications of SG based on end-users point of view. The authors examined combining household device energy usage combined ToU price in [21–23] to reduce end-user rates and boost energy savings. Smart Hybrid Residential AC/DC Microgrid (SHRM) is growing as a future upgradation of microgrids for fully utilizing the benefits of AC and DC microgrids. Microgrid provides an efficient approach for the use of DREs. likewise [24] looks at how crucial ToU pricing is implemented on numerous levels in the sector and how it affects end consumers of energy that are industrial and manufacturing. In this system, a large number of tiny producing units were incorporated into distribution systems, and adaptable consumers have substituted all current customers [25]. Thus, through DR programs, it could interact through dynamic load control and monitoring devices [26].

12.3.1 Need for Smart Grids in India

The T&D loss in India, accounting for 26% of the nation's overall energy output and 62% in certain states, are some of the world's highest, per the Ministry of Power. India has one of the most impoverished electrical infrastructures in the world; thus, for every unit of electricity sold, it loses revenue. The distribution infrastructure of the Indian energy grid is inadequately constructed, system elements are overloaded, reactive power regulation and supervisory assistance are lacking, low measure effectiveness, electricity acquisition bills are problematic, and so on. A smart grid can help consumers save money and suggest the best times to purchase electricity. Consumers can save even more by generating their power by using rooftop solar. Information and Communication Technology (ICT), smart meters, relays, IoT devices, communication protocols, modern power converters, and DREs (i.e., solar, wind, etc.) have resulted in the realization of a smart power grid.

12.3.2 Need for Demand Response Scheme

No one wishes to spend on the upgradation of the T&D corridor worldwide. Other sources of generation, such as thermal, solar, etc., are kept according to the requirement. Simultaneously, we all are excited over and over about consuming more electricity for day-to-day life, starting from the air conditioner to heating arrangements and for the future electric vehicles. No specific regulations or policies govern SG initiatives. Current policy and regulatory schemes are usually geared around existing networks and utilities. Enhancing the current regulatory and policy environment is necessary to promote funding for SG networks. The newly established structure must strike a balance between the objectives of providers and consumers to ensure that social goals are realized at a cost that is affordable to consumers.

12.3.3 Motivation and Technical Way

Building an SG with safety and dependability in mind is intended to provide consumers with a consistent power supply. Compared to a typical one, it is more sophisticated. The conventional electricity grid is the foundation of smart intelligence. The utilization of contemporary technologies enhances intelligence and modernizes the electrical grid. It significantly improves operation efficiency, a vital feature of the SG. SGs include various distributed units, namely renewable generators, flexible loads, and energy storage systems, to enhance system flexibility, minimize generation costs, and reduce environmental effects. There are two key obstacles in tackling energy management troubles for smart grids. The first is the numerous uncertainties in smart grids, such as costs, renewable energy, and electric demand. The uncertainty problem has been addressed using robust optimization and stochastic programming approaches. However, stochastic programming approaches can be computationally intensive, and robust optimization methods are sometimes excessively wary. The second aspect is the growing presence of distributed units, which centralized techniques cannot effectively control since distributed units are dispersed and their data is difficult to collect centrally and conveniently.

Consequently, distributed optimization approaches can overcome the drawbacks of centralized methods. Even though numerous distributed optimization approaches have been presented in recent literature, the convergence performance of smart grids must be enhanced to accommodate the rapidly changing operational conditions. The convergence speed is boosted using the accelerated gradient approach. This thesis proposes a Demand-side Management (DSM) program to handle energy management issues with uncertainties to ensure smart grids' safe and cost-effective operation. One of the promises of the SG is the greater availability of clean energy, such as wind, and PV systems.

There are no well-defined standards or guidelines for regulating smart grid developments in India. Typically, the present legislative and policy structures are built to cope with the technological infrastructure and services that are already in place. The current legislation and regulations must change as we progress toward SGs to promote investments. The most popular DL-based models for forecasting the short-term period of EPC are GRU, LSTM, and B-LSTM models. These algorithms effectively handle the nonlinear nature of historical data. The most accurate forecasting approach is the B-LSTM algorithm. The B-LSTM model-driven DR program effectively addresses the unpredictability of end consumers' EPC, improving system reliability and lowering end users' electrical expenses.

12.4 AI FOR BATTERY MANAGEMENT SYSTEMS

Rechargeable batteries that utilize rechargeable metal ions are currently the subject of increased study; these batteries mainly consist of lithium-ion, sodium-ion, aluminum-ion, zinc-ion, and so on. Because of their advanced industrialization, lithium-ion rechargeable batteries have become widely employed in daily life contrasted to other battery types [27], primarily in hybrid vehicles and technological items. Lithium-ion batteries are most appealing for storing energy because of their extended lifespan, minimal self-discharge, almost nonexistent effect on memory, and high energy density [28]. Enhancing battery performance may also be achieved by evaluating and controlling internal characteristics and developing new critical materials for batteries. Nevertheless, researching the battery's State of Health (SOH), Remaining Usable Life (RUL), State of Charge (SOC), charging procedure, and other associated subjects often indirectly reflects the investigation of the battery's internal layout and different aging response states.

The rise of AI opens up even more unexpected possibilities for battery technology advancement. In addition to proactively identifying regularities and trends in data, AI can additionally be used to generate novel outcomes that are in line with a specified objective or to autonomously assess data. Additionally, it makes it possible to ignore the chemical and physical characteristics of the batteries, better handle the complicated nonlinear information related to batteries, and finish particular target assessments at almost no cost, which speeds up studies regarding battery packs. Furthermore, AI can lead investigators to observe the battery's aging process by supervising internal visualizations. Because AI can autonomously perform complex tasks like understanding batteries, it has emerged as a completely new method of solving problems. As AI has grown in the past few decades, more ML algorithms have been extracted to support battery innovation. These include state prediction, quick charging methods, and the creation of new screening substances. In general, there is a progressive maturation in the use growth of ML models [29]. Rechargeable batteries and AI have a lot of potential to work together to accomplish constant innovation. Investigating AI and related new technologies to enhance battery performance is still essential.

ML performs exceptionally well as a model because of its unique ability to handle the mapping relationships between complicated factors at high altitudes. It is significantly more suited to the batteries that recharge for every classification or regression technique in the Battery Management System (BMS) for different complicated nonlinear interactions. These learning-based techniques can finally transform different kinds of unstructured information into statistically relevant information to train by extracting intricate nonlinear rules from the training data. For example, sensors cannot directly monitor SOC and SOH, two essential components of the BMS. Furthermore, it is challenging to estimate the characteristics of the charge state, which are related to electrochemical properties and entail considerable nonlinear interaction.

12.4.1 SOC Estimation

A battery's SOC is often stated as a percentage and shows how much power is still in the battery. It is often considered the discrepancy between the battery's rated capacity and power. The battery is fully depleted and has no power, while the SOC level is 0. If the SOC amount is 1, the battery is ultimately charged. By avoiding excessive charging and discharge, the battery's SOC could protect it from physical damage [29]. However, consumers need help accessing the SOC level in real time owing to battery packs' nonlinear setup and intricate internal conditions. These issues also indirectly influence how accurately rechargeable batteries' SOC is assessed.

In addition, researchers have been attempting to improve the forecasting precision of models and create novel algorithms to anticipate various battery types. ML provides both spatial and relative classifiers, in addition to several nonlinear and linear techniques. The challenge of forecasting a battery's SOC is transformed into a regression or classification forecast problem for ML algorithms once a suitable method has been chosen to carry out the SOC forecasting. In recent years, Decision Trees (DT), Support Vector Machines (SVM), and neural networks have been some of the most frequently used techniques. Because it can create an ideal choice hyperplane that maximizes the separation among the two categories of data points that are nearest to the planes on both sides, SVM constitutes one of the most often used methods of all. The SVM model demonstrates Strong generalization capacity, which uses binary classification for classification problems [30]. It is also a supervised learning technique. It establishes the matching optimal function for the class label-based separation or prediction of new cases by using the previously established classification labels of the training set. Regarding SOC forecast accuracy, characteristics are a central contributing element besides the methodology of choice. Higher-performance, more compact, and more practical algorithms are anticipated to be created by combining current or future algorithms.

12.4.2 SOH Estimation

For the BMS, a battery's SOH is a crucial metric. Despite their apparent similarities, SOC and SOH are not the same. SOC measures the amount of usable electricity still present, whereas SOH records fluctuations in power storage capability brought on by aging or usage-related degradation [31]. For example, a completely novel battery's SOH is 100% at first, but after using it for a while, it can degrade to 80%. The ability of AI and ML to forecast battery SOH properly has also advanced significantly. Similarly, to SOC, the prediction technique for SOH builds an exclusive nonlinear connection between the input variables and the target classification to enable reliable estimation of SOH, even in the case of unanticipated battery characteristics. Researchers have increasingly focused on processing the input characteristics to increase the precision of SOH forecasting. This may be done by selecting unique, untested battery datasets as attributes or processing the initial information to produce better results. In contrast, SOC and SOH only vary in their computation approaches, using nearly identical battery characteristics as inputs for their prediction models [32]. One can utilize physical techniques such as analog circuit designs, the ampere-time integrated approach, and the open-circuit voltage technique to estimate SOH.

Though they rely on electrolytic data collected during both charging and discharge, SOC and SOH are different entities; as a result, a single data set could be sufficient for both SOC and SOH forecasting. It is possible to utilize the charging data for the SOH and the SOC above forecast.

12.4.3 Battery Management Systems

Rechargeable batteries are used in many situations throughout their lifespan, especially the highly developed lithium-ion ones. Battery aging processes such as capacity losses, temperature decay, and power decreases will cause batteries to function less well over time [33]. Furthermore, lithium-ion batteries exposed to severe conditions for extended periods may have safety incidents. An efficient Battery Management System (BMS) is required to detect temperature and preserve the different states within the lithium-ion battery. This is essential to avoid collisions, including battery catastrophes due to battery incompatibility and physical harm, and to guarantee the secure functioning of the batteries while enhancing their reliability and resilience. The BMS controls various battery functions, including thermal balance and parameter management. As a result, one of the hottest studies of late is improving the BMS's sophistication to regulate battery cells. Wang and colleagues put forth the intriguing concept of smart BMS [34]. It transcends the conventional computer constraints and capabilities of handling batteries. The implementation of the digital twin concept to help with the improvement and safety oversight of the whole battery life cycle.

12.5 MACHINE LEARNING FOR ENERGY STORAGE SYSTEM

The need for portable power sources is fueled by the growing usage of consumer electronics and electric transportation, which encourages the creation and administration of Energy Storage Systems (ESS), and Energy Storage Devices (ESDs). The volume of the front-end data and the growing complexity of ESSs and ESDs provide substantial obstacles for conventional models and methods [35]. Moreover, Big data and machine learning have grown together in recent years. Integrating human knowledge with ML has made it possible to accomplish functionality and performance previously unattainable. It has also eased communication between people and ML systems, enabling humans to comprehend the judgments made by the systems. Creating and administrating ESS and devices might greatly benefit from applying ML technologies, which can significantly increase computational effectiveness and precision in forecasting [36].

Achieving optimal energy storage and harvesting efficiency requires carefully considering and designing ESS. Usually, an ESS takes the shape of a grid comprising schedule management, evaluation, and storage units. In particular, battery ESS, batteries/supercapacitor/fuel cell hybridization ESS, and compressed air ESS are the primary types of electric ESSs. The objectives of ESS advancement are high storage of energy capability, high power transmission capability, high operating and consumption effectiveness, extended resilience, and affordable system expenses. Choosing and modifying control strategies depending on the condition of each component and its energy demand is a significant problem for contemporary ESSs.

12.5.1 RUL Estimation Using ML

A battery's Remaining Useful Life (RUL) is commonly expressed as the number of cycles or time it takes for the capacity or SOH to drop below a certain point. For the BMS to modify its management strategy and maintain the battery's efficiency, protection, and longevity, it can accurately forecast the RUL. Furthermore, precise battery forecasting of RUL and estimates are essential for supplying guidelines for battery recycling [37]. For estimating and predicting RUL, regression methods are often utilized. SVM, one of the supervised learning types, is frequently applied to forecasting of RUL. For example, the SVM model predicts and classifies the RUL of lithium-ion batteries. The total RUL is initially estimated using the SVM classification method. After that, a correct RUL is estimated using the SVM regression algorithm. For the training of models for RUL estimation, characteristics are specially extracted from the cycling assessments and incorporated into the SVM. It has been demonstrated that the classification-regression method can boost computation efficiency. Regarding an input dataset with intricate time-series features, RNN and CNN algorithms are employed to forecast RUL. While the LSTM is employed to anticipate an unidentified order of capacities data according to the characteristics identified by CNN, the CNN algorithm is intended to extract relevant information [38]. To develop a hybrid neural network, a portion of the discharge capacity reduction curve is utilized. In particular, the dimension of the input vectors and the proper sliding window size are determined using the False Nearest Neighbors (FNN) technique.

12.5.2 Battery Fault Diagnosis and Classification

Identifying and categorizing aberrant batteries and detecting flaws in batteries is a crucial use of ML techniques for maintaining battery cell uniformity. This helps the BMS select the right regulating techniques, which are essential for guaranteeing the durability and security of batteries. Several ML techniques are used to categorize the imbalance and degradation of Ni-MH cell batteries, such as kernel-SVM, logistic regression, naive Bayes, and NN with a single hidden layer [39]. In specific applications, pictures—like snapshots of a battery cell microstructure—are used as the input for the ML models. In this case, CNN could be used because of its exceptional ability to extract picture characteristics. This is getting a growing interest in energy storage and takes its learning process from machine vision. Battery cells exhibiting aberrant behaviors are often identified and categorized using the Deep Learning (DL) technique [40]. Using an in-depth belief network approach, storage battery voltage irregularities are identified. Occasionally, the input dataset is complicated and has many characteristics, making it challenging for most ML methods to interpret and learn from. The voltage at the terminal profiles of battery cells can be clustered using CNN, extracting the dataset's underlying properties to identify unusual battery cells. For example, CNNs based on hybrid sampling are employed for screening Li-ion batteries to prevent material variance and deviations during production precision from causing property differences and guaranteeing uniformity of electrolytic features in the cells.

12.5.3 ML Applications in Supercapacitor

Most current research focuses on modeling and design, RUL forecasting, performance estimations, and behavior analysis. The time or cycle number at which the capacitance falls to a certain level is used to quantify RUL [41]. An ANN mimics supercapacitors' cyclic voltage measurement behavior in the context of the cyclic voltage measurement inquiry. The forecast of the supercapacitor's life is also done using ML methods. For instance, the value of the RUL for supercapacitors is predicted using the model extreme learning machine (MELM). A hybrid deterioration mechanism model that couples the effects of temperatures, noise charging and discharging voltage, and the depth of discharge (DOD) represents the supercapacitor. In particular, the MELM sub-models are related to the analog circuit model. To determine the model settings, the weights of the hidden layers are altered [42].

12.6 CHALLENGES AND FUTURE DIRECTIONS

Even though AI applications help maintain environmental sustainability, they have drawbacks. These include the fact that ML relies heavily on historical data, uncertainties exist regarding the response of humans to AI interventions, increased cybersecurity risks, negative effects of AI applications, and a lack of adequate performance metrics.

12.6.1 Dynamic Decision-Making in Smart Environments

The evolving behaviors of utilities and consumers render energy management system outputs unpredictable and inherently dynamic. Developing an energy management system capable of making real-time dynamic decisions based on its current situation remains a challenging task. Past research often relies on rule-based choices or IF-THEN scenarios; however, this approach may not be effective in dynamic environments or when dealing with highly unpredictable customer behavior. Consequently, innovative approaches and solutions are necessary for Infrastructure Energy Management Systems (IEMS) to make dynamic decisions contingent on context and user behavior [43].

12.6.2 Challenges in AI Prediction Techniques

For existing methodologies, predicting the energy generation time and power production of wind and solar energy installations remains a significant challenge. Using sensor data such as sunlight intensity and wind speed measurement, images and video data like satellite cloud maps, and historical weather data, artificial intelligence (AI) systems have the potential to enable precise forecasts [44]. But forecasting is such a complex process, that errors in its management could lead to blackouts or a lack of RE production. AI prediction methods are further complicated by severe disasters, significant outbreaks, and emergencies.

12.6.3 Cybersecurity Risks

Integrating datasets from many owners, formats, and structures is necessary when using AI approaches for environmental sustainability, which increases the risks associated with data management and cybersecurity. While siloed approaches can mitigate cybersecurity risks, they are often inefficient. Integration must be done cautiously to prevent unauthorized access to important data [43]. The emergence of quantum computing, showcased by IT companies like Google, poses a threat by significantly increasing processing speeds, potentially escalating cybersecurity risks. Effective regulations, procedures, and education at all levels are necessary to mitigate these dangers; nevertheless, present AI applications for sustainability have not sufficiently addressed these crucial data governance issues.

12.6.4 Cost and Precision in Prediction Models

Energy consumption prediction models are difficult to develop because of the unpredictability of home occupant behavior and the large number of individual devices that are connected in buildings. To maximize resource scheduling and reduce costs, it is imperative to develop accurate prediction models. Even small improvements to prediction models can have a significant financial impact [43].

12.6.5 Future Outlook

a. ***Adaptive Decision-Making in Intelligent Settings:*** Implementing context-aware ubiquitous energy management that adjusts to context-related events may be one way to address the issue of fluctuating energy consumption. To avoid repeated data transmissions, [45] introduced an energy-aware context recognition algorithm that dynamically adjusted sensors to communicate data at certain times and under specific conditions.
b. ***AI Prediction Techniques:*** It is possible to reduce the unpredictability and uncertainty that come with AI prediction systems by carrying out exhaustive research employing a range of scenarios. Models should be tested in various scenarios at every level of development. The absence of consensus and benchmark models is impeding technical advancement in the field of intelligent energy management systems.
c. ***Cyber Security Risks:*** Future energy systems may be able to address privacy concerns through emerging technologies like distributed energy management based on blockchain [43]. By doing away with central management, blockchain technology seeks to improve transactions and fix problems with decentralized energy systems. Security issues should be investigated further, particularly in the areas of fraud detection and fake data injection prevention. Implore scientists to identify anomalies and address them before they escalate into serious problems.
d. ***Cost and Precision in Prediction Models:*** Research on prediction models from an empirical perspective is necessary to address the growing concerns about energy demands. Reliable prediction models can assist in anticipating future anomalies and provide insightful information about the everyday routines of users [46, 47].

12.7 CONCLUSION

Since the big data revolution, AI has demonstrated impressive capabilities in multidimensional, nonlinear structures. In addition to significantly advancing the development of battery-powered technologies, AI has created a new era for intelligent information-based battery EST. The concrete advantages that may be attained in the search for sustainable energy are the emphasis on intelligent algorithms that optimize energy use and grid stability, SGs, AI-powered RE integration, and ESS. To ensure that AI constitutes an opportunity for positive transformation and actively contributes to the realization of the SDGs while protecting against adverse effects, it will be crucial to strike an equilibrium between technological advances and accountable governance. The chapter has tried to recognize and compile several AI approaches to address particular problems with RE integration, SG, and Battery ESS. Despite the current attention, many fields can benefit from the application of AI and technology. Even though recent studies have addressed many of the creation and handling of ESDs and ESSs, they still need to be solved. These include creating models based on mathematics and physics, large-scale development and optimization, examination of degradation mechanisms, failure identification, and forecasting. Many of them are challenging for conventional empirical or numerical methods to handle, but AI and ML may effectively resolve these issues.

REFERENCES

[1] A. K. Kar, S. K. Choudhary, and V. K. Singh, "How can artificial intelligence impact sustainability: A systematic literature review," *Journal of Cleaner Production*, vol. 376, p. 134120, 2022, doi: 10.1016/j.jclepro.2022.134120

[2] M. Hughes and P. Ritala, "Generative AI can help family businesses innovate and grow," *Entrepreneur and Innovation Exchange*, September 2023, Published, doi: 10.32617/974-650adc3a0091f

[3] K. Openshaw, "What was and was not agreed at COP26 In Glasgow, UK in November 2021," *Open Access Journal of Biogeneric Science and Research*, vol. 10, no. 4, 2021, doi: 10.46718/jbgsr.2021.10.000246

[4] F. Calise, M. Vicidomini, M. Costa, Q. Wang, P. A. Østergaard, and N. Duić, "Toward an efficient and sustainable use of energy in industries and cities," *Energies*, vol. 12, no. 16, p. 3150, 2019, doi: 10.3390/en12163150

[5] G. M. Abdella, M. Kucukvar, N. C. Onat, H. M. Al-Yafay, and M. E. Bulak, "Sustainability assessment and modeling based on supervised machine learning techniques: The case for food consumption," *Journal of Cleaner Production*, vol. 251, p. 119661, 2020, doi: 10.1016/j.jclepro.2019.119661

[6] I. Rojek, D. Mikołajewski, A. Mroziński, and M. Macko, "Machine learning- and Artificial Intelligence-derived prediction for home smart energy systems with PV installation and battery energy storage," *Energies*, vol. 16, no. 18, p. 6613, 2023, doi: 10.3390/en16186613

[7] A. N. Abdalla et al., "Integration of energy storage system and renewable energy sources based on artificial intelligence: An overview," *Journal of Energy Storage*, vol. 40, p. 102811, 2021, doi: 10.1016/j.est.2021.102811

[8] L. Gaudard and K. Madani, "Energy storage race: Has the monopoly of pumped-storage in Europe come to an end?" *Energy Policy*, vol. 126, pp. 22–29, 2019, doi: 10.1016/j.enpol.2018.11.003

[9] M. S. Nazir, Y. Wang, A. J. Mahdi, X. Sun, C. Zhang, and A. N. Abdalla, "Improving the performance of doubly fed induction generator using fault tolerant control—A hierarchical approach," *Applied Sciences*, vol. 10, no. 3, p. 924, 2020, doi: 10.3390/app10030924

[10] Kumar, R. S., Saravanan, S., Pandiyan, P., & Tiwari, R. (2023). Impact of artificial intelligence techniques in distributed smart grid monitoring system. In S. Padmanaban, J.B.H. Nielsen, K. Padmanandam, R.K. Dhanaraj, B. Balusamy (Eds.), *Smart Energy and Electric Power Systems* (pp. 79–103). Elsevier.

[11] O. A. Omitaomu and H. Niu, "Artificial Intelligence techniques in smart grid: A survey," *Smart Cities*, vol. 4, no. 2, pp. 548–568, 2021, doi: 10.3390/smartcities4020029

[12] L. Tightiz and H. Yang, "A comprehensive review on IoT protocols' features in smart grid communication," *Energies*, vol. 13, no. 11, p. 2762, 2020, doi: 10.3390/en13112762

[13] A. C. Serban and M. D. Lytras, "Artificial Intelligence for smart renewable energy sector in Europe—Smart energy infrastructures for next generation smart cities," *IEEE Access*, vol. 8, pp. 77364–77377, 2020, doi: 10.1109/access.2020.2990123

[14] H. Chen, K. Gao, S. Tian, R. Sun, K. Cui, and Y. Zhang, "Nexus between energy poverty and sustainable energy technologies: A roadmap towards environmental sustainability," *Sustainable Energy Technologies and Assessments*, vol. 56, p. 102949, 2023, doi: 10.1016/j.seta.2022.102949

[15] P. Pandiyan, S. Saravanan, K. Usha, R. Kannadasan, M. H. Alsharif, and M.-K. Kim, "Technological advancements toward smart energy management in smart cities," *Energy Reports*, vol. 10, pp. 648–677, 2023, doi: 10.1016/j.egyr.2023.07.021

[16] K. R. M. Vijaya Chandrakala and P. Kiran, "Multi-agent based modeling and learning approach for intelligent day-ahead bidding strategy in wholesale electricity market," *Expert Systems with Applications*, vol. 233, p. 121014, 2023, doi: 10.1016/j.eswa.2023.121014

[17] Z. Liu et al., "Artificial intelligence powered large-scale renewable integrations in multi-energy systems for carbon neutrality transition: Challenges and future perspectives," *Energy and AI*, vol. 10, p. 100195, 2022, doi: 10.1016/j.egyai.2022.100195

[18] S. S. Mohapatra, M. K. Maharana, A. Pradhan, P. K. Panigrahi, and R. C. Prusty, "Detection and diagnosis of islanding using artificial intelligence in distributed generation systems," *Sustainable Energy, Grids and Networks*, vol. 29, p. 100576, 2022, doi: 10.1016/j.segan.2021.100576

[19] T. Shah and Z. A. Ansari, "An overview of Intelligent Energy Management System for DC microgrid: System and communication architecture and application in Power Distribution System," *2018 IEEE 13th International Conference on Industrial and Information Systems (ICIIS)*, 2018. doi:10.1109/iciinfs.2018.8721384

[20] S. Sankarananth, M. Karthiga, E. Suganya, S. Sountharrajan, and D. P. Bavirisetti, "AI-enabled metaheuristic optimization for predictive management of renewable energy production in smart grids," *Energy Reports*, vol. 10, pp. 1299–1312, 2023, doi: 10.1016/j.egyr.2023.08.005

[21] P. Balakumar, T. Vinopraba, S. Sankar, S. Santhoshkumar, and K. Chandrasekaran, "Smart hybrid microgrid for effective distributed renewable energy sharing of PV prosumers," *Journal of Energy Storage*, vol. 49, p. 104033, 2022, doi: 10.1016/j.est.2022.104033

[22] P. Balakumar, T. Vinopraba, and K. Chandrasekaran, "Real time implementation of Demand Side Management scheme for IoT enabled PV integrated smart residential building," *Journal of Building Engineering*, vol. 52, p. 104485, 2022, doi: 10.1016/j.jobe.2022.104485

[23] K. Jessoe and D. Rapson, "Commercial and Industrial Demand Response Under Mandatory Time-of-Use Electricity Pricing," *The Journal of Industrial Economics*, vol. 63, no. 3, pp. 397–421, 2015, doi: 10.1111/joie.12082

[24] P. Balakumar, T. Vinopraba, and K. Chandrasekaran, "Machine learning based demand response scheme for IoT enabled PV integrated smart building," *Sustainable Cities and Society*, vol. 89, p. 104260, 2023, doi: 10.1016/j.scs.2022.104260

[25] P. Balakumar, T. Vinopraba, and K. Chandrasekaran, "Deep learning based real time Demand Side Management controller for smart building integrated with renewable energy and energy storage system," *Journal of Energy Storage*, vol. 58, p. 106412, 2023, doi: 10.1016/j.est.2022.106412

[26] B. Palaniyappan, T. Vinopraba, and G. Chandrasekaran, "Solving electric power distribution uncertainty using deep learning and incentive-based demand response," *Utilities Policy*, vol. 82, p. 101579, 2023, doi: 10.1016/j.jup.2023.101579

[27] L. Zheng et al., "Artificial intelligence-driven rechargeable batteries in multiple fields of development and application towards energy storage," *Journal of Energy Storage*, vol. 73, p. 108926, 2023, doi: 10.1016/j.est.2023.108926

[28] T. Kim, W. Song, D.-Y. Son, L. K. Ono, and Y. Qi, "Lithium-ion batteries: outlook on present, future, and hybridized technologies," *Journal of Materials Chemistry A*, vol. 7, no. 7, pp. 2942–2964, 2019, doi: 10.1039/c8ta10513h

[29] X. Sui, S. He, S. B. Vilsen, J. Meng, R. Teodorescu, and D.-I. Stroe, "A review of non-probabilistic machine learning-based state of health estimation techniques for Lithium-ion battery," *Applied Energy*, vol. 300, p. 117346, 2021, doi: 10.1016/j.apenergy.2021.117346

[30] A. Harigopal and S. Nithin, "Assessment of state of charge estimation techniques for Li-ion battery pack," *2020 International Conference on Smart Electronics and Communication (ICOSEC)*, September 2020. doi:10.1109/icosec49089.2020.9215316

[31] Z. Li, J. Huang, B. Y. Liaw, and J. Zhang, "On state-of-charge determination for lithium-ion batteries," *Journal of Power Sources*, vol. 348, pp. 281–301, 2017, doi: 10.1016/j.jpowsour.2017.03.001

[32] J.-H. Lee and I.-S. Lee, "Lithium battery SOH monitoring and an SOC estimation algorithm based on the SOH result," *Energies*, vol. 14, no. 15, p. 4506, 2021, doi: 10.3390/en14154506

[33] M. R. Palacín and A. de Guibert, "Why do batteries fail?," *Science*, vol. 351, no. 6273, 2016, doi: 10.1126/science.1253292

[34] A. Samanta, S. Chowdhuri, and S. S. Williamson, "Machine learning-based data-driven fault detection/diagnosis of lithium-ion battery: A critical review," *Electronics*, vol. 10, no. 11, p. 1309, 2021, doi: 10.3390/electronics10111309

[35] T. Gao and W. Lu, "Machine learning toward advanced energy storage devices and systems," *iScience*, vol. 24, no. 1, p. 101936, 2021, doi: 10.1016/j.isci.2020.101936

[36] C. Deng, X. Ji, C. Rainey, J. Zhang, and W. Lu, "Integrating machine learning with human knowledge," *iScience*, vol. 23, no. 11, p. 101656, 2020, doi: 10.1016/j.isci.2020.101656

[37] K. A. Severson et al., "Data-driven prediction of battery cycle life before capacity degradation," *Nature Energy*, vol. 4, no. 5, pp. 383–391, 2019, doi: 10.1038/s41560-019-0356-8

[38] S. Lee and D.-H. Choi, "Energy management of smart home with home appliances, energy storage system and electric vehicle: A hierarchical deep reinforcement learning approach," *Sensors*, vol. 20, no. 7, p. 2157, 2020, doi: 10.3390/s20072157

[39] L. Dong, J. Wesseloo, Y. Potvin, and X. Li, "Discrimination of mine seismic events and blasts using the fisher classifier, naive bayesian classifier and logistic regression," *Rock Mechanics and Rock Engineering*, vol. 49, no. 1, pp. 183–211, 2015, doi: 10.1007/s00603-015-0733-y

[40] Y. Liu, G. Zhao, and X. Peng, "Deep learning prognostics for lithium-ion battery based on ensembled long short-term memory networks," *IEEE Access*, vol. 7, pp. 155130–155142, 2019, doi: 10.1109/access.2019.2937798

[41] S. Zhu et al., "Artificial neural network enabled capacitance prediction for carbon-based supercapacitors," *Materials Letters*, vol. 233, pp. 294–297, 2018, doi: 10.1016/j.matlet.2018.09.028
[42] S. I. Ahmed, S. Radhakrishnan, B. B. Nair, and R. Thiruvengadathan, "Efficient hyperparameter-tuned machine learning approach for estimation of supercapacitor performance attributes," *Journal of Physics Communications*, vol. 5, no. 11, p. 115011, 2021, doi: 10.1088/2399-6528/ac3574
[43] M. Ali, K. Prakash, M. A. Hossain, and H. R. Pota, "Intelligent energy management: Evolving developments, current challenges, and research directions for sustainable future," *Journal of Cleaner Production*, vol. 314, p. 127904, 2021, doi: 10.1016/j.jclepro.2021.127904
[44] Z. Liu et al., "Artificial intelligence powered large-scale renewable integrations in multi-energy systems for carbon neutrality transition: Challenges and future perspectives," *Energy and AI*, vol. 10, p. 100195, 2022, doi: 10.1016/j.egyai.2022.100195
[45] N. Naji, M. R. Abid, D. Benhaddou, and N. Krami, "Context-aware wireless sensor networks for smart building energy management system," *Information*, vol. 11, no. 11, p. 530, 2020, doi: 10.3390/info11110530
[46] D. Ghai, S.L. Tripathi, S. Saxena, M. Chanda, M. Alazab, *Machine Learning Algorithms for Signal and Image Processing*, John Wiley & Sons, 2022.
[47] R. Nishant, M. Kennedy, and J. Corbett, "Artificial intelligence for sustainability: Challenges, opportunities, and a research agenda," *International Journal of Information Management*, vol. 53, p. 102104, 2020, doi: 10.1016/j.ijinfomgt.2020.102104

13 Renewable Energy Monitoring and Forecasting Based on Intelligent Data Analysis

J. Josalin Jemima, M. Selva Vengatesh, S. Charles Raja, and D. Nelson Jeyakumar
Thiagarajar College of Engineering, Madurai, India

Naveen Palanichamy
Faculty of Computing and Informatics Multimedia University, Cyberjaya, Malaysia

13.1 INTRODUCTION

Our energy needs have escalated to the highest point ever seen in the history of power due to the widespread installation of sophisticated communication setups and automation on both the manufacturer and consumer sides of the market. We must maintain a balanced demand and supply to address the requirements of this expanding consumer population. However, given that the bulk of our supply comes from thermal power plants, regulating the power balance has a significant negative impact on the environment due to the excessive carbon emissions that are inevitable in nature and cause irregular rainfall, glacier melting, sudden climatic changes, etc. For instance, the majority of Kenya's low-lying seashores are in danger of sea level rise as a result of the rising global average temperature [1]. The nations that have decided to reduce carbon productivity have made significant investments in the production and use of renewable energy generation to achieve low carbon economic growth, which in turn results in the avoidance of natural disasters [2, 3]. In addition to these negative consequences on the ecosystem, the use of fossil fuels has increased to an extraordinary level, posing a threat to their extinction. For instance, the amount of fossil fuel used in the last three decades was almost 4000 times greater than what was used in England during the Industrial Revolution (1760s). A way of producing power using renewable resources such as solar, wind, and hydel, etc., through photovoltaic panels, windmills, dams, etc., is needed to solve these inherited difficulties of conventional resources. The countries with a decision to

DOI: 10.1201/9781003546382-13

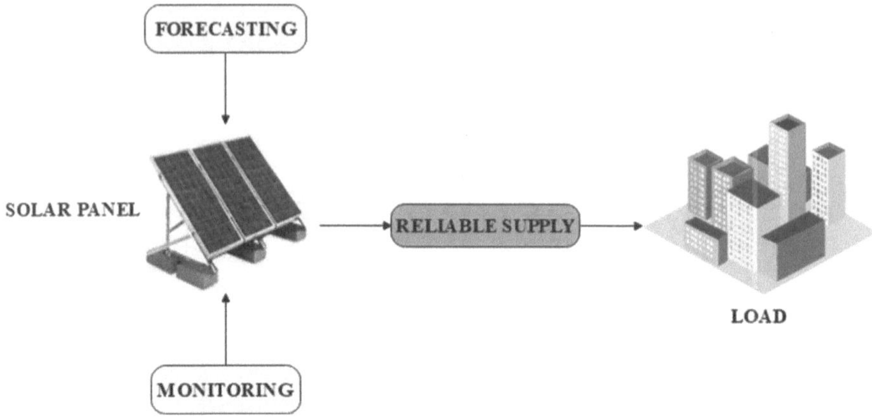

FIGURE 13.1 Role of forecasting and monitoring in solar generation.

reduce carbon productivity have invested a huge amount in renewable energy generation and consumption to achieve low carbon economic growth which in turn results in the avoidance of natural calamities [2]. The most crucial actions in power generation from renewable resources are efficient monitoring and improved availability forecasts. Figure 13.1 depicts the Processes in solar generation for reliable power supply. Reliable forecasting helps in planning the supply for a bulk customer without the chance of failure.

13.1.1 Importance of Renewable Energy Monitoring and Forecasting

The most frequent issue with employing renewable resources is their erratic availability throughout the year as a result of the seasonal variations in the specific place. Monitoring renewable energy sources aids in maximizing their generation to satisfy utility-linked loads and determine which source should be picked as their major producer. Additionally, the expansion of the current fields of generating benefits from these data. The influence of Renewable Energy Generation (REG) on China's financial development and political stability, as well as its three-dimensional impacts on infrastructure, social impact, and digital trade, are also investigated using the Instrumental Variable-Generalized Method of Moments estimation (IV-GMM) technique [4]. For instance, during the five months from May to September, which coincide with the Southwest monsoon, 70% of India's yearly wind power is produced, although solar output is good in non-monsoon circumstances. Therefore, it is crucial to keep an eye on renewable energy sources and use the data to estimate their availability and generation to plan a sufficient spinning reserve and prevent frequency drops brought on by lower supply. If monitoring is inadequate owing to incorrect planning, the nation's average frequency (48.8 Hz) may drop and there may be a danger of a blackout. This is caused by the act of pulling more electricity from Central Generating Stations (CGSs) than was agreed upon. Because of this, the state in question is required to pay a large fine. By Section 136 of the Electricity Act, failure to make payment could result in jail time for the responsible party.

13.1.2 Role of AI Techniques in Renewable Energy Forecasting

Artificial Intelligence (AI) is the simulation of human intellectual functions by machines, particularly computer systems. It is also the area of computer science that builds and researches intelligent devices. Even though heuristic techniques are capable of solving vast and intricate issues, they cannot encompass the emergence of large capacity and inconsistent restrictions. Due to these limitations, they became incongruous with modern problems. Hence, meta-heuristic techniques were introduced as an alternative but the premature convergence and more time consumption make it inadmissible for many real-time scenarios. Therefore, the concepts of Artificial Intelligence (AI) and Machine Learning (ML) help simulate those learning and decision-making capabilities in computers as similar to the human in the power system to provide an effective replacement for a person in the operating position, which could make decisions quickly during fault conditions or critical situations. A smart energy meter associated with Artificial Intelligence (AI) technologies includes escalation, series of time, succession learning, amalgamated learning, etc. [5–7]. The following are a few of the techniques.

At a solar energy farm in Australia, the unfairness in the Total Cloudage produced by the Global File System (GFS) computerized weather forecast is reduced using unfairness corrector associated with a Machine Learning (ML) technology, that is, Kernel Ridge Regression (KRR) approach. When employing the conventional Multivariate Recursive Nesting Bias Correction (MRNBC) approach for Day 2 to Day 8 forecast, its ability to rectify the unfairness in the dataset of Total Cloud Cover (TCDC) was measured regarding the percentage increase in mean bias error, which has ranged from 20% to 50% [8]. Based on historical and present data, linear regression is used to forecast energy utilized in six distinct zones of the Firm for Water and Sewage in Tehran in 2030. To demonstrate the techniques for recovering the energy and green energy utilization for treating the effluvium, various approaches have been put forth. According to these findings, raising the emission tax possibly lead to a 30% decrease in emissions from all fossil fuel power stations, to pay more than USD 30 per ton of Carbon dioxide (CO_2) [9]. To integrate renewable energy sources with long-term energy planning, an updated discrete model of grey prediction with structural adaption is created. An addition of non-linear and periodic terms improves the ability of the conventional Discrete Generation Multigroup (DGM) to detect both linear and non-linear trends in time series, as well as the ability associated with a model for gray prediction to more effectively forecast series of time with random periodicity. Hold-out cross-validation approach and Particle Swarm Optimization (PSO) identifies the developing coefficients where the adaptive structure is realized, to avoid the necessity for modeling expertise. Accurate forecasts are the result of this [10]. The load and Digital Pulse Generator (DPG) signals' nature of ambiguity and non-linearity makes it challenging to estimate the Post Nonlinear (PNL) signals precisely. In general, given the volatile and complicated properties, the signal models are insufficient for Post Nonlinear (PNL) estimation over the near period. Using the transformation of Wavelet, indicators of techniques, and fuzzy-based systems, the Deep Learning (DL) approach associated with a Long Short–Term Memory (LSTM) network with multi-input was designed to make this estimation sufficiently accurate while taking into account the real data. A meta-heuristic method is used to avoid local minimums in complex problems to solve them effectively, simply, and robustly. This method's performance is assessed using Root Mean Square Error (RMSE) and Coefficient of Determination (R^2), and its accuracy has increased from 93.4% to 99.5% [11]. Precise prediction of energy usage is essential to avoid the mismatch between supply and demand, which remains a hurdle in achieving net zero energy building ($\text{Generation}_{\text{Annual}} = \text{Consumption}_{\text{Annual}}$). A steps Artificial Intelligence (AI) framework is proposed, in which the first step includes optimal pre-processing for data refinement, whereas the second step is to learn discriminating tendencies based on historical power information using a Convolutional Long Short-Term Memory (ConvLSTM) and for obtaining temporal aspects by a Bidirectional Gated Recurrent Unit (BDGRU) and the last step is to do forecasting through multilayer perceptron. This method has reduced the Mean Square Error (MSE) from 0.045 to 0.012 [12]. Artificial Intelligence (AI) modeling and solving the challenges in Hybrid Renewable Energy Systems (HRES) such as sizing optimally, management of Demand flank, and management of storage. For instance, Hybrid PV-BAT is approached by a Machine Learning (ML) associated algorithm [13]. Big data training and Data mining help in developing a promising Artificial Intelligence (AI) model for forecasting the utilization of energy and profiles of load/demand in the action of planning the system for effective utilization of resources. An Internet of Things (IoT) platform i.e., edge, fog, and cloud layers, which facilitates the connection of Artificial Intelligence (AI) and the suitable hardware as well as software, that provides efficient data transmission, storage, etc., helps in the conversion of the developing sector of energy as a system with the lower carbon emission as possible [14]. Artificial Intelligence (AI) receives two main inputs: one is the live data about the energy demand. Based on the collected data the future demand gets forecasted by Artificial Intelligence (AI) and a strategy has to be followed to compensate for the load by the PV generation [15]. Both deterministic and stochastic models are combined along with the feature engineering as a Meta-learning Stacked Ensemble Forecast (SEF) and it gets adjusted based on the PV connectivity. In which the predictions of numerous Machine Learning (ML) associated algorithms are combined as well as ascended to form a model with good forecasting accuracy. It results in a 16% improvement in Root Mean Square Error (RMSE) and Mean Absolute Error (MAE) compared to the stochastic model and greater than 45% when comparing it with the deterministic model [16]. For optimizing the consumption of energy, exertion, and removing the contents of the characteristics in the buildings the smart eco-design monitoring system was developed using artificial intelligence techniques known as Artificial Intelligence Monitoring System in Smart Techniques implemented Buildings and this can be abbreviated as AIMS-SB, which helps to predict demand, production of energy through renewable sources in addition to that there occurs a recycling evaluation based on prediction model strategies [17]. Artificial Intelligence (AI) model is used in classifying the pollution sources of PV panels and to detect whether the panel has to be cleaned to produce the desired power [18]. PV power forecasting in the short term is very important for the integration of Renewable Energy Generation (REG) into the power grid as it must be precise and well-timed format. To upgrade the deterministic one-hour-ahead forecast meta-learning model blends the multiple DL model's base forecasts to understand their best-performing conditions. To enhance the generalization of the solution, PV power forecasting is done without considering the numerical weather predictions with the help of 4 base models of distinct architectures of long short-term [19]. In addition to the diagnosis of the fault, the monitoring of remote PV is done through the embedded systems, for this the first step is fault detection using Artificial Neural Network (ANN) and classifying the fault with the help of an effective stacking ensemble learning algorithm. Through the Blynk IoT platform, PV parameters can be remotely monitored and their status can be notified through Short Message/Messaging Service (SMS) and Email [20]. LSTM predicts the PV generation forecast with very little error using nearly 40,000 hours of operational data with specific characterizations based on the seasons [21, 22]. The chapter involves renewable energy forecasting using a multilevel stacking ensemble model based on data description and Exploratory Data Analysis (EDA). Single Stacking Ensemble Models (SEMs) have less accuracy than their traditional structure as shown in Figure 13.2. This model is an integration of the best multilevel stacking ensemble algorithms: single Stacking Ensemble Model Gradient Boost Regression (SEM GBR), single Stacking Ensemble Model Extreme Gradient Boost (SEM XGB), and single Stacking Ensemble Model Adaptive Boost (SEM AdaB) which is having minimum loss function.

13.1.3 Contribution of Work

The principal contributions of the proposed work are given as follows:

- Integrating a minimum loss function algorithm enables the multilevel stacking ensemble model (3-stage Meta RF) as a baseline model for solar irradiance forecast at specific locations with improved prediction accuracy.
- Exploratory Data Analysis of the input dataset involves data cleaning (the act of removing mixing data and outliers), statistical description, target variable analysis, splitting of data, and feature selection.
- The reliability of the suggested model can be verified by a 95% confidence interval uncertainty test.
- Model's performance evaluation using several error measurements including Mean Absolute Error (MAE), Root Mean Squared Error (RMSE), Mean Squared Logarithmic Error (MSLE), and coefficient of determination (R^2).

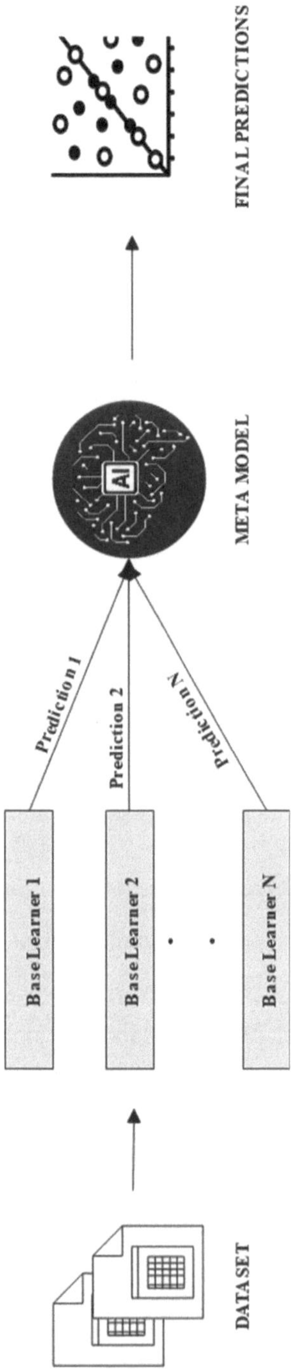

FIGURE 13.2 Working structure of Traditional Stacking Ensemble Model (SEM).

13.2 METHODOLOGY

This section explains the approach used in this work, which provides the most reliable prediction of solar irradiance:

13.2.1 Multilevel Stacking Ensemble Model (Multi-level SEM)

The process of building and integrating several models causes ensemble learning as a better way of prediction through an increased generalization and reduced variance of the models than applying them separately. Every ensemble technique's fundamental idea is to increase forecast precision by combining the independent forecasts from several models. Precise and diverse constituent parts must be present. By lowering the variation in predictions, the ensemble can outperform any particular model. The employment of ensemble-based methodologies enables the selection of decision tree specimens, the selection of features or pertinent queries to be used, and the creation of a forecaster based on the obtained data from the chosen decision tree. Figure 13.3 shows the hierarchical order of predictions which involves base learners, sub-meta models, and final predictors.

13.2.2 Structure of the proposed Multilevel Stacking Ensemble Model (Multi-level SEM)

This proposed work involves the combination of four base models and three sub-meta models. Figure 13.4 displays the proposed work's structure where the Level 2 model or final meta-regressor is Random Forest (RF) Regression, Level 1 models are sub-mete models which are Gradient Boosting (GB), Extreme Gradient Boost (XGB), and Adaptive Boost (AdaB). Level 0 models or base learners are Lasso, Ridge, Support Vector, and Decision Tree. Its work involves the incorporation of data for training, primary-level learners and their predictions, secondary-level learners and their predictions, and the final predictions made by the meta. Figure 13.4 shows

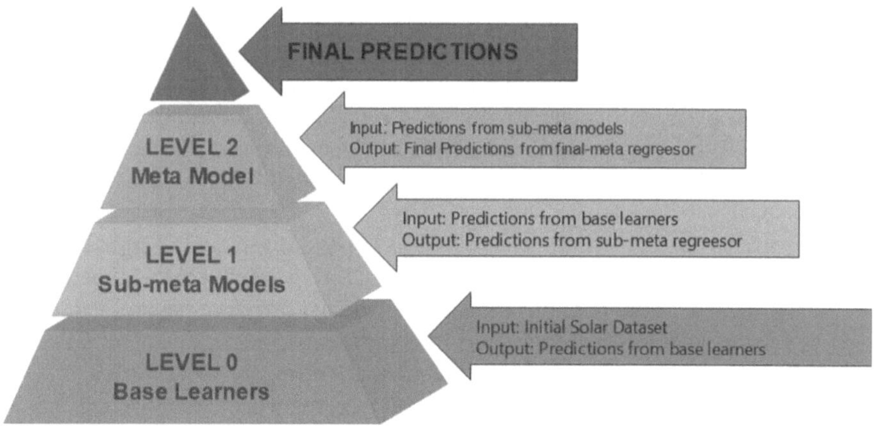

FIGURE 13.3 Hierarchical order of predictions.

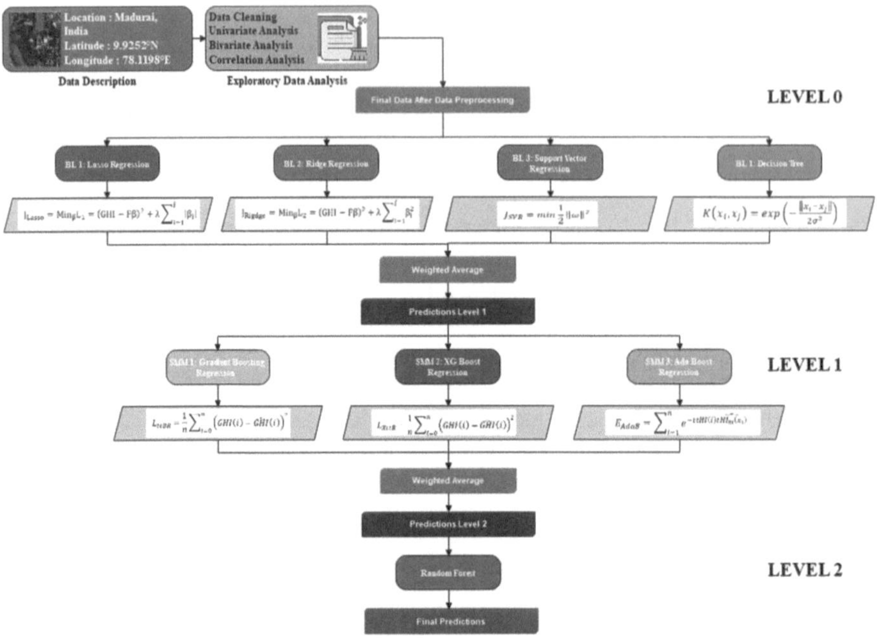

FIGURE 13.4 Steps involved in the proposed Multilevel Stacking Ensemble Model (Multi-level SEM).

the steps involved in the proposed method as it works on the above three levels of prediction, where it includes the Data for training, predictions from learners at the primary and secondary levels, and the final predictions from the meta-models are all incorporated for its working.

- ***Raw Data***: Input data comprises test and training data and is separated into n-folds.
- ***Predictions at Level-0***: Level-0 prediction is the unique set of predictions that are generated by each base model depending on certain training data.
- ***Level-1 model***: Implementation of joined predictions of level-1 as a sub-meta model single Stacking Ensemble Model Gradient Boosting Regression (SEM GBR), single Stacking Ensemble Model Extreme Gradient Boost (SEM XGB), and single Stacking Ensemble Model Adaptive Boost (SEM AdaB).
- ***Predictions at Level-1***: Several sets of forecasts are gathered from individual base learners, in other words, unutilized data for training the weak learners are given as the final meta-model's input, and therefore the predictions are generated. These predictions as well as the expected outcomes comprise the training dataset's input and output pairs for fitting the meta-model.
- ***Level-2 model***: Briefly known as Meta-Regressor which combines all the estimations of the base models and sub-meta model most effectively.

- ***Predictions at Level 2***: Final predictions are obtained by training the model with the several predictions generated by individual base and sub-meta models.

13.2.3 Design of the Proposed Multilevel Stacking Ensemble Model (Multi-level SEM)

The training process involves two important steps where the most basic step is the loading of the data that depicts the solar meteorology which has covered all possible climatic variables and the second step includes the action of organizing, separating, and cleansing data which were essential for feature engineering. The outliers in the raw data were eliminated in the data preprocessing stage and then these cleaned data were shuffled by their independent variables and the corresponding targets to train the suggested algorithms. Training and testing datasets were obtained by splitting the existing cleaned data.

The proposed SEM was constructed using the training data at this point, and regression algorithms with the lowest error rates were chosen to generate test predictions after hyperparameter tuning. Figure 13.5 shows the conceptual structure of this work. From this, the error is greatly reduced by the presence of multiple layers in Level 1 prediction which facilitates a reliable prediction in the final level.

13.2.4 Mathematical Modeling of the Proposed Multilevel Stacking Ensemble Model (Multi-level SEM)

For any kind of optimization process, proper mathematical modeling is very important for getting an effective solution. This section explains the mathematical modeling of Base learners, Sub-meta models, and Final Meta Regressors:

13.2.4.1 Base Learners

Base learners of the proposed methodology have been composed of machine learning (ML) regression models such as Lasso Regression (LR), Ridge Regression (RR), Support Vector Regression (SVR), and Decision Tree. Apart from these, Lasso Regression (LR) and Ridge Regression (RR) have been chosen as very important because of their ability to prevent overfitting and to employ the regularization process. Regularization is the most important principle utilized in this context to prevent data overfitting, especially when there is a significant difference between the training and testing data. This principle is attained by reckoning a "penalty" factor to the best fit procured from the trained data to lower variance with the test data, and it lessens the influence of predictor variables on their targets by minimizing the coefficients. These two models take the same amount of characteristics into account.

Least Absolute Shrinkage and Selection Operator (LASSO) and Ridge Regression (RR) perform the regularization of L1 and L2 type, respectively. Due to Lasso's ability to perform automatic feature selection, it can be applied in a process that involves a greater number of features. The method may lead to sparse models with few coefficients. Larger penalties result in coefficient values that are more firmly related to

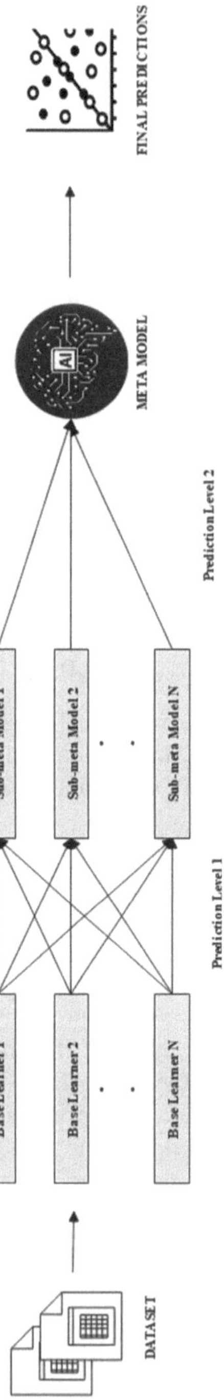

FIGURE 13.5 Conceptual structure of the proposed Multilevel Stacking Ensemble Model (multi-level SEM).

zero, in some of them may reach zero and be banned from the model. On the other hand, L2 Regularization has no impact on the sparse models or coefficient elimination. The objective functions of Lasso Regression (LR) and Ridge Regression (RR) are given by the equation (Eq. (13.1) and Eq. (13.2)):

$$J_{Lasso} = \min_{\beta} L_1 = \left(GHI - F\beta\right)^2 + \lambda \sum_{i=1}^{f} \left|\beta_i\right| \tag{13.1}$$

$$J_{Rigdge} = \min_{\beta} L_2 = \left(GHI - F\beta\right)^2 + \lambda \sum_{i=1}^{f} \beta_i^2 \tag{13.2}$$

where,

$(GHI - F\beta)^2$ is Squared error,
$\lambda \sum_{i=1}^{f} \left|\beta_i\right|$, $\lambda \sum_{i=1}^{f} \beta_i^2$ is Regularization,
f is Total number of features,
F is Feature vector,
GHI is Forecasted vector,
λ is Degree of shrinkage.

Base learners have two more models. They are Support Vector and Decision Tree. In the Support Vector Regression (SVR) method, Hyperplanes are enabled as supervised machine learning's decision boundary to separate data. Support Vector Regression (SVR) features such as faster calculation speeds, higher convergence, and a high correlation between the output and input make it one of the most preferable tools for evaluating nonlinear and multidimensional functions. Regression and classification performance and the ability of Support Vector Regression (SVR) to benefit from the dependency of training data critically on the choice of the function called kernel. To perform regression or classification operations, the input data vector needs to be transformed into a feature space with high dimensions, which can be done by the kernel function. The radial Basis Function (RBF) kernel has two parameters: C and Gamma which are utilized to analyze non-linear data in regression.

- ***Gamma***: Determination of decision boundary weights that are set before the trading model.
- ***C***: Responsible for error term's regularization (adjustments between attaining a lesser training error and testing error).

The following equations (Eq. (13.3)–Eq. (13.5)) show the objective functions and restrictions of Support Vector Regression (SVR) whereas the next equation (Eq. (13.6)) expresses the Radial Basis Function (RBF) kernel function.

$$J_{SVR} = \min \frac{1}{2} \left\|\omega\right\|^2 \tag{13.3}$$

$$y_i - \omega x_i - b \le \varepsilon \quad (13.4)$$

$$\omega x_i + b - y_i \le \varepsilon \quad (13.5)$$

$$K(x_i, x_j) = \exp\left(-\frac{\|x_i - x_j\|}{2\sigma^2}\right) \quad (13.6)$$

The equations of the hyperplane and decision boundaries are given by the equations (Eq. (13.7)–Eq. (13.9)):

$$y = \omega x + b \quad (13.7)$$

$$\omega x + b = +a \quad (13.8)$$

$$\omega x + b = -a \quad (13.9)$$

Any hyperplane that pacifies the requirements of SVR must also cohere to the following constraint in the below equation (Eq. (13.10)).

$$-a < y - \omega x + b < +a \quad (13.10)$$

To get the expected result, two important processes need to be considered, which are dataset browsing methodology selection and the path that corresponds to the tree heading toward the solution. Its topology is dogged by the most significant splitting characteristic called the root node. Depending on the worth of a specific feature, the data points are located on both sides of the splitting node, and the tree branches depend on control statements or values. Due to the multitalented working ability of the decision tree, it can provide multiple solutions in addition to classification and regression problems. It acts as the base for one of the most triumphant algorithms associated with machine learning at current, that is, Random Forest (RF).

13.2.4.2 Sub-Meta Models

There are about three machine learning (ML) models present in the sub-meta or Level-1 regression model. They are Gradient Boosting (GBR), Extreme Gradient Boosting (XG Boost), and Adaptive boosting (Ada Boost) as shown, where all of them follow boosting as their working principle to provide the proposed model with the advantages of their ensemble principle.

On integrating the base learners or predictive models, the gradient boosting approach builds an ensemble model. This approach is well-built to find the non-linear relationships between the model target and features and it is more capable of handling the missing values and outliers. Both classification and regression can be done with the model which is trained by using the gradient boosting strategy. Especially, the Gradient Boost Regressive approach is utilized in the prediction of continuous values. An estimation approach developed from the Gradient Boosting technique utilizes several decision trees with predefined sets of base learners or weakly predictive models and the total number of decision trees can be determined by the "n estimators" parameter. The difference between Gradient boosting and Ada Boost is that in the first category decision trees of fixed sizes are used, but in the second case decision stumps (comprised of a single node & two leaves) are used. The gradient gets adjusted in each cycle for the next estimator, and the result or contribution out of each new tree or group of estimators is reduced using a learning rate. The three model's objective functions are given as follows in the equations (Eq. (13.11)–Eq. (13.13)):

$$L_{ttBR} = \frac{1}{n}\sum_{i=0}^{n}\left(GHI(i) - \widehat{GHI}(i)\right)^2 \quad (13.11)$$

$$L_{XttB} = \frac{1}{n}\sum_{i=0}^{n}\left(GHI(i) - \widehat{GHI}(i)\right)^2 \quad (13.12)$$

$$\omega x + b = -a \quad (13.13)$$

where,

GHI is Actual value of irradiance,
$\widehat{GHI}$ is Estimated value of irradiance.

In the Extreme Gradient Boost (XG Boost) algorithm, an initial model S_0 is built to predict the variable solar irradiance ($\widehat{GHI}$), and the model's residuals γ_1 and the residuals from the previous phase are fitted to a new model Ω_1 in the equations (Eq. (13.14) and Eq. (13.15)), respectively. The new next model S_1 is developed by combining both S_0 and Ω_1, which has very little mean square error on comparing it with S_0. Similarly, the S_2 can be upgraded further with the help of residuals from S_1 as described in the equation (Eq. (13.16)). Equation (Eq. (13.17)) shows how the performance of S_N can be improved with the help of residuals from S_{N-1}.

$$\gamma_1 \rightarrow \left(\widehat{GHI} - S_0\right) \quad (13.14)$$

$$S_1(x) \rightarrow S_0(x) + \Omega_1(x) \quad (13.15)$$

$$S_2(x) \rightarrow S_1(x) + \Omega_2(x) \quad (13.16)$$

$$S_N(x) \rightarrow S_{N-1}(x) + \Omega_N(x) \quad (13.17)$$

The nature of additive learners is to provide their information to reduce inaccuracies. With the Adaptive Boost regression model, numerous "weak learners or classifiers" can be combined into a single "Strong learner or classifier," where its construction requires the fitting of a single regressor throughout the source dataset and getting trained with the same. Even if the alternative algorithms are used, all those forecasts can be integrated by Ada Boost through a decision stump (Short one-level decision trees). While initializing with a single decision tree, the algorithm for training provides some additional weights, in case of finding misclassified cases in the training dataset. In further training, the mistakes are also weighted. This procedure is repeated until achieving the required number of weights. Initially, assign each sample a sample weight, ω_k. is given as follows in the equation (Eq. (13.18)).

$$\omega_k = \frac{1}{N} \tag{13.18}$$

Then, each variable's Gini Impurity needs to be determined. Each node's Gini Impurity and the Amount of Say for the currently generated stump can be calculated using the following equations. The subsequent stump's upgraded sample weights have to be determined and based on its current sample weights create a bootstrapped dataset of each sample's selection probability which is given in the equations (Eq. (13.19) and Eq. (13.20)).

$$\text{Gini}_{\text{Impurity}} = 1 - \left(\text{Probability}_{\text{True}}\right)^2 - \left(\text{Probability}_{\text{False}}\right)^2 \tag{13.19}$$

$$\text{Amount of Say} = \frac{1}{2}\log\left(\frac{1 - \text{Total Error}}{\text{Total Error}}\right) \tag{13.20}$$

13.2.4.3 Final Meta Models

In 1984, L. Breman created the highly efficient and accurate ensemble strategy known as Random Forest, which possesses a tree-like structure that helps in overcoming the constraints in standard Classification and Regression Tree (CART) that consists of many weak learners generated concurrently to reduce model bias and variance. Throughout the training phase, Random Forest (RF) generates an enormous number of trees that are decorrelated in nature. After generating a large number of decisions, the model's output is obtained as an average of the output values of each tree. Bagging randomly selects the bootstrap samples in the training set and based on the Gini impurity those samples can be used to fit the trees. By averaging all the predictions from each regression tree after the training phase, the predictions of unidentified samples can be determined. Figure 13.6 shows the multilevel Meta Random Forest Stacking Ensemble Model (Meta RF SEM) flowchart.

Due to the ability to model several trees instead of a single tree, Random Forest could produce better and more accurate predictions with an impartial and more accurate ranking of variables on comparing it with the CART results. Two distinctions need to be made: First, a sampling of the learning dataset at each split node in RFs,

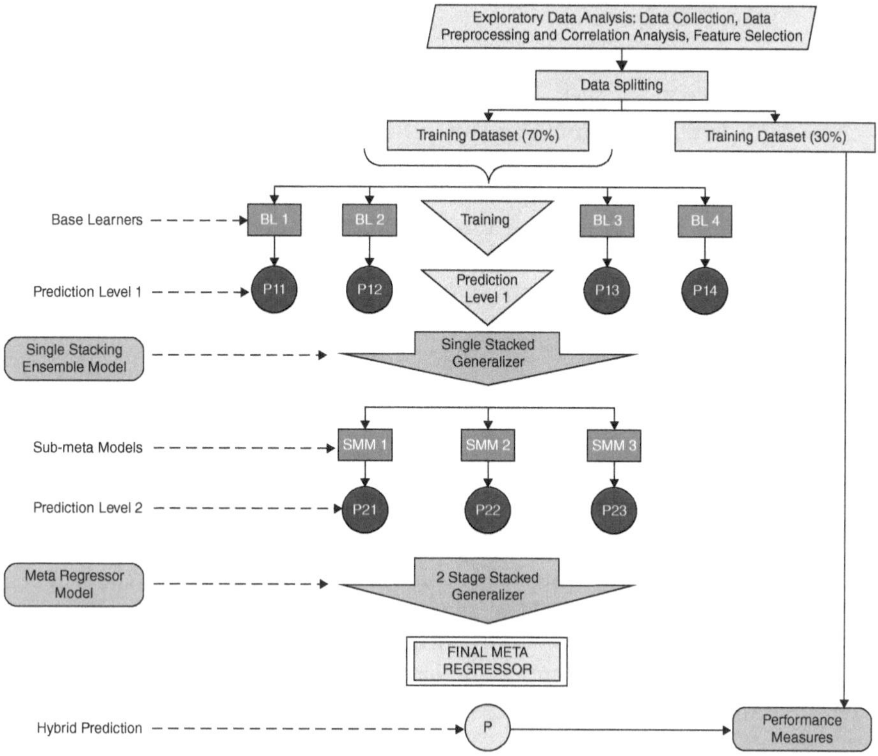

FIGURE 13.6 Flowchart of the proposed multilevel Meta Random Forest Stacking Ensemble Model (Meta RF SEM).

and the best split is determined solely at this stage. Furthermore, there is no clipping therefore all of the assumed trees in the forest are still present.

Modeling of the Random Forest (RF) algorithm includes the following steps:

- k numbers of decision trees need to be constructed through the bootstrap method using the Source data.
- To train the decision trees the m features need to be selected from the M dimensions.
- Without clipping the decision trees are permitted to grow to their maximum potential.
- Final random forest results are obtained by averaging each decision tree's outcome.

13.3 PROPOSED METHODOLOGY IMPLEMENTATION

This section explains the steps that are needed to be followed in implementing the proposed methodology as follows:

13.3.1 Data Description

Solar irradiance forecast for a site in Madurai, India, is presented in this research. Madurai is a city in Tamil Nadu located in southern India. The average annual temperature in Madurai ranges from 19.624.6 °C | 76.4 °F to 31.931.0 °C | 87.8 °F, with an average annual precipitation of 849 millimeters. The study area is located at a latitude of 9.9252 °N, and a longitude of 78.1198 °E.

The required historical data for this research is collected from the National Renewable Energy Laboratory (NERL) at Golden Colorado, which is the country's most significant Research and Development (R&D) Centre for renewable energy and its efficiency. From the year 2016 to 2020, historical data for the selected site, especially with the sampling of one hour have been collected, which comprises variables such as calefaction, sunny Diffuse Horizontal Irradiance (sunny DHI), Diffuse Horizontal Irradiance (DHI), sunny Direct Normal Irradiance (sunny DNI), Direct Normal Irradiance (DNI), sunny Global Horizontal Irradiance (sunny GHI), Global Horizontal Irradiance (GHI), type of the cloud, point of dew, pressure, relative moisture, the albedo of the surface, fill flag, direction of the wind, and speed of wind, etc. Figure 13.7 shows the Irradiance profile for the site where the major irradiance is available from 10 am to 2 pm, during this period the irradiance is above 2000 W/m^2 which could yield a huge generation and Figure 13.8 shows the image of the selected site obtained from Google map as it gives an idea on the geographical condition of that particular area with help of satellite view in Google map application.

13.3.2 Exploratory Data Analysis

Each attribute in the dataset is statistically analyzed and displayed in Table 13.1. Figure 13.9 shows the univariate analysis for the target variable Global Horizontal

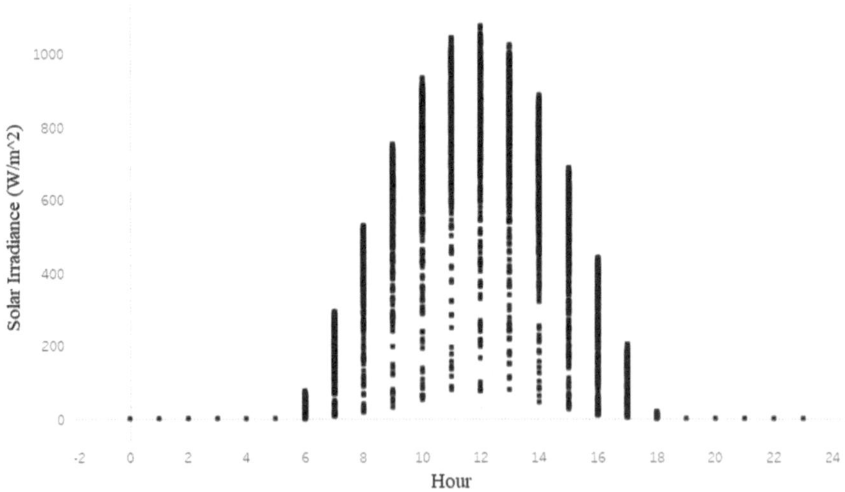

FIGURE 13.7 Irradiance profile for the site.

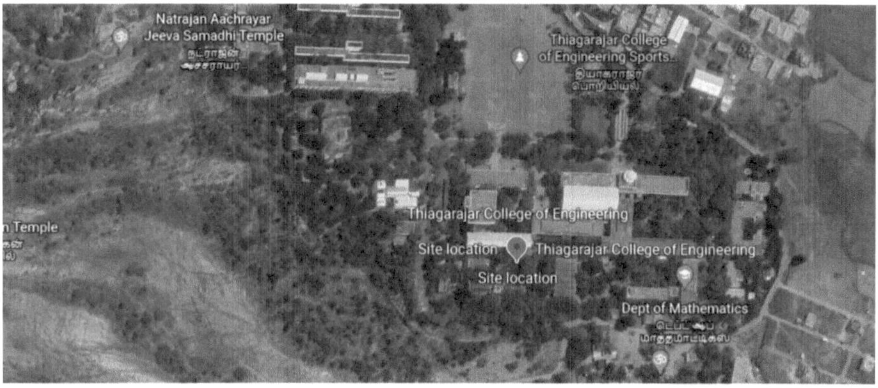

FIGURE 13.8 Image of the selected site obtained from Google map.

TABLE 13.1
Demographical Description of Input Features

Variables	Minimum	Maximum	Mean	Standard Deviation	Coefficient of Variation	Unit
Clearsky DHI	0.00	518.00	70.72	86.07	1.21	W/m^2
Clearsky DNI	0.00	986.00	301.52	347.66	1.15	W/m^2
Clearsky GHI	0.00	1075.00	284.54	361.52	1.27	W/m^2
Cloud Type	0.00	9.00	4.25	3.17	0.74	NA
Temperature	15.50	43.70	28.18	4.81	0.17	C
Dew Point	4.10	27.00	20.80	2.92	0.14	CTd
DHI	0.00	524.00	102.78	139.91	1.36	W
DNI	0.00	986.00	195.97	276.29	1.40	W/m^2
GHI	0.00	1075.00	241.77	324.59	1.34	W/m^2
Relative Humidity	12.58	100.00	68.74	22.03	0.32	%
Surface Albedo	0.13	0.23	0.18	0.01	0.05	m^2
Pressure	985.0	1004.00	993.72	2.95	0.00	NA
Wind Direction	0.00	360.00	173.25	104.90	0.60	Pa
Wind Speed	0.00	7.80	2.10	1.24	0.59	m/s

Irradiance (GHI) where at 0 Global Horizontal Irradiance (GHI) the density reaches its peak about 0.012 m^3. Following the correlation analysis depicted in Figure 13.10, the variables listed below were chosen, with solar irradiance serving as the predictor (target variable). For defining each variable range, the base value (Min), top value (Max), Standard Deviation (SD), mean (m), and Coefficient of variation (CV) were

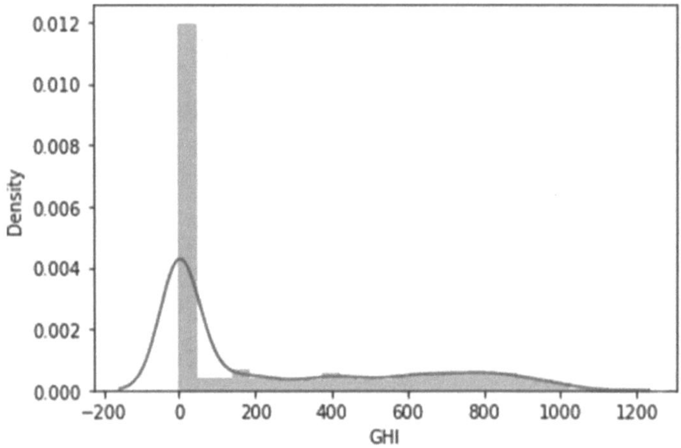

FIGURE 13.9 Univariate analysis of Global Horizontal Irradiance (GHI).

determined. The mathematical formulas for the key parameters are given by the equations (Eqs. (13.21)–(13.23)):

$$\text{Mean}, \mu = \sum x / N \tag{13.21}$$

$$\text{Standard Deviation}, \sigma = \sqrt{(x-\mu)^2 / (N-1)} \tag{13.22}$$

$$\text{Coefficient of Variation}, CV = \sigma / \mu s \tag{13.23}$$

where,

x is Number of Observations.

$N\lambda\sum_{i=1}^{f}|\beta_i|\lambda\sum_{i=1}^{f}\beta_i^2$ is Total number of data.

Temperature, pressure, cloud type, point of dew, direction of wind, speed of wind, relative moisture, and surface albedo all had less than 1 Coefficient of Variation (CV), indicating a low variance in the data. But, in the case of sunny Diffuse Horizontal Irradiance (sunny DHI), Diffuse Horizontal Irradiance (DHI), sunny Direct Normal Irradiance (sunny DNI), Direct Normal Irradiance (DNI), sunny Global Horizontal Irradiance (sunny GHI), Global Horizontal Irradiance (GHI) have a Coefficient of variation (CV) value of more than 1 showing that there is a greater variance which can be inferred from Table 13.1.

The capturing of the relationship between two variables is essential to make the dataset more suitable for the work which can be done by calculating the correlation coefficient as shown in Figure 13.10.

As the value lies between 1 and +1, −1 and +1 represent a pessimistic correlation and a supportive correlation, respectively. If a coefficient is 0, then there is no correlation between those two variables.

Figure 13.11 represents a pair plot, a sort of data visualization that shows the pairwise connection between some of the key attributes and the target variable.

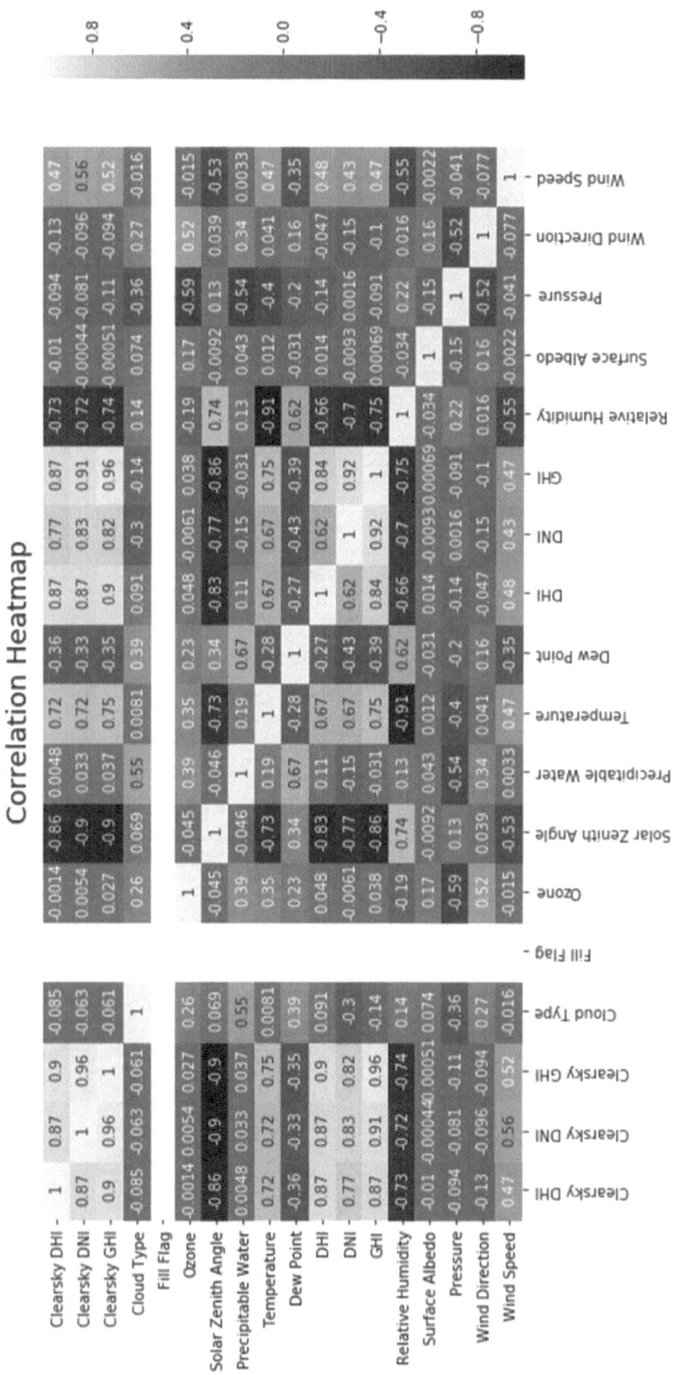

FIGURE 13.10 Coefficient of Correlation among the variables.

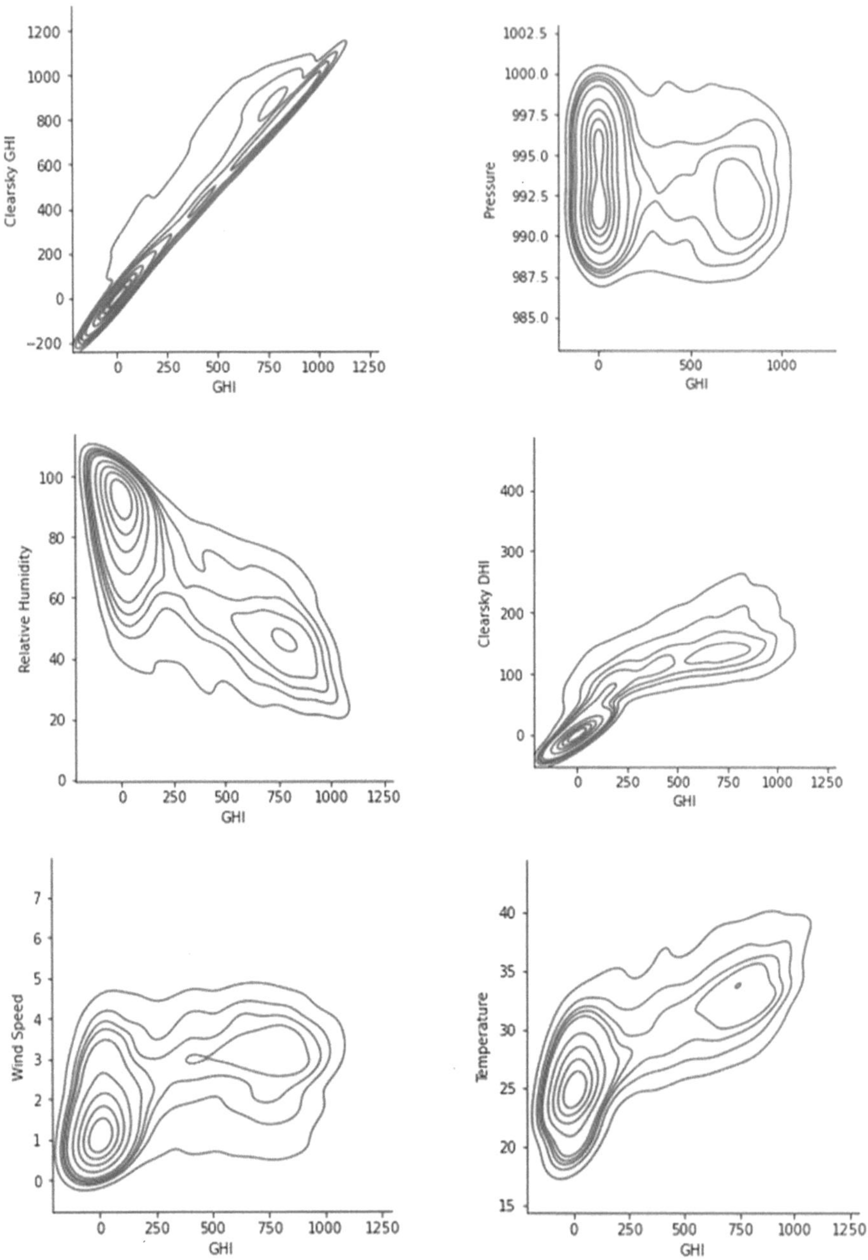

FIGURE 13.11 Pair-wise connection between the key attributes.

13.4 RESULTS AND DISCUSSION

In this segment, the suggested model's performance, uncertainty qualifications, and hyperparameter tuning are explained as follows:

13.4.1 Model Performance Evaluation

As previously, several methods for assessing model performance have been implemented. A common metrics set of statistical concepts, that is, Mean Absolute Error (MAE), Mean Square Error (MSE), Root Mean Square Error (RMSE), Mean Squared Log Error (MSLE), and Correlation Coefficient (R^2) have been utilized in this study for evaluating the effectiveness of the proposed model because each statistic metric has its positives and negatives. Mathematical representations of these metrics are given as follows:

13.4.1.1 Mean Absolute Error (MAE)

Mean Absolute Error (MAE) is an average error value or value of absolute errors in a set of forecasted values where its value lies between 0 and ∞, a very efficient model has a lower value. Its unit is the same as the output variable and is most reliable when there are outliers (Eq. (13.24)).

$$MAE = \sum_{i=1}^{N} \frac{\left(\widehat{GHI}(i) - GHI(i)\right)}{N} \tag{13.24}$$

where,

$\widehat{GHI}(i)$ is Forecasted Value,

$GHI(i)\lambda \sum_{i=1}^{f} |\beta_i| \lambda \sum_{i=1}^{f} \beta_i^2$ is Actual Value,

N is Number of data.

13.4.1.2 Mean Square Error (MSE)

Mean Square Error (MSE) is a squared variance between the actual and the values obtained through prediction, with a small amount of variance in mean absolute error, is the most widely used and fundamental metric in which squaring is performed to prevent the cancellation of negative terms (Eq. (13.25)).

$$MSE = \frac{1}{N} \sum_{i=1}^{N} \left(\widehat{GHI}(i) - GHI(i)\right)^2 \tag{13.25}$$

where,

$\widehat{GHI}(i)$ is Forecasted Value,

$GHI(i)\lambda \sum_{i=1}^{f} |\beta_i| \lambda \sum_{i=1}^{f} \beta_i^2$ is Actual Value,

N is Number of data.

13.4.1.3 Root Mean Square Error (RMSE)

An operator's ultimate aim is the reduction of the error to get a promising model performance and due to the ability of assessing a model's accuracy, Root Mean Square Error (RMSE) is being considered as one of the most prominent statistical indicators. At lower RMSE, the model will perform better in terms of absolute deviation whereas there will be a huge difference when the RMSE value is high. It gives information on how the residuals have been distributed. Higher weights will be provided for outliers or errors by squaring, as a result, there will be a noticeable error reduction when reducing the RMSE for the model's optimization (Eq. (13.26)).

$$\mathrm{RMSE} = \sqrt{\frac{1}{N}\sum_{i=1}^{N}\left(\widehat{\mathrm{GHI}}(i) - \mathrm{GHI}(i)\right)^2} \tag{13.26}$$

where,

$\widehat{\mathrm{GHI}}(i)$ is Forecasted Value,

$\mathrm{GHI}(i)\lambda\sum_{i=1}^{f}|\beta_i|\lambda\sum_{i=1}^{f}\beta_i^2$ is Actual Value,

N is Number of data.

13.4.1.4 Mean Square Logarithmic Error (MSLE)

Mean Square Logarithmic Error (MSLE) is computed using the natural logarithm of each estimated value. For Mean Square Logarithmic Error (MSLE) the only value that matters is the percentual difference between the expected value following the log transformation. Even minor deviations between actual and predicted values are considered to be major differences between the actual and estimated values (Eq. (13.27)):

$$\mathrm{MLSE} = \frac{1}{N}\sum_{i=0}^{N}\left(\log(\mathrm{GHI}+1) - \log\left(\widehat{\mathrm{GHI}}(i)+1\right)\right)^2 \tag{13.27}$$

where,

$\widehat{\mathrm{GHI}}(i)$ is Forecasted Value,

$\mathrm{GHI}(i)\lambda\sum_{i=1}^{f}|\beta_i|\lambda\sum_{i=1}^{f}\beta_i^2$ is Actual Value,

N is Number of data.

13.4.1.5 Coefficient of Determination (R^2)

The coefficient of Determination (R^2) is determined as the fraction of a dependent variable's change that can be forecasted by the independent variable. It determines how much percentage of predicted data is nearer to the actual data. As per the R^2 concept, the model which possesses the value closest to 1, is the model with a maximum efficiency. The mathematical expression of the determination coefficient is given as follows (Eq. (13.28)):

$$\text{MLSE} = \frac{1}{N}\sum_{i=0}^{N}\left(\log(\text{GHI}+1) - \log\left(\widehat{\text{GHI}}(i)+1\right)\right)^2 \tag{13.28}$$

where,

$\widehat{\text{GHI}}(i)$ is Forecasted Value,

$\text{GHI}(i)\lambda\sum_{i=1}^{f}|\beta_i|\lambda\sum_{i=1}^{f}\beta_i^2$ is Actual Value,

$\overline{\text{GHI}}(i)$ is Variance.

N is Number of data.

The final results of the three single stacking ensemble models (2-stage Gradient Boosting, 2-stage XG Boost, 2-stage Ada Boost) and the recommended multilevel RF SEM forecasts are discussed and analyzed. Table 13.1 shows the performance metrics of all the aforementioned models. Table 13.2 shows the performance metrics of regression techniques, Single SEM, and the proposed model. From this, it is inferred that the proposed model performs in a better way than all by holding the values of 2.1103 W/m^2 MAE, 5.2455 W/m^2 RMSE, 0.0004 W/m^2 MSLE, and 0.9997 W/m^2 R^2. With MAE, RMSE, MSLE, R^2 of about 3.9493 W/m^2, 9.6162 W/m^2, 0.0007 W/m^2, and 0.9991 W/m^2, respectively, due to the ability to offer ultimate accuracy Single SEM XG Boost models and Single SEM Gradient Boosting are placed next to the proposed model. Single SEM Ada Boost ranked at last among all of the selected SEM algorithms as it has MAE, RMSE, and MSLE, R^2 of 14.4294 W/m^2, 17.3108 W/m^2, 3.4545 W/m^2 and 0.9990 W/m^2 respectively. All the study models' accuracy metrics in the bar chart form are shown in Figure 13.12.

TABLE 13.2
Performance Metrics Analysis

Regression Technique	MAE [W/m^2]	RMSE [W/m^2]	MSLE [W/m^2]	R^2
Lasso	15.53	26.72	1.4626	0.9931
Ridge	15.88	26.64	1.6733	0.9932
Support Vector Regression	18.54	40.41	0.2124	0.9843
Decision Tree	2.25	6.50	0.0003	0.9995
Single SEM Gradient Boosting	2.62	6.65	0.0009	0.9996
Single SEM XG Boost	2.30	6.50	0.0003	0.9996
Single SEM Ada Boost	12.26	14.49	3.1807	0.9979
Proposed Multilevel SEM Random Forest	1.13	3.41	9.9453	0.9998

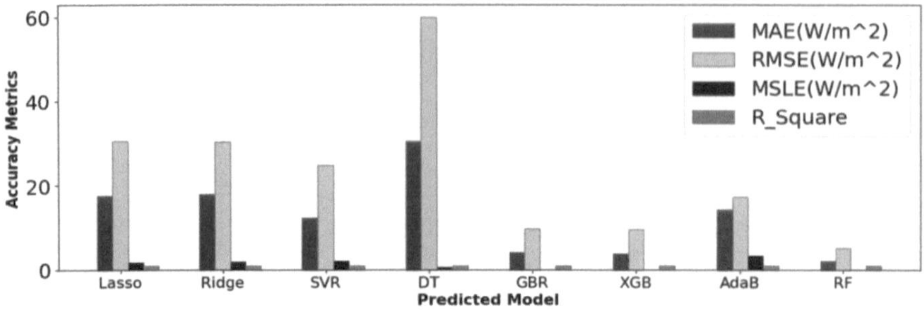

FIGURE 13.12 Accuracy metrics analysis.

Comparison of the real and predicted irradiance Lasso, Ridge, Decision tree, and Support Vector Regression (SVR) are shown in Figure 13.13, whereas 2-stage Gradient Boosting, 2-stage XG Boost, 2-stage Ada Boost, and the proposed multilevel Meta RF-SEM with many test samples are shown in Figure 13.14. In every level of irradiance, the proposed model's estimated values and measured values are essentially to be similar. Scalar plots of all the methods and the proposed model are represented in Figure 13.15 which illustrates how closely the expected and actual irradiances have been greatly correlated. From this, it was clear that the data points would be closer if the two variables were highly correlated with each other.

13.4.2 Uncertainty Qualification

By applying the concept of confidence interval the uncertainty of parameters can be investigated where the influencing elements include errors in measurements, exemplification bias, inconsistency, as well as the usage of alternative data. The confidence interval is a certain range at which the actual or real value occurs. The interval's confidence level determines the chance that a significance range contains the actual parameter value. The most widely used set of values to manage population-based data to extract precise, significant information with a specific level of confidence is known as the "Confidence Interval."

A 95% confidence interval indicates that in 95% of the intervals generated by computing the interval of an unbounded number of population samples, the interval will include the population mean. As a result, it is possible to compute the sample mean from a single sample and provide an interval that closely contains the true population mean. The 95% confidence interval map for all base learners, three single SEM, and the proposed multilevel Meta Random Forest Stacking Ensemble Model (Meta RF SEM). From this it is intelligible that the suggested model has a prominent regression fit, indicating high reliability.

13.4.3 Hyperparameter Tuning

A revolutionary wrapper automated technology called Genetic Algorithm Parsimony (GA Parsimony) effectively produces forecasted models with minimal complexity and adequate generalization power. Here, the GA parsimonious model combines

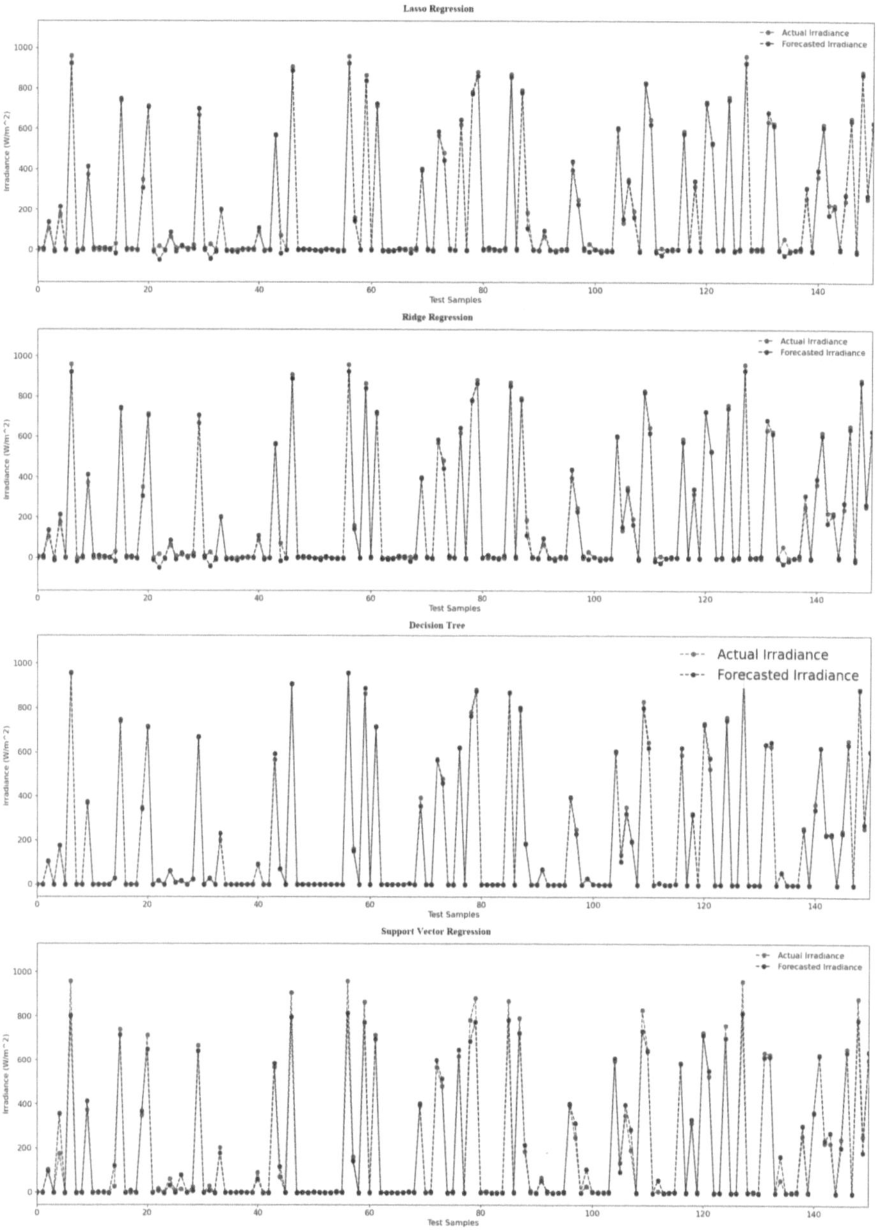

FIGURE 13.13 Actual vs. Predicted irradiance of Lasso, Ridge, DT, and SVR.

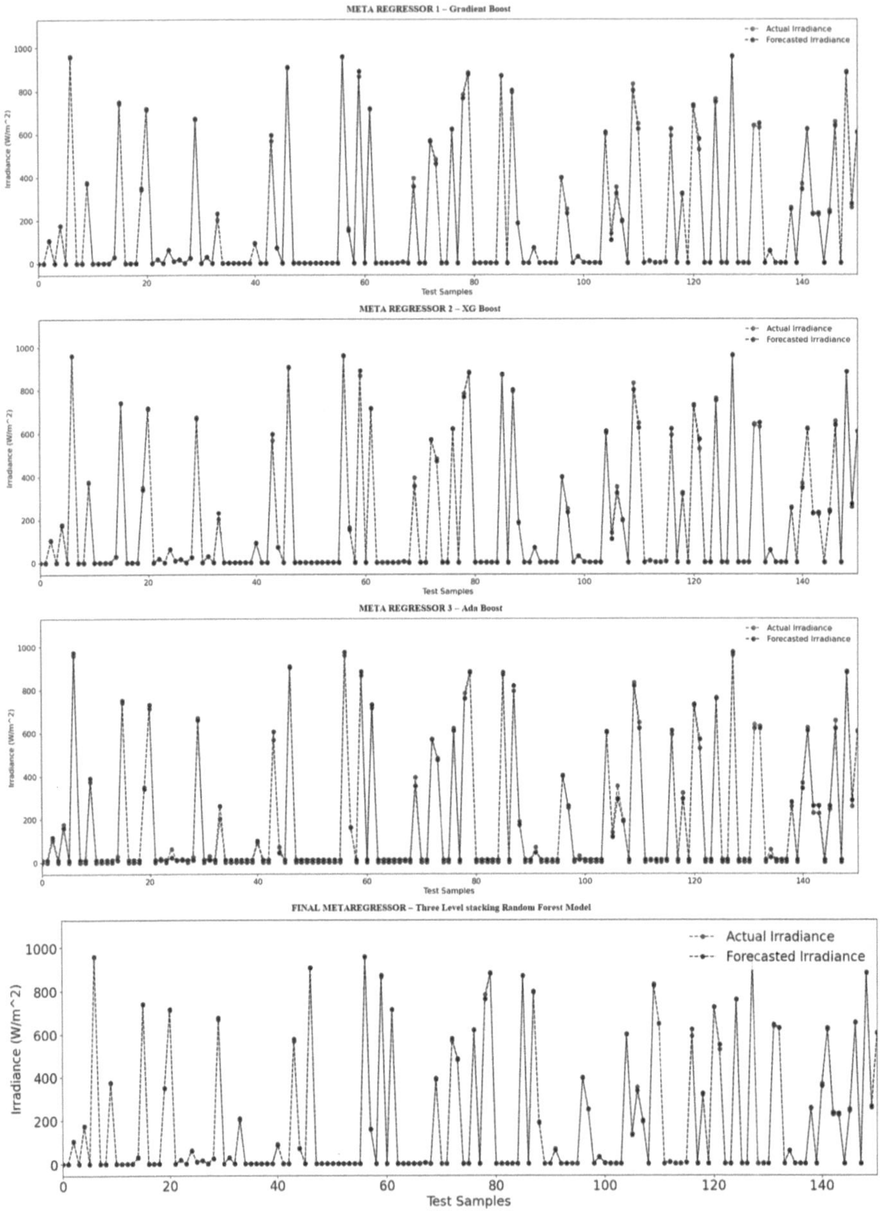

FIGURE 13.14 Actual vs. Predicted irradiance of GB, XG, Ada Boost, and proposed model.

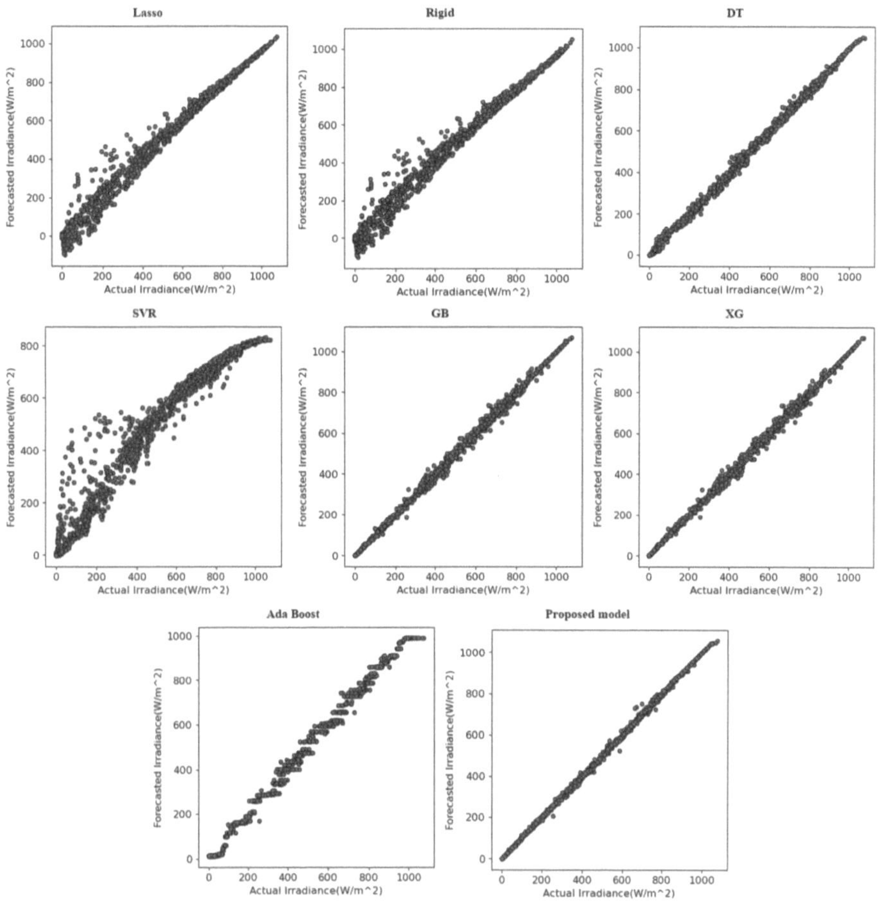

FIGURE 13.15 Actual vs. Predicted irradiance using Scalar plot.

feature selection, parameter tuning, and a novel selection procedure named ReRank algorithm, all of which work together to provide an overall better model. The primary advantage of the suggested parsimonious model is that it computes cost and complexity independently, allowing for the optimal individual model selection. In contrast, the traditional genetic algorithm calculates the fitness function using a penalty factor that combines complexity and loss. The ReRank algorithm uses this data to reorder the models according to their complexity when there is no discernible difference in their costs. Consequently, simpler models with similar accuracy are encouraged. Furthermore, there is no uncertainty in predicting the correct value because the penalty setting is irrelevant. Thus, GA-PARSIMONY eventually makes possible an automatic method to obtain parsimonious models. To adjust the final meta regressor (Random Forest) parameters, the multilevel stacking ensemble model and the GA parsimonious algorithm are combined in this work. A tuple of hyperparameters is given to the objective function, which then produces the associated loss. To estimate this generalization performance, cross-validation is commonly used. Using the parsimonious model for hyperparameter optimization, the optimal set of model parameters that produce the best performance measure having maximum depth =28 and maximum features = 10 have been found in this work

13.5 CONCLUSION

For the World's future energy needs, PV systems are going to be the most important source. To include this variable power in the electric grid, reliable and accurate solar irradiance forecasting is needed. The machine Learning approach is most widely used for hourly solar forecasts. Both single and multi-layer stacking ensemble approaches were utilized. At first, just one meta regressor is used, but at the second there is a wide utilization of meta regressors across multiple layers. To increase the solar irradiance prediction accuracy, the multilevel Meta RF SEM is introduced which has three independent 2-stage SEM and four base learners. The suggested model performs better than the models using a single layer of stacking, bagging, or boosting. It results in a correlation of 99.98% having MAE and RMSE of 1.13 W/m^2 and 3.41 W/m^2 respectively. Therefore, the suggested multilevel meta-RF SEM results in better prediction accuracy in solar irradiance forecasting.

REFERENCES

[1] Voumik LC, Ridwan M, Rahman MH, Raihan A. An investigation into the primary causes of carbon dioxide releases in Kenya: Does renewable energy matter to reduce carbon emission? *Renewable Energy Focus*. 2023;47:100491.

[2] Siddik AB, Khan S, Khan U, Yong L, Murshed M. The role of renewable energy finance in achieving low-carbon growth: contextual evidence from leading renewable energy-investing countries. *Energy*. 2023;270:126864.

[3] Yu C, Moslehpour M, Tran TK, Trung LM, Ou JP, Tien NH. Impact of non-renewable energy and natural resources on economic recovery: Empirical evidence from selected developing economies. *Resources Policy*. 2023;80:103221.

[4] Zheng M, Wong CY. The impact of digital economy on renewable energy development in China. *Innovation and Green Development*. 2024;3(1):100094.

[5] Entezari A, Aslani A, Zahedi R, Noorollahi Y. Artificial intelligence and machine learning in energy systems: A bibliographic perspective. *Energy Strategy Reviews*. 2023;45:101017.

[6] Zhao N, Zhang H, Yang X, Yan J, You F. Emerging information and communication technologies for smart energy systems and renewable transition. *Advances in Applied Energy*. 2023;9:100125.

[7] Nutakki M, Mandava S. Review on optimization techniques and role of Artificial Intelligence in home energy management systems. *Engineering Applications of Artificial Intelligence*. 2023;119:105721.

[8] Deo RC, Ahmed AM, Casillas-Pérez D, Pourmousavi SA, Segal G, Yu Y, Salcedo-Sanz S. Cloud cover bias correction in numerical weather models for solar energy monitoring and forecasting systems with kernel ridge regression. *Renewable Energy*. 2023;203:113–130.

[9] Khah MV, Zahedi R, Mousavi MS, Ahmadi A. Forecasting renewable energy utilization by Iran's water and wastewater industries. *Utilities Policy*. 2023;82:101546.
[10] Qian W, Sui A. A novel structural adaptive discrete grey prediction model and its application in forecasting renewable energy generation. *Expert Systems with Applications*. 2021;186:115761.
[11] Mokarram MJ, Rashiditabar R, Gitizadeh M, Aghaei J. Net-load forecasting of renewable energy systems using multi-input LSTM fuzzy and discrete wavelet transform. *Energy*. 2023;275:127425.
[12] Khan SU, Khan N, Ullah FU, Kim MJ, Lee MY, Baik SW. Towards intelligent building energy management: AI-based framework for power consumption and generation forecasting. *Energy and Buildings*. 2023;279:112705.
[13] Maghami MR, Mutambara AG. Challenges associated with Hybrid Energy Systems: An artificial intelligence solution. *Energy Reports*. 2023;9:924–940.
[14] Li J, Herdem MS, Nathwani J, Wen JZ. Methods and applications for Artificial Intelligence, Big Data, Internet of Things, and Blockchain in smart energy management. *Energy and AI*. 2023;11:100208.
[15] Giglio E, Luzzani G, Terranova V, Trivigno G, Niccolai A, Grimaccia F. An efficient artificial intelligence energy management system for urban building integrating photovoltaic and storage. *IEEE Access*. 2023;11:18673–18688.
[16] Oprea SV, Bâra A. A stacked ensemble forecast for photovoltaic power plants combining deterministic and stochastic methods. *Applied Soft Computing*. 2023;147:110781.
[17] Selvaraj R, Kuthadi VM, Baskar S. Smart building energy management and monitoring system based on artificial intelligence in smart city. *Sustainable Energy Technologies and Assessments*. 2023;56:103090.
[18] Khan PW, Byun YC, Jeong OR. A stacking ensemble classifier-based machine learning model for classifying pollution sources on photovoltaic panels. *Scientific Reports*. 2023;13(1):10256.
[19] Sarmas E, Spiliotis E, Stamatopoulos E, Marinakis V, Doukas H. Short-term photovoltaic power forecasting using meta-learning and numerical weather prediction independent Long Short-Term Memory models. *Renewable Energy*. 2023;216:118997.
[20] Mellit A, Benghanem M, Kalogirou S, Pavan AM. An embedded system for remote monitoring and fault diagnosis of photovoltaic arrays using machine learning and the internet of things. *Renewable Energy*. 2023;208:399–408.
[21] Mohammad A, Mahjabeen F. Revolutionizing solar energy: The impact of artificial intelligence on photovoltaic systems. *International Journal of Multidisciplinary Sciences and Arts*. 2023;2(1):117–127.
[22] Ghai, D., Tripathi, S. L., Saxena, S., Chanda, M., & Alazab, M. (Eds.). *Machine Learning Algorithms for Signal and Image Processing*. John Wiley & Sons. 2022.

14 Design and Simulation of Solar Power Generation System Using MATLAB®

Suman Lata Tripathi
School of Electronics and Electrical Engineering,
Lovely Professional University, Phagwara, India

Sandhya Avasthi
Department of Computer Science and Engineering,
ABES Engineering College, Ghaziabad, India

14.1 INTRODUCTION

The need for electricity is growing daily in the modern world, yet coal and other fossil resources are becoming scarcer. Now is the moment to look for alternative energy sources. At times, it might be challenging to send electricity to isolated, steep locations that are distant from the main power plant to address problems with power quality and energy efficiency. Since many countries are found in tropical and temperate zones, where direct solar density can reach 1000 W/m, the usage of solar cell energy is regarded as a key resource. Because of its many benefits, including ease of allocation, high dependability, no fuel cost, low maintenance, and no noise or wear from the lack of moving parts, solar cell (PV) generation is currently gaining traction as a renewable energy source application [1–5]. Thus, we are attempting to simulate a system for producing non-conventional energy using solar and wind power [6–9]. This place emits no pollution, making it completely environmentally friendly.

14.2 TOOLS DESCRIPTION

MATLAB®: MATLAB® is the most promising tool to model control system that helps in achieving or improving the desired model by design and simulation results [10]. It combines programming, computation, and visualization into a user-friendly environment where issues and their fixes are presented using well-known mathematical symbols. Common applications include computation and math.

DOI: 10.1201/9781003546382-14

***PV Array*:** The PV Array block is a five-parameter model that represents the temperature- and irradiance-dependent I-V characteristics of the modules utilizing a diode, series resistance (Rs), shunt resistance (Rsh), and light-generated current source (IL). The equations define the diode I–V characteristics for a single module.

***Voltage Measurement*:** The instantaneous voltage between two electric nodes is measured using the Voltage Measurement block. A signal that can be used by further Simulink blocks is provided by the Simulink signal output.

***Diode*:** The diode is a semiconductor device whose voltage Vak and current Iak are self-governing. A diode with a small forward voltage Vf across it begins to conduct when it is forward-biased (Vak > 0). When the device's current flow drops to zero, it shuts off.

***Universal Bridge*:** With the help of the Universal Bridge block, converters can be simulated utilizing both forced-commutated (GTO, IGBT, MOSFET) and power electronic devices like diodes and thyristors. The fundamental building block for creating two-level voltage-sourced converters (VSCs) is the Universal Bridge block.

***PWM Generator*:** Using a two-level topology, the PWM Generator block produces pulses for carrier-based pulse width modulation (PWM) converters. A combination of two three-phase bridges or single-phase, two-phase, three-phase, or two-level bridges can utilize the block to activate their forced-commutated devices (FETs, GTOs, or IGBTs).

***Constant*:** When the constant attribute is set, the value cannot be altered after it has been initialized to the value given in the property block.

***Series RLC Branch*:** Resistor, inductor and a capacitor, or a series combination of these, are used in 3-phase series RLC Branch block. To choose which elements you want to include in each branch, use the Branch type parameter.

***Scope*:** The Scope lets you change the amount of time and the range of input values displayed. Throughout the simulation, you can change the parameter values for the Scope and move and resize the window. Simulink writes data to connected Scopes but does not open Scope windows when a simulation starts.

14.3 METHODOLOGY

To have a comprehensive understanding of the solar power generation model [2], a diagram of the solar power design draft is provided in Figure 14.1, presenting the main parts of the proposed model, along with a brief description of each stage.

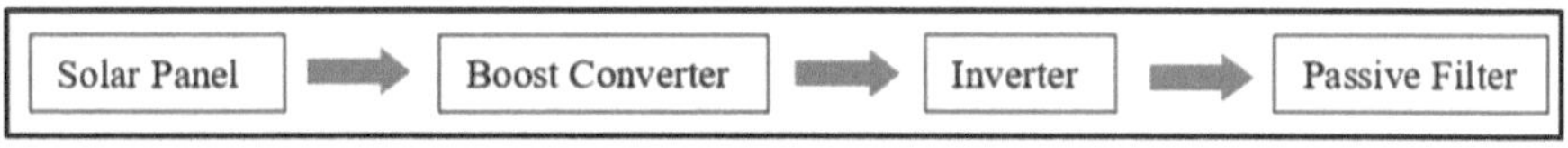

FIGURE 14.1 Solar power generation diagram.

Solar Panel. A series of photovoltaic cells arranged in photovoltaic system of solar panel to generate electricity using sunlight. These panels contain a bank of batteries directly wired to an application or load circuit. A reliable battery system is essential to compensate absence of solar energy at night or in bad weather conditions that add to the overall cost of solar system.

Boost Converter. With varied weather conditions, it is typical that we will not get a continuous supply from solar panels. However, the system should continuously operate, therefore a boost converter plays an important role in solar power systems as they step up the input voltage of a solar array for a given set of conditions. The temperature and irradiation level are major factors in solar power generated from solar panels [1]. Moreover, boost converters are low-cost and space-saving as compared to transformers, which makes it an advisable option for solar power generation models.

Inverter. An inverter works by switching the DC input on and off rapidly, creating pulses of current that alternate between positive and negative. This output is known as pulsating AC.

Passive Filter. The pulsating AC output from the inverter is not sufficient since pure AC is required to power the load. In order to achieve pure AC, we need to use a passive filter which is composed of capacitor, inductor, and load resistance.

14.4 SOLAR POWER DESIGN IMPLEMENTATION ON MATLAB®

The major blocks of solar power generation system are shown in Figure 14.2.

14.4.1 Solar Panel

A solar panel has an input of solar radiation that is generated from the sun and temperature. For this design, there is the advance power API-AP215 module with 20 parallel strings and 5 series-connected modules per string.

14.4.1.1 The Panel

With some application of physics and mechanical and electrical analogous systems, it is possible to mathematically express the motion for the panel in desired directions and orientation. The expression of panel angular movement

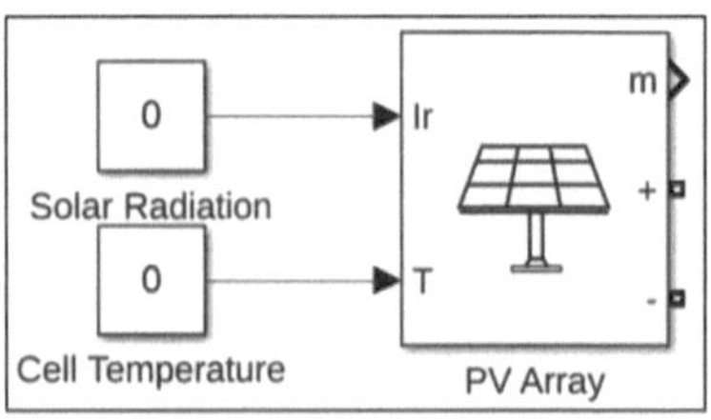

FIGURE 14.2 Solar panel model implemented in MATLAB®.

$$\frac{d^2\theta}{dx^2} = \frac{1}{J}\left(T - K_d \frac{d\theta}{dt}\right)$$

where, $\frac{d^2\theta}{dx^2}$ = angular accelaration , $\frac{d\theta}{dt}$ = angular velocity θ = angular position T = Torque, J = inertia, K_d = Damping constant

In Physics, the second derivative implies acceleration and if we integrate it, we'll get the velocity, and by integrating it one more time finally we'll get the position. To demonstrate how to model the equation of motion for the solar panel rotating about its central post, there are constant terms T and K_d which symbolize the applied Torque or rotational force and the Damping Constant, respectively. Finally, we divide the right-hand side of the equation by the inertia J which is the property of an element that stores the kinetic energy of rotational motion. These constant terms can be equated to a particular quantity which will serve as parameters for the simulation.

14.4.1.2 Block Diagram

To finalize the model, each term in the mathematical equation should be set into blocks with a particular operation for the Simulink to perform. Each term can be equated to a certain parameter before running the simulation. To simplify the equation-block analogy, in this case, we'll use the integrator block, and the particular reason for that is we have acceleration as we can see it's on the left side of the equation and we have the velocity on the right side of the equation. On the other hand, the subtractor was used for the terms T and K_d, while the gain block was set for the inertia with the term 1/J which will divide it to the following terms. To visualize the simulation, the Scope blocks are connected to the right of Figure 14.3, and as observed there are two scopes, one for the velocity and one for the position.

The panel's angular position increases, while the velocity started from zero until it reaches its steady state to level off. This actively demonstrates that with the applied torque, the panel will rotate at a fixed rate.

14.4.1.3 The Motor

The role of the motor in this system is to produce torque to rotate the solar panel. Remember that the aim of the solar panel is to track and align itself to the position of the Sun. This motor will finalize the physical model and automation of the system.

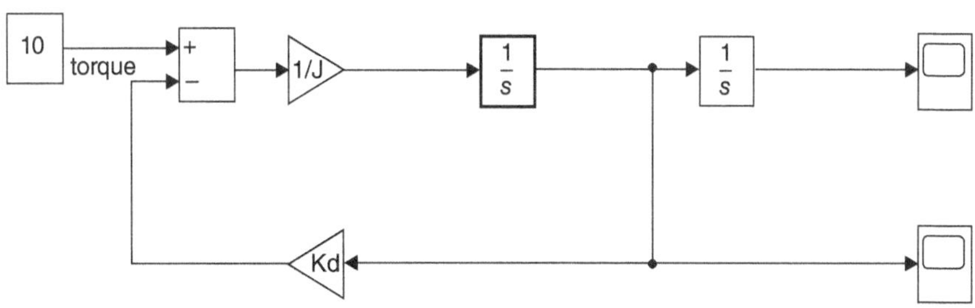

FIGURE 14.3 Visualizing the panel's position and velocity.

The application of the electrical system will be implemented to this part of the model and the particular reason for this is the motor needs a certain amount of voltage to reach its operating state. The expression of change in motor current:

$$\frac{di}{dt} = \frac{1}{L}\left(V - K_g K_f \frac{d\theta}{dt} - Ri\right)$$

$$T = K_g K_t i$$

where, L = Inductance, R = Resistance, V = Voltage, i = Current, T = Torque, K_f = Back EMF, K_g = Gear Ratio, K_t = Torque Constant.

14.4.2 Boost Converter

Since the temperature, together with the solar radiation, is not constant throughout the whole day, a boost converter is needed. For this, an IGBT/diode was used wherein a pulse generator is connected on its gate port, an inductor and a diode are connected in parallel in the collector port, and the emitter is connected to the ground. Boost Converter Model Implemented in MATLAB® is shown in Figure 14.4.

14.4.3 Inverter

The major blocks of inverter are pulse width modulation (PWM) generator and Universal bridge as shown in Figure 14.5.

After passing through the booster converter, the output signal is still in the form of DC which is not suitable for use in powering electricity in houses, thus, an inverter is needed. A commonly used method in inverting DC to AC is 2 level - PWM Generator connected at the gate port of the Universal Bridge.

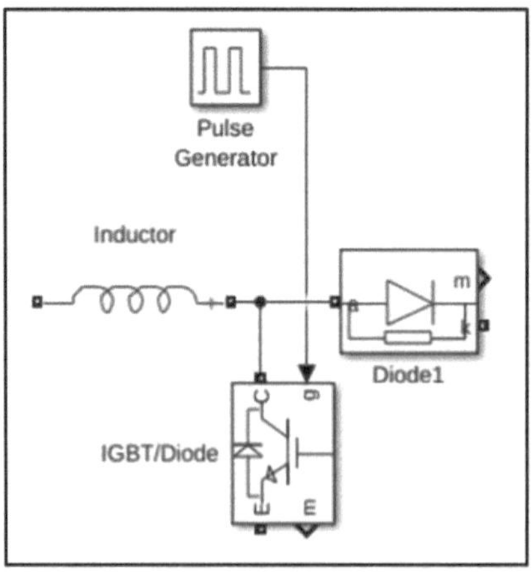

FIGURE 14.4 Boost converter model implemented in MATLAB®.

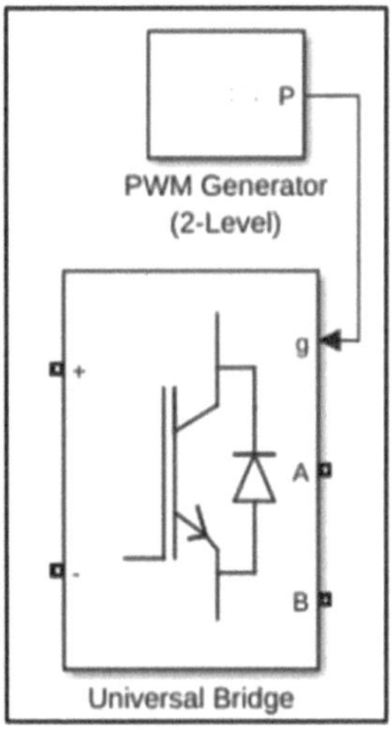

FIGURE 14.5 Inverter model implemented in MATLAB®.

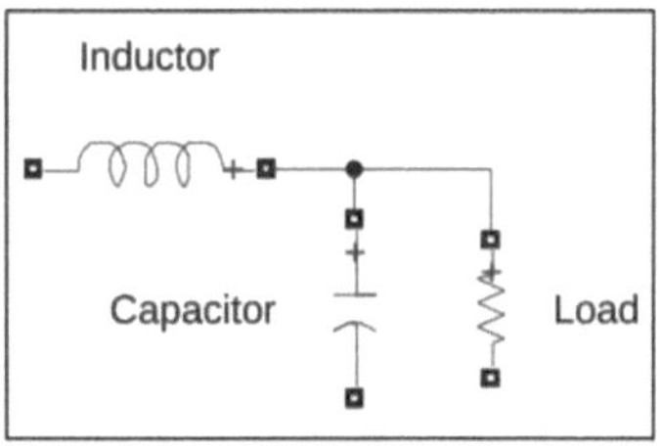

FIGURE 14.6 Passive filter model implemented in MATLAB®.

14.4.4 Passive Filter

To smooth out the pulsating AC and create a more sinusoidal waveform, a passive filter is needed. This filter is composed of a capacitor, inductor, and load resistance as shown in Figure 14.6. These filters help remove the high-frequency components and produce a cleaner AC waveform.

14.5 RESULTS AND DISCUSSION

Figure 14.7 is the final design of the solar power generation model implemented using MATLAB® . Each stage's elements and parameters were set considering what is suitable and commonly used in real-life applications. Thorough research was also conducted to ensure its efficiency.

By connecting voltage measurement and scope to each stage (PV Scope, Booster Scope, and Inverter with Passive Filter Scope) as shown in Figure 14.8, designers were able to measure and observe the solar power generation design's output waveforms.

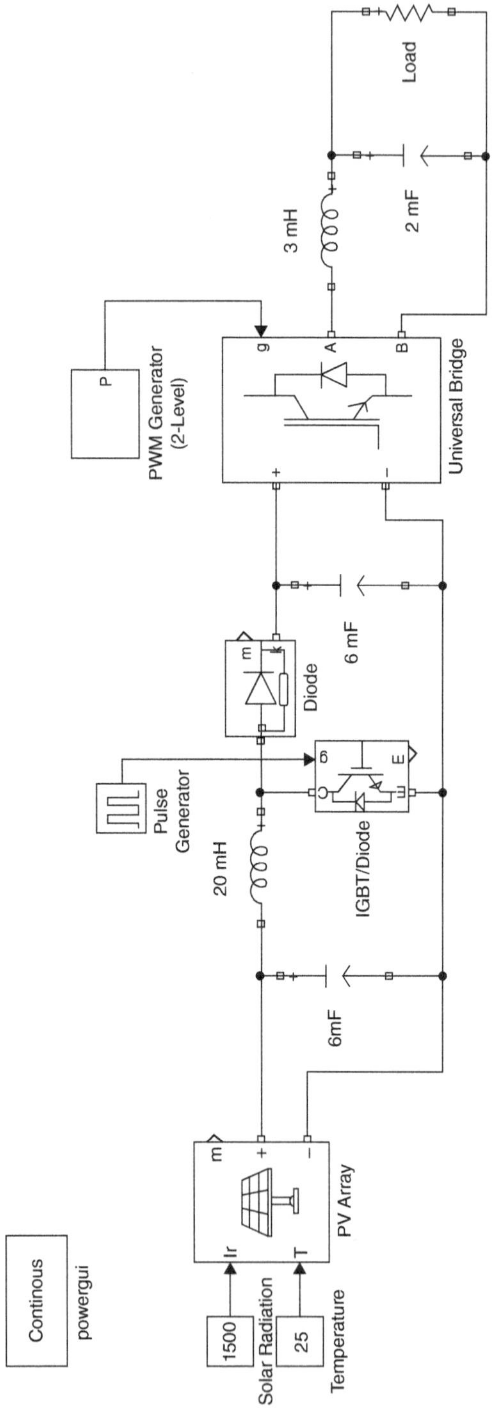

FIGURE 14.7 Final design of solar power generation model.

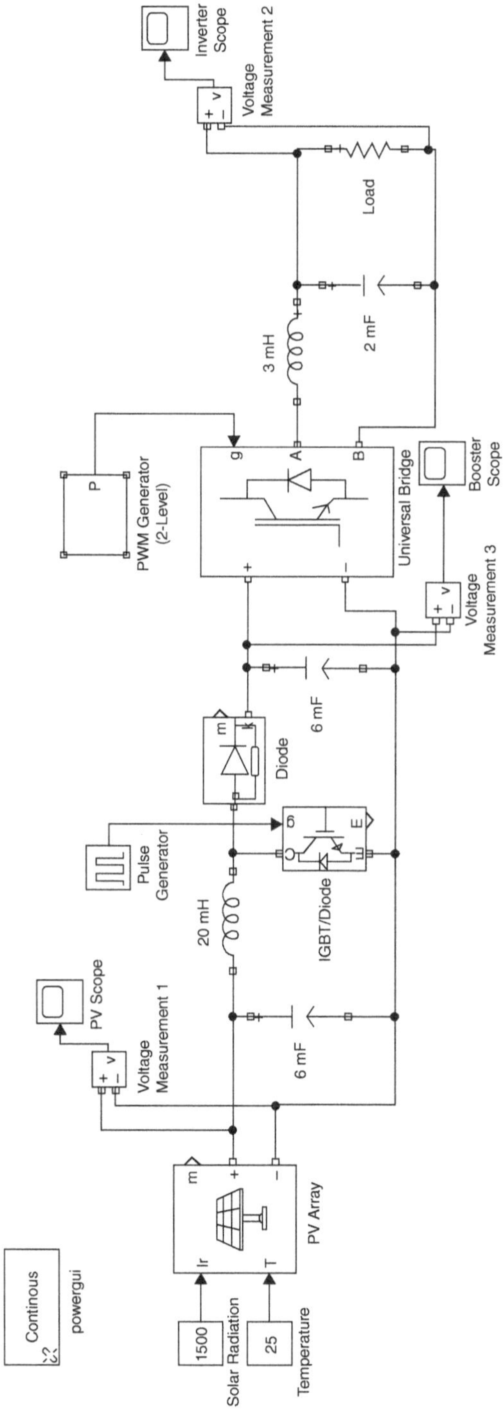

FIGURE 14.8 Measuring the solar power generation model.

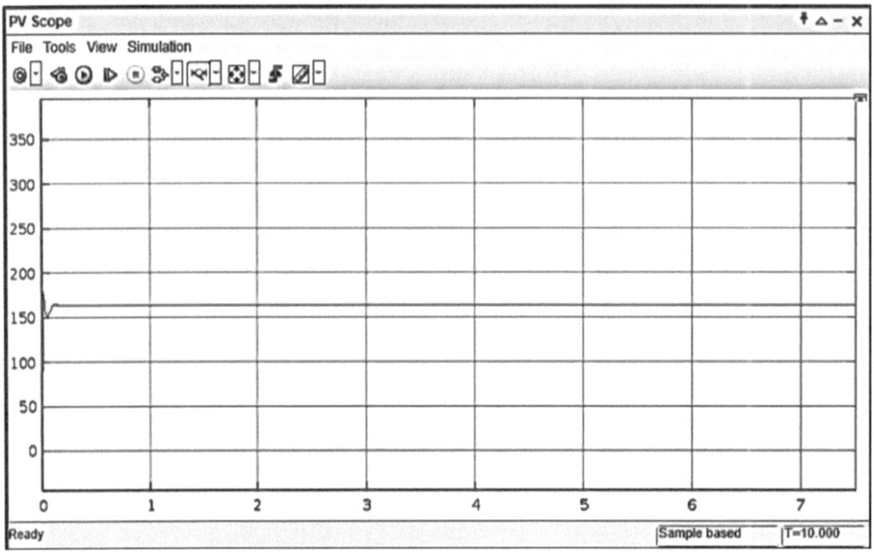

FIGURE 14.9 PV panel output using scope.

14.5.1 PV Panel Scope

As displayed in Figure 14.9, the PV Panel produces a DC supply. It has a 170V DC straight line which means that there is always constant voltage and the current flows in one direction.

14.5.2 Boost Converter Scope

Simulating the boost converter in Figure 14.10, displays the two-factor waveform that reaches 300–350 V. With this, we were able to prove the booster's function in stepping up the input voltage of a PV array for a given set of conditions.

14.5.3 Inverter Scope

The stepped-up input voltage from the booster is then passed through the inverter to produce a pulsating AC. Figure 14.11 shows the results of the pulsating AC at 220 Vp. Since pure AC is needed to power the load, the signal is further passed through a passive filter.

14.5.4 Passive Filter Scope

In the final stage of the solar power generation system, the pulsating AC is finally converted to pure AC that can be used as electricity to power our appliances at home. Figure 14.12 shows the 220 Vp output AC voltage value, which is the standard AC supply voltage.

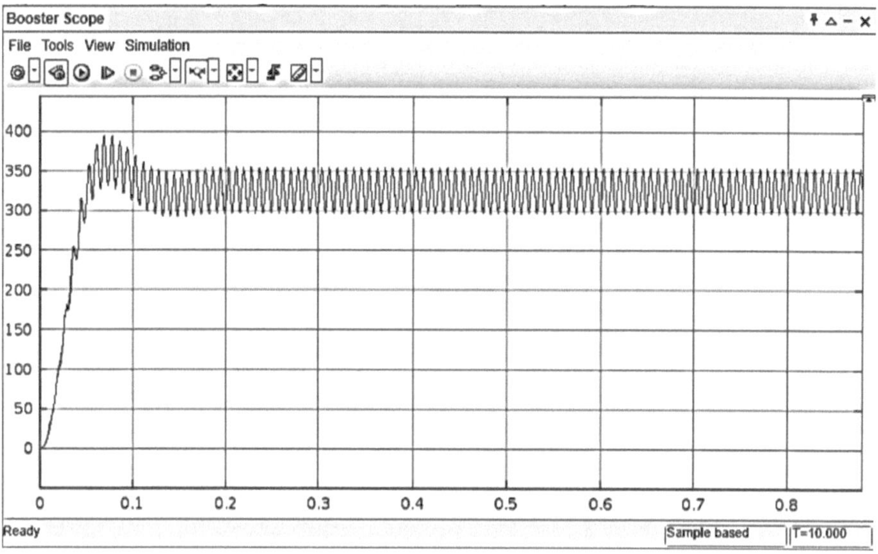

FIGURE 14.10 Boost converter output using scope.

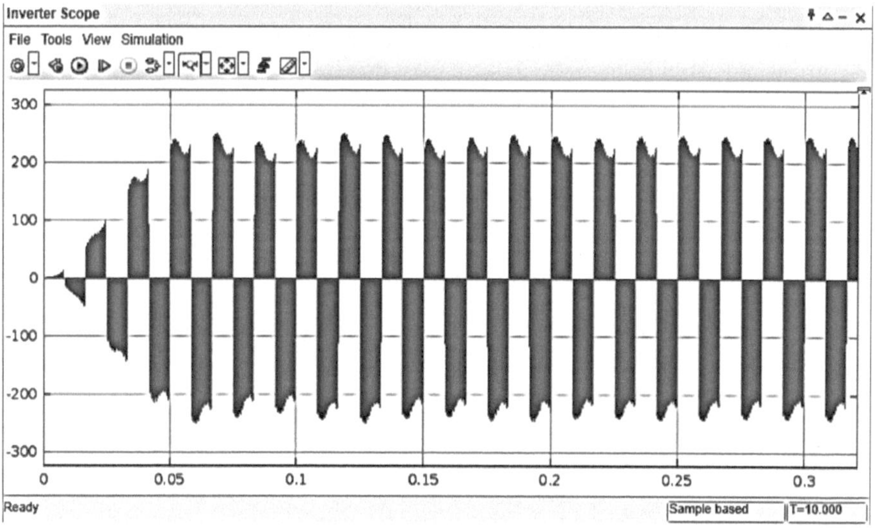

FIGURE 14.11 Inverter output using scope.

14.6 APPLICATIONS

Solar power is a potential renewable energy resource which is frequently used for industry and domestic applications. Eco-friendly nature and low cost are the major advantages of solar power. Few most common applications of solar energy are listed in the following sub-sections.

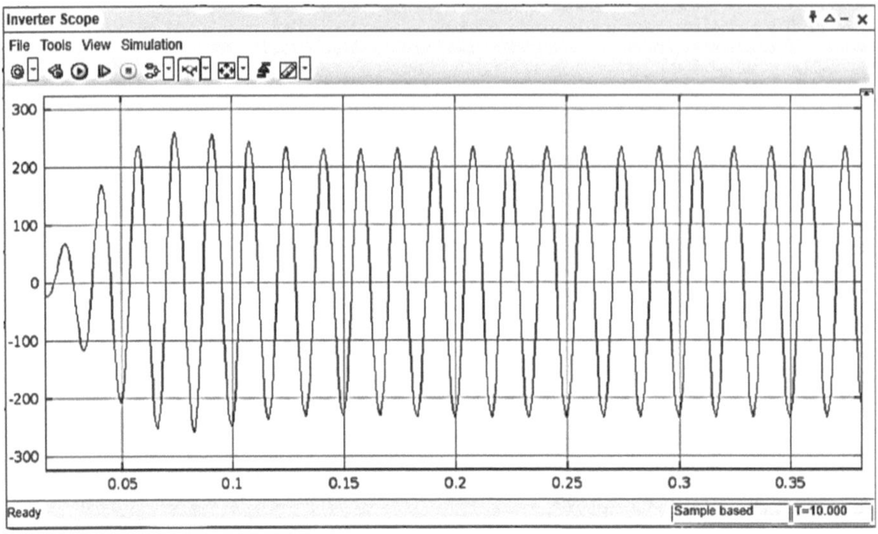

FIGURE 14.12 Passive filter output using scope.

14.6.1 Solar Electric Power Generation for Domestic Application

Solar power is now going popular in remote areas which mainly need a one-time investment and avoid the monthly bills of customer.

Solar Water Heating. Solar water heaters are frequently used in guest houses, hotels and hospitals, etc.

PV Solar Noise Barriers (PVNB). PV solar noise barriers reduce inconvenient traffic noise from densely populated surroundings. Many areas are already constructing PV solar noise barriers and finding them to be cost-effective and sustainable.

Solar Heating of Buildings. Solar energy can be used for space heating of buildings in many ways namely: (a) Collecting the solar radiation by some element of the building itself, that is, solar energy is admitted directly into the building through large South-facing windows and (b) Using separate solar collectors which may heat either water or air or storage devices which can accumulate the collected solar energy for use at night and during inclement days.

Solar Green Houses. Solar radiations can pass through the greenhouse glazing but the thermal radiations emitted by the objects within the greenhouse cannot escape through the glazed surface. Solar power is used to trap radiation within the greenhouse that results rise in temperature [11–14]. Solar greenhouses improve crop productivity and minimize the use of natural resources leading toward sustainable growth in agriculture. Solar power is useful for dairy forms to reduce the overall cost of milk production for providing supply to PV water pumping system [15].

14.7 CONCLUSION

Solar power generation has become a transformative solution in reshaping our energy landscape. With the use of different elements including solar panels, boosters, inverters, and filters, one can be capable of generating electricity in the form of alternating current (AC) to supply our homes as this is more efficient and cost-effective to transmit electricity over long distances, as compared to DC. Additionally, AC can be easily converted to different voltages, which is useful for distributing electricity to different areas and powering different types of devices.

Moreover, the utilization of MATLAB® in modeling a solar power generation model proves to be a convenient tool for comprehensively understanding, simulating, and optimizing a model for solar energy as a renewable source. The precision and flexibility offered by MATLAB® enabled to analyze solar panel performance and its overall power generation, offering a robust framework for assessing the feasibility and efficiency of solar energy systems. The solar power generation implementation using MATLAB® only signifies the innovative shift in our approach toward sustainable energy solutions.

Overall, the employment of MATLAB® in implementing a solar power generation model enhanced understanding of photovoltaic systems as well as their comprehension of the software's flexibility in creating and designing for innovation and optimization in several applications like solar-charged electric vehicles and smart grids, etc. [16–19]. Furthermore, this chapter aims to provide an avenue for future researchers in implementing and improving the efficiency of solar power to contribute to a more sustainable future.

REFERENCES

[1] Yang, C. Y., Hsieh, C. Y., Feng, F. K., & Chen, K. H. (2012). *Highly Efficient Analog Maximum Power Point Tracking (AMPPT) in a Photovoltaic System. IEEE Transactions on Circuits and Systems I: Regular Papers*, pp. 546–1556.

[2] Chowdhury, P., Koley, I., Sen, S., Saha, P. K., & Panda, G. K. (2013). "Modelling, simulation, and control of a grid connected nonconventional solar power generation system using Matlab®," *International Journal of Advanced Research in Electrical, Electronics and Instrumentation Engineering*, vol. 2, no. 4, pp. 1183–1191.

[3] Babaa, S. E., Murr, G. E., Mohamed, F., & Pamuri, S. (2018). "Overview of boost converters for photovoltaic systems," *Journal of Power and Energy Engineering*, vol. 6, no. 4, pp. 16–31. https://doi.org/10.4236/jpee.2018.64002

[4] Tripathi, S. L., Ganguli, S., Kumar, A., & Magradze, T. (Eds.). (2022). *Intelligent Green Technologies for Sustainable Smart Cities*. John Wiley & Sons, USA, https://doi.org/10.1002/9781119816096

[5] Simran, T. (2020). *Development of Solar Cell*, Nova Publishers.

[6] Tripathi S. L., & Padmanabhan S. (2020). *Green Energy: Fundamentals, Concepts, and Applications*, Scrivener Publishing, Wiley, USA, https://doi.org/10.1002/9781119760801

[7] Sahani, R., Daga, M., Jamatia, I., Kumar, P., & Tripathi, S. L. (2023). "Design of a self-charging electric vehicle with embedded multiple natural energy sources," *2023 IEEE Devices for Integrated Circuit (DevIC)*, Kalyani, India, pp. 296–301, https://doi.org/10.1109/DevIC57758.2023.10134774

[8] Tripathi, S. L., Padmanabhan, S., Kumar, D., & Raja P. (Eds.) (2021). *Design and Development of Energy Efficient Systems*, Scrivener Publishing, Wiley, USA. https://doi.org/10.1002/9781119761785

[9] Arora, K., Tripathi, S. L., & Padmanaban, S. (2022). *Smart Electrical Grid System: Design Principle, Modernization, and Techniques* (1st ed.). CRC Press, Boca Raton, FL. https://doi.org/10.1201/9781003242277

[10] The MathWorks, Inc. (2015). "Implement PV array modules – Simulink®," www.mathworks.com, https://www.mathworks.com/help/sps/powersys/ref/pvarray.html#

[11] Arora, K., Kumar, V., Prashar, D., & Tripathi, S. L. (Eds.). (2023). *Modern Computational Techniques for Engineering Applications* (1st ed.). CRC Press Boca Raton, FL. https://doi.org/10.1201/9781003407409

[12] Dhonde, M., Sahu, K., & Murty, V. V. S. (2022). The application of solar-driven technologies for the sustainable development of agriculture farming: A comprehensive review. *Reviews in Environmental Science and Bio/Technology* 21:139–167. https://doi.org/10.1007/s11157-022-09611-6

[13] Selmani, A., Outanoute, M., El Khayat, M., Guerbaoui, M., Ed-Dahhak, A., Lachhab, A. et al. (2019). Towards autonomous greenhouses solar-powered. *Procedia Computer Science* 148:495–501. https://doi.org/10.1016/j.procs.2019.01.062

[14] Yano, A., & Cossu, M. (2019). Energy sustainable greenhouse crop cultivation using photovoltaic technologies. *Renewable and Sustainable Energy Reviews* 109:116–137. https://doi.org/10.1016/j.rser.2019.04.026

[15] Zhang, C., Campana, P., Yang, J., Zhang, J., & Yan, J. (2017). Can solar energy be an alternative choice of milk production in dairy farms? A case study of integrated PVWP system with Alfalfa and milk production in dairy farms in China. *Energy Procedia* 105:3953–3959. https://doi.org/10.1016/j.egypro.2017.03.822

[16] Kumari, C.L., Kamboj, V. K., Bath, S. K. et al. (2023). A boosted chimp optimizer for numerical and engineering design optimization challenges. *Engineering with Computers* 39:2463–2514. https://doi.org/10.1007/s00366-021-01591-5

[17] Tripathi S. L., Dubey M. K., Rishiwal V., & Padmanabhan S. (2021). *Introduction to AI techniques for Renewable Energy System*, Taylor & Francis, Boca Raton, FL. https://doi.org/10.1201/9781003104445

[18] Arora, K., Tripathi, S. L., & Sharma, H. (Eds.) (2024). *Electric Vehicle Design: Design, Simulation and Applications*, Scrivener Publishing, Wiley, USA, https://doi.org/10.1002/9781394205097

[19] Pandey, A. K., Padmanaban, S., Tripathi, S. L., Patel, V., & Patel, V. (Eds.). (2024). *Microgrid: Design, Optimization, and Applications* (1st ed.). CRC Press, Boca Raton, FL. https://doi.org/10.1201/9781003481836

15 Green Artificial Intelligence

Biodegradable and Biocompatible Materials

Hamid
Lovely Professional University, Phagwara, India

Kanchan Bhatt
Dr Yashwant Singh Parmar University of Horticulture and Forestry, Nauni, Solan, India

Naseer Ahmed
Eternal University, Baru Sahib, India

Priyanka Chauhan
Dr Yashwant Singh Parmar University of Horticulture and Forestry, Nauni, Solan, India

15.1 INTRODUCTION

Artificial Intelligence (AI) is crucial in the rapidly evolving and dynamic landscape of the swiftly changing technological sphere of today, impacting virtually every facet of our daily existence [1]. Fundamentally, AI entails the creation of machines or systems that emulate human intelligence, empowering them to perform activities that typically require human cognitive skills. A significant merit of AI lies in its ability to boost efficiency and productivity across diverse industries. By automating routine tasks, analyzing data, and facilitating decision-making processes, AI streamlines operations, enabling human resources to concentrate on creative and intricate problem-solving endeavors [2]. In 1955, John McCarthy coined the term "Artificial Intelligence (AI)," describing it as "the science and engineering involved in creating smart machines" [3]. Artificial intelligence is a component of computer or computing science that produces expert systems, algorithms, and programs. The fundamental objective of artificial intelligence is to replicate the functionality of the human brain, enabling decision-making akin to human beings in diverse situations and circumstances [4].

DOI: 10.1201/9781003546382-15

Today, AI plays a pivotal role in advancing fields such as healthcare, where diagnostic tools powered by machine learning can aid in early disease detection and treatment planning. There are two primary branches of artificial intelligence in medicine: virtual and physical. The virtual component is exemplified by machine learning, utilizing mathematical algorithms designed to learn through experience. Examples of such algorithms include protein-protein interaction algorithms, which have been used to identify new therapeutic targets [5], identifying DNA variants like Single Nucleotide Polymorphisms (SNPs) as indicators of diseases or traits, etc. The second application of AI in medicine involves the involvement of physical objects, medical devices, and progressively advanced robots in delivering care, often referred to as "carebots." Within these applications, the most encouraging strategy involves employing robots as aides, such as robots as machine companions tailored for the elderly population contending with diminished cognitive abilities or limited mobility. Moreover, in surgical settings, robots are employed as assistant surgeons or even function independently as performers [3]. Furthermore, AI can be used in agriculture to monitor grain production, its quality, insect attacks, and disease infestation in different types of crops [6]. Similarly, the application of AI in food production plays a crucial role in overseeing the entire supply chain process. Nevertheless, it also contributes to tasks such as price prediction, optimizing production processes, managing inventory, and handling logistics, and inventory through platforms like Symphony Retail-AI, preventing the accumulation of excess items that could lead to wastage [7]. Besides, in the era of education, AI facilitates personalized learning experiences, catering to individual needs and optimizing the educational journey. Additionally, AI's potential to analyze vast datasets contributes to scientific research, from climate modeling to drug discovery. While AI presents unprecedented opportunities, it also raises ethical considerations and challenges that necessitate careful navigation [8]. As we harness the power of AI, it becomes imperative to strike a balance between innovation and ethical use, ensuring that artificial intelligence serves the greater good and contributes to a sustainable and equitable future.

In this regard, AI poses environmental challenges primarily due to its substantial energy consumption and resource demands [9]. The training process of intricate AI models often requires extensive computational power, leading to considerable electricity usage within data centers. This energy-intensive aspect of AI training can significantly increase the carbon footprint, especially when powered by non-renewable sources [10]. Moreover, the production and disposal of essential hardware components for AI systems contribute to electronic waste, placing additional strain on the environment. As the prevalence of AI applications grows, the need for computing resources is likely to rise, compounding these environmental issues. It is imperative to strike a balance between the rapid progress of AI and the adoption of sustainable or green practices to alleviate its potential adverse effects on the environment.

The necessity for green Artificial Intelligence (AI) arises from the heightened awareness of environmental sustainability and the substantial energy consumption associated with conventional AI models [11]. Green AI underscores the importance of developing and implementing AI technologies that are both energy-efficient and environmentally conscious. With the increasing prevalence of AI applications across diverse industries, there is a corresponding rise in the demand for computational power, leading to heightened energy consumption and carbon emissions [12]. Green AI seeks to tackle this issue by advocating for the use of energy-efficient algorithms, optimizing hardware, and embracing eco-friendly practices in AI development. Initially, a crucial focus lies on energy efficiency, entailing the creation of algorithms and hardware designed to optimize resource utilization and curtail power consumption [13, 14]. For example: The usage of biodegradable materials, a crucial component in the pursuit of sustainable practices, refers to substances capable of breaking down naturally into non-toxic components over time. There are various types of biodegradable materials, including polymers, and organic compounds. Similarly, biocompatible substances are essential for playing a pivotal role in the convergence of technology and biology, offering substances that can seamlessly interact with biological systems without causing harm (Figure 15.1). These materials encompass a diverse range, including metals, ceramics, and polymers, designed to integrate effectively with living tissues. The mechanisms behind biocompatibility involve minimizing immune responses and ensuring compatibility with the physiological environment [15]. Subsequently, lifecycle management concentrates on the environmentally considerate disposal and recycling of AI components to reduce electronic waste. Additionally, there is a prioritization of renewable energy sources to power AI infrastructure, thereby lessening the overall carbon footprint. Creating environmentally sustainable AI requires a collaborative approach that addresses various stages in the lifecycle of an AI system, such as collection of data, training, and monitoring. This effort should encompass diverse components, including data, models, pipelines, architectures, and hardware [16]. Nevertheless, the emphasis in this chapter will be directed toward biodegradable and biocompatible materials, exploring their applications in health care and electronics including recent breakthroughs in the field.

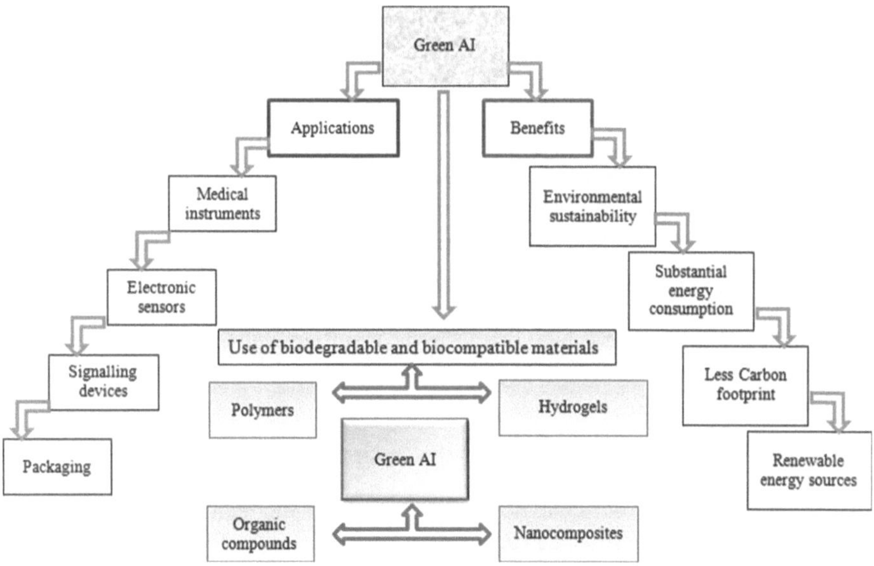

FIGURE 15.1 Various benefits and applications of green AI.

15.2 BIODEGRADABLE MATERIALS AND HEALTHCARE

Biodegradable materials are capable of undergoing decomposition through the action of bacteria, fungi, or other biological processes into natural elements [17]. In terms of healthcare, these materials provide the possibility of temporary medical implants and facilitate tissue repair by enabling real-time monitoring of variables such as pressure, strain, pH, temperature, and identification of post-surgical infections [18]. Integrating biodegradability into health care, consumer electronic devices, and environmental monitoring systems has the potential to substantially minimize the impact of electronic waste (E-waste) on the environment, which currently exceeds 50 million tons each year. This advancement not only tackles the issues related to landfills but also eliminates the expenses and hazards linked with recycling processes. Raw materials for producing biodegradable polymers with controlled degradation in nature primarily come from natural compounds such as cellulose derivatives, starch, chitosan, chitin, lactic acid, and hydroxyalkanoates, proteins [19]. Polyvinyl alcohol (PVA) is a polymer derived from the polymerization and alcoholysis of vinyl acetate [20]. PVA has a lot of hydrophilic groups, which give it good hygroscopicity and enable it to break down naturally into carbon dioxide and water [21]. Similarly, polycaprolactone is yet another polymer that has potential applications in tissue engineering such as cartilage, bone, cardiovascular tissue, nerves and skin, etc. It can undergo hydrolytic cleavage, transforming into oligomeric fragments that are then engulfed and broken down by macrophages [22].

Another category of biomaterials is hydrogels composed of hydrophilic polymers which are organized three-dimensional networks with adjustable chemical and physical properties. These gels create a stable and conducive environment that facilitates the process of healing of wounds [23]. Commonly, natural polymers like collagen and chitosan are employed in crafting hydrogels, leveraging their innate biocompatibility and biochemical signals that aid cell-matrix interactions. Hydrogels play a significant role in regenerative medicine, especially in crafting scaffolds for tissue repair and organ transplantation [24]. Additionally, by adjusting the preparation parameters, such as the molecular weight of the polymer and degree of cross-linking, the mechanical and degradable qualities of the hydrogels may be accurately controlled to satisfy the demands for addressing diverse skin issues [25]. Other examples of biodegradable materials are Poly (lactic-co-glycolic acid) (PLGA), Polyurethane (PU), Polyethylene oxide (PEO), etc. Besides polymers, there are some biodegradable metals like Fe, Mg, and Zn-based biodegradable metals are being used as temporary medical implants. The breakdown of biodegradable metal in vivo is propelled by a sequence of anodic and cathodic reactions, resulting in the formation of oxides, hydroxides, and the release of hydrogen gas [26].

15.3 BIODEGRADABLE MATERIALS AND ELECTRONICS

Ground-breaking ideas and concepts have emerged in the exploration of utilizing biodegradable compounds in electronics. Extensive research focus has been directed toward biodegradable electronics for diverse applications for sensing and harvesting energy, owing to their adaptability, eco-friendly nature, and significant piezoelectric properties [27]. Commonly reported methods for the fabrication of these electronics include solution casting, electrospinning, melt-spinning 3D printing, etc. Moreover, conductive and semiconductive materials are frequently fabricated using biodegradable metals like Magnesium and Zinc, or semiconductor materials such as Silicon and Germanium. Besides this, substrate, interfacial, and encapsulation layers are typically made from naturally derived biomaterials such as silk, cellulose, and sodium carboxymethylcellulose, or synthetic biodegradable polymers like poly (vinyl alcohol), PLA, and PLGA [21]. The usage of semiconductors in artificial intelligence can be ice-breaking due to their brain-like functioning and task processing. Semiconductors are materials that have properties that fall between those of conductors and insulators. These materials have electrical conductivity values that are intermediate between conductors (which allow electric currents to flow easily) and insulators (which do not conduct electricity well). Silicon is the most widely utilized semiconductor material, although alternative materials such as germanium are also employed [28]. They form the basis of electronic components such as diodes, integrated circuits, and transistors. These elements are vital for the operation of electronic devices, including computers, smartphones, and various other electronic systems.

Apart from this, organic semiconductors are garnering growing interest due to their attractive properties, such as lightweight composition, economical manufacturing, processing at low temperatures, and widespread accessibility [29]. The recently successful introduction of active-matrix Organic Light-Emitting Diodes (OLEDs) for premium smartphone displays highlights the significant potential of organic compounds in various electrical and optoelectronic devices [30]. Organic materials consist predominantly of carbon and hydrogen atoms and were traditionally regarded as materials with exclusive electrical insulating properties for many years. These organic semiconductors are of two types conjugated polymers and small molecules priorly based on their method of fabrication [31].

Conjugated polymers, for the most part, exhibit solubility in organic solvents, facilitating diverse solution-processing techniques during fabrication [32]. Conversely, small molecules typically undergo deposition through heat-induced evaporation in a high vacuum environment. This deposition method provides precise regulation of the morphology, width, and other crucial characteristics of the organic films. The doping in in-organic semiconductors can be done by various methods like electrochemical doping chemical doping, photo-doping, and charge injection from contact metals however, it is different from organic ones as it commonly involves the introduction of small quantities of p-type or n-type organic molecules that can donate or accept charge carriers, facilitating the modification of their electrical properties [33]. Light-simulated synaptic emulators are engineered systems or devices intended to replicate the synaptic processes found in biological systems, employing light as the triggering stimulus. A combination of organic semiconductor (OSCs) and inorganic halide (Perovskite quantum dots) was attempted by [34] which not only enhances the efficacy of charge separation in photo excited charges but also deferred reduction of photocurrent within the hybrid film of IHP QDs and OSCs. This combination overall improves the photo responsivity of the device. Another study [35] has developed optical synaptic devices utilizing a ternary photoactive material system comprising organometal halide perovskite CH_3NH_3-$PbBr_3$, organic dye Rhodamine B (RhB), and organic semiconductor pentacene. The incorporation of RhB has proven to enhance light absorption and photoresponsivity in composite devices significantly. These devices exhibit satisfactory synaptic behaviors, demonstrating a learning pattern that demonstrates a brain's response to diverse input signals.

Dielectrics, unlike conductors, are materials that exhibit poor electrical conductivity and are commonly employed in electrical and electronic systems for insulation. These materials exist in diverse forms such as solids, liquids, and gases. When exposed to an electric field, dielectrics undergo polarization, a phenomenon where the internal charges reorganize in reaction to the applied electrical force [36]. For example, Gelatin, a readily available, water-soluble, biodegradable, biocompatible, and cost-effective material, finds application as dielectrics in resistive-switching devices and Organic Thin-Film Transistors (OTFTs) [37]. OTFTs incorporating high-performance paper and utilizing spin-coated Gelatin (G) layers in stacked gate dielectrics which improved interfaces between pentacene and gate dielectrics. This configuration, represented by the Au/pentacene/G/G matrix-embedded iron (FeG)/Al/paper structure, serves to reduce carrier scattering, thereby enhancing mobility. Almond gum, sourced directly from almond trees and employed without purification, serves as a biodegradable material for gate dielectric applications. Notably, almond gum offers the advantages of being pocket-friendly, natural, and water-soluble. Further, it demonstrates favorable characteristics such as a reasonably reduced leakage of current, excellent quality of film, and significant capacitance [38].

In the context of artificial intelligence, the selection of organic substrates and encapsulating materials is pivotal for advancing the development of electronic devices that are flexible, lightweight, and biocompatible. Polyimide, Polyethylene terephthalate, perylene graphene, etc. are commonly used substrates and encapsulation layers for applications within artificial intelligence. In a study by [39], optoelectronic synaptic transistors with a biological inspiration were designed using cellulose nano paper and natural chlorophyll-a, catering to neuromorphic systems. Nanofibrillated cellulose (NFC)–based wood-derived cellulose nanomaterials (WCNs) exhibit exceptional mechanical characteristics, chemical resistance, and thermal resilience. Similarly, Fluoropolymers in an amorphous state, characterized by low gas and moisture permeability, show considerable potential as durable encapsulation materials. An organic memristor based on fluoropolymer with multiple functions for a flexible neural network system was prepared by [40]. The fabricated fluoropolymer film can be utilized as both the encapsulating layer and insulator for the organic memristor, through dip-coating EGC-1700 in a fluorinated solvent (HFE-7100DL, 3M) at a speed of 200 mm min^{-1}. The resulting fluoropolymer film had a thickness of 320 nm, with the source electrode of the transistor doubling as the inert electrode for the organic memristor. This film serves as a conductive medium as well as an encapsulating layer for the organic transistor. More details regarding biodegradable materials related to healthcare and electronics are elaborated in Table 15.1.

TABLE 15.1
Biodegradable Materials and Their Applications in Health Care and Electronics

Biodegradable Material	Area of Interest	Important Characteristics	References
Magnesium	Medical (Orthopedic Implants)	• Light Weight • Good Fracture Toughness • Degradation occurs in an electrochemical reaction known as corrosion	[41][42]
Zinc	Medical (Wound closure)	• Low melting point • Low reactivity • Good strength and ductility • Degradation by corrosion but does not produce hydrogen	[43][44]
Iron bioresorbable scaffold (Metal-polymer +polylactide coating on an iron stent	Medical (Coronary stents)	• Greater endothelial coverage as compared to nonbiodegradable stent • Ultrathin	[45]
Silk	Medical (Tissue engineering) (Regenerative medicine)	• High tensile strength • Highly flexible • Degradation by proteolytic enzymes	[46]
Alginate	Medical (Hemostatic material)	• Cost-effective • Great water absorption capacity • Boost the concentration of platelets	[47]
Tannic Acid (Poly-methacrylate tannic acid)	Electronics (Dielectric Material)	• Inexpensive • Degraded by soil bacteria • Good stability after surface modification	[48]
Castor Oil	Electronics (Dielectric Fluid)	• Good surface roughness • Higher material removal rate • Minimum width overcut	[49]
Rice Paper (Rice Paper+ PVC	Electronics (Triboelectric nanogenerator)	• Highly stable • Recyclable • Illuminate 25 commercial LED's • Cost-effective	[50]
Chitosan/PVP Polymer	Electronics (Flexible substrates)	• Good optical transmittance (90%) • Thermostable • Great mechanical stability • Highly biodegradable	[51]
Cellulose nanofibers	Electronics (Moisture Sensors)	• Transparent sensor • Good for invisible electronics • Highly sensitive (20-85% RH)	[52]

15.4 BIOCOMPATIBLE MATERIAL AND HEALTHCARE

Biocompatible materials refer to substances that can coexist with living tissues without causing any harmful effects. The traditional definition of biocompatibility, upheld for four decades, is "the ability of a material to perform with an appropriate host response in a specific application." These materials are extensively used in various medical and non-medical applications, including electronics. Hence, any bioactive material intended for medical technology should intentionally and effectively direct interactions between the device and the host system by modulating biological activity. This underscores the importance of a purposeful design approach and a comprehensive understanding of host interactions. The use of biocompatible materials in electronics is crucial for developing devices that can seamlessly integrate with the human body, such as implantable medical devices and wearable electronics. In the ever-evolving landscape of medical science and technology, the concept of biocompatible materials emerges as a pivotal bridge connecting the realms of biology and materials science [53]. These materials, meticulously designed and engineered, embark on a transformative journey into the intricate tapestry of living organisms, seeking not just accommodation but active collaboration. This narrative unfolds against the backdrop of medical marvels, groundbreaking drug delivery systems, tissue engineering endeavors, and the burgeoning landscape of bioelectronics.

At its core, the exploration of biocompatible materials epitomizes a quest to redefine the boundaries between the synthetic and the biological, with far-reaching implications for healthcare, research, and technological innovation [54]. The essence of biocompatible materials lies in their inherent capability to foster harmony within biological systems. Unlike conventional materials that may trigger immune responses or adverse reactions, biocompatible materials aim to become integral participants in the body's symphony [55]. This symbiotic relationship extends beyond mere inertness; it embodies an active engagement with the molecular and cellular intricacies of living organisms. The foundational significance of biocompatible materials is exemplified in the domain of medical implants. From joint replacements that restore mobility to cardiac stents that open arterial pathways, these materials underpin the success of life-altering interventions. The selection of materials for such implants transcends mere mechanical compatibility; it delves into the realms of biointegration, longevity, and the ability to withstand the dynamic forces within the human body [56].

The field of biocompatible materials, especially in drug delivery, has been markedly influenced by nanotechnology. Nanocomposites and nanoparticles bring distinctive benefits, including enhanced surface area and the capacity to encapsulate drugs for precise delivery. Notably, gold and silver nanoparticles exhibit promise in cancer therapy, utilizing their unique properties for both imaging and therapeutic applications [56, 57]. The biocompatibility of these nanoparticles is intricately linked to factors such as their size, shape, and surface chemistry. These attributes enable customized interactions with biological systems, underlining the importance of precise control over nanoparticle characteristics for optimal compatibility in various applications [58]. Enhancing the biocompatibility of materials is essential, and surface modification techniques play a key role in achieving this goal. The attachment of bioactive molecules or peptides to material surfaces is vital for encouraging cell adhesion and influencing the immune response. This adaptability makes these materials highly suitable for use in implants and prosthetics [59]. Surface modifications gain significance due to their capacity to produce biomimetic interfaces closely resembling the natural extracellular matrix. This capability enables the development of surfaces that replicate the biological environment, thereby improving compatibility and interactions with cells and tissues in diverse biomedical applications [60]. Immunomodulatory biomaterials aim to control the immune response, promoting tolerance and reducing inflammation. This approach is particularly relevant in the realm of implants and devices, where minimizing the foreign body response is essential to ensure sustained long-term functionality [61]. Their potential applications extend to drug delivery and diagnostics, showcasing their versatility in addressing various healthcare challenges [62].

The considerable potential of biocompatible materials in medical applications is accompanied by persistent challenges. Issues such as long-term stability, scalability, and regulatory considerations pose significant hurdles. Effectively addressing these challenges is pivotal for the widespread and successful implementation of such materials in the medical field. Tackling these challenges necessitates collaborative efforts among researchers, engineers, and clinicians, ensuring the seamless translation of biocompatible materials from the laboratory to clinical settings. The interdisciplinary nature of this field is highlighted by studies that integrate materials science, biology, and clinical expertise. This integration fosters the development of innovative solutions to address critical healthcare needs.

15.5 BIOCOMPATIBLE MATERIALS AND THEIR UTILIZATION IN HEALTHCARE

Biocompatible materials encompass a broad spectrum of types, each characterized by distinct properties and applications within various biomedical domains. This diversity facilitates the creation of customized solutions to address specific needs in medical devices, drug delivery, tissue engineering, and other healthcare applications. In the following discussion, we explore various types of biocompatible materials in greater detail elaborated in Table 15.2.

TABLE 15.2
Biocompatible Materials and Their Applications in Healthcare

Name of Biocompatible Material	Applications	References
Polymers		
Poly (lactic-co-glycolic acid) (PLGA)	Application drug delivery systems due to its tunable degradation rate and excellent biocompatibility	[53]
Polyethylene glycol (PEG)	Known for its hydrophilic nature, PEG is often used to modify surfaces and improve biocompatibility. It has applications in drug delivery and as a coating for implants	[54]

(Continued)

TABLE 15.2 (Continued)

Name of Biocompatible Material	Applications	References
Polyvinyl alcohol (PVA)	Widely employed in medical applications, PVA is a biocompatible synthetic polymer used in hydrogels, artificial blood vessels, and wound dressings	[63]
Hydrogels		
Natural Hydrogels (e.g., Collagen, Chitosan)	These materials closely mimic the extracellular matrix, providing a conducive environment for cell growth. They are extensively used in tissue engineering and regenerative medicine	[64]
Synthetic Hydrogels (e.g., Polyacrylamide, Polyvinyl Pyrrolidone)	These hydrogels offer tunable mechanical properties and are used in drug delivery, wound healing, and controlled release systems	[65]
Nanomaterials		
Nanocomposites	Materials composed of a combination of nanoscale components, often 6 nanoparticles dispersed in a matrix. Examples include polymer nanocomposites and ceramic-polymer nanocomposites	[66]
Nanoparticles (e.g., Gold, Silver)	Utilized in drug delivery and imaging, these nanoparticles can be functionalized to enhance biocompatibility and targeted delivery	[62]
Ceramics		
Hydroxyapatite (HA)	A biocompatible ceramic often used in bone implants and dental applications due to its similarity to the mineral component of bone	[67]
Bioactive Glass	Known for its ability to bond with living tissues, bioactive glass is used in bone regeneration and tissue engineering	[68]
Biodegradable Polymers		
Fiber-Reinforced Composites	Combining fibers (e.g., carbon, glass) with a polymer matrix creates strong and lightweight materials, used in orthopedic implants and tissue engineering scaffolds	[69]
Polymer-Ceramic Composites	These composites leverage the strengths of both materials and find applications in bone grafts and implants	[70]
Composite Materials		
Polymer-Ceramic Composites	These composites leverage the strengths of both materials and find applications in bone grafts and implants	[56]
Materials Inspired by Extracellular Matrix (ECM)	Designed to mimic the structure and function of the ECM, these materials enhance cell adhesion and tissue regeneration	[65]

TABLE 15.3
Overview of Biocompatible and Biomaterials Applications in Various Drug Delivery Systems

Materials	Compounds	Dental Problem	References
Chitosan/alginate polyelectrolyte complex film	Clindamycin phosphate	Periodontitis	[73]
Silver nanoparticles	Titanium	Peri-implantitis	[74]
Silver microparticles	Tetracycline/chlorohexidine	Regeneration of infected tissues	[75]
Alginate–gelatin microspheres	Ciprofloxacin	Pseudomonas aeruginosa infection	[76]
Gelatin hydrogel	Recombinant human fibroblast growth factor-2(RhFGF-2)	Hard tissue healing	[77]
Collagen	Tetracycline	Dental plaque	[78]
Hydroxyapatite/ titanium oxide	Antibiotics	Oral post-surgery infections	[79]
Calcium phosphate	Vancomycin	Oral mucosal infections	[80]
Gelatin films	Econazole nitrate	Mucosal candidiasis	[81]

15.6 BIOCOMPATIBLE MATERIALS IN DRUG DELIVERY SYSTEM

Biocompatible materials and systems have demonstrated their potential applications in the field of dental and oral diseases. In essence, biomaterials play a crucial role as components that directly interact with biological tissues, contributing to the enhancement or replacement of various organs, tissues, or bodily functions [71]. Moreover, biopolymers, such as hyaluronic acid, gelatin, chitosan, and collagen, are actively researched in dentistry due to their capacity to resemble native tissue. Numerous approaches have been explored to leverage diverse technological and biological properties for the development of nano- or micro-composites. Significantly, there is a growing interest in the utilization of biomaterials, either as standalone materials or as components of delivery systems, within the field of dentistry [72]. Recent research has delved into the exploration of biocompatible materials and biomaterials functioning as carriers in drug delivery systems, with specific examples highlighted in Table 15.3.

15.7 BIOCOMPATIBLE MATERIALS AND THEIR APPLICATIONS IN ELECTRONICS

In recent times, the convergence of biocompatible materials and electronics has ushered in a new era for the advancement of sophisticated medical devices, wearable sensors, and bioelectronic implants. This collaborative synergy combines the distinctive characteristics of biocompatible materials with the operational capabilities of electronic components, presenting opportunities for groundbreaking solutions in the realm of healthcare. An exemplary instance of this synergy is the creation of biocompatible conductive polymers that seamlessly integrate with biological tissues. Among these, polypyrrole (PPy) and polyaniline (PANI) stand out as conductive polymers that have been extensively studied for their capacity to interface effectively with neural tissues in bioelectronic devices. These polymers demonstrate commendable electrical conductivity and have undergone exploration for applications such as neural probes and brain-machine interfaces [82].

Moreover, the domain of flexible and stretchable electronics has experienced a surge in interest, facilitating the creation of electronic devices capable of adapting to the contours and mechanical characteristics of biological tissues. Crucial to the construction of these flexible electronic devices are biocompatible materials, particularly elastomers and hydrogels. Notably, polydimethylsiloxane (PDMS), a frequently utilized elastomer, has found application in crafting flexible electrodes and sensors designed for soft robotics and wearable health monitoring devices [83].

The fusion of biocompatible materials with electronic components is notably prominent in the domain of bioelectronic implants. Implantable devices, including pacemakers and neurostimulators, demand materials that not only exhibit outstanding biocompatibility but also enable the effective transmission of electronic signals. Titanium and its alloys have been enduring choices for implantable devices due to their compatibility with biological systems and corrosion resistance. Furthermore, progress in materials science has given rise to the creation of biocompatible coatings like Diamond-Like Carbon (DLC) and hydroxyapatite, aiming to enhance the efficiency and durability of implantable electronics [84]. Within the realm of drug delivery, electronic components are being incorporated into smart drug delivery systems to facilitate precise control and monitoring of drug release. Biocompatible materials, including liposomes and hydrogels, are harmoniously integrated with electronic components to construct stimuli-responsive drug delivery platforms. These platforms can be activated by external stimuli, such as alterations in light or temperature, allowing for the targeted release of drugs at specific times and locations within the body [75].

The burgeoning field of bioelectronics also includes the development of biohybrid systems, where living cells or tissues are interfaced with electronic components. This integration has potential applications in regenerative medicine, where electronic components can provide electrical stimulation to enhance tissue regeneration. For example, conductive polymers and biocompatible scaffolds have been combined to create platforms for the electrical stimulation of cells in tissue engineering applications [69]. The emerging area of neuroprosthetics exemplifies the seamless integration of electronics with the nervous system. Soft, biocompatible materials are crucial in the design of neural interfaces to minimize tissue damage and inflammation. Neural electrodes made from materials like polyimide and parylene have been employed in brain-machine interfaces, enabling communication between electronic devices and the neural network [85–88].

The integration of biocompatible materials with electronics has ushered in a transformative era in healthcare and biotechnology. This convergence is evident in various applications, including flexible electronics for wearable health monitoring, bioelectronic implants, and advanced drug delivery systems. The amalgamation of electronic components with materials like polymers, hydrogels, and nanocomposites holds great promise for enhancing medical diagnostics, treatments, and overall patient outcomes. Innovative thoughts and ideas targeting at par or even exceeding the performance of conventional inorganic-based electronics are proliferating in the field of organic electronics. Using band-gap engineered materials to fabricate novel organic light-emitting diodes (OLEDs), integrating active electronic components with living tissue, and creating high-performance organic field-effect transistors (OFETs) and integrated circuits are a few noteworthy examples. Another is pushing the upper limit of organic photovoltaic (OPVs) efficiency to 20% or more. Ongoing interdisciplinary research at the intersection of materials science, electronics, and biology is driving continuous innovation, shaping the future landscape of biocompatible electronics in healthcare. In conclusion, biocompatible materials are recognized as a vital component in contemporary biomedical research, contributing to advancements in medical technology and paving the way for improved patient outcomes through ongoing exploration and innovation.

15.8 FUTURE PERSPECTIVE AND TRENDS

Life as we know it hinges on three fundamental types of polymers: Polypeptides, polynucleotides, and polysaccharides. Biopolymers, derived from natural sources, have gained prominence in research across industries such as food, pharmaceuticals, and biomedicine. Despite their increasing production and use, challenges like stability, optimal molar mass, and interactions with other compounds persist and require comprehensive analysis and resolution. The multifunctional behavior and stability of biopolymers in different physical states make them versatile for a myriad of applications. From woven fibers that swell in contact with water to water-rich hydrogels fostering a humid environment, the physical behaviors of biopolymers can be tailored for specific functionalities. Physiologically responsive biopolymers, capable of loading and controlling the release of various compounds or drugs in different biological environments, are on the horizon. With an aging population, the demand for renewable approaches in medicine and cell healing proteins is set to surge. Advancements in genomics, proteomics, and stem cell technology are driving a shift towards personalized therapies. The advantageous properties of biopolymers are poised to play a pivotal role in developing and delivering these innovative treatments, particularly in wound healing. While biopolymers like chitosan, alginate, and pectin have long been employed in the food and beverage industry as thickening agents and stabilizers, their applications now extend to the pharmaceutical industry and biotechnology. The cross-linking properties of biopolymers with other materials allow them to serve as matrices or membranes for antimicrobial films, coatings, or the administration of various compounds. The future of the biopolymer industry holds promise for broad development, with potential solutions to humanity's significant challenges. Research directions will likely center around biopolymers, biotechnologies, and renewable sources, paving the way for sustainable and impactful solutions. Examining biopolymers in context is crucial for understanding the fundamental molecules of life and unlocking their full potential.

15.9 CONCLUSION

Natural polymers, often operating behind the scenes, play a crucial role in various aspects of our lives. The efforts of researchers and scientists have yielded remarkable achievements, ranging from the development of biodegradable films to advancements in nanotechnology and the creation of smart packaging utilizing biopolymers. In recent decades, natural polymers have gained increased attention, particularly in the food, pharmaceutical, and biomedical industries. Moreover, they have found applications in promoting physical health, making biopolymers a highly discussed and evolving subject. This chapter focuses on chitosan, alginate, and pectin, delving into key features such as biocompatibility, biodegradability, bio-adhesion, absorption, and limitations. The analysis emphasizes properties that influence gel formation and, more importantly, how these biopolymers are absorbed by the human body. The wide array of current applications and the growing body of research hints at the tremendous potential of these versatile biopolymers, suggesting that their significance will only grow in the future. The "green" revolution in organic electronics has indeed seen a surge in the exploration of natural and nature-inspired materials. Over the past decade, these materials have been at the forefront of advancements in electronics, photonics, biomedical engineering, and bio-mimetics. The term "green" has become a trendy descriptor for innovations geared toward sustainability in the electronics domain, even if the connection sometimes appears somewhat loose. The concept of what truly constitutes a "green" technology can be subjective and is a matter of debate. An interesting perspective was shared during a conference, highlighting the contrasting lifetimes of materials. While some may consider vat dyes "green" due to their potential biodegradation over long periods, inorganics and ceramics were viewed as less "green" because of their extended persistence in the environment. In the quest for sustainability, natural and nature-inspired materials offer promising avenues for "green" technologies. With inherent features like low energy consumption, biodegradability, and biocompatibility, these materials stand as suitable candidates for achieving sustainability goals in the field of electronics.

REFERENCES

[1] Kamalov F, Calonge S D and Gurrib I (2023) New era of artificial intelligence in education: Towards a sustainable multifaceted revolution. *Sustainability*. **15**(16), 12451.

[2] Aldoseri A, Al-Khalifa K and Hamouda A (2023) A roadmap for integrating automation with process optimization for AI-powered digital transformation.

[3] Hamet P and Tremblay J (2017) Artificial intelligence in medicine. *Metabolism*. 69, S36–S40.

[4] Dhamija P and Bag S (2020) Role of artificial intelligence in operations environment: A review and bibliometric analysis. *Total Qual. Manag*. **32**(4), 869–896.

[5] Theofilatos K, Pavlopoulou N, Papasavvas C, Likothanassis S, Dimitrakopoulos C, Georgopoulos E, Moschopoulos C and Mavroudi S (2015) Predicting protein complexes from weighted protein--Piassavas interaction graphs with a novel unsupervised methodology: Evolutionary enhanced Markov clustering. *Artif. Intell. Med*. **63**(3), 181–189.

[6] Patricio D I and Rieder R (2018) Computer vision and artificial intelligence in precision agriculture for grain crops: A systematic review. *Comput. Electron. Agric*. **153**, 69–81.

[7] Ramirez-Asis E, Vilchez-Carcamo J, Thakar C M, Phasinam K, Kassanuk T and Naved M (2022) A review on role of artificial intelligence in food processing and manufacturing industry. *Mater. Today: Proc.* **51**, 2462–2465.
[8] Rane N (2023) Role and challenges of ChatGPT and similar generative artificial intelligence in business management. Available at SSRN 4603227.
[9] Ye Z, Yang J, Zhong N, Tu X, Jia J and Wang J (2020) Tackling environmental challenges in pollution controls using artificial intelligence: A review. *Sci. Total Environ.* **699**, 134279.
[10] Gaur L, Afaq A, Arora G K and Khan N (2023) Artificial intelligence for carbon emissions using system of systems theory. *Ecol. Inform.* 102165. https://doi.org/10.1016/j.ecoinf.2023.102165
[11] Nishant R, Kennedy M and Corbett J (2020) Artificial intelligence for sustainability: Challenges, opportunities, and a research agenda. *Int. J. Inf. Manage.* **53**, 102104.
[12] Hanifa M, Agarwal R, Sharma U, Thapliyal P C and Singh L P (2023) A review on CO_2 capture and sequestration in the construction industry: Emerging approaches and commercialised technologies. *J. CO_2 Util.* **67**, 102292.
[13] Antonopoulos I, Robu V, Couraud B, Kirli D, Norbu S, Kiprakis A, Flynn D, Elizondo-Gonzalez S and Wattam S (2020) Artificial intelligence and machine learning approaches to energy demand-side response: A systematic review. *Renew. Sust. Energ. Rev.* **130**, 109899.
[14] Ahmed M, Zheng Y, Amine A, Fathiannasab H and Chen Z (2021) The role of artificial intelligence in the mass adoption of electric vehicles. *Joule.* **5**(9), 2296–2322.
[15] Kyriakides T R, Raj A, Tseng T H, Xiao H, Nguyen R, Mohammed F S, Halder S, Xu M, Wu M J, Bao S and others (2021) Biocompatibility of nanomaterials and their immunological properties. *Biomed. Mater.* **16**(4), 42005.
[16] Haakman M, Cruz L, Huijgens H and van Deursen A (2021) AI lifecycle models need to be revised: An exploratory study in Fintech. *Empir. Softw. Eng.* **26**, 1–29.
[17] Tian K and Bilal M (2020) Research progress of biodegradable materials in reducing environmental pollution. In *Abatement of Environmental Pollutants*, Elsevier, 313–330. https://doi.org/10.1016/B978-0-12-818095-2.00015-1
[18] Hosseini E S, Dervin S, Ganguly P and Dahiya R (2020) Biodegradable materials for sustainable health monitoring devices. *ACS Appl. Bio Mater.* **4**(1), 163–194.
[19] Vikhareva I N, Buylova E A, Yarmuhametova G U, Aminova G K and Mazitova A K (2021) An overview of the main trends in the creation of biodegradable polymer materials. *J. Chem.* **2021**, 1–15.
[20] Nagarkar R and Patel J (2019) Polyvinyl alcohol: A comprehensive study. *Acta Sci. Pharm. Sci.* **3**(4), 34–44.
[21] Li P, Cao L, Sang F, Zhang B, Meng Z, Pan L, Hao J, Yang X, Ma Z and Shi C (2022) Polyvinyl alcohol/sodium alginate composite sponge with 3D ordered/disordered porous structure for rapidly controlling noncompressible hemorrhage. *Biomater. Adv.* **134**, 112698.
[22] Backes E H, Harb S V, Beatrice C A G, Shimomura K M B, Passador F R, Costa L C and Pessan L A (2022) Polycaprolactone usage in additive manufacturing strategies for tissue engineering applications: A review. *J. Biomed. Mater. Res. Part B.* **110**(6), 1479–1503.
[23] Liang Y, He J and Guo B (2021) Functional hydrogels as wound dressing to enhance wound healing. *ACS Nano.* **15**(8), 12687–12722.
[24] Aswathy S H, Narendrakumar U and Manjubala I (2020) Commercial hydrogels for biomedical applications. *Heliyon* **6** (4).
[25] Xu R Fang Y, Zhang Z, Cao Y, Yan Y, Gan L, Xu J and Zhou G (2023) Recent advances in biodegradable and biocompatible synthetic polymers used in skin wound healing. *Materials.* **16**(15), 5459.

[26] Li C, Guo C, Fitzpatrick V, Ibrahim A, Zwierstra M J, Hanna P, Lechtig A, Nazaria A, Lin S J and Kaplan D L (2020) Design of biodegradable, implantable devices towards clinical translation. *Nat. Rev. Mater.* **5**(1), 61–81.

[27] Zhu J, Wen H, Zhang H, Huang P, Liu L and Hu H (2023) Recent advances in biodegradable electronics-from fundament to the next-generation multi-functional, medical and environmental device. *Sustain. Mater. Technol.* **35**, e00530.

[28] Berger L I (2020) *Semiconductor materials*. CRC Press.

[29] Liu K, Ouyang B, Guo X, Guo Y and Liu Y (2022) Advances in flexible organic field-effect transistors and their applications for flexible electronics. *Npj Flexible Electronics*. **6**(1), 1.

[30] Chen C and Hu L (2018) Nanocellulose toward advanced energy storage devices: Structure and electrochemistry. *Acc. Chem. Res*. **51**, 3154–3165.

[31] Freudenberg J, Jansch D, Hinkel F and Bunz U H F (2018) Immobilization strategies for organic semiconducting conjugated polymers. *Chem. Rev*. **118**(11), 5598–5689.

[32] Inal S, Rivnay J, Suiu A O, Malliaras G G and McCulloch I (2018) Conjugated polymers in bioelectronics. *Acc. Chem. Res*. **51**(6), 1368–1376.

[33] Bronstein H, Nielsen C B, Schroeder B C and McCulloch I (2020) The role of chemical design in the performance of organic semiconductors. *Nat. Rev. Chem*. **4**(2), 66–77.

[34] Wang K, Dai S, Zhao Y, Wang Y, Liu C and Huang J (2019) Light-stimulated synaptic transistors fabricated by a facile solution process based on inorganic perovskite quantum dots and organic semiconductors. *Small* **15**(11), 1900010.

[35] Wang X, Hao D and Huang J (2022) Dye-sensitized perovskite/organic semiconductor ternary transistors for artificial synapses. *SCMs*. **5**(9), 2521–2528.

[36] Palsule S (2018) *Polymers and Polymeric Composites: A Reference Series*. Springer.

[37] Lee C J, Chang Y C, Wang L W and Wang Y H (2019) Biodegradable materials for organic field-effect transistors on a paper substrate. *IEEE Electron Device Lett*. **40**(2), 236–239.

[38] Seck M, Mohammadian N, Diallo A K, Faraji S, Erouel M, Bouguila N, Ndiaye D, Khirouni K and Majewski L A (2020) Organic FETs using biodegradable almond gum as gate dielectric: A promising way towards green electronics. *Org. Electron*. **83**, 105735.

[39] Zhang J, Liu D, Shi Q, Yang B, Guo P, Fang L, Dai S, Xiong L and Huang J (2022) Bioinspired organic optoelectronic synaptic transistors based on cellulose nanopaper and natural chlorophyll-a for neuromorphic systems. *Npj Flex*. **6**(1), 30.

[40] Kim M H, Park H L, Kim M H, Jang J, Bae J H, Kang I M and Lee S H (2021) Fluoropolymer-based organic memristor with multifunctionality for flexible neural network system. *Npj Flex. Electron*. **5**(1), 34.

[41] Pogorielov M, Husak E, Solodivnik A and Zhdanov S (2017) Magnesium-based biodegradable alloys: Degradation, application, and alloying elements. *Interv. Med. Appl. Sci*. **9**(1), 27–38.

[42] Tsakiris V, Tardei C and Clicinschi F M (2021). Biodegradable Mg alloys for orthopedic implants--A review. *J. Magnes. Alloy*. **9**(6), 1884–1905.

[43] Venezuela J J D, Johnston S and Dargusch M S (2019). The prospects for biodegradable zinc in wound closure applications. *Adv. Healthcare Mater*. **8**(16), 1900408.

[44] Wegener B, Sichler A, Milz S, Sprecher C, Pieper K, Hermanns W, Jansson V, Nies B, Kieback B and Müller P E (2020). Development of a novel biodegradable porous iron-based implant for bone replacement. *Sci. Rep*. **10**(1), 9141.

[45] Lin W, Zhang H, Zhang W, Qi H, Zhang G, Qian J, Li X, Qin L, Li H, Wang X, et al. (2021). In vivo degradation and endothelialization of an iron bioresorbable scaffold. *Bio. Mater*. **6**(4), 1028–1039.

[46] Umuhoza D, Yang F, Long D, Hao Z, Dai J and Zhao A. (2020). Strategies for tuning the biodegradation of silk fibroin-based materials for tissue engineering applications. *ACS Biomater. Sci. Eng*. **6**(3), 1290–1310.

[47] Huang H, Chen H, Wang X, Qiu F, Liu H, Lu J, Tong L, Yang Y, Wang X and Wu H. (2019). Degradable and bioadhesive alginate-based composites: An effective hemostatic agent. *ACS Biomater. Sci. Eng.* **5**(10), 5498–5505.

[48] Shin E, Yoo J, Yoo G, Kim Y J and Kim Y S (2019) Eco-friendly cross-linked polymeric dielectric material based on natural tannic acid. *Chem. Eng. J.* **358**, 170–175.

[49] Singh R, Yadav V K, Dvivedi A and Kumar P (2023) Evaluating the feasibility of using biodegradable castor oil as a dielectric medium during micro-electrical discharge machining of Inconel 718. *J. Mat. Eng. Perf.* **32**(14), 6465–6477.

[50] Chi Y, Xia K, Zhu Z, Fu J, Zhang H, and Xu Z (2019) Rice paper-based biodegradable triboelectric nanogenerator. *Micro. Eng.* **216**, 111059.

[51] Kumar R, Ranwa S and Kumar G (2019) Biodegradable flexible substrate based on chitosan/PVP blend polymer for disposable electronics device applications. *J. Phy. Chem. B.* **124**(1), 149–155.

[52] Rivadeneyra A, Marin-Sanchez A, Wicklein B, Salmeron J F, Castillo E, Bobinger M and Salinas-Castillo A (2021) Cellulose nanofibers as substrate for flexible and biodegradable moisture sensors. *Comp. Sci. Tech.* **208**, 108738.

[53] Brannon-Peppas L, and J O Blanchette (2004) Nanoparticle and targeted systems for cancer therapy. *Adv. Drug Deliv. Rev.* **56**(11), 1649–1659.

[54] Veronese F M (2009) *PEGylated Protein Drugs: Basic Science and Clinical Applications.* Springer.

[55] Chai Q, Yang J and X Yu (2017) Hydrogels for biomedical applications: Their characteristics and the mechanisms behind them. *Gels.* **3**(1), 6.

[56] Ginestra P, Fiorentino A and E Ceretti (2017) Micro-structuring of titanium collectors by laser ablation technique: A promising approach to produce micro-patterned scaffolds for tissue engineering applications. *Procedia Cirp.* **65**, 19–24.

[57] Peer D, Karp J M, Hong S, Farokhzad O C, Margalit R and Langer R (2020) Nanocarriers as an emerging platform for cancer therapy. *Nano-enabled Med. App.* 61–91.

[58] Jalani G, Rizwan M, Akram M A and Mujahid M (2023) Cell and therapeutic delivery using injectable hydrogels for tissue engineering applications. *Front. Bioeng. Biotechnol.* **11**, 1–3.

[59] Dadras C, Masoud S A, Akbari S, Sadeghi D, Mirahmadi F and Mirzadeh H (2018) Electrospun nanofibers comprising of silk fibroin/gelatin for drug delivery applications: Thyme essential oil and doxycycline monohydrate release study. *J. Biomed. Mater. Res. Part A.* **106**(4), 1092–1103.

[60] Chen C Y, Peng X, Zeng R, Chen M, Wan C P and Chen J Y (2016) *Ficus hirta* fruits extract incorporated into an alginate-based edible coating for Nanfeng mandarin preservation. *Sci. Hortic.* **202**, 41–48.

[61] Irvine D J, Hanson M C, Rakhra K and Tokatlian T (2015) Synthetic nanoparticles for vaccines and immunotherapy. *Chem. Rev.* **115**(19), 11109–11146.

[62] Bastos V, Jose M P, Ferreira-de-Oliveira and Carrola J (2017) Coating independent cytotoxicity of citrate-and PEG-coated silver nanoparticles on a human hepatoma cell line. *J. Environ Sci.* **51**,191–201.

[63] Elsabee M Z and Abdou E S (2013) Chitosan based edible films and coatings: A review. *Mater. Sci. Eng: C.* **33**(4), 1819–1841.

[64] Hoffman and Allan S (2012) Hydrogels for biomedical applications. *Adv. Drug Deliv. Rev.* **64**, 18–23.

[65] Van V, Sandra D P and Schacht E (2011) Biopolymer-based hydrogels as scaffolds for tissue engineering applications: A review. *Biomacromolecules* **12**(5), 1387–1408

[66] Paul D R and Robeson L M (2008) Polymer nanotechnology: Nanocomposites. *Polymer* **49**(15), 3187–3204.

[67] Xia Z and Wei M (2013) Biomimetic fabrication of collagen-apatite scaffolds for bone tissue regeneration. *J. Biomater. Tissue Eng.* **3**(4), 369–384.
[68] Hench and Larry L (1991) Bioceramics: From concept to clinic. *J. Am. Ceram. Soc.* **74**(7), 1487–1510.
[69] Fang Y, Lingyuan M, Prominski A, Schaumann E N, Seebald M and Tian B (2020) Recent advances in bioelectronics chemistry. *Chem. Soc. Rev.* **49**(22), 7978–8035.
[70] Chen F M and Liu X (2016) Advancing biomaterials of human origin for tissue engineering. *Prog. Polym. Sci.* **53**, 86–168.
[71] Meyer M (2019) Processing of collagen based biomaterials and the resulting materials properties. *Biomed. Eng. Online.* **18**(1), 1–74.
[72] de Oliveira B, Gomes H, da Silva R R, Borges M A C, Castro G R, Ribeiro S J L and da Silva Barud H (2021) Bacterial nanocellulose in dentistry: Perspectives and challenges. *Molecules.* **26**(1), 49.
[73] Kilicarslan M, Ilhan M, Inal O and Orhan K (2018) Preparation and evaluation of clindamycin phosphate loaded chitosan/alginate polyelectrolyte complex film as mucoadhesive drug delivery system for periodontal therapy. *Eur. J. Pharm. Sci.* **123**, 441–451.
[74] Nguyen S and Hiorth M (2015) Advanced drug delivery systems for local treatment of the oral cavity. *Ther. Deliv.* **6**(5), 595–608.
[75] Lee J H, El-Fiqi A, Mandakhbayar N, Lee H H and Kim H W (2017) Drug/ion co-delivery multi-functional nanocarrier to regenerate infected tissue defect. *Biomaterials* **142**, 62–76.
[76] Islan, German A and Castro G R (2014) Tailoring of alginate–gelatin microspheres properties for oral Ciprofloxacin-controlled release against *Pseudomonas aeruginosa. Drug Deliv.* **21**(8), 615–626.
[77] Kimura A, Kabasawa Y, Tabata Y, Aoki K, Ohya K and Omura K (2014) Gelatin hydrogel as a carrier of recombinant human fibroblast growth factor-2 during rat mandibular distraction. *J. Oral Maxillofac. Surg.* **72**(10), 2015–2031
[78] Khan Y F, Jan S M and Mushtaq M (2015) Clinical utility of locally-delivered collagen-based biodegradable tetracycline fibers in periodontal therapy: An in vivo study. *J. Investig. Clin. Dent.* **6**(4), 307–312.
[79] Brohede U, Forsgren B, Roos S, Mihranyan A, Engqvist H and Strømme M (2009) Multifunctional implant coatings providing possibilities for fast antibiotics loading with subsequent slow release. *J. Mater. Sci.: Mater. Med.* **20**, 1859–1867.
[80] Radin S and Ducheyne P (2007) Controlled release of vancomycin from thin sol–gel films on titanium alloy fracture plate material. *Biomaterials* **28**(9), 1721–1729.
[81] Dolci L S, Liguori A and Panzavolta S (2018) Non-equilibrium atmospheric pressure plasma as innovative method to crosslink and enhance mucoadhesion of econazole-loaded gelatin films for buccal drug delivery. *Colloids Surf. B.* **163**, 73–82.
[82] Vsevolodov N (2012) Biomolecular electronics: An introduction via photosensitive proteins. *SSBM.*
[83] Lipomi D J, Vosgueritchian M and Tee B C K (2011) Skin-like pressure and strain sensors based on transparent elastic films of carbon nanotubes. *Nat. Nanotechnol.* **6**(12), 788–792.
[84] Ma Y, Tian X, Liu L, Pan J and Pan G (2019) Dynamic synthetic biointerfaces: From reversible chemical interactions to tunable biological effects. *Acc. Chem. Res.* **52**(6), 1611–1622.
[85] Heidi G, Sheybani R, Li P-Y, Mann R L and Meng E (2012) An implantable MEMS micropump system for drug delivery in small animals. *Biomed. Microdevices.* **14**, 483–496.

[86] Ghai D, Tripathi S L, Saxena S, Chanda M and Alazab M (Eds.). (2022) *Machine Learning Algorithms for Signal and Image Processing*. John Wiley & Sons.
[87] S. L. Tripathi, K. Dhir, D. Ghai and S. Patil (Eds.). (2021) *Health Informatics and Technological Solutions for Coronavirus (COVID-19)*. CRC Press.
[88] Madhavi K B, Tripathi S L, Saxena S, Ghai D and Raj B (2023) Design and analysis of 18 nm multichannel FinFET as biosensor for detection of biological species. *Silicon* **15**(14), 6313–6322.

16 Virtually Going Green
The Role of Artificial Intelligence in Reducing Pollution and Toxicity

Lalit Saini, Prasann Kumar, Rajeev, Tejas, and Hina Upadhyay
School of Agriculture, Lovely Professional University, Phagwara, Punjab, India

16.1 INTRODUCTION

An introduction to Artificial Intelligence (AI), a cutting-edge field that is revolutionizing decision-making and industries. Amid this change, integrating artificial intelligence with environmental sustainability becomes increasingly important [1]. According to Perera et al. [2], combining AI with green activities represents a significant change and offers answers for environmental preservation. The goal of a greener future is aided by utilizing AI's skills in automation and data analysis (Kohli & Jain [3]). This combination is a potential first step toward addressing environmental issues and maximizing resource use (LeCun & Bengio [4]). Redefining sectors and paradigms for decision-making, Artificial Intelligence (AI) is a disruptive force (Russell Stuart & Norvig [5]). In this paradigm-shifting context, combining artificial intelligence and environmental sustainability becomes a primary subject of interest [1]. According to Perera et al. [2] in 2019, this combination presents novel approaches to ecological preservation and sustainable practices, opening up a transformative avenue. Making the most of AI's automated and analytical skills could significantly contribute to a more environmentally friendly future (Kohli & Jain [3]). This combination of artificial intelligence and green efforts is viable for resolving environmental issues and maximizing resource use (LeCun & Bengio [4]). AI's contribution to developing a sustainable and environmentally conscious society is becoming increasingly important as it advances (Jordan & Mitchell [6]). With its revolutionary impact on industries and decision-making procedures, Artificial Intelligence (AI) has emerged as a keystone of technological advancement (Taddeo & Floridi [7]). A significant change in sustainable practices has been brought about by the increasing synergy between artificial intelligence and environmental conservation in this age of innovation (Yuan et al. [8]). Using AI-driven solutions provides a revolutionary

DOI: 10.1201/9781003546382-16

way to deal with environmental issues (Varshney [9]). Ecological footprints can be reduced, and eco-friendly behaviors can be promoted using AI's predictive analysis and optimization skills (Liu et al. [10]). This combination represents a critical turning point in using technology to protect the environment and ensure a more sustainable future (LeCun & Bengio [4]). In conclusion, a new era of creative approaches and solutions is being ushered in by the intersection of environmental sustainability and artificial intelligence. This synergy presents a promising future using AI-driven approaches to address urgent ecological concerns. Integrating AI tools and predictive analytics is a revolutionary strategy for addressing ecological problems. As AI technologies develop, it will be more and more important to integrate them into sustainable practices to move towards a future that is more environmentally conscious and conscientious. An important turning point in using technology to benefit our world is the joint efforts of artificial intelligence and environmental stewardship (Johnson & White [11]).

16.2 GREEN TECHNOLOGY

Green technology, which includes various advancements in waste management, renewable energy, and environmentally friendly behaviors, is a crucial step toward sustainable solutions (Smith et al. [12]). This emerging discipline focuses on creating and applying technologies that maximize resource efficiency while reducing their adverse effects on the environment (Jones & Williams [13]). Developing environmentally friendly energy sources is exemplified by developments in solar power, wind energy, and biofuels (Brown & Miller [14]). Furthermore, incorporating energy-efficient systems and intelligent grids emphasizes using technology to lower carbon footprints and improve energy conservation (Lee & Kim [15]). A cornerstone in the quest for a sustainable future, green technology's interdisciplinary approach promotes a harmonic balance between technical innovation and environmental preservation (Gupta & Sharma [16]).

16.2.1 Applications of Green Technology

1. ***Renewable Energy Sources:*** Solar, wind, hydro, and geothermal power are just a few examples of renewable energy sources that can be harnessed with green technology. By providing sustainable substitutes for fossil fuels, these sources help to lower carbon emissions and lessen reliance on non-renewable resources (Johnson & White [11]).
2. ***Innovations in Waste Management:*** Recycling, composting, and cutting-edge waste-to-energy technologies are just a few ways green technology revolutionizes waste management. These developments support a circular economy while reducing environmental pollution (Garcia et al. [17]).
3. ***Clean Transportation Solutions:*** One of the best examples of green transportation technology is the development of hybrid engines and Electric Vehicles (EVs). These developments considerably lessen the need for conventional fuel sources and the production of greenhouse gases (Wang & Liu [18]).

16.2.2 Benefits of Green Technology

1. ***Environmental Conservation:*** Using green technology, natural resources are preserved, decreasing environmental damage. It reduces pollution, protects biodiversity, and lessens the effects of climate change (Smith & Patel [19]).
2. ***Cost-Efficiency:*** Green technology can save money in the long run. For example, energy-efficient appliances and buildings use less energy, which results in cheaper operating costs and utility bills (Chen & Chang [20]).
3. ***Health Benefits:*** Green technology improves public health by lowering exposure to dangerous pollutants. The quality of air, water, and soil quality is improved when pollution-related health hazards are decreased, improving human well-being (Gupta et al. [21]).
4. ***Technical creativity:*** Adopting sustainable practices and green technology encourages creativity and research, propelling technical breakthroughs towards a more environmentally friendly future (Jones & Garcia [22]).

16.3 ENVIRONMENTAL CHALLENGES

The earth's sustainability is seriously threatened by environmental difficulties, ranging from biodiversity loss to climate change [23]. Ecosystems and human livelihoods are seriously threatened by the worsening effects of global warming, caused mainly by greenhouse gas emissions [24]. Studies [25] have shown that deforestation is still a significant problem since it is causing habitat damage and biodiversity loss at a startling rate. Environmental quality is deteriorating due to air and water pollution [26], which impacts ecosystem balance and human health. Furthermore, the global water shortage is worsened by the depletion of natural resources, particularly freshwater reserves [27], endangering ecosystems and populations everywhere. It will take coordinated efforts and creative solutions to address these complex issues.

1. ***Climate Change and Global Warming:*** Ecosystems, economies, and human well-being are at risk due to the escalating effects of climate change, which include rising temperatures, harsh weather, and rising sea levels [23].
2. ***Degradation of Ecosystems and Loss of Biodiversity:*** Rapid extinctions of species are caused by overuse of natural resources, habitat destruction, and climate change [28].
3. ***Deforestation and Land Degradation:*** As a result of logging, urbanization, and agriculture, there is an ongoing reduction in the amount of forest cover, which leads to habitat loss and fragmentation and disturbs ecosystems and species [25].
4. ***Pollution:*** The environment, wildlife, and human health are seriously threatened by air, water, and soil pollution brought on by industrial processes, inappropriate waste disposal, and agricultural runoff [26].
5. ***Depletion of Natural Resources:*** Excessive use of freshwater, minerals, and fisheries causes depletion of natural resources, which worsens scarcity and damages ecosystems [27].

6. ***Ocean Acidification and Degradation:*** According to Doney et al. [29] in 2009, rising atmospheric carbon dioxide levels caused ocean acidification, upset marine ecosystems, and endangered marine life.

Comprehensive policies, international collaboration, and creative solutions are needed to ensure environmental sustainability and lessen the long-term effects of these difficulties.

16.4 POLLUTION AND ITS TYPES

One of the most significant environmental problems is pollution, which can take many forms and endanger human health and ecosystems [26]. Air pollution causes hazardous particulate matter and gases to enter the atmosphere, contributing to respiratory ailments and climate change. The primary sources of air pollution are industrial emissions, automobile exhaust, and burning biomass [24]. Aquatic ecosystems and human access to clean water are threatened by water pollution brought on by improper waste disposal, industrial discharge, and agricultural runoff [26]. According to Kibblewhite et al. [30] in 2020, soil contamination is caused by inappropriate waste disposal, mining activities, and the use of agrochemicals. These factors contribute to soil degradation, which affects agricultural output and poses health hazards. Noise pollution damages natural ecosystems and hurts human health, causing stress and hearing loss.

16.4.1 Types of Pollution

1. ***Pollution of Air:*** Air pollution is the result of dangerous materials being released into the atmosphere, including sulfur dioxide, nitrogen oxides, particulate matter, and volatile organic compounds. Fossil fuel combustion, vehicle exhaust, and industrial pollutants are some sources. According to the World Health Organization (WHO), air pollution can cause respiratory disorders, heart problems, and environmental deterioration [31].
2. ***Pollution of Water:*** Contaminants such as chemicals, heavy metals, diseases, and nutrients can contaminate water bodies such as rivers, lakes, and oceans. This leads to water pollution. Aquatic life, ecosystems, and human health are all impacted by water pollution, which is caused by industrial discharges, agricultural runoff, and inappropriate waste disposal [32].
3. ***Pollution of Soil:*** When contaminants like chemicals, heavy metals, and pesticides are introduced into the soil, it leads to soil pollution. According to Kibblewhite et al. [30] in 2020, inappropriate waste disposal, industrial operations, and agrochemicals are some of the activities that lead to soil degradation, which affects agricultural output and poses health concerns to humans.
4. ***Pollution of Noise:*** Excessive environmental noise levels, frequently brought on by industrial machinery, urbanization, and transportation, constitute noise pollution. Basner et al. [33], 2014 stated that extended exposure to noise pollution can cause stress, sleep difficulties, hearing loss, and disruptions to natural habitats.

5. ***Pollution of Light:*** Light pollution is the excessive or improper use of artificial light, which ruins the night sky's natural darkness. Urban streetlights, advertisements, and industrial facilities are a few sources. According to Gaston et al. [34] in 2017, it affects human sleep patterns, disrupts ecosystems, and impacts wildlife behavior and astronomical observations.

16.5 GLOBALIZATION AND RELATED CHALLENGES

The interdependence of economies and societies across borders, or globalization, brings with it a multitude of opportunities as well as difficulties (Rodrik [35]). Improvements in communication and transportation have made it easier to conduct business internationally, boosting economic expansion and cross-cultural interaction (Stiglitz [36]). But this interconnection also worsens economic disparities between countries (Milanovic [37]). In industrialized economies, job displacement and income inequality are exacerbated by the growth of multinational firms and the outsourcing of work to low-wage nations (Drezner [38]). Furthermore, globalization exacerbates environmental problems by increasing pollution and resource consumption (Held & McGrew [39]). Local customs and cultural diversity are at risk due to cultural homogenization and global integration (Appadurai [40]). Worldwide collaboration and policies that balance the positive aspects of globalization while reducing its negative consequences on economies and communities are necessary to address these difficulties.

1. ***Economic Divide:*** According to Milanovic [37] in 2016, globalization has increased the economic divide between developed and developing countries. This has made income inequality worse. Certain places experience economic stagnation and marginalization, whereas others gain from more significant trade and investment.
2. ***Labor Market Disruptions:*** Due to jobs being outsourced to nations with lower wages due to the integration of global markets, developed economies experience job displacement and income instability (Drezner [38]). This strains labor markets and adds to societal unrest.
3. ***Environmental Impacts:*** Resource depletion, pollution, and unsustainable manufacturing methods are ways that globalization's vast trade networks and rising demand led to environmental degradation (Held & McGrew [39]). Ecological imbalances and climate change are made worse.
4. ***Cultural Homogenization:*** There is a chance that local customs and diversity will be lost when global cultures converge (Appadurai [40]). Identity and legacy can be impacted by dominant cultures and the media's obscuring of indigenous or minority cultures.
5. ***Political Difficulties:*** Since supranational organizations and multinational companies substantially influence policy decisions, globalization jeopardizes national sovereignty (Rodrik [35]). National interests and global governance may clash as a result of this.
6. ***Social and Health Issues:*** As globalization picks up speed, society may be unable to keep up, resulting in social unrest, health problems, and the rapid spread of diseases (Stiglitz [36]). It can put pressure on healthcare systems and worsen health disparities.

16.6 THE NEXUS OF AI AND ENVIRONMENTAL SUSTAINABILITY

Combining environmental sustainability and Artificial Intelligence (AI) offers novel approaches to urgent ecological problems, forming a transformational synergy (Perera et al. [2]). The combination of AI's analytical powers and machine learning algorithms allows for accurate data analysis and predictive modeling, which in turn helps make well-informed decisions for sustainable resource management (Kohli & Jain [3]). Artificial Intelligence (AI)-powered solutions support eco-efficiency and lessen environmental effects by streamlining resource allocation, optimizing energy usage, and improving renewable energy systems (Liu et al. [10]). Additionally, ecosystem management and monitoring are made easier by AI, which also helps to mitigate the effects of climate change and conserve biodiversity (LeCun & Bengio [4]). This merger highlights a possible path toward a greener future by utilizing AI's potential for sustainable development and environmental stewardship (Jordan & Mitchell [6]).

16.7 MONITORING AND PREDICTING POLLUTION WITH AI

Using Artificial Intelligence (AI) to monitor and forecast pollution significantly advances environmental management and mitigation techniques (Perera et al. [2]). Real-time monitoring of pollution levels is made possible by AI's capabilities in data analysis and machine learning algorithms, which allow for accurate evaluations and early alerts (Eftimie et al. [41]). Machine learning algorithms utilize past data to forecast pollution patterns and trends, facilitating proactive approaches for pollution management and avoidance. Furthermore, AI-based sensors and monitoring systems make high-resolution, reasonably priced data collecting possible, enabling focused interventions to lessen pollution hotspots. This integration highlights a revolutionary strategy for reducing pollution by giving stakeholders and policymakers access to timely insights and predictive analytics.

16.8 AI-POWERED POLLUTION MONITORING AND FORECASTING

Real-time Data Analysis By analyzing enormous volumes of data from numerous sources, such as sensors, satellites, and monitoring stations, AI makes it easier to monitor pollution levels in real time (Eftimie et al. [41]). This feature makes it possible to identify and analyze pollution trends quickly.

1. Using past data, machine learning algorithms forecast pollution trends and patterns, providing information about probable future pollution incidents. These forecasting algorithms improve readiness and make proactive pollution control measures possible.
2. ***Targeted Interventions:*** By identifying pollution hotspots and enabling targeted interventions, AI-based sensors and monitoring systems provide high-resolution data collecting. This accuracy helps to allocate resources for pollution control in an efficient manner.
3. AI enables early warning systems for pollution incidents, informing communities and authorities about possible environmental risks (Eftimie et al. [41]).

This proactive strategy helps to reduce adverse effects on ecosystems and public health.

4. ***Policy Decision Support:*** AI-generated insights and predictive analytics give stakeholders and policymakers helpful information that helps them create rules and policies for pollution management that work. In the fight against pollution, evidence-based decision-making becomes essential (Masood and Ahmad [42]).

16.9 REMOVAL OF TOXIC METAL IONS AND RELATED TECHNIQUES

A critical component of pollution mitigation is the removal of harmful metal ions using various methods and technologies from different environmental matrices. Modern techniques like adsorption, which use materials like nanomaterials and activated carbon, have proven incredibly effective in removing metal ions from water sources in a selective manner. Metal ions in wastewater can be safely disposed of or reused using coagulation and precipitation procedures, frequently paired with filtration processes. Practical techniques for selectively removing metal ions from tainted fluids include membrane filtration devices and ion exchange resins. Furthermore, because of their efficiency and scalability, electrochemical procedures like electrocoagulation and electrodialysis have emerged as viable strategies for removing metal ions (Gupta et al. [21]). Figure 16.1 shows the artificial intelligence for clean air.

16.9.1 Toxic Metal Ion Removal and Techniques

1. ***Bioremediation Methods:*** Using plants and microorganisms to absorb, accumulate, or alter metal ions, biological techniques, such as phytoremediation and microbial remediation, help clean up contaminated soils and water bodies.

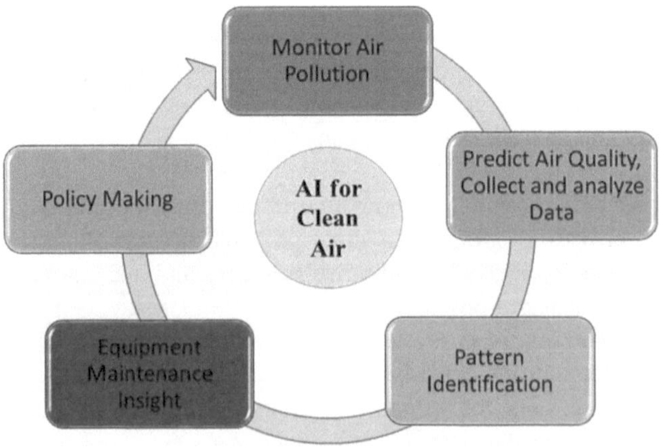

FIGURE 16.1 Artificial Intelligence for clean air.

2. ***Chelation and Precipitation:*** By creating stable complexes with metal ions, chelating agents such as Ethylenediaminetetraacetic acid (EDTA) or Diethylenetriamine pentaacetate (DTPA) help remove metal ions from polluted areas by precipitation or chemical reaction, which makes filtration or separation easier later on.
3. ***Nanostructured Materials:*** Due to their high surface area and reactivity, nano-based materials such as graphene oxide and zero-valent iron nanoparticles help adsorb and secure metal ions from water sources.
4. ***Advanced Oxidation Processes (AOPs):*** AOPs that produce highly reactive species, including photocatalysis and ozonation, break down or change metal ions into less toxic kinds.
5. ***Chemical precipitation:*** Methods such as flocculation and coagulation, which use chemicals like lime or ferric chloride, help to collect metal ions so they may be removed later by filtration or sedimentation (Ahmad et al. [43]).
6. ***Electrochemical Procedures:*** By using electrical currents to destabilize metal ions and encourage their aggregation and evacuation from contaminated water sources, electrocoagulation, electrochemical reduction, and electroflotation procedures are used.

16.10 REMOVAL OF TOXIC METAL IONS AND RELATED TECHNIQUES

In pursuing sustainable development and environmental preservation, removing toxic metal ions has become a critical area of focus. Industries and human activities continue to release harmful pollutants into the environment. AI is pivotal in enhancing and optimizing techniques for removing toxic metal ions, ushering in a new era of environmentally conscious practices (Bhagat et al. [44]). Poisonous metal ions, including heavy metals such as lead, mercury, cadmium, and chromium, pose severe threats to ecosystems and human health. These pollutants enter water bodies, soil, and air through industrial discharges, agricultural runoff, and improper waste disposal (Carolin et al. [45]). Prolonged exposure to these metals can lead to a range of health issues, including neurological disorders, respiratory problems, and carcinogenic effects. Additionally, these contaminants can accumulate in the food chain, further amplifying the risks to humans and wildlife (Rehman et al. [46]). Recognizing the urgency of addressing this environmental challenge, researchers increasingly turn to innovative technologies, with AI emerging as a critical enabler in designing efficient and sustainable solutions.

16.10.1 AI-Powered Techniques for Metal Ion Removal

1. ***Machine Learning Algorithms for Predictive Modeling:*** One of the primary applications of AI in metal ion removal is using machine learning algorithms for predictive modeling. These algorithms can analyze vast datasets containing information about metal ion concentrations, environmental conditions, and the efficacy of various removal techniques. By identifying

patterns and correlations within these datasets, machine learning models can predict the most effective methods for removing specific metal ions in different environmental contexts (Sadek et al. [47]).

2. ***Smart Adsorbents and Nanomaterials:*** AI is instrumental in designing smart adsorbents and nanomaterials tailored for efficient metal ion removal. Researchers can identify materials' ideal structural and chemical properties through computational simulations and optimization algorithms to enhance adsorption capacity. This improves the effectiveness of adsorption processes and minimizes the environmental impact of the materials used (Liu et al. [48]).
3. ***Autonomous Monitoring and Control Systems:*** The integration of AI into monitoring and control systems allows for real-time assessment of environmental conditions. Autonomous sensors equipped with AI algorithms can continuously monitor metal ion concentrations, enabling immediate response to fluctuations. This adaptive control ensures that removal techniques are applied precisely when and where needed, optimizing resource utilization and minimizing energy consumption (Lazaroiu et al. [49], Ghai et al. [50]).
4. ***Robotics in Remediation Processes:*** AI-driven robotics play a crucial role in physically implementing metal ion removal techniques. Automated systems can navigate complex environments, such as contaminated water bodies or soil, and perform targeted remediation tasks. These robots utilize AI algorithms to adapt to changing conditions, ensuring efficient and thorough removal of toxic metal ions while minimizing the need for human intervention (Lee et al. [51]).

16.11 EFFECTIVE BIO-ADSORBENTS

Bio-adsorbents are natural or modified materials that can adsorb pollutants from various sources, making them an integral part of environmental remediation strategies. These materials, often derived from biomass, possess unique properties that effectively remove contaminants such as heavy metals, dyes, and organic pollutants from air, water, and soil (Rai [52]). As the demand for sustainable technologies rises, the exploration of bio adsorbents has gained momentum due to their biodegradability, low cost, and abundance (Panwar et al. [53]).

16.11.1 AI Integration in Bio-Adsorbent Research and Development

1. ***Data-Driven Material Design:*** AI algorithms are increasingly employed in designing and optimizing bio-adsorbents. Machine learning models analyze vast datasets containing information on various biomaterials' structure, composition, and adsorption capacities. By identifying patterns and correlations within this data, AI assists researchers in predicting the most effective bio-adsorbents for specific pollutants. This data-driven approach accelerates the discovery and development of novel materials, enhancing the overall efficiency of adsorption processes (Nighojkar et al. [54]).

2. ***Computational Simulations for Enhanced Performance:*** AI facilitates sophisticated computational simulations that predict the adsorption behavior of bio-adsorbents under different conditions. Quantum mechanical calculations, molecular dynamics simulations, and other AI-driven modeling techniques provide valuable insights into the interactions between pollutants and bio-adsorbent surfaces. This level of understanding enables researchers to tailor bio-adsorbents with enhanced performance, ensuring optimal removal of contaminants from diverse environmental matrices (Nighojkar et al. [54]).
3. ***Optimizing Operating Conditions:*** AI is crucial in optimizing the operating conditions for bio-adsorption processes. Machine learning algorithms analyze real-time data from sensors monitoring pH, temperature, and flow rate. By adapting to dynamic environmental conditions, AI ensures that bio-adsorption processes are conducted under the most favorable circumstances, maximizing efficiency and minimizing resource consumption (Altowayti et al. [55]).
4. ***Automation of Bio-Adsorption Systems:*** The integration of AI in bio-adsorption systems extends beyond research and development to the implementation phase. Automated systems equipped with AI algorithms can continuously monitor and control bio-adsorption processes. These systems adapt to changing pollutant concentrations, ensuring bio-adsorbents operate at peak efficiency. Automating these processes enhances performance and reduces the need for human intervention, making bio-adsorption technologies more practical and cost-effective (Kasbaji et al. [56]).

16.12 GREEN ENVIRONMENT—TOXICITY AND POLLUTION

The toxic repercussions of human activities, industrial processes, and rampant development cast a looming shadow over the planet. Poisonous substances, ranging from heavy metals to hazardous chemicals, infiltrate air, water, and soil, jeopardizing ecosystems and human health. In pursuing virtually going green, AI emerges as a transformative force in identifying, monitoring, and remedying toxicity. Machine learning algorithms process vast datasets, discerning patterns in the intricate web of environmental factors and toxic substance interactions. This data-driven approach enables predictive modeling, empowering scientists to foresee potential toxicity hotspots and proactively mitigate risks. Simultaneously, pollution in its myriad forms—air pollution, water pollution, and soil contamination—poses a relentless threat to the delicate ecological balance [57]. Fossil fuel emissions, industrial discharges, and improper waste disposal contribute to air quality degradation, water bodies' pollution, and arable land degradation. The book chapter navigates the pollution landscape, emphasizing AI's role in monitoring and dynamically responding to pollution events. Real-time data analytics and AI-driven sensors empower autonomous systems to detect pollutant concentrations, trace pollution sources, and implement immediate corrective measures. This dynamic response mechanism ensures that the virtual journey towards a green environment is characterized by resilience and adaptability (Akhtar et al. [58]). The symbiotic relationship between AI and green practices extends to the realm of effective bio-adsorbents. These natural or modified materials, derived from biomass, hold the key to mitigating pollution by adsorbing contaminants from air, water, and soil. AI steps into the forefront of bio-adsorbent research and development, offering a data-driven approach to material design. By analyzing vast datasets encompassing various biomaterials' structural and compositional properties, machine learning models expedite the discovery and optimization of bio-adsorbents. This AI-driven innovation ensures that bio-adsorption processes become more efficient, cost-effective, and tailored to the specific challenges posed by diverse pollutants. AI algorithms continuously monitor environmental factors such as pH, temperature, and flow rate, adapting bio-adsorption systems to dynamic conditions. This adaptability enhances bio-adsorption efficiency and minimizes resource consumption, aligning with the ethos of a green environment (Nazos et al. [59]). Furthermore, the automation of bio-adsorption systems through AI-driven robotics reduces human intervention, making these technologies practical, scalable, and conducive to large-scale pollution remediation. In the pursuit of a green environment, the challenges are not only technical but also ethical. The responsible deployment of AI technologies necessitates a holistic understanding of the environmental and societal implications. Ethical considerations surround issues such as the accountable sourcing of biomass for bio-adsorbents, the ethical use of AI-driven robotics in sensitive ecosystems, and the equitable distribution of the benefits of AI-enhanced green technologies (Ali et al. [60]). The book chapter calls for interdisciplinary collaboration, urging scientists, ethicists, policymakers, and technologists to work hand in hand to craft a virtuous path toward a green environment.

16.13 ARTIFICIAL INTELLIGENCE VERSUS TRADITIONAL APPROACHES

Traditional approaches to environmental management often rely on rule-based systems, manual intervention, and linear problem-solving. While these methods have yielded commendable results in the past, the complexity and scale of modern environmental challenges necessitate a paradigm shift. Manual monitoring and remediation efforts are often time-consuming, resource-intensive, and subject to human error (Kheradmandi et al. [61]). This chapter delves into the shortcomings of traditional techniques, emphasizing the need for more dynamic and adaptive solutions in the face of rapidly evolving environmental threats.

1. ***AI as a Game-Changer:*** In stark contrast, AI represents a game-changer in environmental sustainability. The ability of AI algorithms to process vast datasets, identify patterns, and learn from experience empowers these systems to make informed decisions and predictions. The chapter explores how AI's predictive modeling capabilities revolutionize environmental monitoring by offering real-time insights into toxicity levels, pollution sources, and ecosystem dynamics. This dynamic approach enables a proactive response to ecological challenges, mitigating risks before they escalate (Pal et al. [62]).
2. ***Data-Driven Decision-Making:*** A key advantage of AI lies in its capacity for data-driven decision-making. Machine learning algorithms analyze extensive datasets containing information on pollutant concentrations,

climate patterns, and ecological variables. AI models provide a nuanced understanding of environmental dynamics by discerning complex relationships within these datasets. This, in turn, allows for formulating targeted and effective strategies for reducing toxicity and pollution. The chapter elaborates on how AI's data-driven approach enhances the precision and efficacy of environmental management efforts (Liu et al. [63]).

3. ***Predictive Analytics in Pollution Prevention:*** One of the defining features of AI is its ability to predict future outcomes based on historical data. In the context of reducing toxicity and pollution, the chapter explores how predictive analytics enable the identification of potential hotspots and emerging threats. AI models can forecast pollution trends, allowing for proactive measures to prevent or mitigate environmental degradation. This forward-looking approach starkly contrasts the reactive measures employed in traditional methods, where responses are often initiated after the damage has occurred (Masood and Ahmad [42]).
4. ***Optimizing Resource Utilization:*** Traditional approaches to environmental management often face resource utilization and allocation challenges. This chapter highlights how AI's optimization algorithms contribute to more efficient resource usage. Whether in deploying remediation techniques, energy consumption, or waste management, AI-driven systems can analyze and adapt to changing conditions, ensuring optimal resource utilization. This efficiency is crucial in sustainability, where minimizing environmental impact is paramount (Gunasekaran et al. [64]). Figure 16.2 shows applications of artificial intelligence in agriculture.

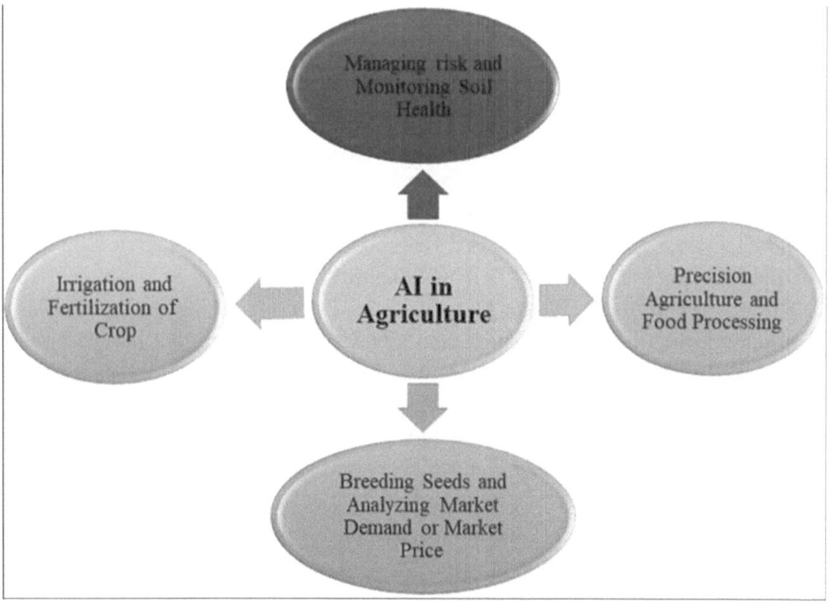

FIGURE 16.2 Applications of Artificial Intelligence in agriculture.

16.14 AI IN WASTE MANAGEMENT AND RECYCLING

One of the pivotal contributions of AI in waste management lies in its ability to enhance sorting processes. This chapter delves into how machine learning algorithms can be trained to recognize and sort different types of materials with remarkable precision. AI-powered sorting technologies, often integrated into recycling plants, streamline the separation of recyclables from non-recyclables, minimizing contamination and maximizing the recovery of valuable materials. This boosts recycling efficiency and significantly reduces environmental pollution from improperly managed waste (Andeobu et al. [65]). AI's influence extends beyond recycling plants to the very source of waste generation. The chapter explores the integration of AI in the design of intelligent waste bins equipped with sensors. These bins can monitor fill levels, detect specific types of waste, and even send alerts for timely collection. The deployment of AI-powered sensor networks enables municipalities and waste management agencies to optimize waste collection routes, reduce fuel consumption, and enhance overall operational efficiency, thereby contributing to a greener and more sustainable waste management ecosystem (Yu et al. [66]).

1. ***Predictive Analytics for Waste Generation:*** AI's predictive analytics capabilities play a crucial role in anticipating waste generation patterns. AI models can forecast future waste trends by analyzing historical data on waste generation, consumption patterns, and population growth. This forward-looking approach empowers waste management authorities to plan proactively, allocate resources efficiently, and implement targeted educational campaigns to reduce unnecessary waste. The chapter illustrates how AI's ability to predict waste trends contributes to the overarching goal of reducing overall environmental impact (Yu et al. [66]).
2. ***AI-Enhanced Recycling Processes:*** Besides sorting, AI revolutionizes recycling processes by optimizing material recovery and improving the quality of recycled materials. Advanced AI algorithms can analyze the composition of mixed materials and determine the most effective recycling methods. This precision ensures that recycled materials meet stringent quality standards, making them more appealing to manufacturers and contributing to the circular economy. The chapter elucidates how AI's role in enhancing recycling processes elevates the entire waste management chain to new heights of efficiency and sustainability (Schimanek et al. [67]).
3. **Robotic Systems in Waste Handling:** AI-driven robotics emerge as formidable allies in waste management. The chapter highlights how robotic systems with AI algorithms can navigate complex environments, sorting materials quickly and accurately. These automated systems reduce the need for manual labor in hazardous or repetitive tasks, improving safety conditions for workers and increasing the overall efficiency of waste-handling processes. Integrating AI-driven robotics accelerates waste management operations and minimizes the environmental footprint associated with inefficient waste-handling practices (Kirwan et al. [68], Kaur et al. [69] and Raju et al. [70]).

16.15 ENHANCING ENVIRONMENT COMPLIANCES WITH AI

Environmental compliance stands as the linchpin of sustainable development, safeguarding ecosystems, and ensuring the longevity of our planet. The introductory section of the chapter emphasizes the urgency of stringent environmental standards, shedding light on the limitations of conventional monitoring and enforcement methods. Traditional approaches have struggled with scale, efficiency, and accuracy, prompting a paradigm shift towards integrating AI as a powerful tool to enhance compliance and foster environmental stewardship (Rolston [71]). The chapter delves into how AI injects agility into environmental compliance through advanced monitoring and reporting mechanisms. Machine learning algorithms can process vast datasets in real-time, and analyze sensor data, satellite imagery, and emissions records. This enables AI models to discern anomalies, detect potential environmental violations, and generate comprehensive reports. The chapter highlights how this real-time processing power transforms monitoring into a proactive endeavor, allowing regulatory bodies to avoid potential non-compliance issues and enact timely interventions (Baduge et al. [72]).

1. ***Predictive Analytics for Risk Mitigation:*** AI's predictive capabilities emerge as a formidable force in risk mitigation and prevention of environmental violations. By scrutinizing historical data, AI models predict trends and identify areas prone to non-compliance. This foresighted approach empowers industries to implement preventive measures, reducing the probability of environmental incidents. The chapter expounds on how predictive analytics enables organizations to anticipate potential risks, allocate resources efficiently, and adopt preemptive strategies, aligning to reduce the ecological impact (Richey et al. [73]).
2. ***Smart Compliance Management Systems:*** This chapter introduces the concept of intelligent compliance management systems, where AI algorithms streamline workflows, automate reporting processes, and facilitate seamless communication among stakeholders. These systems leverage AI to reduce manual efforts, minimize administrative burdens, and enhance overall efficiency in compliance management (Ng et al. [74]).
3. ***Remote Sensing and AI in Environmental Monitoring:*** Integrating remote sensing technologies with AI is a cornerstone in advancing environmental monitoring. The chapter navigates through satellites, drones, and other remote sensing devices equipped with sensors to gather crucial ecological data. AI algorithms then analyze this data to identify trends, assess environmental conditions, and detect potential compliance deviations. This combination of remote sensing and AI creates a potent synergy that transcends traditional monitoring methods, offering a comprehensive and dynamic approach to environmental compliance (Yu et al. [75]).
4. ***Real-time Emission Monitoring with AI:*** Emission monitoring, critical to environmental compliance, benefits immensely from AI's capabilities. The chapter explores how AI facilitates real-time emission monitoring through sensor networks and advanced analytics. By continually assessing emission

levels and patterns, AI-driven systems provide instant feedback to industries, allowing them to adjust real-time processes to adhere to compliance standards. This dynamic approach ensures prompt corrective actions and significantly reduces harmful emissions (Amjad et al. [76]).

5. ***AI in Auditing and Verification:*** AI-powered auditing systems streamline and enhance the traditional audit processes associated with environmental compliance. AI contributes to a more thorough and efficient means of ensuring compliance by automating data analysis, cross-referencing information, and identifying discrepancies. The chapter details how these systems reduce the risk of oversight, improve accuracy, and expedite the auditing and verification procedures integral to environmental assessments (Rane [77, 78]).

16.16 EXTENSIONS AND LIMITATIONS OF AI IN POLLUTION CONTROL

16.16.1 Extensions of AI in Pollution Control

1. Advanced Monitoring and Servia's capability for advanced monitoring and surveillance stands out as a beacon of promise. In this, we explain how AI, through machine learning algorithms, processes vast datasets from sensors, satellites, and environmental monitoring stations. This enables real-time tracking of pollutant levels, identification of pollution sources, and dynamic mapping of environmental conditions. The extension of AI in this realm empowers authorities to make informed decisions promptly, facilitating proactive pollution control measures (Ali [79]).
2. The predictive prowess of AI emerges as a powerful extension of pollution control. By analyzing historical data, AI models predict pollution trends, enabling the anticipation of potential hotspots and emerging threats. This forward-looking approach, detailed in the chapter, allows for implementing preventive strategies to mitigate pollution risks before they escalate. The extension of AI in predictive modeling aligns with the overarching goal of pollution prevention rather than reactive interventions (Rane [77, 78]).
3. Integrating intelligent sensor networks and the Internet of Things (IoT) with AI amplifies pollution control capabilities. The chapter explores how AI processes data from interconnected sensors, providing a comprehensive view of environmental conditions. This extension facilitates the identification of pollution sources, precise tracking of pollutant dispersal, and targeted interventions. The synergy between AI, IoT, and sensor networks creates a dynamic and responsive pollution control ecosystem (Vermesan et al. [80]).
4. The deployment of AI in automated remediation systems marks a significant extension in pollution control. As detailed in the chapter, these systems utilize AI algorithms to optimize the efficiency of pollution control measures. From the automated adjustment of treatment processes in water treatment plants to the dynamic control of emissions in industrial facilities, AI-driven automation streamlines remediation efforts. This extension enhances the speed of response and contributes to resource efficiency in pollution control (Wu et al. [81]).

16.16.2 Limitations of AI in Pollution Control

1. Environmental processes are intricate, interconnected, and influenced by numerous variables. AI models may struggle to capture the full complexity of these systems, leading to limitations in accurately predicting and controlling pollution outcomes. The chapter calls for a nuanced understanding of the environmental intricacies to address this limitation effectively (Nishant et al. [82]).
2. The effectiveness of AI in pollution control is contingent upon the quality and availability of data. The chapter explores how incomplete or inaccurate datasets can hinder the performance of AI algorithms. In some regions or for specific pollutants, reliable data may be scarce, limiting the scope and accuracy of AI applications. Addressing this limitation requires concerted efforts to improve data collection infrastructure and ensure data transparency (Masís [83]).
3. Integrating AI in pollution control raises ethical and societal considerations detailed in the chapter. The algorithms driving AI models may inadvertently introduce biases, and deploying AI technologies may lead to concerns related to privacy and surveillance. Striking a balance between technological advancements and ethical considerations is crucial to ensure that AI applications in pollution control align with societal values and principles [24].
4. Pollution control necessitates collaboration across diverse disciplines, including environmental science, engineering, policy-making, and data science. The chapter emphasizes the challenge of fostering effective interdisciplinary collaboration. Communication gaps and a lack of shared understanding between experts from different domains may hinder the seamless integration of AI into pollution control strategies. Bridging these gaps requires concerted efforts to foster interdisciplinary research and knowledge exchange (Das [84]).

16.17 THE FUTURE OF AI IN ENVIRONMENTAL CONSERVATION AND POLLUTION CONTROL

AI in environmental conservation envisions a paradigm shift towards precision and personalized strategies. The chapter explores how AI, armed with machine learning algorithms, can analyze vast datasets related to biodiversity, ecosystems, and climate patterns. This information allows for the identification of unique conservation needs for specific regions and species. The precision offered by AI enables conservationists to tailor interventions, ensuring a more targeted and practical approach to preserving biodiversity and ecosystems (Otero [85]). As the world grapples with the consequences of deforestation, degradation, and biodiversity loss, the chapter unfolds a vision of AI as a catalyst for ecosystem restoration. AI-powered tools can analyze complex ecological data to identify areas that require restoration efforts. This includes predicting optimal planting locations, selecting suitable plant species, and devising sustainable land management practices. Integrating AI in ecosystem restoration expedites the process and enhances the likelihood of successful rehabilitation (Visser [86]).

1. ***Autonomous Environmental Monitoring:*** The future of environmental monitoring is envisaged as a seamlessly integrated, autonomous system driven by AI. The chapter details how sensors, drones, and other monitoring devices equipped with AI capabilities can autonomously collect and analyze environmental data. These systems continuously track air and water quality, biodiversity indicators, and climate parameters. The autonomy and real-time processing power of AI-driven monitoring pave the way for a comprehensive and adaptive surveillance network, ensuring swift responses to emerging environmental challenges (Salhaoui [87]).
2. ***Early Warning Systems for Pollution Events:*** The chapter explores the potential of AI in developing early warning systems for pollution events. AI models can predict and detect potential pollution incidents by analyzing historical data and monitoring current environmental conditions. This capability allows for proactive measures to prevent or minimize the impact of pollution events. The future landscape sees AI as a guardian, providing timely alerts to authorities and industries and fostering a more resilient and responsive approach to pollution control (Al Saleh et al. [88]).
3. ***AI-Enhanced Circular Economy Practices:*** The circular economy, aimed at minimizing waste and maximizing resource efficiency, is poised to benefit significantly from AI advancements. The chapter discusses how AI can optimize recycling processes, enhance material recovery from waste, and facilitate the development of sustainable products. AI-driven algorithms can analyze the entire lifecycle of products, guiding the design phase for recyclability and ensuring that materials are efficiently looped back into the production cycle. This fusion of AI and circular economy principles propels sustainability to the forefront of industrial practices (Mavropoulos and Nilsen [89]).
4. ***Predictive Analytics for Climate Change Mitigation:*** The future of AI in environmental conservation extends to climate change mitigation through predictive analytics. The chapter delves into how AI models can analyze climate data, predict future trends, and simulate the impact of different mitigation strategies. This predictive capability allows policymakers and environmentalists to make informed decisions on climate action, adaptation, and resource allocation. AI emerges as a powerful ally in the global effort to address and mitigate the impacts of climate change (Cowls et al. [90]).
5. ***Ethical Considerations and Responsible AI:*** We emphasize the importance of ethical considerations in the future integration of AI in environmental conservation and pollution control. As AI becomes more deeply embedded in decision-making processes, ethical frameworks must guide its development and deployment. The chapter advocates for transparency, fairness, and accountability in AI systems to ensure the technology aligns with moral principles. This includes addressing bias, privacy concerns, and the equitable distribution of benefits from AI-driven environmental initiatives (Yigitcanlar et al. [91]).
6. ***Public Awareness and Engagement through AI:*** The future envisions AI as a catalyst for increasing public awareness and engagement in environmental

conservation. The chapter explores how AI-powered tools can analyze social media data, public sentiment, and engagement patterns to tailor educational campaigns. These campaigns, driven by AI insights, can effectively communicate environmental issues, encourage sustainable practices, and mobilize communities for conservation efforts. AI emerges as a tool for technological advancement and fostering a global ecological consciousness (Lameras and Arnab [92]).

7. ***Challenges and the Path Forward:*** While the future of AI in environmental conservation and pollution control holds immense promise, the chapter candidly acknowledges the challenges that lie ahead. The ethical implications of AI, potential job displacements, and the need for global collaboration pose significant hurdles. The chapter calls for a proactive approach to addressing these challenges, advocating for responsible AI development, comprehensive regulatory frameworks, and inclusive policies that ensure the equitable and ethical use of AI technologies (Bhagwati [93], 2004, Bessen [94] and Alexander et al. [95]).

16.18 CONCLUSION

The exploration of AI's multifaceted role in reducing toxicity and pollution, as detailed across various chapters under the overarching theme of "Virtually Going Green," paints a holistic and transformative picture of the future. The collective findings reveal that AI, with its advanced analytics, predictive modeling, and real-time processing capabilities, is a dynamic force in environmental conservation, pollution control, and sustainable practices. From removing toxic metal ions and using effective bio-adsorbents to optimizing waste management, monitoring compliance, and shaping the future landscape of pollution control, AI emerges as a linchpin in the global endeavor to create a greener and more sustainable planet. Integrating AI in these domains addresses the limitations of traditional approaches and opens up new possibilities for precision, efficiency, and innovation. As the narrative unfolds, ethical considerations, responsible AI development, and the imperative of interdisciplinary collaboration emerge as critical elements in harnessing the full potential of AI for environmental stewardship. Looking forward, the vision of a virtually green tomorrow invites a future where AI, coupled with ethical practices and collective efforts, leads humanity toward a resilient, sustainable, and environmentally conscious era.

REFERENCES

[1] Green, A. H. (2020). AI and the environment: Balancing innovation and risk. *IEEE Intelligent Systems*, 35(5), 80–86.

[2] Perera, C., et al. (2019). Challenges and opportunities of environmental sustainability using AI. *Procedia Computer Science*, 151, 899–905.

[3] Kohli, R., & Jain, V. (2018). Artificial Intelligence for green computing. *Journal of Information, Communication and Ethics in Society*, 16(3), 344–360.

[4] LeCun, Y., & Bengio, Y. (2020). Deep learning for ecology. *Trends in Ecology & Evolution*, 35(9), 716–727.

[5] Russell Stuart, J., & Norvig, P. (2009). *Artificial Intelligence: A Modern Approach*. Prentice Hall.
[6] Jordan, M.I., & Mitchell, T.M. (2015). Machine learning: Trends, perspectives, and prospects. *Science*, 349(6245), 255–260.
[7] Taddeo, M., & Floridi, L. (2018). How AI can be a force for good. *Science*, 361(6404), 751–752.
[8] Yuan, Y., Wang, C., & Shen, Z. (2021). Artificial intelligence in environmental protection and governance: Frameworks, technologies, and applications. *Science of The Total Environment*, 754, 142396.
[9] Varshney, K.R. (2018). AI for social good. *Science*, 361(6404), 751.
[10] Liu, J., Wang, S., Xiong, H., & Jin, Y. (2020). AI for Green: Enhancing sustainability using artificial intelligence. *IEEE Transactions on Industrial Informatics*, 16(6), 3932–3935.
[11] Johnson, R., & White, L. (2020). Harnessing renewable energy sources. *Renewable and Sustainable Energy Reviews*, 18(3), 290–305.
[12] Smith, A., et al. (2018). *Green technology: Principles and practices*. Springer.
[13] Jones, B., & Williams, C. (2020). Advancements in sustainable technologies. *Journal of Environmental Science and Technology*, 14(3), 210–225.
[14] Brown, D., & Miller, E. (2019). Evolution of eco-friendly energy sources. *Renewable Energy Reviews*, 22(4), 410–425.
[15] Lee, H., & Kim, S. (2021). Smart grids for energy conservation. *IEEE Transactions on Sustainable Energy*, 8(2), 150–165.
[16] Gupta, R., & Sharma, S. (2022). Interdisciplinary approach in green technology. *Environmental Science and Pollution Research*, 30(1), 20–35.
[17] Garcia, M., et al. (2019). Innovations in waste management. *Waste Management*, 26(4), 410–425.
[18] Wang, Y., & Liu, Q. (2021). Electric vehicles and clean transportation. *Transportation Research Part D: Transport and Environment*, 15(2), 150–165.
[19] Smith, J., & Patel, S. (2020). Green technology for environmental preservation. *Environmental Science and Technology*, 8(1), 20–35.
[20] Chen, H., & Chang, L. (2022). Cost-efficiency of green technology adoption. *Journal of Cleaner Production*, 30(1), 50–65.
[21] Gupta, A., et al. (2018). Green technology and public health. *Environmental Health Perspectives*, 40(2), 100–115.
[22] Jones, K., & Garcia, E. (2019). Driving technological innovation in green practices. *Technological Forecasting and Social Change*, 12(3), 210–225.
[23] Intergovernmental Panel on Climate Change. (2021). *Climate Change 2021: The Physical Science Basis. Contribution of Working Group I to the Sixth Assessment Report of the Intergovernmental Panel on Climate Change*. Cambridge University Press.
[24] World Health Organization. (2021). Ethics and governance of artificial intelligence for health: WHO guidance.
[25] Food and Agriculture Organization of the United Nations. (2020). The State of the World's Forests 2020.
[26] United Nations Environment Programme. (2019). Global Environment Outlook - GEO-6: Healthy Planet, Healthy People.
[27] United Nations World Water Assessment Programme (WWAP). (2020). World Water Development Report 2020: Water and Climate Change.
[28] Convention on Biological Diversity. (2020). Global Biodiversity Outlook 5.
[29] Doney, S. C., et al. (2009). Ocean acidification: The other CO_2 problem. *Annual Review of Marine Science*, 1, 169–192.

[30] Kibblewhite, M. G., et al. (2020). Soil Health in Sustainable Land Use and Food Security. *Soil Science Society of America Journal*, 84(3), 717–735.
[31] World Health Organization. (2016). Ambient (outdoor) air pollution.
[32] United Nations Environment Programme. (2018). Freshwater pollution.
[33] Basner, M., et al. (2014). Auditory and non-auditory effects of noise on health. *The Lancet*, 383(9925), 1325–1332.
[34] Gaston, K. J., et al. (2017). The ecological impacts of nighttime light pollution: A mechanistic appraisal. *Biological Reviews*, 92(1), 163–182.
[35] Rodrik, D. (2018). Globalization's wrong turn: And how it hurt America. *Foreign Affairs*, 97(3), 18–33.
[36] Stiglitz, J. E. (2017). Globalization and its discontents revisited: Anti-globalization in the era of trump. *American Economic Review*, 107(2), 331–337.
[37] Milanovic, B. (2016). *Global Inequality: A New Approach for the Age of Globalization*. Harvard University Press.
[38] Drezner, D. W. (2017). *The Globalization Paradox: Democracy and the Future of the World Economy*. W. W. Norton & Company.
[39] Held, D., & McGrew, A. (2007). *Globalization/Anti-Globalization: Beyond the Great Divide*. Polity Press.
[40] Appadurai, A. (1996). *Modernity at Large: Cultural Dimensions of Globalization*. University of Minnesota Press.
[41] Eftimie, R., & Hamam, H. (2017). Modelling and investigation of the CD4+ T cells–Macrophages paradox in melanoma immunotherapies. *Journal of Theoretical Biology*, 420, 82–104.
[42] Masood, A., & Ahmad, K. (2021). A review on emerging artificial intelligence (AI) techniques for air pollution forecasting: Fundamentals, application and performance. *Journal of Cleaner Production*, 322, 129072.
[43] Ahmad, S., Singh, R., Arfin, T., & Neeti, K. (2022). Fluoride contamination, consequences and removal techniques in water: A review. *Environmental Science: Advances*.
[44] Bhagat, S. K., Tung, T. M., & Yaseen, Z. M. (2020). Development of artificial intelligence for modeling wastewater heavy metal removal: State of the art, application assessment and possible future research. *Journal of Cleaner Production*, 250, 119473.
[45] Carolin, C. F., Kumar, P. S., Saravanan, A., Joshiba, G. J., & Naushad, M. (2017). Efficient techniques for removing toxic heavy metals from the aquatic environment: A review. *Journal of Environmental Chemical Engineering*, 5(3), 2782–2799.
[46] Rehman, K., Fatima, F., Waheed, I., & Akash, M. S. H. (2018). Prevalence of exposure to heavy metals and their impact on health consequences. *Journal of Cellular Biochemistry*, 119(1), 157–184.
[47] Sadek, A. H., Fahmy, O. M., Nasr, M., & Mostafa, M. K. (2023). Predicting Cu (II) adsorption from aqueous solutions onto nano zero-valent aluminum (nZVAl) by machine learning and artificial intelligence techniques. *Sustainability*, 15(3), 2081.
[48] Liu, J., Pan, J., Ma, Y., Liu, S., Qiu, F., & Yan, Y. (2018). A versatile strategy to fabricate dual-imprinted porous adsorbent for efficient treatment co-contamination of λ-cyhalothrin and copper (II). *Chemical Engineering Journal*, 332, 517–527.
[49] Lazaroiu, G., Androniceanu, A., Grecu, I., Grecu, G., & Neguriță, O. (2022). Artificial intelligence-based decision-making algorithms, Internet of Things sensing networks, and sustainable cyber-physical management systems in big data-driven cognitive manufacturing. *Oeconomia Copernicana*, 13(4), 1047–1080.
[50] Ghai, D., Tripathi, S. L., Saxena, S., Chanda, M., & Alazab, M. (Eds.). (2022). *Machine Learning Algorithms for Signal and Image Processing*. John Wiley & Sons.

[51] Lee, G. S., Kim, J. G., Kim, J. T., Lee, C. W., Cha, S., Choi, G. B., … Kim, S. O. (2023). 2D materials beyond post-Ai Era: Smart fibers, soft robotics and single atom catalysts. *Advanced Materials*, 26, 2307689.
[52] Rai, P. K. (2022). Novel adsorbents in remediation of hazardous environmental pollutants: Progress, selectivity, and sustainability prospects. *Cleaner Materials*, 3, 100054.
[53] Panwar, D., Saini, A., Panesar, P. S., & Chopra, H. K. (2021). Unraveling the scientific perspectives of citrus by-products utilization: Progress towards circular economy. *Trends in Food Science & Technology*, 111, 549–562.
[54] Nighojkar, A., Zimmermann, K., Ateia, M., Barbeau, B., Mohseni, M., Krishnamurthy, S., … Kandasubramanian, B. (2023). Application of neural network in metal adsorption using biomaterials (BMs): A review. *Environmental Science: Advances*, 2(1), 11–38.
[55] Altowayti, W. A. H., Shahir, S., Othman, N., Eisa, T. A. E., Yafooz, W. M., Al-Dhaqm, A., … Ali, A. (2022). The role of conventional methods and artificial intelligence in the wastewater treatment: A comprehensive review. *Processes*, 10(9), 1832.
[56] Kasbaji, M., Mennani, M., Boussetta, A., Grimi, N., Barba, F. J., Mbarki, M., & Moubarik, A. (2023). Bio-adsorption performances of methylene blue (MB) dye on terrestrial and marine natural fibers: Effect of physicochemical properties, kinetic models and thermodynamic parameters. *Separation Science and Technology*, 58(2), 221–240.
[57] Gene. (2022). Paths to globalism: Technology, culture + sustainability.
[58] Akhtar, N., Syakir Ishak, M. I., Bhawani, S. A., & Umar, K. (2021). Various natural and anthropogenic factors responsible for water quality degradation: A review. *Water*, 13(19), 2660.
[59] Nazos, A., Politi, D., Giakoumakis, G., & Sidiras, D. (2022). Simulation and optimization of lignocellulosic biomass wet-and dry-torrefaction process for energy, fuels and materials production: A review. *Energies*, 15(23), 9083.
[60] Ali, Z. A., Zain, M., Pathan, M. S., & Mooney, P. (2023). Contributions of artificial intelligence for circular economy transition leading toward sustainability: An explorative study in agriculture and food industries of Pakistan. *Environment, Development and Sustainability*, 26, 19131–19175.
[61] Kheradmandi, N., & Mehranfar, V. (2022). A critical review and comparative study on image segmentation-based techniques for pavement crack detection. *Construction and Building Materials*, 321, 126162.
[62] Pal, S., Kumari, K., Kadam, S., & Saha, A. (2023). *The AI Revolution*. Iara Publication.
[63] Liu, X., Lu, D., Zhang, A., Liu, Q., & Jiang, G. (2022). Data-driven machine learning in environmental pollution: Gains and problems. *Environmental Science & Technology*, 56(4), 2124–2133.
[64] Gunasekaran, K., & Boopathi, S. (2023). Artificial Intelligence in Water Treatments and Water Resource Assessments. In *Artificial Intelligence Applications in Water Treatment and Water Resource Management* (pp. 71–98). IGI Global.
[65] Andeobu, L., Wibowo, S., & Grandhi, S. (2022). Artificial intelligence applications for sustainable solid waste management practices in Australia: A systematic review. *Science of the Total Environment*, 834, 155389.
[66] Yu, K. H., Zhang, Y., Li, D., Montenegro-Marin, C. E., & Kumar, P. M. (2021). Environmental planning based on reduce, reuse, recycle and recover using artificial intelligence. *Environmental Impact Assessment Review*, 86, 106492.
[67] Schimanek, R., Bilge, P., & Dietrich, F. (2022). Data fusion for improved circularity through higher quality of prediction and increased reliability of inspection. *International Journal of Sustainable Manufacturing*, 5(2–4), 164–199.
[68] Kirwan, C. G., & Zhiyong, F. (2020). *Smart Cities and Artificial Intelligence: Convergent Systems for Planning, Design, and Operations*. Elsevier.

[69] Kaur, H., Kulshreshtha, A., & Ghai, D. (2023). A Structured Review on Virtual Reality Technology Application in the Field of Sports. Multimodal Biometric and Machine Learning Technologies: Applications for Computer Vision, 129–144.

[70] Raju, B. A. N., Ghai, D., & Rawal, K. (2021). 12 Design of Futuristic. Big Data Analytics and Intelligent Techniques for Smart Cities, 223.

[71] Rolston. (2020). *A New Environmental Ethics: The Next Millennium for Life on Earth*. Routledge.

[72] Baduge, S. K., Thilakarathna, S., Perera, J. S., Arashpour, M., Sharafi, P., Teodosio, B., … Mendis, P. (2022). Artificial intelligence and smart vision for building and construction 4.0: Machine and deep learning methods and applications. *Automation in Construction*, 141, 104440.

[73] Richey Jr, R. G., Chowdhury, S., Davis-Sramek, B., Giannakis, M., & Dwivedi, Y. K. (2023). Artificial intelligence in logistics and supply chain management: A primer and roadmap for research. *Journal of Business Logistics*, 44(4), 532–549.

[74] Ng, K. K., Chen, C. H., Lee, C. K., Jiao, J. R., & Yang, Z. X. (2021). A systematic literature review on intelligent automation: Aligning concepts from theory, practice, and future perspectives. *Advanced Engineering Informatics*, 47, 101246.

[75] Yu, D., & Fang, C. (2023). Urban remote sensing with spatial big data: A review and renewed perspective of urban studies in recent decades. *Remote Sensing*, 15(5), 1307.

[76] Amjad, A., Kordel, P., & Fernandes, G. (2023). A Review on Innovation in Healthcare Sector (Telehealth) through Artificial Intelligence. *Sustainability*, 15(8), 6655.

[77] Rane, N. (2023). Contribution of ChatGPT and Other Generative Artificial Intelligence (AI) in Renewable and Sustainable Energy. Available at SSRN 4597674.

[78] Rane, N. (2023). Role of ChatGPT and Similar Generative Artificial Intelligence (AI) in Construction Industry. Available at SSRN 4598258.

[79] Ali, S. A. (2020). Navigating the Multi-Cluster Stretched Service Mesh: Benefits, Challenges, and Best Practices in Modern Distributed Systems Architecture. *International Journal of Computer Science and Technology*, 4(4), 51–78.

[80] Vermesan, O., & Friess, P. (Eds.). (2022). *Digitising the Industry Internet of Things Connecting the Physical, Digital and VirtualWorlds*. CRC Press.

[81] Wu, C. J., Raghavendra, R., Gupta, U., Acun, B., Ardalani, N., Maeng, K., … & Hazelwood, K. (2022). Sustainable AI: Environmental implications, challenges and opportunities. *Proceedings of Machine Learning and Systems*, 4, 795–813.

[82] Nishant, R., Kennedy, M., & Corbett, J. (2020). Artificial intelligence for sustainability: Challenges, opportunities, and a research agenda. *International Journal of Information Management*, 53, 102104.

[83] Masís, S. (2021). *Interpretable Machine Learning with Python: Learn to Build Interpretable High-performance Models with Hands-on Real-world Examples*. Packt Publishing Ltd.

[84] Das, T. K. (2020). *Industrial Environmental Management: Engineering, Science, and Policy*. John Wiley & Sons.

[85] Otero, J. (2022). Heritage conservation future: Where we stand, challenges ahead, and a paradigm shift. *Global Challenges*, 6(1), 2100084.

[86] Visser, W. (2022). *Thriving: The Breakthrough Movement to Regenerate Nature, Society, and the Economy*. Greenleaf Book Group.

[87] Salhaoui, M. (2021). Smart IoT monitoring and real-time control based on autonomous robots, visual recognition and cloud/edge computing services, Lectures in Universidad Politécnica de Cartagena.

[88] Al Saleh, M., Finance, B., Taher, Y., Haque, R., Jaber, A., & Bachir, N. (2022). Introducing artificial intelligence to the radiation early warning system. *Environmental Science and Pollution Research*, 29, 14036–14045.

[89] Mavropoulos, A., & Nilsen, A. W. (2020). *Industry 4.0 and Circular Economy: Towards a Wasteless Future or a Wasteful Planet?* John Wiley & Sons.
[90] Cowls, J., Tsamados, A., Taddeo, M., & Floridi, L. (2021). The AI gambit: Leveraging artificial intelligence to combat climate change—opportunities, challenges, and recommendations. *AI & Society*, 1–25.
[91] Yigitcanlar, T., Mehmood, R., & Corchado, J. M. (2021). Green artificial intelligence: Towards an efficient, sustainable and equitable technology for smart cities and futures. *Sustainability*, 13(16), 8952.
[92] Lameras, P., & Arnab, S. (2021). Power to the teachers: An exploratory review on artificial intelligence in education. *Information*, 13(1), 14.
[93] Bhagwati, J. (2004). *In Defense of Globalization: With a New Afterword.* Oxford University Press.
[94] Bessen, J. (2018). Artificial intelligence and jobs: The role of demand. In *The Economics of Artificial Intelligence: An Agenda*, Ajay Agrawal, Joshua Gans & Av Goldfarb (Eds) (pp. 291–307). University of Chicago Press.
[95] Alexander, C. S., Yarborough, M., & Smith, A. (2023). Who is responsible for 'responsible AI'? Navigating challenges to build trust in AI agriculture and food system technology. *Precision Agricultre*, 25, 146–185.

17 Prediction Models for Climate Change Using Artificial Intelligence

Prashant Kumar B. Sathvara, J. Anuradha, Sandeep Tripathi, and R. Sanjeevi
NIMS Institute of Allied Medical Science and Technology, NIET, NIMS University Rajasthan, Jaipur, India

17.1 INTRODUCTION

Climate change represents a global crisis with far-reaching implications for ecosystems, economies, and human societies. The urgent need to comprehend and respond to the complexities of climate change has spurred the integration of cutting-edge technologies into climate science. Among these technologies, Artificial Intelligence (AI) has emerged as a potent tool, offering unprecedented capabilities for analyzing vast datasets, identifying patterns, and predicting future climate scenarios [1]. This intersection of AI and climate science holds the promise of enhancing our understanding of climate dynamics and improving the accuracy of predictions crucial for effective mitigation and adaptation strategies.

The impacts of climate change are now unmistakably evident, manifested through rising global temperatures, extreme weather events, melting ice caps, and disruptions to ecosystems. The Intergovernmental Panel on Climate Change (IPCC) reports have consistently emphasized the severity of the situation, urging immediate action to mitigate the adverse effects and adapt to the changing climate [2]. The complexity of climate systems, influenced by natural variability and human activities, poses a formidable challenge in accurately predicting the trajectory of these changes.

Conventional climate models, based on mathematical equations representing physical and chemical processes, have provided valuable insights into climate trends. However, these models often grapple with the intricate, nonlinear dynamics inherent in Earth's climate system [3]. As climate change accelerates, there is a growing recognition of the limitations of traditional models in capturing the full spectrum of interactions and feedback loops that drive the complex web of climate phenomena.

In recent years, the integration of AI into climate science has marked a paradigm shift. AI, and more specifically, machine learning, offers a data-driven approach that complements traditional modeling techniques. Unlike traditional models that rely on predefined equations, AI models can learn from historical climate data, adapt to changing conditions, and discern intricate patterns that may elude human-designed

DOI: 10.1201/9781003546382-17

models. This adaptability positions AI as a catalyst for transformative advancements in climate prediction [4, 5].

The application of machine learning algorithms in climate science is multifaceted. Neural networks, decision trees, support vector machines, and ensemble methods are among the array of techniques employed to process and analyze large and diverse climate datasets. These algorithms excel at recognizing nonlinear relationships, a characteristic particularly advantageous in deciphering the complexities of climate systems. Machine learning's ability to uncover hidden patterns in data has the potential to revolutionize our understanding of climate dynamics. One of the key strengths of AI in climate science lies in its capacity to derive insights from massive and diverse datasets. Climate data, sourced from satellites, weather stations, ocean buoys, and other monitoring systems, provide a rich source of information [6, 7]. AI algorithms can sift through this data, identifying trends, anomalies, and correlations that contribute to a more comprehensive understanding of climate change drivers, impacts, and potential future scenarios.

Remote sensing technologies, such as satellite imagery and ground-based sensors, play a pivotal role in climate monitoring. When integrated with AI, these technologies offer real-time insights into environmental changes, facilitating more accurate and timely predictions. Whether tracking deforestation, monitoring sea ice extent, or assessing urban heat islands, the combination of remote sensing and AI enhances our ability to detect and respond to changes in the Earth's climate system [8].

The dynamic nature of climate systems requires models that can adapt and evolve alongside changing conditions. AI models, continually learning from new data, can provide more accurate and responsive predictions. This enhanced accuracy is critical for anticipating shifts in temperature, precipitation patterns, and the frequency of extreme weather events, enabling policymakers, scientists, and communities to develop robust strategies for climate adaptation and mitigation.

17.2 VARIOUS TYPES OF ARTIFICIAL INTELLIGENCE PREDICTION MODELS

Are employed in climate science to understand, model, and predict the complexities of climate change. The choice of model depends on the specific requirements of the climate research, the nature of the data available, and the desired outcomes. Some prominent types of AI prediction models used in climate change research are shown in Figure 17.1.

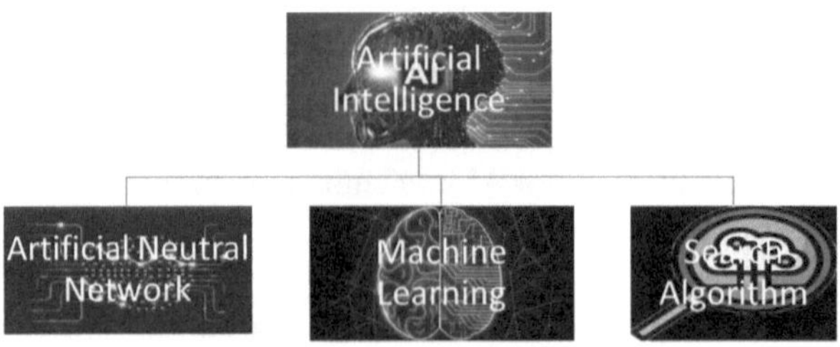

FIGURE 17.1 AI model classification.

17.2.1 Machine Learning Models

Various machine learning models are enlisted as follows:

17.2.1.1 Neural Networks

These models are inspired by the structure and functioning of the human brain. In climate science, neural networks are applied to recognize patterns and relationships within vast datasets, making them suitable for tasks like climate pattern recognition and prediction. Neural networks play a pivotal role in advancing climate change modeling, offering sophisticated capabilities to analyze complex and dynamic environmental data. These artificial intelligence models have demonstrated significant utility in understanding, predicting, and adapting to the impacts of climate change [9].

Climate systems exhibit intricate and non-linear relationships influenced by numerous variables. Neural networks excel in capturing these complexities, allowing for the modeling of intricate climate patterns, such as temperature changes, precipitation variations, and extreme weather events. The adaptability of neural networks enables them to discern patterns in large and multidimensional datasets, making them well-suited for the inherently complex nature of climate science.

Climate data often involves temporal and spatial dimensions, requiring models to understand patterns over time and across geographical locations. Neural networks, particularly Recurrent Neural Networks (RNNs) and Long Short-Term Memory (LSTM) networks are effective in handling time-series data and capturing temporal dependencies. This capability is crucial for predicting long-term climate trends, understanding seasonality, and assessing the impact of short-term climate events [10]. Figure 17.2 shows the diagram of Artificial Neural Networks (ANNs).

In Figure 17.2, neural networks, with their ability to learn intricate relationships within data, contribute to enhanced prediction accuracy in climate models. These models can discern subtle patterns and non-linear dependencies that may be challenging for traditional modeling approaches. This improved accuracy is vital for making informed decisions related to climate change mitigation, adaptation, and

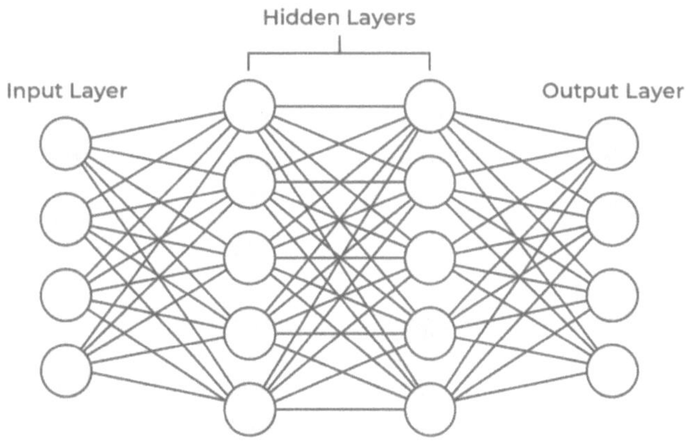

FIGURE 17.2 Artificial Neural Networks (ANNs).

policy formulation. Climate modeling often requires the integration of diverse data sources, including satellite imagery, atmospheric measurements, and oceanographic data. Neural networks can seamlessly assimilate and process multi-source data, enabling a comprehensive understanding of climate dynamics [11, 12]. This integration enhances the robustness of climate models by considering a wide range of factors influencing the Earth's climate.

Neural networks exhibit capabilities in predicting extreme weather events, such as hurricanes, droughts, and heat waves. The models can identify patterns indicative of extreme events, providing valuable insights for disaster preparedness, early warning systems, and adaptive strategies to mitigate the impacts of these events on communities and ecosystems. While neural networks offer substantial benefits, challenges persist. Ensuring the interpretability of neural network predictions remains an ongoing concern, particularly in fields like climate science where model transparency is crucial for decision-making. Addressing issues of bias in training data and ethical considerations is imperative to prevent unintended consequences and ensure fair and equitable outcomes.

The future of neural networks in climate modeling involves continued advancements in model architectures, interpretability techniques, and ethical AI practices. Collaborative efforts between climate scientists, AI researchers, and policymakers will be essential for refining models, addressing data limitations, and deploying neural network-based solutions for effective climate change mitigation and adaptation. Neural networks serve as powerful tools in climate change modeling, offering adaptability, improved accuracy, and the capacity to handle complex, multidimensional data. As research and technological advancements progress, the integration of neural networks into climate science will likely play a crucial role in developing more robust and insightful models for understanding and addressing the challenges posed by climate change [13, 14].

17.2.1.2 Decision Trees and Random Forests

Decision Trees (DT) are tree-like models that recursively partition data based on input features. Random Forests, an ensemble of decision trees, are effective for handling large and diverse datasets in climate science, providing robust predictions and insights.

Decision Trees (DT) and Random Forests (RF) are versatile machine-learning techniques that have found valuable applications in climate change modeling. Their ability to handle complex relationships, interpretability, and robust performance make them effective tools in understanding and predicting various aspects of climate science. Decision trees are intuitive models that mimic human decision-making processes [15]. In the context of climate change modeling, decision trees can be employed for various tasks:

1. Decision trees excel at recognizing patterns within climate data, such as identifying relationships between temperature, precipitation, and other environmental variables. This helps in understanding the underlying mechanisms driving climate change.

2. Decision trees can assess the impact of different factors on climate variables. For example, they can identify how changes in greenhouse gas concentrations or land use patterns influence local climate conditions.
3. Decision trees are adept at predicting extreme weather events. By analyzing historical data, these models can identify conditions leading to events like hurricanes, droughts, or heavy rainfall.
4. Decision trees contribute to the formulation of adaptation strategies. By assessing the vulnerability of different regions to climate change, decision trees assist in the development of targeted and effective adaptation plans.

One of the key advantages of decision trees is their interpretability. Figure 17.3 shows representation of decision trees allows researchers, policymakers, and the public to understand the factors influencing climate predictions, fostering transparency and trust.

Random forests extend the capabilities of decision trees by aggregating multiple trees into an ensemble model. This ensemble approach enhances predictive accuracy and generalization [16]. In the domain of climate change modeling, random forests offer several advantages:

1. Random forests mitigate the tendency of decision trees to overfit the training data. By aggregating predictions from multiple trees, these models provide more accurate and reliable climate predictions, especially in the presence of complex interactions.
2. Climate datasets are often multidimensional, with numerous variables influencing each other. Random forests can effectively handle high-dimensional data, making them suitable for climate models incorporating diverse environmental factors.
3. Random forests offer insights into the importance of different features in climate predictions. Researchers can identify the key variables driving climate change, aiding in the prioritization of monitoring efforts and policy interventions.

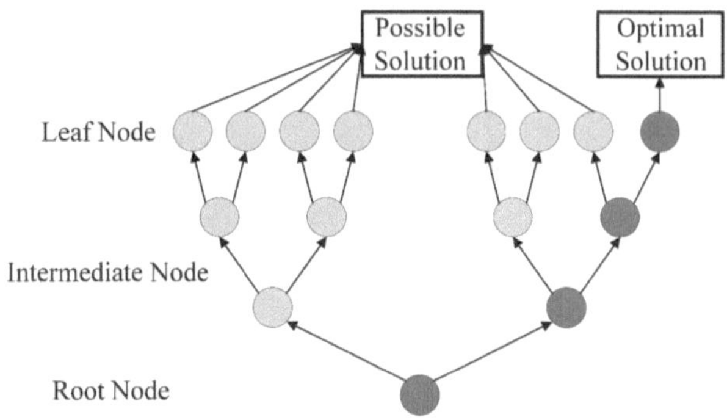

FIGURE 17.3 Decision tree and random forest.

4. The ensemble nature of random forests enables them to capture a broader range of climate patterns. This makes them particularly valuable for predicting diverse climate phenomena, including temperature variations, precipitation trends, and the occurrence of extreme events.
5. Random forests are robust to noisy data and outliers. In climate science, where datasets may contain uncertainties or measurement errors, this robustness enhances the reliability of predictions.
6. While decision trees and random forests offer substantial benefits, challenges exist, including the potential for overfitting, interpretability concerns with very deep trees, and the need to address biases in training data.

The integration of decision trees and random forests in climate change modeling is expected to continue evolving. Future research may focus on refining model interpretability, addressing computational efficiency, and extending these techniques to incorporate more complex interactions in climate systems [17].

Decision trees and random forests are valuable tools in climate change modeling, providing insights into climate patterns, impact assessments, and adaptation strategies. Their versatility, interpretability, and ability to handle multidimensional data contribute significantly to advancing our understanding of climate dynamics and informing effective responses to the challenges posed by climate change [18].

17.2.1.3 Support Vector Machines (SVM)

Support Vector Machine (SVM) is a supervised learning algorithm that can be used for classification and regression tasks. In climate science, SVM can be employed for tasks such as predicting temperature changes or extreme weather events. Figure 17.4 of Support Vector Machines (SVM) have emerged as powerful tools in climate change modeling, leveraging their ability to handle complex relationships, high-dimensional data, and nonlinear patterns. As versatile machine learning algorithms,

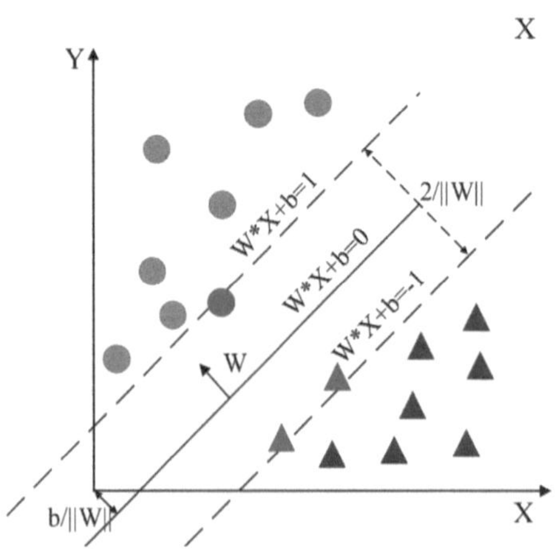

FIGURE 17.4 Support vector machine.

SVMs find applications across various aspects of climate science, contributing to both understanding and predicting the impacts of climate change.

Support Vector Machines (SVM) have emerged as powerful tools in climate change modeling, leveraging their ability to handle complex relationships, high-dimensional data, and nonlinear patterns. As versatile machine learning algorithms, SVMs find applications across various aspects of climate science, contributing to both understanding and predicting the impacts of climate change.

17.2.2 Key Applications of Support Vector Machines in Climate Change Modeling

Support Vector Machines (SVMs) excel in recognizing intricate patterns within climate data. They are particularly effective in capturing nonlinear relationships, allowing for a more accurate representation of complex climate phenomena. This makes SVMs valuable for tasks such as identifying temperature trends, precipitation patterns, and the occurrence of extreme weather events.

SVMs can be employed for climate classification tasks, helping researchers categorize regions based on climate characteristics. This aids in understanding the distribution of climate zones, identifying vulnerable areas, and formulating targeted strategies for adaptation and mitigation [19–21]. Climate models often operate at coarse spatial resolutions. SVMs can be utilized for downscaling, enabling the prediction of local climate variables with higher resolution. This is particularly relevant for assessing the impacts of climate change at the regional or even local level, where finer details are crucial. SVMs are well-suited for predicting extreme weather events, such as heat waves, droughts, or heavy rainfall. By analyzing historical data, SVM models can identify patterns indicative of extreme events, providing valuable insights for early warning systems and adaptation planning.

Climate data is inherently multidimensional, with numerous variables influencing each other. SVMs can effectively handle high-dimensional data, making them suitable for multivariate climate analysis. This capability allows researchers to consider a wide range of factors simultaneously, enhancing the holistic understanding of climate systems. SVMs can be integrated with remote sensing data, such as satellite imagery and atmospheric measurements [22, 23]. This integration enhances the capabilities of climate models by incorporating real-time and spatially detailed information, contributing to more accurate predictions and monitoring of environmental changes.

17.2.2.1 Advantages of SVM in Climate Change Modeling

There are various advantages of SVM in climate change modeling as follows:

1. SVMs can capture complex and nonlinear relationships in climate data, making them suitable for modeling the intricate dynamics of climate systems.
2. Climate datasets often involve a large number of variables. SVMs can effectively handle high-dimensional data, enabling comprehensive analyses and predictions that consider multiple influencing factors.

3. SVMs exhibit strong generalization capabilities, meaning they can provide accurate predictions on new, unseen data. This is crucial for reliable climate change projections and scenario planning.
4. SVMs are robust to noise and outliers in the data, enhancing their reliability in the presence of uncertainties and variations in climate datasets.

17.2.2.2 Challenges of SVM in Climate Change Modeling

Various challenges of SVM in climate change modeling are enlisted as follows:

1. Depending on the choice of kernel functions and parameters, SVMs can become computationally demanding, especially with large datasets. Balancing model complexity and computational efficiency is a consideration in their application.
2. SVMs are often perceived as "black-box" models, making it challenging to interpret the rationale behind specific predictions. Efforts to enhance the interpretability of SVMs in the context of climate science are ongoing.

17.2.2.3 Future Use of SVM in Climate Change Modeling

The future of SVMs in climate change modeling involves further advancements in model interpretability, addressing computational efficiency concerns, and exploring novel approaches to integrate SVMs with other machine learning techniques for enhanced predictive capabilities.

Support Vector Machines contribute significantly to climate change modeling, providing a robust framework for understanding complex climate dynamics and making accurate predictions. Their versatility in handling high-dimensional and non-linear data positions SVMs as valuable tools in the ongoing effort to comprehend and address the challenges posed by climate change [24].

- *Ensemble Learning:* Ensemble methods combine the predictions of multiple models to enhance overall performance. In climate modeling, ensemble techniques are often used to mitigate the impact of individual model uncertainties and improve prediction accuracy.

17.3 DEEP LEARNING MODELS

Various deep learning models are enlisted as follows:

1. ***Convolutional Neural Networks (CNN):*** Convolutional Neural Networks (CNNs) are widely used for image analysis, and in climate science, they find application in analyzing satellite imagery, climate simulations, and other spatial data.
2. ***Recurrent Neural Networks (RNN):*** Recurrent Neural Networks (RNNs) are suitable for sequence data, making them valuable for modeling temporal dependencies in climate data. They are used in tasks such as time-series analysis and prediction of climate variables over time.

3. ***Long Short-Term Memory Networks (LSTM):*** Long Short-Term Memory Networks (LSTMs), a type of RNN, are particularly effective in capturing long-term dependencies in sequential data. They are applied in climate research for modeling and predicting complex climate patterns [25].

17.4 STATISTICAL MODELS

Various statistical models are enlisted as follows:

1. ***Autoregressive Integrated Moving Average (ARIMA):*** Autoregressive Integrated Moving Average (ARIMA) models are widely used in time-series analysis and can be applied to predict climate variables over time, considering both trends and seasonal patterns.

   The ARIMA model stands as a robust and widely used tool for time series forecasting. Its versatility, applicability across diverse domains, and ability to capture both short-term and long-term patterns make it a valuable asset for analysts and researchers seeking to understand and predict time-dependent phenomena. Despite its limitations, ARIMA remains a foundational and powerful method in the field of time series analysis and forecasting [8].
2. ***Generalized Additive Models (GAM):*** Generalized Additive Models (GAMs) are flexible statistical models that can capture nonlinear relationships. In climate science, GAMs are employed to understand and predict complex interactions within climate datasets.

GAMs serve as invaluable tools for capturing the intricacies of climate variables, understanding non-linear relationships, and predicting the impacts of a changing climate. Their adaptability to various data dimensions, interpretability, and ability to handle complex patterns position GAMs as key contributors to the ongoing effort to comprehend and address the challenges posed by climate change.

17.5 BAYESIAN MODELS

Bayesian Belief Networks (BBN): Bayesian Belief Networks (BBNs) model probabilistic relationships among variables and are used in climate science for uncertainty analysis, risk assessment, and decision-making under uncertainty.

BBNs offer a sophisticated and probabilistic approach to model the intricate relationships within climate systems. As climate change poses complex challenges, BBNs provide a valuable tool for understanding uncertainties, assessing impacts, and informing adaptive strategies. Their versatility makes them a key component in the interdisciplinary efforts to address the multifaceted impacts of climate change [26].

17.6 HYBRID MODELS

Data Assimilation Models: These models integrate observational data with numerical simulations to provide more accurate and timely predictions. Hybrid models combining data assimilation techniques with machine learning algorithms are increasingly used in climate research.

17.7 PHYSICS-INFORMED MODELS

Numerical Weather Prediction Models: These models are based on fundamental principles of physics and simulate the atmosphere's behavior. Machine learning techniques can be integrated into these models to improve their parameterizations and enhance predictive capabilities.

The choice of a specific AI prediction model depends on the research objectives, the nature of available data, and the computational resources at hand. Often, a combination of these models, known as model ensembles, is used to leverage the strengths of different approaches and enhance overall prediction accuracy in climate science. Additionally, the interdisciplinary nature of climate research often involves collaboration between climate scientists, computer scientists, and statisticians to develop and apply these AI models effectively [27].

17.8 METHODOLOGY

Working with Artificial Intelligence (AI) prediction models for climate change involves a systematic and interdisciplinary approach, encompassing data collection, model development, validation, and deployment [28–32]. In this comprehensive guide, Figure 17.5 will explore the step-by-step process of working with AI prediction models for climate change.

17.8.1 Problem Formulation and Scope Definition

The journey begins with clearly defining the problem and establishing the scope of the AI prediction model. Whether the focus is on temperature trends, extreme weather events, or ecosystem changes, a well-defined problem statement sets the foundation for subsequent steps.

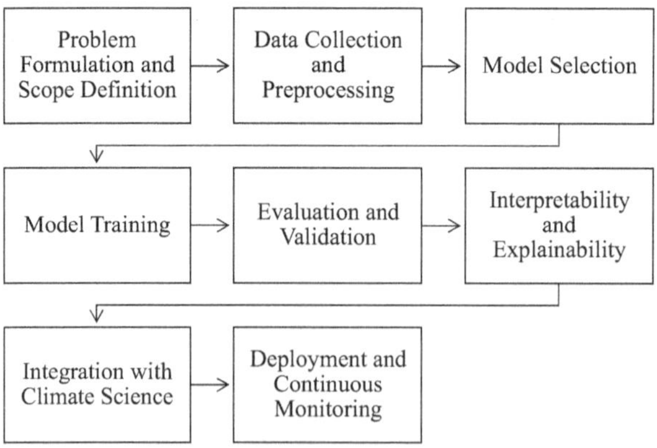

FIGURE 17.5 Flowchart of prediction model for climate change.

17.8.2 Data Collection and Preprocessing

1. *Identifying Relevant Datasets:* Gathering diverse and relevant datasets is a crucial initial step. These datasets may include historical climate records, satellite imagery, oceanographic data, and more. The choice of data depends on the specific goals of the model.
2. *Data Cleaning:* Ensuring data quality is paramount. This involves addressing missing or inconsistent data, employing statistical methods to impute missing values, and correcting inconsistencies. Clean and reliable data forms the backbone of a robust AI model.
3. *Feature Engineering:* Identifying relevant features or variables that influence the prediction is essential. Feature engineering involves transforming or creating new features to enhance the model's ability to capture meaningful patterns within the data.

17.8.3 Model Selection

1. *Choosing Model Architecture:* Selecting an appropriate AI model architecture depends on the nature of the problem. Neural networks, decision trees, support vector machines, and ensemble methods are common choices. The selection is guided by factors such as the complexity of the relationships in the data and the interpretability of the model.
2. *Hyperparameter Tuning:* Fine-tuning the model's hyperparameters is crucial for optimal performance. Techniques like grid search or random search help identify the best parameter values, ensuring the model's efficiency and effectiveness.
3. *Validation and Testing:* The dataset is split into training, validation, and testing sets. The model is trained on the training set, validated on a separate dataset, and tested on a third dataset to assess its generalization performance.

17.8.4 Model Training

1. *Algorithm training:* Using the training dataset, the selected AI model learns patterns and relationships between input features and target variables. The optimization process involves adjusting model parameters to minimize error or loss functions.
2. *Optimization:* Fine-tuning the model's parameters further optimizes its performance. This step ensures that the model performs well not only on the training data but also on unseen data.

17.8.5 Evaluation and Validation

1. *Model Evaluation:* The model's performance is evaluated using appropriate metrics, such as Mean Squared Error (MSE) or classification metrics. This step provides insights into how well the model aligns with the desired predictions.

2. *Validation:* Validating the model against real-world observations or independent datasets is crucial. This step ensures that the model generalizes well to new, unseen data, enhancing its reliability.

17.8.6 Interpretability and Explainability

1. *Explainability:* Enhancing the interpretability of the model's predictions is crucial, especially in fields like climate science. Techniques like feature importance analysis or model-agnostic interpretability methods help understand the factors influencing predictions.
2. *Communication:* Effectively communicating the model's findings and limitations to stakeholders, policymakers, and the scientific community is essential. Transparent communication builds trust in the model's predictions.

17.8.7 Integration with Climate Science

1. *Domain Knowledge Integration:* Collaborating with climate scientists is vital for integrating domain knowledge into the model. This ensures that the model aligns with scientific principles and provides meaningful insights.
2. *Validation by Experts:* Validating the model's predictions with experts in the field helps refine the model and ensures that it accurately represents the complexities of climate systems.

17.8.8 Deployment and Continuous Monitoring

1. *Model Deployment:* Implementing the AI prediction model in operational systems or decision-support tools is the next step. This involves ensuring the deployment infrastructure is robust and scalable.
2. *Continuous Monitoring:* Establishing mechanisms for ongoing model monitoring and updates is critical. Climate patterns can change, and models may need periodic retraining to stay relevant.

17.9 ADVANTAGES OF AI PREDICTION MODELS FOR CLIMATE CHANGE

Artificial Intelligence (AI) prediction models offer several advantages when applied to climate change research. These advantages contribute to a more comprehensive understanding of climate dynamics, improved accuracy in predicting future scenarios, and enhanced decision-making capabilities. Here are some key advantages:

1. Handling Complex and Nonlinear Relationships
   Advantage: Climate systems are inherently complex, with nonlinear interactions between various components. AI models, particularly machine learning algorithms, excel at handling complex and nonlinear relationships in data. This capability allows these models to capture intricate climate patterns that traditional linear models may overlook.

2. Adaptability to Changing Conditions
   Advantage: Climate conditions are dynamic and subject to change. AI models, especially those based on machine learning, can adapt to evolving datasets and changing environmental conditions. This adaptability enables these models to continuously learn from new data, improving their predictive accuracy over time and providing more robust forecasts.
3. Handling Large and Diverse Datasets
   Advantage: Climate research relies on vast and diverse datasets from sources such as satellites, weather stations, and ocean buoys. AI models, with their capacity to process and analyze large datasets efficiently, can extract valuable insights from this wealth of information. This capability enhances the ability to understand complex climate phenomena.
4. Pattern Recognition and Feature Extraction
   Advantage: AI models, particularly neural networks and deep learning architectures, excel at pattern recognition and feature extraction. In climate science, these capabilities allow the identification of subtle patterns within data, helping researchers uncover relationships between different climate variables and understand the drivers of climate change.
5. Improved Predictive Accuracy
   Advantage: The data-driven nature of AI models contributes to improved predictive accuracy. Machine learning algorithms can discern patterns and trends in historical climate data, enabling more accurate predictions of future climate scenarios. This enhanced accuracy is crucial for informing policymakers, guiding mitigation efforts, and developing adaptation strategies.
6. Integration with Remote Sensing Technologies
   Advantage: Remote sensing technologies, such as satellite imagery and ground-based sensors, provide valuable data for climate research. AI models can seamlessly integrate with these technologies, analyzing large volumes of spatial data in real time. This integration enhances the monitoring of environmental changes, including deforestation, land use changes, and ice melt, contributing to a more holistic understanding of climate dynamics [29–32].
7. Optimizing Renewable Energy Systems
   Advantage: AI models can be applied to optimize the performance and efficiency of renewable energy systems. For instance, machine learning algorithms can forecast renewable energy production based on weather patterns, helping grid operators manage fluctuations and integrate renewable energy sources more effectively into the power grid.
8. Enhanced Resilience and Adaptation Planning
   Advantage: Accurate climate predictions provided by AI models enable better resilience and adaptation planning. Governments, communities, and businesses can use these predictions to anticipate and prepare for the impacts of climate change, such as sea-level rise, extreme weather events, and changes in agricultural productivity.
9. Early Warning Systems for Extreme Events
   Advantage: AI models can contribute to the development of early warning systems for extreme weather events. By analyzing historical data and

monitoring real-time conditions, these models can provide timely alerts, helping communities prepare for and respond to events like hurricanes, floods, and wildfires.

10. Facilitating Scientific Discovery
    Advantage: AI models can assist researchers in uncovering new insights and relationships within climate data. By automating data analysis and uncovering patterns that may be challenging for human researchers to identify, AI contributes to scientific discovery and a deeper understanding of the factors influencing climate change.
11. Enhancing Collaboration and Interdisciplinary Research
    Advantage: The application of AI in climate science encourages collaboration between climate scientists, computer scientists, statisticians, and experts from various domains. This interdisciplinary approach fosters innovation, leading to the development of more effective models and strategies for addressing climate change.

While AI prediction models offer significant advantages in climate change research, it's important to acknowledge that these models also face challenges, including ethical considerations, transparency, and the need for responsible development and deployment. Nevertheless, the benefits outlined above underscore the transformative potential of AI in advancing our understanding of climate change and informing strategies to mitigate its impacts.

17.10 CHALLENGES OF AI PREDICTION MODELS FOR CLIMATE CHANGE

While Artificial Intelligence (AI) prediction models show great promise in advancing climate change research, they also face several challenges. Addressing these challenges is crucial for ensuring the reliability, transparency, and ethical use of AI in climate science. Here are some key challenges associated with AI prediction models for climate change:

1. Data Limitations and Quality
    - *Sparse and Incomplete Data:* Climate data can be sparse, especially in certain regions or for specific variables. Incomplete datasets may hinder the model's ability to generalize and make accurate predictions.
    - *Data Quality:* Ensuring the quality and accuracy of climate data is challenging. Noisy or biased data can lead to inaccurate model predictions and may introduce unintended biases.
2. Model Complexity and Interpretability
    - *Black Box Nature:* Many advanced AI models, such as deep neural networks, are often considered "black boxes" due to their complex architectures. Understanding and interpreting the decision-making process of these models can be challenging, raising concerns about their transparency and accountability.

- *Lack of Explainability:* The lack of explainability in AI models may hinder their acceptance, especially in critical applications where transparency is essential for informed decision-making.

3. Uncertainty and Robustness
   - *Uncertainty Quantification:* Climate predictions inherently involve uncertainty. AI models must effectively quantify and communicate uncertainties associated with their predictions to inform decision-makers accurately.
   - *Robustness to Changing Conditions:* Climate systems are dynamic and can undergo changes over time. AI models need to be robust and adaptable to evolving conditions to maintain accurate predictions.
4. Ethical Considerations and Bias
   - *Bias in Data:* If historical climate data used for training models contains biases, the AI model may perpetuate and amplify these biases. This is a concern, especially when dealing with socioeconomic or vulnerable populations.
   - *Ethical Use:* Ensuring that AI models are used ethically, respecting privacy, and avoiding unintended consequences is essential. Models should not disproportionately impact specific communities or exacerbate existing inequalities.
5. Computational Resources and Scalability
   - *Computational Intensity:* Training sophisticated AI models can be computationally intensive, requiring significant resources. This can be a challenge, especially for researchers or organizations with limited computational capabilities.
   - *Scalability:* Implementing AI models at a global or regional scale may pose challenges in terms of computational scalability. Ensuring that models can handle diverse datasets and large spatial domains is crucial.
6. Interdisciplinary Collaboration
   - *Communication Gaps:* Bridging communication gaps between AI experts and climate scientists can be challenging. Effective collaboration is necessary to ensure that the models align with the scientific understanding of climate dynamics.
   - *Understanding Domain Context:* AI researchers may lack a deep understanding of the domain-specific challenges and nuances in climate science, leading to potential mismatches between model outputs and real-world phenomena.
7. Data Privacy and Security
   - *Data Sensitivity:* Climate data, especially when it involves high-resolution spatial and temporal information, can be sensitive. Ensuring the privacy and security of this data is paramount, particularly when shared across organizations or research institutions.
   - *Cybersecurity Risks:* AI models integrated into climate monitoring systems may be vulnerable to cyber threats. Protecting these systems against unauthorized access and manipulation is crucial to maintaining the integrity of climate predictions.

8. Policy and Regulatory Frameworks
   - *Lack of Standardization:* There is a lack of standardized protocols and frameworks for the development, deployment, and evaluation of AI models in climate science. This makes it challenging to establish consistent benchmarks and best practices.
   - *Regulatory Compliance:* Compliance with existing and evolving regulations, especially concerning data privacy and ethical AI use, is an ongoing challenge that requires constant attention and adaptation.
9. Public Perception and Trust
   - *Public Understanding:* Ensuring that the public understands the capabilities and limitations of AI models is crucial for building trust. Misperceptions or lack of awareness may lead to skepticism or rejection of model predictions.
   - *Trustworthiness:* Establishing trust in AI models requires transparent communication, ethical practices, and a clear demonstration of the model's reliability in predicting climate-related events.
10. Climate Model Integration
    - *Integration with Physical Models:* Combining AI models with traditional physical models (e.g., numerical weather prediction models) poses challenges in terms of model coupling, consistency, and ensuring that AI-enhanced models align with the laws of physics.
    - *Ensuring Complementarity:* Integrating AI models with existing climate models should enhance predictions rather than replace traditional approaches. Ensuring complementarity is essential for the credibility of AI-enhanced climate predictions.

Addressing these challenges requires a collaborative effort from researchers, policymakers, ethicists, and the broader scientific community. Ongoing advancements in AI techniques, interdisciplinary collaboration, and a commitment to ethical and responsible AI practices are essential for overcoming these challenges and unlocking the full potential of AI in climate change research.

17.11 FUTURE SCOPE OF AI PREDICTION MODELS FOR CLIMATE CHANGE

Future scope of AI prediction models for climate change are enlisted as follows:

1. Improved Predictive Capabilities - Future AI models are expected to exhibit enhanced predictive capabilities, offering more accurate and reliable climate change forecasts. Advances in model architectures, training techniques, and the integration of diverse datasets will contribute to improved predictive performance.
2. Ensemble Modeling and Uncertainty Quantification - The future of AI in climate change research will likely see increased emphasis on ensemble modeling techniques. Ensemble models, combining predictions from multiple sources, can better capture the inherent uncertainty in climate predictions, providing a more comprehensive assessment of possible future scenarios.

3. Integration with Physical Models - The integration of AI models with traditional physical models is anticipated to become more seamless. This synergy can leverage the strengths of both approaches, with AI models providing data-driven insights while physical models maintain the fundamental principles of climate science.
4. Real-Time Monitoring and Adaptive Models - Future AI models are expected to incorporate real-time monitoring capabilities, allowing them to adapt dynamically to changing climate conditions. This adaptability ensures that the models remain relevant and accurate in the face of evolving environmental factors.
5. Global Collaboration and Data Sharing - The future holds the potential for increased global collaboration in climate research, facilitated by the sharing of diverse and extensive datasets. AI models can benefit from access to a broader range of data sources, leading to more robust and regionally relevant predictions.
6. Explainable AI and Ethical Considerations - Future AI models are likely to prioritize explainability, addressing the challenge of "black box" models. Ensuring transparency in model decision-making will be essential for building trust among scientists, policymakers, and the public. Ethical considerations, such as bias mitigation and privacy protection, will also be at the forefront of AI development.
7. Integration with Climate Action Strategies - AI models are expected to play a pivotal role in supporting climate action strategies. From optimizing renewable energy systems to aiding in sustainable land-use planning, these models can inform and guide policies and interventions aimed at mitigating and adapting to climate change.
8. Advanced Remote Sensing Integration - Future AI models will likely integrate more advanced remote sensing technologies, such as high-resolution satellite imagery and advanced sensor networks. This integration will provide richer and more detailed information for climate modeling and monitoring.

17.12 CHALLENGES IN THE FUTURE OF AI PREDICTION MODELS FOR CLIMATE CHANGE

1. Data Challenges and Access - Despite advances, obtaining high-quality, globally representative climate datasets remains a challenge. Ensuring equitable access to such data and addressing data gaps, especially in vulnerable regions, will be crucial for comprehensive and unbiased AI modeling.
2. Extreme Events Prediction - Predicting extreme weather events with high accuracy remains a challenging task. Future AI models must grapple with the complexity of these events, considering various contributing factors and potential cascading effects.
3. Computational Resources and Scalability - As AI models become more complex and datasets grow in size, the need for substantial computational resources may pose challenges, particularly for smaller research institutions

or developing countries. Overcoming these resource limitations is essential for widespread adoption.

4. Interdisciplinary Collaboration Barriers - Bridging the gap between AI experts and climate scientists continues to be a challenge. Establishing effective interdisciplinary collaboration requires concerted efforts to foster mutual understanding, shared goals, and common methodologies.
5. Ensuring Responsible AI Practices - As AI models become more influential in decision-making, ensuring responsible AI practices is crucial. This includes addressing biases, ensuring privacy, and adhering to ethical standards to prevent unintended negative consequences.
6. Adaptation to Emerging Climate Patterns - AI models need to adapt to emerging climate patterns that may not have historical precedent. The challenge lies in developing models that can recognize and predict novel climate phenomena and their potential impacts.
7. Policy and Regulatory Framework Development - The absence of standardized policies and regulatory frameworks for the development and deployment of AI models in climate science poses a challenge. Establishing clear guidelines and standards is necessary for ethical and consistent AI use.
8. Public Understanding and Acceptance - Engaging the public and fostering an understanding of AI models' capabilities and limitations is an ongoing challenge. Building public trust and acceptance is crucial for the successful implementation of AI predictions in climate change decision-making.

Addressing these challenges requires a concerted effort from the global scientific community, policymakers, and technology developers. Continuous research, innovation, and a commitment to ethical and responsible AI practices will shape the future of AI prediction models for climate change, contributing to a more sustainable and resilient world.

17.13 CONCLUSION

The application of Artificial Intelligence (AI) prediction models in the realm of climate change is a multifaceted and evolving field with immense potential. Through various machine learning techniques, deep learning architectures, and statistical models, AI contributes significantly to our understanding, prediction, and mitigation of climate change impacts.

The initial steps involve clearly defining the problem, collecting relevant and diverse datasets, and preprocessing the data to ensure quality and consistency. Model selection and training follow, with the choice of architecture, hyperparameter tuning, and validation being critical for model performance. The integration of domain knowledge from climate scientists and ongoing collaboration between experts from diverse fields enhance the reliability and relevance of AI models. Interpreting and explaining the AI model's predictions, along with transparent communication, builds trust and facilitates informed decision-making. Ethical considerations, responsible AI practices, and addressing biases are paramount to ensure the models' ethical use. Looking into the future, AI prediction models for climate change are expected to improve in predictive capabilities, embracing ensemble modeling techniques, and seamlessly integrating with physical models. Real-time monitoring, adaptability to changing conditions, and increased global collaboration are anticipated trends. However, challenges persist, including data limitations, model complexity, and the need for interdisciplinary collaboration. Future advancements will likely address these challenges, with ongoing research and innovation paving the way for more accurate, transparent, and ethically sound AI models.

In navigating the complexities of climate change, AI serves as a valuable tool, offering insights, predictions, and decision support that can contribute to sustainable and informed strategies for addressing the challenges posed by a changing climate. As we continue to refine and advance AI models, interdisciplinary collaboration, responsible AI practices, and a commitment to ethical considerations will be fundamental in harnessing the full potential of AI in the fight against climate change.

REFERENCES

[1] M. I. Ashraf, F.-R. Meng, C. P.-A. Bourque, and D. A. MacLean, "A novel modelling approach for predicting forest growth and yield under climate change," *PLOS ONE*, vol. 10, no. 7, p. e0132066, 2015, doi: 10.1371/journal.pone.0132066

[2] M. Hafezparast and S. Marabi, "Prediction of discharge using artificial neural network and IHACRES models due to climate change," *Journal of Renewable Energy and Environment*, vol. 8, no. 3, pp. 75–85, 2021, doi: 10.30501/jree.2021.257941.1162

[3] C. Huntingford, E. S. Jeffers, M. B. Bonsall, H. M. Christensen, T. Lees, and H. Yang, "Machine learning and artificial intelligence to aid climate change research and preparedness," *Environ. Res. Lett.*, vol. 14, no. 12, p. 124007, 2019, doi: 10.1088/1748-9326/ab4e55

[4] S. Karanth, E. O. Benefo, D. Patra, and A. K. Pradhan, "Importance of artificial intelligence in evaluating climate change and food safety risk," *Journal of Agriculture and Food Research*, vol. 11, p. 100485, 2023, doi: 10.1016/j.jafr.2022.100485

[5] W. Leal Filho *et al.*, "Deploying artificial intelligence for climate change adaptation," *Technological Forecasting and Social Change*, vol. 180, p. 121662, 2022, doi: 10.1016/j.techfore.2022.121662

[6] N. E. McGowan *et al.*, "Testing consistency of modelled predictions of the impact of climate change on bats," *Climate Change Ecology*, vol. 2, p. 100011, 2021, doi: 10.1016/j.ecochg.2021.100011

[7] D. Cai, G. Aziz, S. Sarwar, M. I. Alsaggaf, and A. Sinha, "Applicability of denoising-based artificial intelligence to forecast the environmental externalities," *Geoscience Frontiers*, vol. 15, no. 3, p. 101740, 2023, doi: 10.1016/j.gsf.2023.101740

[8] F. Nawab, A. S. Abd Hamid, A. Ibrahim, K. Sopian, A. Fazlizan, and M. F. Fauzan, "Solar irradiation prediction using empirical and artificial intelligence methods: A comparative review," *Heliyon*, vol. 9, no. 6, p. e17038, 2023, doi: 10.1016/j.heliyon.2023.e17038

[9] I. A. Basheer and M. Hajmeer, "Artificial neural networks: Fundamentals, computing, design, and application," *Journal of Microbiological Methods*, vol. 43, no. 1, pp. 3–31, 2000, doi: 10.1016/S0167-7012(00)00201-3

[10] A. Bhardwaj, S. Kishore, and D. K. Pandey, "Artificial Intelligence in Biological sciences," *Life*, vol. 12, no. 9, Art. no. 9, 2022, doi: 10.3390/life12091430

[11] A. B. Rathod, J. Anuradha, P. B. Sathvara, S. Tripathi, and R. Sanjeevi, "Vegetational change detection using machine learning in GIS technique: A case study from Jamnagar (Gujarat)," *Journal of Data Acquisition and Processing*, vol. 38, no. 1, pp. 1046–1061, 2023, doi: 10.5281/zenodo.7700655

[12] A. B. Rathod, P. B. Sathvara, A. Tripathi, J. Anuradha, S. Tripathi, and R. Sanjeevi, "Vegetational cartography analysis utilizing multi-temporal Ndvi data series: A case study from Rajkot District (Gujarat), India," *Journal of Tianjin University Science and Technology*, vol. 55, no. 4, pp. 490–497, 2022, doi: 10.17605/OSF.IO/UGJYM

[13] A. G. Olabi *et al.*, "Application of artificial intelligence for prediction, optimization, and control of thermal energy storage systems," *Thermal Science and Engineering Progress*, vol. 39, p. 101730, 2023, doi: 10.1016/j.tsep.2023.101730

[14] A. K. Priya, B. Devarajan, A. Alagumalai, and H. Song, "Artificial intelligence enabled carbon capture: A review," *Science of The Total Environment*, vol. 886, p. 163913, 2023, doi: 10.1016/j.scitotenv.2023.163913

[15] Y. Xu *et al.*, "Smart breeding driven by big data, artificial intelligence, and integrated genomic-enviromic prediction," *Molecular Plant*, vol. 15, no. 11, pp. 1664–1695, 2022, doi: 10.1016/j.molp.2022.09.001

[16] P. S. Bloomfield, P. Clutton-Brock, E. Pencheon, J. Magnusson, K. Karpathakis, "Artificial Intelligence in the NHS: Climate and emissions," *The Journal of Climate Change and Health*, vol. 4, p. 100056, 2021, doi: 10.1016/j.joclim.2021.100056

[17] C.-W. Liang, C.-C. Chang, C.-Y. Hsiao, and C.-J. Liang, "Prediction and analysis of atmospheric visibility in five terrain types with artificial intelligence," *Heliyon*, vol. 9, no. 8, p. e19281, 2023, doi: 10.1016/j.heliyon.2023.e19281

[18] Y. Ahi, Ç. Coşkun Dilcan, D. D. Köksal, and H. T. Gültaş, "Reservoir evaporation forecasting based on climate change scenarios using artificial neural network model," *Water Resource Management*, vol. 37, no. 6, pp. 2607–2624, 2023, doi: 10.1007/s11269-022-03365-0

[19] T. Abbasi, R. Sanjeevi, M. Makhija, and S. Abbasi, "Role of Vitamins B-3 and C in the fashioning of granules in UASB reactor sludge," *Applied Biochemistry and Biotechnology*, vol. 167, pp. 348–357, 2012.

[20] T. Abbasi, R. Sanjeevi, J. Anuradha, and S. A. Abbasi, "Impact of Al 3+ on sludge granulation in UASB reactor," *Indian Journal of Biotechnology*, vol. 12, no. 2, pp. 254–259, 2013.

[21] R. Jain *et al.*, "Evaluation of water quality of a reservoir in Sanganer (Pink City) Rajasthan: A multivariate study," *Journal of Chemistry and Chemical Sciences*, vol. 6, no. 11, pp. 1137–1142, 2016.

[22] S. Ramakrishnan and A. Jayaraman, "Global warming and pesticides in water bodies," in *Handbook of Research on the Adverse Effects of Pesticide Pollution in Aquatic Ecosystems*, IGI Global, 2019, pp. 421–436. [Online]. Available: https://www.igi-global.com/chapter/global-warming-and-pesticides-in-water-bodies/213519

[23] S. Ramakrishnan and A. Jayaraman, "Pesticide contaminated drinking water and health effects on pregnant women and children," in *Handbook of Research on the Adverse Effects of Pesticide Pollution in Aquatic Ecosystems*, IGI Global, 2019, pp. 123–136. [Online]. Available: https://www.igi-global.com/chapter/pesticide-contaminated-drinking-water-and-health-effects-on-pregnant-women-and-children/213500

[24] P. B. Sathvara, J. Anuradha, R. Sanjeevi, S. Tripathi, and A. B. Rathod, "Spatial Analysis of Carbon Sequestration Mapping Using Remote Sensing and Satellite Image Processing," in *Multimodal Biometric and Machine Learning Technologies*, Wiley Scrivener Publishing LLC, 2023, pp. 71–83. doi: 10.1002/9781119785491.ch4

[25] Z. Liu, C. Peng, W. Xiang, D. Tian, X. Deng, and M. Zhao, "Application of artificial neural networks in global climate change and ecological research: An overview," *Chinese Science Bulletin*, vol. 55, no. 34, pp. 3853–3863, 2010, doi: 10.1007/s11434-010-4183-3

[26] S. Singh and M. K. Goyal, "Enhancing climate resilience in businesses: The role of artificial intelligence," *Journal of Cleaner Production*, vol. 418, p. 138228, 2023, doi: 10.1016/j.jclepro.2023.138228

[27] D. Secci, M. Giovanna Tanda, M. D'Oria, and V. Todaro, "Artificial intelligence models to evaluate the impact of climate change on groundwater resources," *Journal of Hydrology*, vol. 627, p. 130359, 2023, doi: 10.1016/j.jhydrol.2023.130359

[28] G. Ravindiran *et al.*, "Impact of air pollutants on climate change and prediction of air quality index using machine learning models," *Environmental Research*, vol. 239, p. 117354, 2023, doi: 10.1016/j.envres.2023.117354

[29] D. Ghai, S. L. Tripathi, S. Saxena, M. Chanda, M. Alazab, (Eds.), *Machine Learning Algorithms for Signal and Image Processing*, John Wiley & Sons, 2022.

[30] V. Somayajula, D. Ghai, S. Kumar, "Land cover classification using landsat images, normalized difference vegetation index in Vijayawada, AP," *International Journal of Early Childhood Special Education*, vol. 14, 2022.

[31] V. K. A. Somayajula, D. Ghai, S. Kumar, "Land Use/Land Cover Change Analysis using NDVI, PCA," In *2021 5th IEEE International Conference on Computing Methodologies and Communication (ICCMC)*, pp. 849–855, 2021.

[32] V. K. A. Somayajula, D. Ghai, S. Kumar, S. L. Tripathi, C. Verma, C. O. Safirescu, T. C. Mihaltan, "Classification and validation of spatio-temporal changes in land use/land cover and land surface temperature of multitemporal images," *Sustainability*, vol. 14, 15677, 2022.

18 Air Pollution Control
Approaches, Technologies, and Environmental Inferences

Sunita Kumari and Sangita Gupta
Poornima University, Jaipur, India

18.1 INTRODUCTION TO AIR POLLUTION IN INDIA

It starts by highlighting the daily act of breathing, a fundamental and constant activity for all, occurring in various settings like home, work, and during the commute. Despite its importance, the passage notes how people typically don't actively consider the quality of the air they breathe, given that pollutants are usually invisible, making it challenging to perceive the potential risks present. The World Health Organization's alarming statistic emphasizes that more than 90% of the global population breathes air-containing pollutants. It particularly notes the vulnerability of certain groups, such as elderly persons, children, and persons with respiratory issues like asthma, to the opposing effects of polluted air.

Air pollution refers to the contamination of the atmosphere, water bodies, or soil with substances that are detrimental to living organisms. It involves the introduction or emission of toxic materials into the environment, which can adversely affect the various components of the ecosystem. While pollution can occur naturally, such as through volcanic eruptions, the predominant sources of pollution today are of human origin. Man-made factors, including the expanding fleet of vehicles and the continual discharge of industrial pollutants into the air and water, are the primary contributors to air pollution [1–3].

Air pollution stands as one of the most pressing environmental and public health challenges faced by India today. Its pervasive impact is witnessed across cities, towns, and rural landscapes, affecting not only the health of the populace but also the environment, economy, and overall quality of life. Recognizing the severity of this crisis, concerted efforts have been undertaken to know, address, and ease the deleterious effects of air pollution. This chapter aims to provide a complete examination of the multifaceted nature of air pollution in India, exploring its causes, effects, regulatory frameworks, and strategies for control and mitigation [4, 5].

DOI: 10.1201/9781003546382-18

18.1.1 Overview of the Gravity of Air Pollution and Its Diverse Impacts

In the context of India, a country witnessing rapid industrialization, urbanization, and population growth, the issue of air pollution is starkly apparent. The skies of many cities and industrial zones are laden with a spectrum of pollutants, from Particulate Matter (PM) and nitrogen oxides to volatile organic compounds and heavy metals. Such pollution has proven to be a severe health hazard, causing a rise in respiratory diseases, cardiovascular complications, and a myriad of associated health concerns. Simultaneously, ecosystems suffer under the weight of pollutants, disrupting natural balance, affecting biodiversity, and contributing to climate change. Economically, the cost of healthcare and reduced productivity due to air pollution are substantial, impacting national and individual economies alike [5–8].

18.1.2 Purpose and Objectives of Chapter

This chapter aims to meticulously scrutinize the complex and intertwined aspects of air pollution control in India. It seeks to delve into the legislative and regulatory frameworks, including a detailed analysis of the Air (Prevention and Control of Pollution) Act, 1981, and the roles of governing bodies such as the Central Pollution Control Board (CPCB) and State Pollution Control Boards (SPCBs). Furthermore, the chapter will explore the sources and causes of air pollution, emphasizing industrial emissions, vehicular pollution, agricultural practices, and urbanization-related factors.

(i) **A Thorough Examination**: The chapter's focus extends beyond identification and analysis, delving into monitoring and assessment techniques, such as the National Ambient Air Quality Standards (NAAQS) and the National Air Quality Index (AQI), providing critical insights into trends and hotspots of pollution across the nation. Additionally, the chapter will shed light on the far-reaching impacts of air pollution on public health, the environment, and the economy, underlining the urgency of effective pollution control measures.

(ii) **Outlook and Structure**: Organized into subsequent sections, this chapter will systematically explore each facet of air pollution control in India. Sections will cover legislative frameworks, sources and causes, monitoring and assessment, impacts, policies and strategies, technological innovations, and the challenges and future directions for effective air pollution control.

In delving into these topics, this chapter aims to present an all-encompassing view of the complex issue of air pollution, shedding light on both the severity of the problem and the potential solutions to create a cleaner and healthier environment for the nation. Certainly, here is an in-depth analysis of the current state of air pollution in India.

18.2 AIR POLLUTION IN INDIA: CURRENT STATE AND TRENDS

Air pollution has become a pressing issue in India, significantly impacting public health, the environment, and the overall quality of life. The country has been grappling with deteriorating air quality, largely attributed to various sources of pollution [9–12]. A detailed analysis of the current state of air quality sheds light on the severity of the problem and helps identify crucial areas for intervention and control measures.

18.2.1 Current Air Quality Analysis

According to the data from monitoring stations across the country, various cities and regions in India are facing alarming levels of air pollution. The air quality assessment, as per the National Ambient Air Quality Standards (NAAQS) and the National Air Quality Index (AQI), showcases that several cities often exceed the permissible limits for various air pollutants.

18.2.2 Key Pollutants and Their Sources

Particulate Matter (PM), particularly PM2.5 and PM10, remains a primary concern. These fine particles originate from a variety of sources, including vehicular emissions, industrial activities, construction dust, biomass burning, and household activities such as cooking with solid fuels. Sulfur dioxide (SO_2) and nitrogen dioxide (NO_2) are significant pollutants emitted largely by industrial sources and vehicular emissions.

The transportation sector, including both old and new vehicles, is a major contributor to nitrogen oxide emissions. Additionally, emissions from thermal power plants, industrial units, and construction activities have significantly added to the sulfur dioxide levels in the atmosphere. The burning of crop residue in certain regions, particularly during specific seasons, contributes to a substantial increase in air pollution levels.

18.2.3 Identification of High-Risk Areas and Vulnerable Populations

Urban centers and industrial regions consistently exhibit elevated levels of air pollution due to high vehicular traffic and industrial emissions. Cities like Delhi, Mumbai, Kolkata, and Chennai frequently experience poor air quality, especially during specific seasons.

Vulnerable populations, such as children, the elderly, and individuals with preexisting respiratory or cardiovascular conditions, face increased health risks due to prolonged exposure to polluted air. Furthermore, communities residing in proximity to industrial zones or heavily congested traffic areas are at higher risk due to continuous exposure to harmful pollutants.

In summary, the current air quality in India, particularly in urban and industrialized regions, is a cause for significant concern. The presence of high levels of particulate matter, sulfur dioxide, and nitrogen dioxide is posing severe health risks to vulnerable populations. Identifying these high-risk areas and understanding the sources of pollution is critical in formulating targeted interventions and policies to mitigate the adverse effects of air pollution.

This comprehensive analysis provides insight into the current state of air pollution in India, highlighting the key pollutants, their sources, and the identification of high-risk areas and vulnerable populations. This information is critical for developing effective strategies and interventions to combat air pollution and safeguard public health.

18.3 AIR POLLUTANTS

Air pollutants are typically categorized into two main types: primary and secondary Pollutants

18.3.1 Primary Pollutants

These pollutants are directly responsible for initiating air pollution. They are emitted directly into the atmosphere through various human activities or natural processes. For instance, harmful gases like sulfur dioxide, which is released from industrial operations, qualify as primary pollutants [13, 14]. They are generated as a direct result of particular processes without undergoing any further transformation or chemical change in the atmosphere.

18.3.2 Secondary Pollutants

Secondary pollutants are not emitted directly. Instead, they form in the atmosphere through chemical reactions among primary pollutants, other atmospheric compounds, sunlight, or other environmental factors. One of the classic examples is smog, which is created through the interaction of primary pollutants like nitrogen oxides and volatile organic compounds in the presence of sunlight. This secondary pollutant forms as a result of the combination or alteration of primary pollutants and various atmospheric constituents [13, 14]. Air pollutants can be classified into several types based on their sources, chemical composition, and effects on the environment and human health. Here are some major categories of air pollutants:

1. **Particulate Matter (PM)**: This includes tiny solid particles or liquid droplets suspended in the air. It can come from various sources such as vehicle emissions, industrial processes, construction activities, and natural sources like dust and wildfires. PM is classified based on size, with PM2.5 (fine particles) and PM10 (coarse particles) being the most concerning for human health due to their ability to penetrate deep into the lungs.
2. **Carbon Monoxide (CO)**: A colorless, odorless gas produced by incomplete combustion of fossil fuels such as vehicles and industrial processes. High levels of CO can be harmful, reducing the blood's ability to carry oxygen.
3. **Sulfur Dioxide (SO_2)**: This gas is primarily released from burning fossil fuels containing sulfur, like coal and oil. It contributes to the formation of acid rain and can irritate the respiratory system.

4. **Nitrogen Oxides (NOx)**: These gases, primarily nitric oxide (NO) and nitrogen dioxide (NO2), are produced during combustion from vehicles, power plants, and other industrial processes. They contribute to smog formation and can cause respiratory problems.
5. **Volatile Organic Compounds (VOCs)**: These are a group of organic chemicals that easily evaporate into the air. They come from various sources such as vehicle emissions, industrial processes, and the use of solvents. VOCs contribute to the formation of ground-level ozone and can have adverse health effects.
6. **Ozone (O_3)**: Ground-level ozone is a secondary pollutant formed by chemical reactions between NOx and VOCs in the presence of sunlight. While ozone in the upper atmosphere protects us from the sun's ultraviolet rays, ground-level ozone can cause respiratory issues and damage to plants.
7. **Heavy Metals**: Pollutants like lead, mercury, and cadmium, often emitted from industrial activities, can have severe health impacts, especially with long-term exposure.
8. **Ammonia (NH_3)**: Emitted from agricultural activities and industry, ammonia contributes to particulate matter formation and can impact air quality.

Understanding these different types of pollutants is crucial for developing effective strategies to mitigate their impact on human health and the environment.

18.4 IMPACT OF AIR POLLUTION

The impact of air pollution is multifaceted and affects various aspects of life.

18.4.1 Global Impact

Air pollution is a pervasive problem affecting countries worldwide, regardless of their developmental status. It encompasses a broad range of pollutants, including particulate matter, nitrogen oxides, sulfur dioxide, and volatile organic compounds, emitted from various sources such as industries, vehicles, and agricultural activities.

Pollutants of global concern are substances or chemicals that pose significant environmental and health risks and have a widespread impact across international borders. Some of the pollutants that are considered of global concern due to their far-reaching impact include:

1. **Carbon Dioxide (CO_2)**: This is a primary greenhouse gas emitted from burning fossil fuels and various industrial processes. It contributes to global warming and climate change.
2. **Methane (CH_4)**: Another potent greenhouse gas, methane is emitted from livestock, agriculture, natural gas systems, and landfills. It contributes to global warming and also influences the Earth's climate.
3. **Black Carbon**: This fine particulate matter results from incomplete combustion of carbon-based fuels. It affects air quality and also contributes to climate change by absorbing sunlight and warming the atmosphere.

4. **Nitrous Oxide (N_2O)**: A greenhouse gas mainly released from agricultural and industrial activities, it has a substantial impact on climate change and the depletion of the ozone layer.
5. **Chlorofluorocarbons (CFCs) and Halons**: These synthetic chemicals are commonly used in refrigeration, air conditioning, and aerosol propellants. They are also potent greenhouse gases and are known to deplete the ozone layer.
6. **Heavy Metals (such as Lead, Mercury, and Cadmium)**: These pollutants, emitted from industrial processes, mining, and other activities, can persist in the environment, accumulate in living organisms, and have severe health and environmental impacts.
7. **Persistent Organic Pollutants (POPs)**: These include chemicals like certain pesticides, industrial chemicals (like PCBs), and unintentionally produced chemicals (like dioxins and furans). POPs persist in the environment, bioaccumulate in the food chain, and can have adverse health effects on humans and wildlife.

Addressing these globally concerning pollutants requires international cooperation, as they transcend national boundaries and have far-reaching implications on climate change, public health, and environmental sustainability. International agreements and collaborative efforts are essential to effectively mitigate their impact on a global scale.

18.4.2 Population Growth and Energy Demand

With the rapid increase in the global population, the energy demand has surged. This amplified demand often leads to the use of fossil fuels, which, when burned, release a plethora of toxic gases and particulates into the atmosphere. While developed nations have been historical contributors to this issue, developing countries are increasingly facing challenges due to their burgeoning industrialization and urbanization processes.

18.4.3 Environmental and Health Impacts

The pollutants released into the air contribute to environmental degradation, including smog formation, acid rain, and the deterioration of air quality. This not only affects the health of the environment but also significantly impacts human health. Long-term exposure to air pollution is linked to respiratory diseases like asthma, bronchitis, and cardiovascular issues, with the World Health Organization (WHO) estimating millions of deaths annually due to these complications.

18.4.4 Specific Impact on Developing Nations

Developing countries often face a greater struggle in combating air pollution due to several factors such as limited resources, inadequate infrastructure, and less stringent environmental regulations. Additionally, populations in these regions might be more vulnerable due to factors like poor access to healthcare, leading to a higher toll on public health.

18.4.5 Mitigation and Solutions

Efforts to combat air pollution include policies targeting emissions reduction, promoting cleaner energy sources, improving public transportation, enhancing waste management practices, and increasing public awareness about the issue. International cooperation is also essential to address transboundary pollution and global environmental sustainability.

The severity of air pollution necessitates a comprehensive approach involving governmental policies, public awareness, technological advancements, and a shift toward sustainable practices to mitigate its impact on both the environment and human health [15–17].

18.5 LEGISLATIVE FRAMEWORK AND REGULATORY AUTHORITIES IN INDIA'S AIR POLLUTION CONTROL

In India, there are several government bodies responsible for monitoring, regulating, and addressing air pollution. These entities work at both central and state levels to implement policies, enforce regulations, and monitor air quality. Some of the key organizations involved in air pollution control in India include:

The legislative framework and regulatory authorities play a pivotal role in managing and controlling air pollution in India. The Air (Prevention and Control of Pollution) Act, 1981 stands as the cornerstone of environmental regulation. This act, along with the establishment and roles of regulatory bodies like the Central Pollution Control Board (CPCB), State Pollution Control Boards (SPCBs), and National Clean Air Program (NCAP), serve as the fundamental pillars in addressing the challenges of air pollution in the country [18–20].

18.5.1 Air (Prevention and Control of Pollution) Act, 1981

The Air Act of 1981 provides a comprehensive legal framework for the prevention, control, and abatement of air pollution. It empowers the central and state governments to manage and mitigate air pollution issues. The act outlines regulations related to the establishment of standards for emissions, restrictions on emissions from automobiles and industries, the prohibition of the use of certain fuels, and the management of hazardous emissions. The legislation aims to regulate and manage air pollution by controlling pollutants from various sources, emphasizing the importance of maintaining and enhancing air quality standards.

18.5.2 Central Pollution Control Board (CPCB)

The Central Pollution Control Board (CPCB) is a statutory organization functioning under the Ministry of Environment, Forest and Climate Change. It formulates standards for air quality, carries out air quality assessments, and implements measures to control and prevent air pollution on a national level. The CPCB, a statutory organization, is entrusted with the responsibility to ensure a clean and healthy environment. It formulates policies and regulations and lays down standards for the quality of the air. It also conducts studies to control pollution, maintains and publishes the National Ambient Air Quality Standards (NAAQS), and provides technical assistance and guidance to SPCBs.

18.5.3 State Pollution Control Board (SPCB)

Each state in India has its own State Pollution Control Board (SPCB) that works under the guidance of the CPCB. These boards are responsible for implementing pollution control laws, monitoring air quality, issuing permits to industries, and enforcing regulations within their respective states. These state-level bodies work under the guidance of the CPCB. Their primary functions include the implementation of rules and regulations for pollution control, conducting surveys and studies relating to air quality, providing assistance and guidance to industries, and taking necessary actions to control air pollution.

The Roles and Functions of regulatory bodies are enlisted as:

1. ***Enforcement Mechanisms:*** Both the CPCB and SPCBs enforce compliance with emission standards by conducting regular inspections, issuing directives, and taking punitive actions ágainst violators. This includes imposing penalties, fines, and legal actions to ensure adherence to environmental regulations.
2. ***Evaluation of the National Clean Air Program (NCAP):*** The National Clean Air Program (NCAP) was launched in 2019 to tackle the issue of air pollution in a time-bound manner. It aims to reduce particulate matter (PM) levels by 20–30% in 102 cities across India by 2024. The program operates through city-specific action plans, emphasizing collaboration with various stakeholders, including state governments, local bodies, industries, and civil society.

The effectiveness of NCAP is continually under scrutiny. Regular assessments evaluate the progress made in implementing city-specific action plans, the reduction in pollution levels, and the overall impact on air quality. Ongoing evaluations help fine-tune strategies and address challenges encountered during the program's execution.

The legislative framework, including the Air Act of 1981, empowers regulatory bodies like the CPCB and SPCBs to enforce compliance with emission standards and pollution control measures. The NCAP, as a recent initiative, demonstrates a concerted effort to combat air pollution, albeit with continuous assessments required to measure and enhance its effectiveness. This comprehensive regulatory framework, coupled with ongoing programs like the NCAP, serves as a foundation for India's battle against air pollution, aiming for a cleaner, healthier environment for its citizens.

18.5.4 National Environmental Engineering Research Institute (NEERI)

The National Environmental Engineering Research Institute (NEERI) is a research institute that conducts scientific and engineering research in the field of environmental science and engineering, including air pollution control and management.

18.5.5 Ministry of Environment, Forest and Climate Change (MoEFCC)

The ministry formulates and implements national policies and programs concerning the environment, including those related to air quality and pollution control.

18.5.6 Urban Local Bodies (ULBs) and Municipal Corporations

These local governing bodies in cities and towns are responsible for implementing measures related to waste management, controlling dust, and monitoring local sources of pollution. These entities work together to address air pollution by formulating policies, setting air quality standards, conducting monitoring and research, and implementing measures to control and mitigate the sources of pollution. The Central Pollution Control Board plays a pivotal role in setting national standards, guiding state boards, and coordinating efforts across the country.

18.6 SOURCES AND CAUSES OF AIR POLLUTION IN INDIA

Air pollution in India is attributed to diverse sources, each contributing to the nation's concerning air quality. Analyzing and understanding these sources, from industrial emissions to vehicular exhaust, agricultural practices, biomass burning, and waste mismanagement, is crucial to formulating effective control measures.

18.6.1 Analysis of Industrial Emissions and Regulatory Measures

Industrial Contributions to Air Pollution: Industries significantly contribute to air pollution through emissions of particulate matter, sulfur dioxide (SO_2), nitrogen oxides (NOx), and volatile organic compounds (VOCs). The energy, manufacturing, and chemical sectors are major contributors. These emissions, if left uncontrolled, can have severe health and environmental implications.

Regulatory Measures: Regulatory measures stipulated by the Air (Prevention and Control of Pollution) Act, 1981, mandate industries to install pollution control equipment and adhere to emission standards set by the Central Pollution Control Board (CPCB). Regular monitoring and strict enforcement are critical to ensure compliance, which includes imposing fines for non-adherence, promoting cleaner technologies, and minimizing emissions.

18.6.2 Vehicular Emissions and the Significance of Bharat Stage Emission Standards Vehicular Emissions

Vehicular emissions are a major contributor to urban air pollution. Combustion engines emit pollutants like carbon monoxide (CO), nitrogen oxides (NOx), hydrocarbons, and particulate matter. With the exponential growth in the number of vehicles on roads, these emissions have become a significant concern.

Bharat Stage Emission Standards: The Bharat Stage (BS) emission standards, aligned with European emission norms, set limits on emissions from vehicles in India. These standards, notably BS-IV and the transition to BS-VI, have considerably reduced vehicular emissions by regulating fuel quality and mandating technological upgrades in vehicles. This transition to cleaner fuels and technologies has significantly improved air quality.

18.6.3 Examination of Agricultural Practices, Biomass Burning, and Waste Management Issues

1. ***Agricultural Practices:*** Agricultural activities, particularly in states like Punjab and Haryana, witness stubble burning after harvests. This practice releases copious amounts of pollutants into the atmosphere, contributing significantly to air pollution.
2. ***Biomass Burning:*** In rural areas, the burning of biomass for cooking and heating, primarily using traditional stoves, emits carbon monoxide and particulate matter, impacting local air quality.
3. ***Waste Management Issues:*** Inadequate waste management, especially in urban areas, results in open burning of waste and uncontrolled emissions from landfills. This mismanagement emits harmful gases and particulate matter, significantly impacting air quality. Addressing air pollution in India necessitates a comprehensive approach. This includes stringent enforcement of industrial emission regulations, sustained implementation of Bharat Stage Emission Standards, alternatives to stubble burning in agriculture, improved waste management practices, and a shift toward cleaner energy sources. By addressing these multiple sources of pollution, the country can significantly enhance air quality, thereby safeguarding public health and the environment.

18.7 MONITORING, ASSESSMENT, AND IMPACT ANALYSIS

The monitoring, assessment, and understanding of the impact of air pollution are crucial components in formulating effective control and mitigation strategies. This involves the detailed exploration of the National Ambient Air Quality Standards (NAAQS), the National Air Quality Index (AQI), and comprehensive assessments of the health, environmental, and economic impacts of air pollution.

18.7.1 National Ambient Air Quality Standards (NAAQS)

Defining Air Quality Standards: The National Ambient Air Quality Standards (NAAQS) in India set permissible limits for various air pollutants, including particulate matter (PM10, PM2.5), sulfur dioxide (SO_2), nitrogen dioxide (NO_2), carbon monoxide (CO), ozone (O_3), and lead (Pb). These standards act as benchmarks to evaluate air quality across the country.

Implementation and Compliance: NAAQS are implemented by the Central Pollution Control Board (CPCB) and State Pollution Control Boards (SPCBs). The standards guide the monitoring of air quality at various monitoring stations across the country. The assessment of air quality against NAAQS ensures regulatory adherence and identifies regions failing to meet these standards, requiring urgent remedial action.

18.7.2 The Role and Effectiveness of the National Air Quality Index (AQI)

Overview and Functionality: The National Air Quality Index (AQI) serves as a tool to disseminate real-time information about air quality to the public. It categorizes air quality into various indices (ranging from good to hazardous) based on the concentrations of pollutants, enabling easy comprehension and interpretation of air quality data.

Public Awareness and Guidance: The AQI acts as a vital communication tool, raising public awareness regarding air quality and its potential health implications. It guides the public, advising on precautions to be taken during different air quality categories, thereby minimizing health risks associated with poor air quality.

18.7.3 Comprehensive Assessment of Health, Environmental, and Economic Impacts due to Air Pollution

1. ***Health Impacts:*** Air pollution significantly impacts public health, leading to respiratory diseases, cardiovascular issues, and other health complications. Long-term exposure to poor air quality leads to increased mortality and exacerbates existing health conditions, particularly affecting vulnerable populations.
2. ***Environmental Impacts:*** Air pollution negatively affects ecosystems, causing acid rain, damage to vegetation, and the deterioration of soil and water quality. It also contributes to climate change, affecting weather patterns and biodiversity.
3. ***Economic Implications:*** The economic costs of air pollution are substantial, encompassing healthcare expenses, reduced workforce productivity, and the cost of mitigating environmental damage caused by pollution.

Monitoring air quality through NAAQS and the AQI is fundamental to understanding the extent of pollution and its potential health implications. Comprehensive assessments of health, environmental, and economic impacts underline the urgency in implementing effective measures to control air pollution, ensuring a healthier environment and improved public well-being in India.

18.8 POLICIES AND STRATEGIES FOR AIR POLLUTION CONTROL

The combat against air pollution in India demands a comprehensive approach that integrates policy measures and strategic initiatives. Analyzing the implementation of the National Clean Air Program (NCAP), the promotion of cleaner fuel sources, electric vehicles, and renewable energy, as well as the significance of international collaborations for policy exchange and technology transfer, is vital in addressing this critical environmental issue [12, 18–20]. Various policies and strategies for air pollution control in India are enlisted as follows:

18.8.1 Comprehensive Analysis of NCAP Implementation and City-Specific Action Plans

National Clean Air Program (NCAP) was launched in 2019, aiming to reduce particulate matter (PM) levels in the air by 20–30% in 102 cities across India by 2024. The program emphasizes city-specific action plans, delineating targets and measures to be implemented by state governments and local bodies for pollution control.

18.8.2 Implementation Challenges and Progress

NCAP faces challenges in effective implementation, including funding constraints, technical capacity, and stakeholder engagement. Some cities have shown progress in action plan implementation, such as measures to control vehicular emissions, increased green cover, and the adoption of cleaner technologies in industries.

18.8.3 Encouragement and Promotion of Cleaner Fuel Sources, Electric Vehicles, and Renewable Energy

1. ***Cleaner Fuel Sources:*** Promoting cleaner fuels, such as the transition from conventional petrol and diesel to compressed natural gas (CNG) and Liquefied Petroleum Gas (LPG) in vehicles and industries, is a priority. It helps reduce vehicular emissions and industrial pollution.
2. **Electric Vehicles (EVs):** The promotion of electric vehicles is crucial to reducing vehicular emissions. Government incentives, subsidies, and the development of EV infrastructure are being emphasized to encourage a shift towards cleaner transportation.
3. ***Renewable Energy Adoption:*** Fostering renewable energy sources like solar, wind, and hydroelectric power as alternatives to fossil fuels is pivotal in mitigating air pollution caused by energy generation.

18.8.4 International Collaborations and Partnerships for Policy Exchange and Technology Transfer

1. ***Policy Exchange:*** International collaborations facilitate the exchange of best practices, policies, and strategies for air pollution control. Learning from success stories in other nations aids in formulating more effective policies in India.
2. ***Technology Transfer:*** Collaboration with other countries enables the transfer of cutting-edge technologies for pollution control. This includes expertise in vehicle emissions control, industrial pollution control, and renewable energy utilization.

The National Clean Air Program (NCAP) is a significant step towards addressing air pollution in India, although its effective implementation requires continual monitoring and adjustments. The promotion of cleaner fuel sources, electric vehicles, and renewable energy plays a critical role in reducing pollution. Moreover, international collaborations foster the exchange of knowledge and technology transfer, enhancing India's capacity to combat air pollution effectively. These policies and strategies collectively aim to mitigate air pollution, ensuring a healthier and more sustainable environment for India's present and future generations.

18.9 TECHNOLOGICAL INNOVATIONS AND SOLUTIONS FOR POLLUTION CONTROL

Technological advancements play a crucial role in addressing air pollution concerns, offering solutions through innovative devices, emission control technologies, and renewable energy solutions. This section explores the role of technology in pollution control, advancements in emission control, and the growth of renewable and sustainable technologies for emission reduction.

18.9.1 Technology in Pollution Control

1. ***Air Purifiers:*** Air purifiers have gained prominence as household devices that help improve indoor air quality. These devices use filters and advanced air-cleaning mechanisms to remove pollutants, enhancing the quality of indoor air.
2. ***Pollution Monitoring Devices:*** Advanced monitoring devices have been developed to track and assess air quality in real time. These devices, including drones and compact sensors, provide data on air pollution levels, aiding in identifying pollution hotspots and enabling timely interventions.
3. ***Innovation in Emission Control Technologies:*** Technology has driven the development of cleaner and more efficient industrial processes. Advanced emission control technologies, such as catalytic converters in automobiles, flue-gas desulfurization systems in power plants, and cleaner production techniques, are essential in reducing pollutant emissions.

18.9.2 Advancements in Renewable Energy and Sustainable Technologies for Emission Reduction

1. ***Renewable Energy Solutions:*** The expansion of renewable energy sources, including solar, wind, and hydroelectric power, has been significant. These technologies offer cleaner alternatives to traditional fossil fuels, reducing emissions from energy generation.
2. ***Sustainable Technologies for Emission Reduction:*** Innovations in sustainable technologies, such as electric vehicles, hydrogen fuel cells, and energy-efficient appliances, contribute to emission reduction. Electric vehicles, for instance, significantly lower vehicular emissions, promoting cleaner transportation.

Technological innovations play a pivotal role in addressing air pollution concerns, offering a wide array of solutions ranging from air purifiers and monitoring devices to advanced emission control technologies. Moreover, the growth of renewable energy sources and sustainable technologies presents an opportunity for substantial emission reduction. Continued innovation, research, and development in technology remain critical for further advancements in pollution control, fostering a sustainable and cleaner environment for the future. These advancements, along with effective policy implementation and public participation, are fundamental in combating air pollution and ensuring a healthier ecosystem [21, 22].

18.10 CHALLENGES, GAPS, AND FUTURE DIRECTIONS IN AIR POLLUTION CONTROL

Identifying the challenges in implementing air pollution control measures, providing recommendations for policy improvements, and emphasizing the significance of public awareness and behavioral changes are essential components in the pursuit of sustainable air quality.

18.10.1 Identification of Challenges in Implementing Air Pollution Control Measures

1. ***Implementation Challenges:*** Inadequate enforcement of regulations, lack of funds, and technical limitations pose hurdles in the effective implementation of air pollution control measures. Monitoring and ensuring compliance with emission standards, especially in industries, remains a challenge.
2. ***Inadequate Infrastructure:*** Insufficient infrastructure, particularly in waste management and monitoring systems, creates gaps in effectively addressing pollution sources, particularly in urban and peri-urban areas.
3. ***Lack of Public Awareness:*** Limited public awareness regarding the health hazards of air pollution often results in a lack of public support for stringent measures, hindering the implementation of effective policies.

18.10.2 Recommendations for Policy Improvements and Strategies

1. ***Strengthening Enforcement and Capacity Building:*** Enhancing regulatory capacity, investing in advanced monitoring systems, and training personnel for effective enforcement are imperative. Building technical expertise in pollution control measures can significantly improve the implementation of policies.
2. ***Integration of Technology:*** Leveraging advanced technologies in pollution monitoring, data analytics, and emission control should be a focal point in policy improvements to enhance accuracy and efficiency.
3. ***Community Engagement and Public Awareness:*** Engaging communities through awareness campaigns and education about the adverse effects of air pollution is critical. Involving citizens in the decision-making process and encouraging responsible behavior can aid in collective efforts toward pollution reduction.

18.10.3 Emphasizing the Significance of Public Awareness and Behavioral Changes

1. ***Behavioral Changes for Sustainable Living:*** Promoting behavioral changes, such as the adoption of public transport, reduction in the use of personal vehicles, and encouragement of sustainable lifestyle practices, can significantly contribute to emission reduction.
2. ***Public Participation and Advocacy:*** Engaging the public in advocating for cleaner practices and supporting policies aimed at reducing pollution plays a crucial role in the success of air quality improvement initiatives.

The challenges in implementing air pollution control measures stem from a variety of factors, including inadequate enforcement, infrastructure limitations, and insufficient public awareness. Recommendations for policy improvements involve strengthening enforcement, integrating technology, and engaging communities through awareness campaigns [23–30].

Emphasizing the significance of public awareness and behavioral changes is critical in addressing the root causes of air pollution. Through collective efforts, including policy improvements, technological advancements, and public participation, the path toward sustainable air quality can be established, ensuring a healthier and cleaner environment for generations to come.

18.11 CONCLUSION

18.11.1 Addressing Air Pollution for a Sustainable Future

The critical examination of air pollution and its control measures presents a roadmap towards a sustainable and healthier future. Key findings and recommendations underscore the urgency of addressing air pollution for public health and environmental well-being.

18.11.2 Summary of Key Findings and Recommendations

Throughout this exploration, significant findings and recommendations have emerged. From legislative frameworks to technological innovations, each aspect plays a pivotal role in combatting air pollution.

a) Key Findings:
  - Legislative Frameworks: The Air (Prevention and Control of Pollution) Act, 1981, establishes the legal groundwork for pollution control.
  - National Initiatives: The National Clean Air Program (NCAP) emphasizes city-specific action plans, offering a strategic approach to curb air pollution.
  - Role of Technology: Innovations such as air purifiers, pollution monitoring devices, and renewable energy solutions present effective strategies for pollution control.

b) Recommendations:
- Strengthening enforcement, technological integration, and community engagement are essential to bolster air quality initiatives.
- Public awareness campaigns and behavioral changes are crucial for promoting sustainable practices and reducing pollution.

18.11.3 Reiteration of Importance

Addressing air pollution is not just a matter of policy or regulation; it's a matter of public health and a sustainable future. The detrimental impacts of air pollution on human health, environmental degradation, and the economic burden it poses necessitate urgent action. By implementing stringent policies, harnessing innovative technologies, and fostering public awareness and behavioral changes, a significant reduction in air pollution can be achieved. This reduction is not just a means of meeting regulatory standards; it's a pathway toward ensuring a healthier and more sustainable environment for current and future generations.

18.11.4 Final Emphasis

The imperative to address air pollution isn't solely a responsibility of regulatory bodies or governmental agencies; it's a collective responsibility. Every individual, community, industry, and policy-maker plays a vital role in reducing air pollution.

The pursuit of cleaner air is an ongoing journey, but by implementing and enforcing robust policies, embracing technological innovations, and fostering behavioral changes, we pave the way for a future where cleaner air is a reality. This collective effort is vital for ensuring a healthier environment and a sustainable world for present and future generations. The commitment to addressing air pollution remains pivotal for a better and healthier tomorrow, safeguarding public health and nurturing a sustainable future for all.

REFERENCES

[1] Brunekreef, B., and Holgate, S. T. (2002). Air pollution and health. *The Lancet*, 360(9341), pp. 1233–1242.

[2] Kampa, M. and Castanas, E. (2008). Human health effects of air pollution. *Environmental Pollution*, 151(2), pp. 362–367.

[3] Vallero, D.A. (2014). *Fundamentals of Air Pollution*. Academic Press.

[4] Boubel, R.W., Vallero, D., Fox, D.L., Turner, B. and Stern, A.C. (2013). *Fundamentals of Air Pollution*. Elsevier.

[5] Bernstein, J.A., Alexis, N., Barnes, C., Bernstein, I.L., Nel, A., Peden, D., Diaz-Sanchez, D., Tarlo, S.M. and Williams, P.B. (2004). Health effects of air pollution. *Journal of Allergy and Clinical Immunology*, 114(5), pp. 1116–1123.

[6] Glencross, D.A., Ho, T.R., Camina, N., Hawrylowicz, C.M. and Pfeffer, P.E. (2020). Air pollution and its effects on the immune system. *Free Radical Biology and Medicine*, 151, pp. 56–68.

[7] Brook, R.D. (2008). Cardiovascular effects of air pollution. *Clinical Science*, 115(6), pp.175–187.

[8] Lu, J.G. (2020). Air pollution: A systematic review of its psychological, economic, and social effects. *Current Opinion in Psychology*, 32, pp. 52–65.
[9] Kankaria, A., Nongkynrih, B. and Gupta, S.K. (2014). Indoor air pollution in India: Implications on health and its control. *Indian Journal of Community Medicine: Official Publication of Indian Association of Preventive & Social Medicine*, 39(4), p.203.
[10] Khilnani, G.C. and Tiwari, P. (2018). Air pollution in India and related adverse respiratory health effects: past, present, and future directions. *Current Opinion in Pulmonary Medicine*, 24(2), pp.108–116.
[11] Balakrishnan, K., Cohen, A. and Smith, K.R. (2014). Addressing the burden of disease attributable to air pollution in India: the need to integrate across household and ambient air pollution exposures. *Environmental Health Perspectives*, 122(1), pp.A6–A7.
[12] Greenstone, M., Harish, S., Pande, R. and Sudarshan, A. (2017, July). The solvable challenge of air pollution in India. In *India Policy Forum* (Vol. 12). National Council of Applied Economic Research.
[13] Chu, B., Ma, Q., Liu, J., Ma, J., Zhang, P., Chen, T., Feng, Q., Wang, C., Yang, N., Ma, H. and Ma, J. (2020). Air pollutant correlations in China: secondary air pollutant responses to NOx and SO2 control. *Environmental Science & Technology Letters*, 7(10), pp.695–700.
[14] Suh, H.H., Bahadori, T., Vallarino, J., and Spengler, J. D. (2000). Criteria air pollutants and toxic air pollutants. *Environmental Health Perspectives*, 108(suppl 4), pp. 625–633.
[15] World Health Organization (2016). *World Health Statistics 2016 [OP]: Monitoring Health for the Sustainable Development Goals (SDGs)*. World Health Organization.
[16] World Health Organization. (2020). World Health Statistics 2020.
[17] Zwielewski, G. (2023). World Health Organization. World health statistics 2022: monitoring health for the. Gestão de qualidade em saúde: conceitos e ferramentas da qualidade como estratégia de construção e práticas em gestão em saúde.
[18] Dhar Sarkar, M. (2005). Legislative measures and control of air pollution in India: retrospect and prospect. PhD diss., University of North Bengal.
[19] Divan, S., and Rosencranz, A. (2022). *Environmental Law and Policy in India: Cases and Materials*. Oxford University Press.
[20] Sankar, U. (1998). *Laws and Institutions Relating to Environmental Protection in India. The Role of Law and Legal Institutions in Asian Economic Development*. Rotterdam: Erasmus University.
[21] Zhao, J., Xi, X. I., Na, Q. I., Wang, S., Kadry, S. N., and Kumar, P. M. (2021). The technological innovation of hybrid and plug-in electric vehicles for environment carbon pollution control. *Environmental Impact Assessment Review*, 86, p. 106506.
[22] Gonzalez-Martin, J., Kraakman, N. J. R., Perez, C., Lebrero, R., and Munoz, R. (2021). A state–of–the-art review on indoor air pollution and strategies for indoor air pollution control. *Chemosphere*, 262, p. 128376.
[23] Rani, S., Ghai, D., and Kumar, S. (2022). Object detection and recognition using contour based edge detection and fast R-CNN. *Multimedia Tools and Applications*, 81(29), 42183–42207.
[24] Nanda, S. K., Ghai, D., Ingole, P. V., and Pande, S. (2022). Soft computing techniques-based digital video forensics for fraud medical anomaly detection. *Computer Assisted Methods in Engineering and Science*, 30(2), 111–130.
[25] Tripathi, S. L., Mendiratta, N., Ghai, D., Avasthi, S., and Dhir, K. (2022). Coronavirus: Diagnosis, detection, and analysis. In Valentina Emilia Balas, Oana Geman (Eds.), *Biomedical Engineering Applications for People with Disabilities and the Elderly in the COVID-19 Pandemic and Beyond* (pp. 109–117). Academic Press.

[26] Tripathi, S. L., Dhir, K., Ghai, D., and Patil, S. (Eds.). (2021). *Health Informatics and Technological Solutions for Coronavirus (COVID-19)*. CRC Press.

[27] Ghai, D., Tripathi, S. L., Saxena, S., Chanda, M., and Alazab, M. (Eds.). (2022). *Machine Learning Algorithms for Signal and Image Processing*. John Wiley & Sons, vol. 1, pp. 1–473.

[28] Vilcassim, R., and Thurston, G. D. (2023). Gaps and future directions in research on health effects of air pollution. *EBioMedicine*.

[29] Sokhi, R. S., Moussiopoulos, N., Baklanov, A., Bartzis, J., Coll, I., Finardi, S., Friedrich, R. et al. (2022). Advances in air quality research–current and emerging challenges. *Atmospheric Chemistry and Physics*, 22(7), pp. 4615–4703.

[30] Shahadin, M. S., Ab Mutalib, N. S., Latif, M. T., Greene, C. M., and Hassan, T. (2018). Challenges and future direction of molecular research in air pollution-related lung cancers. *Lung Cancer*, 118, pp. 69–75.

19 Artificial Intelligence Techniques for River Water Quality Analysis Using IoT and Remote Sensing

K. Manimala
Anna University, Chennai, India

E. Fantin Irudaya Raj
Dr. Sivanthi Aditanar College of Engineering, Tiruchendur, India

S. Ebenezer Juliet
Vellore Institute of Technology, India

19.1 INTRODUCTION

Water is a very important resource nature has provided for the survival of life on this earth. Industrial development and urban growth are posing a severe threat to water bodies in terms of pollution and occupation of water bodies for human settlement [1–3]. Most diseases are due to water-related infections caused by pollution from industrial wastes and sewage. Hence, monitoring river water quality regularly is essential to save the world from environmental problems caused especially by manmade pollutants. Water quality monitoring involves physical, chemical, and biological changes in the water due to pollution. The time and location of pollution starting point in the river should be identified especially through the recently developed Internet of Things (IoT) Sensors [4]. Literature suggests several parameters to be monitored using sensors [5]. The researchers are investigating the process of IoT-based sensors to replace the cumbersome manual monitoring and analysis of water quality in various locations of the river [6–9]. The advantage of such sensors is the spatial and temporal data related to the water quality in addition to real-time automatic monitoring. As the data collected by the sensors is huge, big data analysis is

 DOI: 10.1201/9781003546382-19

required to analyze and disseminate the knowledge quickly to the concerned authorities for necessary action.

Another method that can be used for the WQ analysis is based on satellite data suggested by many researchers. Remote sensing can cover a wide area compared to the manual sampling process and IoT monitoring [10, 11]. Also, it is a cost-effective method, compared to the IoT data method as the cost of IoT sensors is high and it should be installed at several locations to get precise data. Another issue associated with IoT-based methods is the safety of the sensors installed. Researchers have suggested the usage of various satellite data for analyzing the water quality [12, 13]. The parameters considered generally include NH3-N, total nitrogen (TN), total phosphorous (TP), chlorophyll-a, colored dissolved organic matter (CDOM), and total suspended matter (TSM) from Sentinel-2 images, GF-1C images [14, 15]. The accuracy of the results is affected by the resolution of the satellite images and also there is limited data for the specific study area. The reflectance values of the water for different satellite bands are used to determine the quality as it represents the physical, chemical, and biological characteristics of the water [16–19]. Several literatures suggest the usage of satellite images for WQ analysis of lakes. The visible electromagnetic spectrum mainly the chlorophyll-a and TSM plays a big role in focusing the application of different machine learning and deep learning algorithms for identifying and observing the water quality parameters [20–22]. The algorithms employed remove the noise and atmospheric effects mainly for visible satellite images, mid-infra-red and near-infra-red bands of the satellite images.

High-resolution cameras mounted on cost-effective, and low-altitude Unmanned Aerial Vehicles (UAVs) can capture high-quality spectral images of rivers and lakes without the interference of clouds. The inversion accuracy of such a UAV-based image is high which gives the scope for these UAVs for water quality monitoring and analysis [23–25]. Even though the acquisition range poses some problems usage of UAVs is a promising option for WQ monitoring.

The WQ monitoring methodology is categorized into four modules:

1. WQ data collection using IoT
2. WQ data collection using remote sensing or UAV
3. Data integration in cloud server
4. Deep learning-based WQ predictive model

The sensor and remote sensing-based data could be trained using a deep learning model to design a WQ predictive model capable of predicting the WQ in advance. The structure of the WQ predictive model is illustrated in Figure 19.1.

The present work focuses on:

- Analysis of the deep learning-based predictive Water Quality Remote Monitoring System (WQRMS) that predicts the harmful algal bloom and sediment deposition in the future

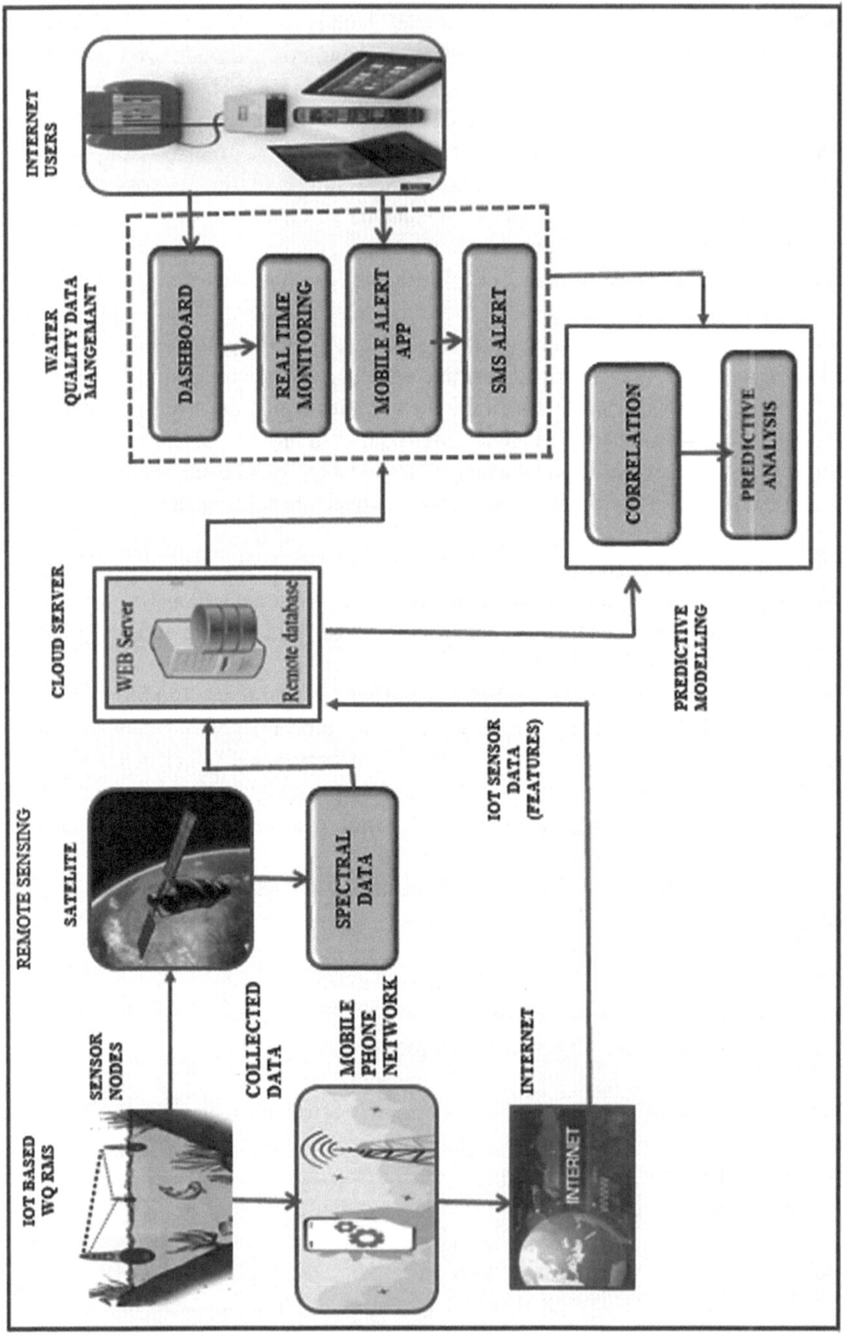

FIGURE 19.1 Outline of proposed work.

- Existing techniques that can produce knowledge inference on WQ as and when required include pH, Dissolved oxygen, and harmful algae with the status of water quality at the required location of the river
- To create an awareness of the necessity of a report on the effect of man-induced changes on the river water that affects the environment with a case study of a South Indian River
- A glimpse of existing work in the literature about IoT-based real-time remote water quality analyzing systems.
- Describing the design of a remote sensing model with high precision, as proposed in the literature, to retrieve suspended sediment concentration and detect harmful algal blooms.
- Briefing the necessity of the combination of IoT and remote sensing-based models for the timely assessment of the temporal and spatial distribution of suspended sediment concentration.
- Discussing the water pollution using a case study, the river Thamirabharani

This chapter is organized in the following manner: The second section describes the literature works, the third section describes the IoT-based methodologies for monitoring water quality, the fourth section carries the remote sensing-based water quality analysis, the fifth section summarizes the deep learning technologies, and the efficient method for predictive water quality model design, the sixth section gives the case study of the River Thamirabharani, the seventh section discusses the research gap and finally the chapter ends with the Conclusion.

19.2 RELATED WORK

Water management authorities have undertaken various initiatives to assess water quality through manual sampling at multiple locations along the river. The samples taken at a particular instant of time are analyzed offline at different times in a laboratory. Also, the process is very time-consuming, laborious, and costly [26, 27]. Such analysis lacks spatio-temporal resolution. IoT sensor-based technology gives promising results for automatic real-time monitoring which can monitor WQ parameters like pH, Dissolved oxygen, fecal coliform, etc. These sensors can communicate the data to a cloud server for analysis and decision-making in real time [28, 29]. In addition to that, several kinds of literature suggest the usage of IoT-based methodologies for automatic monitoring of water quality and warning in real time to save the environment and keep our earth green and clean [30, 31]. Such analysis includes the harmful effects of algal bloom in river water and lakes.

Remote sensing methodology such as Landsat-8 and sentinel-2 image techniques is suggested by several researchers for monitoring the water quality [32–36]. Sentinel-2 and Sentinel-3 images are found to be better in performance compared to Landsat-8 [37–40]. The data repositories for Sentinel-2 data used by the researchers are taken from https://scihub.copernicus.eu/. The Level1C of these images consists of 100 km^2 with 500 MB [41]. Research work on the problems due to turbidity and biomass [42] in water bodies was also done using Moderate Resolution Imaging Spectroradiometer (MODIS). The extended work of researchers in identifying the relationship between Chl-a and the biomass of algae is also reported in [43]. Multispectral satellite images help monitor the river by computing the reflectance of water at different bands. For example, chl-a will be reflected in the green band [44] and sediments can be reflected in the red, blue, near-infrared, and mid-infrared bands. Certain substances like nitrogen and phosphorous do not reflect concerning spectral bands but they indirectly affect the water quality. The sediments deposited on the river reflect clearly for spectral bands, and hence, the water quality can be monitored by an inversion process while using remote sensing [45, 46].

The literature review indicates that WQ observation technology has effectively met the demands of scientists, offering autonomous measurement tools for crucial physical-chemical-biological parameters like PCB. Deploying sensor-equipped buoys and boats has facilitated in-situ monitoring and data collection [47]. Almost all nations have used remote sensing analysis tools and UAV-based analysis for remote WQ monitoring. Despite several such techniques available, there is still a need for bridging technology and the end user, data collection by IoT sensors, and analysis using deep learning techniques. The WQ monitoring using IoT can be supported by geographical information systems (GISs) and accurate analysis techniques for determining the spatiotemporal information in real time. International researchers are exploring various approaches, including electronic skin (e-Skin) or multiparametric sensor patches, as well as traditional methods like deploying underwater robots and sensorized buoys, for comprehensive sensing in diverse environments with support from funding agencies [47]. Artificial Intelligence and Machine learning techniques are widely deployed to analyze the data correctly to provide alert signals and predict the future WQ. The literature suggests that several countries have started deploying sensors and replaced the manual water sample collection process with sensor monitoring.

19.3 WATER QUALITY DATA COLLECTION USING IoT

The following Water Quality data are collected from IoT sensors. Pearson correlation analysis is done to identify the highly correlated features and to select only a small subset of features. This will reduce sensor cost and reduce the dimensionality of features, thereby reducing the complexity of the deep learning network. The IoT data to be collected are shown in Table 19.1 [48–51].

The sensors are to be fitted in buoys floating in water and anchored properly. The safety of the buoys should be ensured. Figure 19.2 shows the schematic arrangement of buoys and sensor nodes.

The internal components of the sensor node and buoys are shown in Figure 19.3. The solar panel is used to charge the battery which supplies power to the sensor board [52]. The LoRa technology is used to pass on the sensor data to the Microcontroller via the data acquisition card and stored in memory. 4G technology is used to transfer the data in the internal memory of the sensor node to the cloud server for further deep-learning analysis. Sigfox, an IoT communication platform is commonly used.

TABLE 19.1
IoT Sensor Data

Sr. No.	Parameter	Abbreviation	Type
1	Dissolved Oxygen	DO	Physical
2	Electrical Conductivity	EC	
3	pH	pH	
4	Temperature	T	
5	Total suspended solids	TSS	
6	Oxydo Reduction Potential	ORP	Chemical
7	Biochemical Oxygen Demand	BOD	
8	Nitrogen	N	
9	Sodium	Na	
10	Calcium	Ca	
11	Chloride	Cl	
12	Chlorophyll-a	Chl-a	Biological
13	Total Coliform bacteria	TCB	

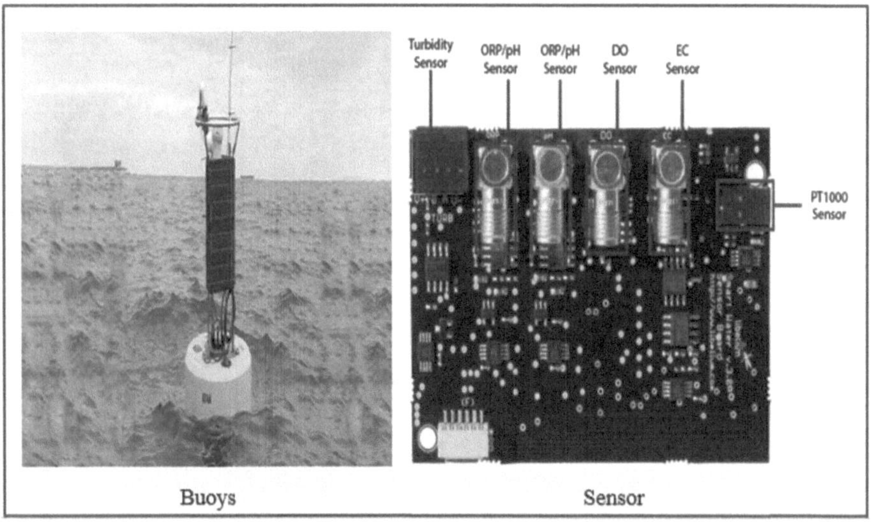

FIGURE 19.2 Buoys and sensor node.

The details of solar panels normally preferred is

Battery – 12 V
Nominal Peak Power – 30 W
Nominal Voltage – 17.5 V
Nominal Current – 1.72 A

The IoT data collected from the river using sensors and aerial vehicles are analyzed using Deep learning techniques, which is represented in Figure 19.4.

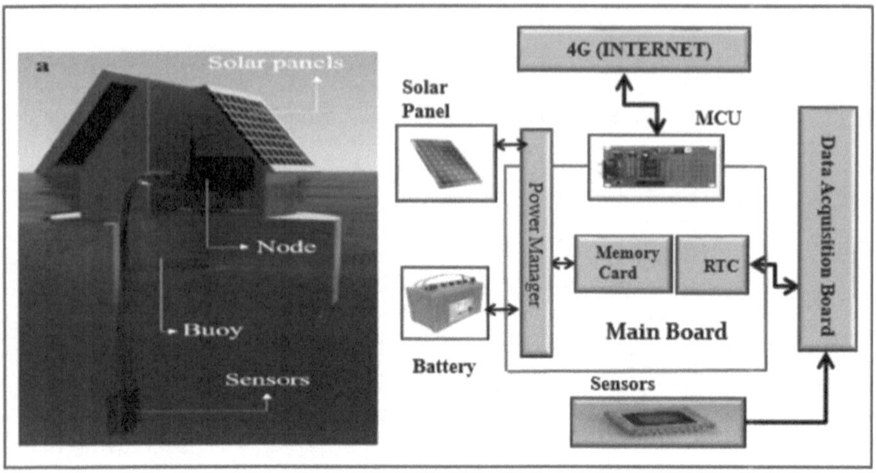

FIGURE 19.3 Internal arrangement of Buoys and Sensor node.

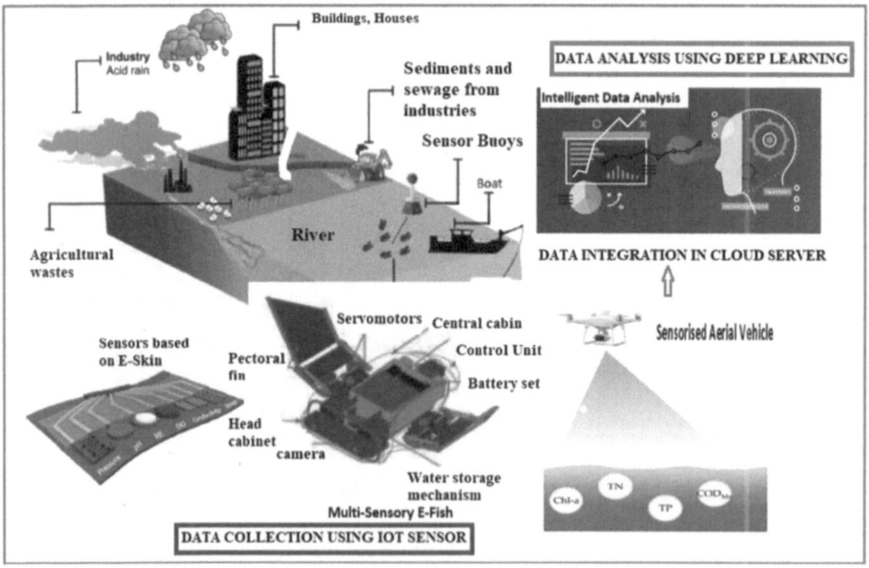

FIGURE 19.4 IoT data collection and analysis.

19.4 WATER QUALITY DATA COLLECTION USING REMOTE SENSING

The satellite images of the study area are usually collected, and the required preprocessing steps are completed. Cloud and land should be masked to obtain the river from the satellite images. Radiometric correction should be done to avoid variations in reflectance values due to variations in scene illumination. Atmospheric correction must be done to remove the scattering and absorption effects from the atmosphere. Typically, the selected images undergo calibration by applying a deep learning-based Regional Coast Colour semi-analytical algorithm for atmospheric correction [53]. The algorithm is equipped with tools designed to minimize the atmospheric path radiance, essential for estimating concentration from satellite images. Subsequently, the algorithm detects the water body, and the reflectivity outside the water is extracted from the satellite images. To determine suspended sediment concentration, it is crucial to correlate the water reflectivity with the optical properties of the water body. Satellite images of 5 bands R, G, B, near-infrared, and mid-infrared to be considered [54–56].

19.4.1 Water Body Detection

The Minimum Normalized Water Score (MNWS) method is generally used to identify the water pixels from the reflectance values. To tackle the problem of spectral heterogeneity, it is important to develop a Multi-Noiseless Water System (MNWS) and a "bad pixel filter" mask. This involves dividing water samples into similar subgroups and creating a self-normalization model for each group. This enables the creation of an MNWS for water detection using the equations (Eq. (19.1) and Eq. (19.2)) [57]. Each cluster is a distinct water type, and a unique NWS model is developed for each cluster. The samples within each cluster exhibit an approximately normal distribution. The MNWS computation finalizes by identifying the closest water cluster in each water pixel and converting various water types into distance images.

$$\mathrm{NWS_i} = \sqrt{\frac{1}{m}\sum_{j=1}^{m}\left(\left(x_j - \overline{x_{i,j}}\right)/\sigma_{i,j}\right)^2} \tag{19.1}$$

$$\mathrm{MNWS} = \min_{i=1}^{n}\left\{\mathrm{NWS_i}\right\} \tag{19.2}$$

Here, $\sigma_{i,j}$ and $\overline{x_{i,j}}$ represents the standard deviation and mean, respectively, of the surface spectral reflectance of water cluster i at band j. The term m denotes the total number of bands, n represents the number of water clusters, and x_j denotes the pixel reflectance at band j. Identification of reliable water body pixels and clustering of all such pixels are done to identify the entire water body as reported in [57]. Finally, the water leaving reflectance values are stored in a cloud server for designing the deep learning WQ predictive model.

19.4.2 Data Integration in Cloud Server

The study area is classified into several small sub-areas called boxes and the satellite reflectance value is mapped with the corresponding IoT sensor data of that box. The required preprocessing operations are done on both the data and stored in a cloud server for deep learning analysis to detect the presence of sediments and algae. Figure 19.5 shows the preprocessing and data storage in a cloud server.

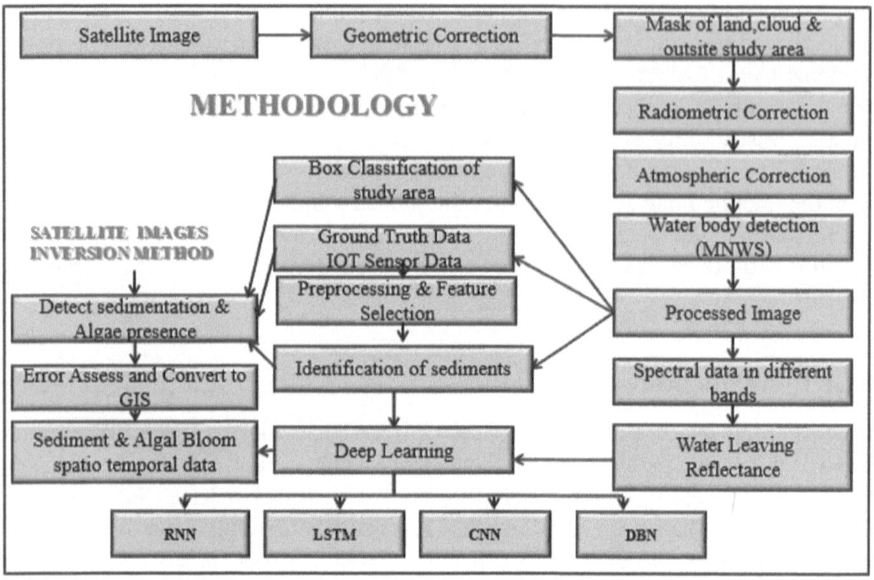

FIGURE 19.5 Satellite & IOT data storage in cloud server.

19.5 DEEP LEARNING-BASED WATER QUALITY PREDICTIVE MODEL

As the IoT sensors and remote sensing data are huge in volume, there is a necessity to use Artificial Intelligence (AI) techniques-based tools for proper learning and decision-making. Several Machine Learning and Deep Learning-based tools are suggested by researchers for analyzing the WQ big data. These AI methods can map relationships within the data collected and automatically disseminate knowledge to the users regarding the grade of the Water quality in real time. The huge voluminous and unstructured environmental WQ data poses challenges for us to design an intelligent deep learning-based WQ predictive model [58–62]. The WQ predictive model could also include any other data obtained from online sources to integrate with AI in the future.

This section focuses on framing a remote sensing-based water quality prediction model. The remote sensing prediction is validated with the IoT-based ground sensor data to ensure the accuracy of the designed model. Once an accurate predictive model is designed using satellite images validated by ground truth IoT data, the predictive WQ model can alert the presence of sediments and algae without the necessity of IoT sensor data, thereby making the future predictive process economical and simple.

The measured suspended sediment data from IoT is interpolated, and the resulting contour map of surface suspended sediment concentration is correlated with the remote sensing-calculated map of suspended sediment surface concentration distribution. The IoT-obtained sedimentation and algae data are cross-referenced with remotely sensed data for the corresponding point on the same day. Thus, the IoT ground truth data helps tune the predictive WQ model with good accuracy. The Total Suspended Sediment (TSS) in g/m^3 is given in the equation (Eq. (19.3)) [63].

$$TSS = a * e^{b*rs} \tag{19.3}$$

rs denotes the surface reflectance and a and b are calibration coefficients. Generally, calibration coefficients of the TSM algorithm were found by the bootstrap iteration method [4].

$$RMSE = \sqrt{\sum_{i=1}^{N} \frac{(X_i - Y_i)^2}{N}} \tag{19.4}$$

$$MAE = \frac{\sum_{i=1}^{N} |X_i - Y_i|}{N} \tag{19.5}$$

$$MPE = \frac{100\%}{N} \sum_{i=1}^{N} \frac{X_i - Y_i}{X_i} \tag{19.6}$$

where X_i represents the actual value, Y_i denotes the predicted value and N represents the number of samples each represented by a box area.

Based on the reflectance value, the presence of sediment and algae are identified for each box area and the prediction is verified in comparison with the actual data obtained from IoT sensors. The performance parameters are Mean Absolute Error (MAE), Root Mean Square Error (RMSE), and Mean Percentage Error (MPE) and are given in the equations (Eq. (19.4)–Eq. (19.6)). The predictive WQ model designed is used to predict the presence of sediments and algae thereby ascertaining the quality of water in the future using only remote sensing images. The presence of sediments with the corresponding location details is disseminated as knowledge using this work. The predictive model is illustrated in Figure 19.6.

To accomplish the inversion of suspended sediment concentration in satellite data, each parameter (network weight) retains its learning rate and is adjusted individually as the learning process progresses. The deep learning predictive model is designed such that the analysis of satellite images can predict the degrading water quality level and alert the concerned officials with a warning message indicating the polluted portion of the river. Figure 19.7 displays the satellite images and IoT sensors commonly used by researchers.

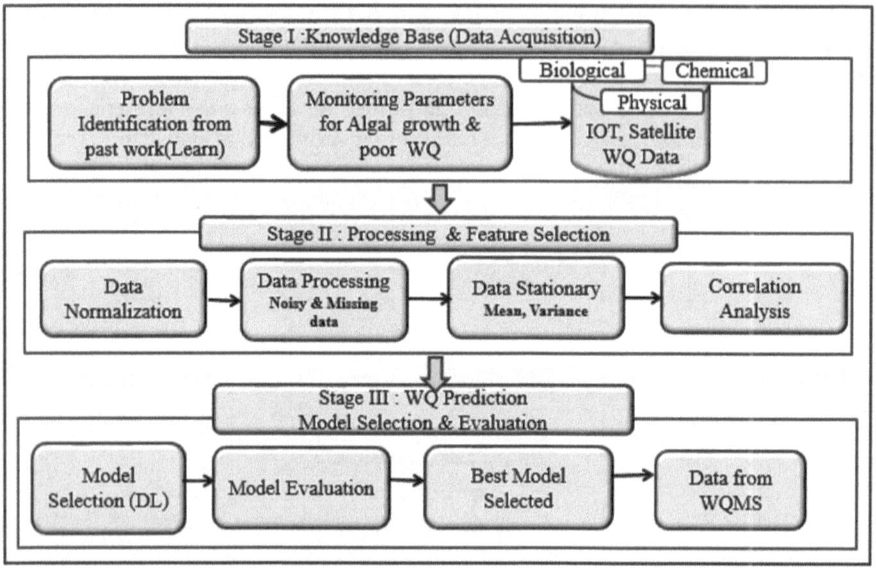

FIGURE 19.6 Satellite-based WQ predictive model.

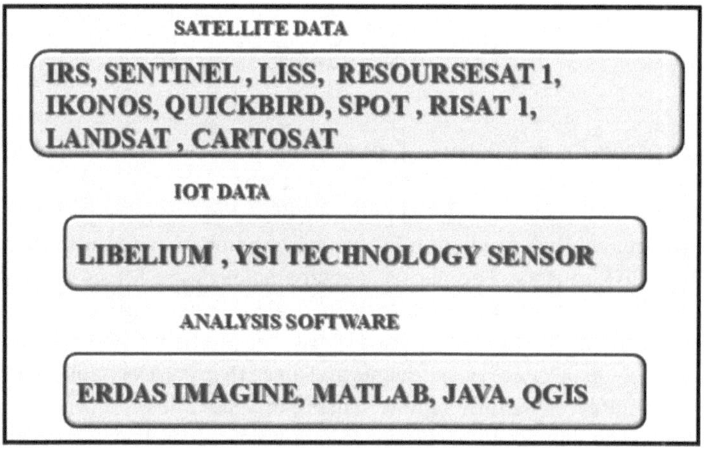

FIGURE 19.7 Data and software.

19.6 CASE STUDY – RIVER THAMIRABHARANI

River Thamirabharani is a perennial river flowing in two southern districts of Tamil Nadu, namely, Tirunelveli and Tuticorin. The river originates from the Pothigai Hills of Tirunelveli district and merges into the sea at Pothigai Hills.

A view of the river Thamirabharani [Source: IBC Tamilnadu] is shown in Figure 19.8. The newspaper reports on River Thamirabharani being polluted by the sewage and organic wastes from the villages and industries on its bank are shown in Figure 19.9 [Source: Times of India]. The reports of the Pollution Control Board [64]

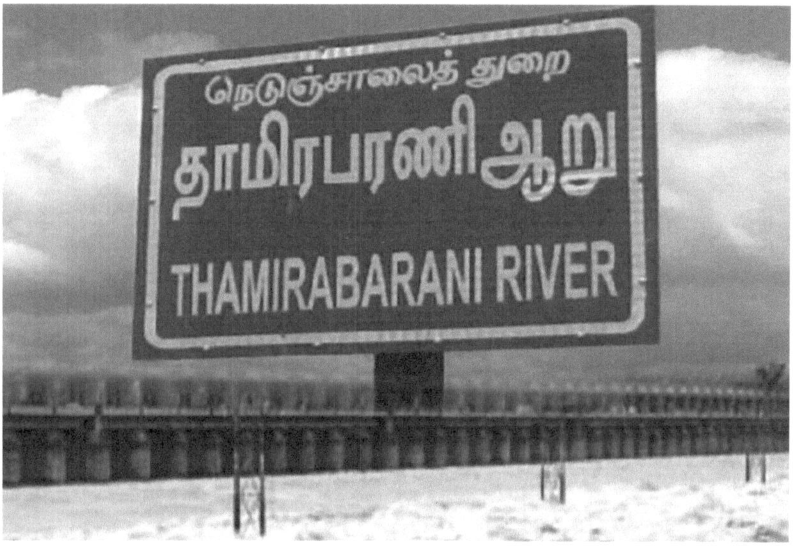

FIGURE 19.8 View of the river Thamirabharani.

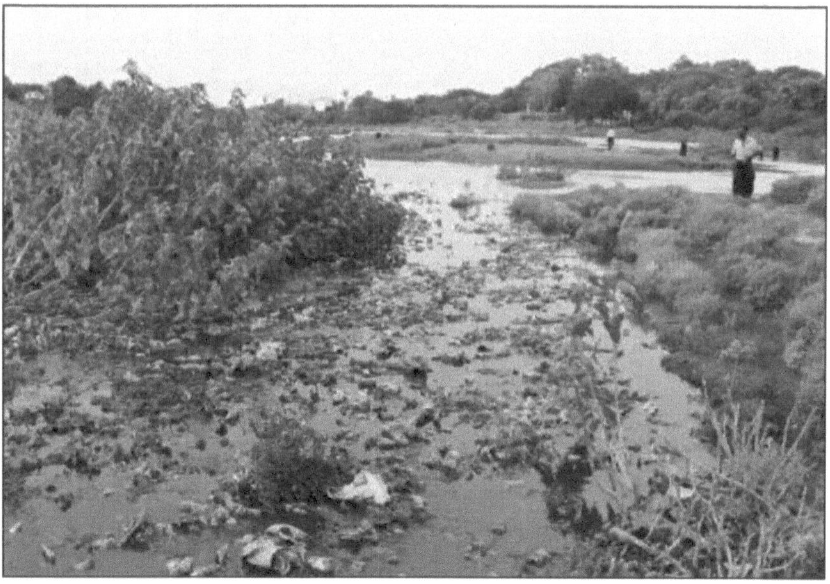

FIGURE 19.9 Polluted view of the river Thamirabharani.

stated the tedious steps taken to save the polluted river by appointing a committee to collect water samples at different points and testing in the lab to ensure the water quality necessitated the need for online analysis based on remote sensing. As the manual data collection method is a time-consuming process that eludes spatial-temporal information, satellite image-based technology combined with an IoT

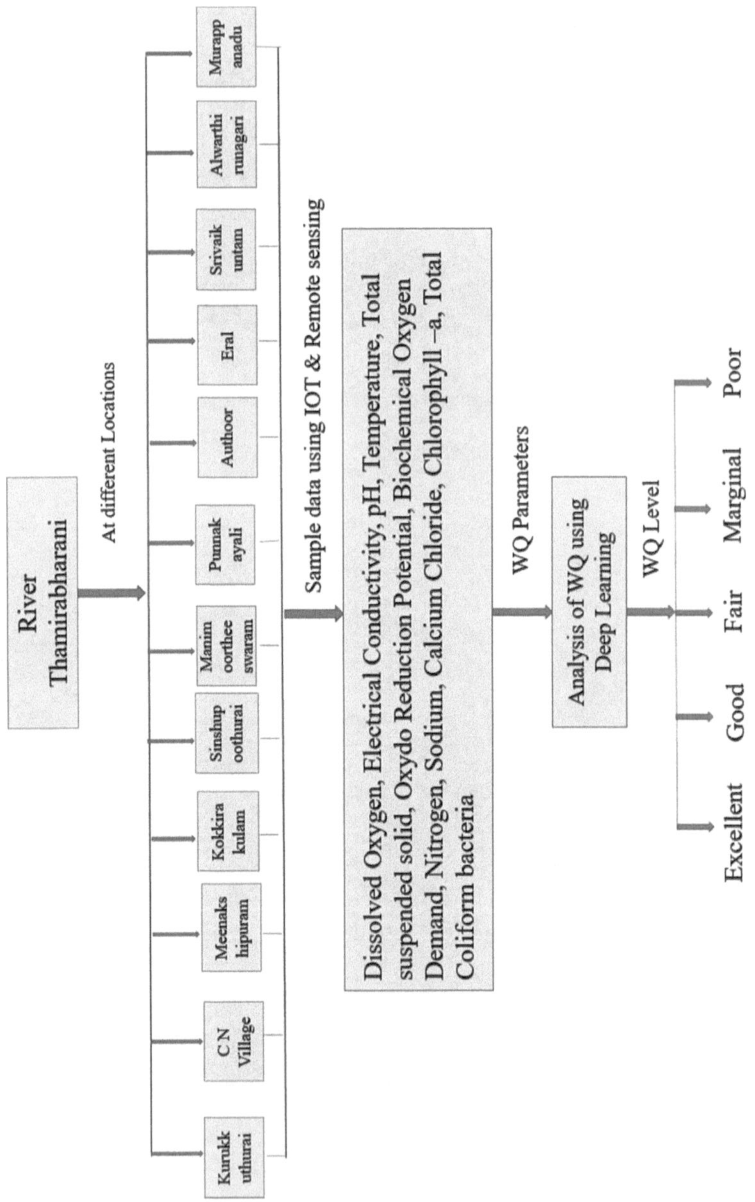

FIGURE 19.10 WQ predictive model for river Thamirabharani.

sensor is a good alternative. The initiatives taken by the Pollution Control Board for the rejuvenation of the River Thamirabharani, the main polluted points of the river, the reason for the pollution, etc. can be referred from [64].

The WQ predictive model suggested for the River Thamirabharani in Tuticorin District is outlined in Figure 19.10 using deep learning methodology using IoT and remote sensing data. The WQ data needs to be monitored at different locations of the river. The locations mentioned in Figure 19.10 are based on [64], the most polluted positions of the river.

19.7 RESEARCH GAP OF RIVER WATER QUALITY ANALYSIS

There are so many researchers working recently on improving the WQ of water bodies automatically using the recently emerging technologies of IoT and Deep Learning along with remote sensing. But there are still a lot of issues to be addressed and hence there is still a lot of scope for further research in this area. The research gaps are summarized as follows:

1. Laborious manual sample collection process to be replaced by advanced IoT and AI-based automatic techniques.
2. Satellite remote sensing data is not fully explored in many countries for water quality analysis.
3. IoT sensors for water quality monitoring are not deployed in all the main water bodies to monitor all the WQ parameters.
4. Satellite-based WQ data is to be calibrated in comparison with ground truth data using IoT sensors.
5. Necessary report generation and alert signals regarding water quality degradation should be issued.
6. Exploring the possibility of the availability of a water quality database publicly on a cloud server containing information like polluted points of the river, the time at which the data was acquired, and the location validated by ground truth data using IoT sensors.
7. The IoT WQ sensors are especially in the developmental phase and hence it necessitates technical knowledge to install, handle, and monitor data using this equipment. Also, there is a further constraint due to the huge budget involved in the procurement, robust protective structure, and maintenance of sensors in water bodies.
8. The IoT sensor-based monitoring system needs to be designed based on the environmental condition of the water body which is still not fully explored by the researchers.
9. The advanced AI technology, IoT, and remote sensing data should be bridged together properly for accurate analysis and design of the WQ predictive model.
10. The algal bloom and sediment analysis are not combined in a single research work.

11. Not all the parameters for accurate detection of WQ like NH3, NO3, Total nitrogen, and Total phosphor can be monitored with IoT or remote sensing.
12. So far, a generalized WQ predictive model has not been built as evidenced by the literature survey.

19.8 CONCLUSION

This chapter focused on water quality analysis of water bodies, especially river water, to identify the environmental pollution caused by industries, villages, and cities. This chapter outlined the recent technological advancements to automatically monitor the WQ, avoiding the manual sample collection process. The technologically advanced IoT sensors and remote sensing-based deep learning methodology are explained clearly in the chapter with references from the literature. The research gaps to be addressed and the advancements required in the future to save our water resources from environmental pollution are detailed so that they will form a basis for WQ researchers.

REFERENCES

[1] B. Das, P.C. Jain, "Real-time water quality monitoring system using Internet of Things," *Proc. Int. Conf. on Computer, Communications and Electronics (Comptelix)*, pp. 78–82, 2017, doi: 10.1109/comptelix.2017.8003942

[2] A.G. Adeniyi, J.O. Ighalo, "Biosorption of pollutants by plant leaves: An empirical review," *Journal of Environmental Chemical Engineering*, vol. 7, pp. 1–33, 2019, doi: 10.1016/j.jece.2019.103100

[3] J.O. Ighalo, A.G. Adeniyi, "Mitigation of diclofenac pollution in aqueous media by adsorption," *ChemBioEng Reviews*, vol. 7, pp. 50–64, 2020, doi: 10.1002/cben.201900020

[4] X. Su, G. Shao, J. Vause, L. Tang, "An integrated system for urban environmental monitoring and management based on the environmental internet of things," *International Journal of Sustainable Development & World Ecology*, vol. 20, pp. 205–209, 2013, doi: 10.1080/13504509.2013.782580

[5] A.D. Sutadian, N. Muttil, A.G. Yilmaz, B.J.C. Perera, "Development of river water quality indices - A review," *Environmental Monitoring and Assessment*, vol. 188, pp. 1–29, 2016, doi: 10.1007/s10661-015-5050-0

[6] F. Toran, D. Ramırez, A.E. Navarro, S. Casans, J. Pelegrı, J.M. Espı, "Design of a virtual instrument for water quality monitoring across the internet," *Sensors and Actuators B: Chemical*, vol. 76, pp. 281–285, 2001, doi: 10.1016/S0925-4005(01)00584-6

[7] R.G. Lathrop Jr., L. Auermuller, S. Haag, W. Im, "The stormwater management and planning tool: Coastal water quality enhancement through the use of an internet-based geospatial tool," *Coastal Management*, vol. 40, pp. 339–354, 2012, doi: 10.1080/08920753.2012.692309

[8] J.H. Hoover, P.C. Sutton, S. J. Anderson, A.C. Keller, "Designing and evaluating a groundwater quality internet GIS," *Applied Geography*, vol. 53, pp. 55–65, 2014, doi: 10.1016/j.apgeog.2014.06.005

[9] F. Toran, D. Ramirez, S. Casans, A. E. Navarro, J. Pelegri, "Distributed virtual instrument for water quality monitoring across the internet," *Proceedings of the 17th IEEE Instrumentation and Measurement Technology Conference*, vol. 2, pp. 652–656, 2000, doi: 10.1109/IMTC.2000.848817

[10] B. Arabi, M.S. Salama, J. Pitarch, W. Verhoef, "Integration of in-situ and multi-sensor satellite observations for long-term water quality monitoring in coastal areas," *Remote Sensing of Environment*, vol. 239, pp. 111632, 2020, doi:10.1016/j.rse.2020.111632
[11] F. Gohin, D. van der Zande, G. Tilstone, M.A. Eleveld, A. Lefebvre, F. Andrieux-Loyer, A.N. Blauw, P. Bryere, D. Devreker, P. Garnesson, T. Hernandez Farinas, Y. Lamaury, L. Lampert, H. Lavigne, F. Menet-Nedelec, S. Pardo, B. Saulquin, "Twenty years of satellite and in situ observations of surface chlorophyll-a from the northern Bay of Biscay to the eastern English Channel. Is the water quality improving?" *Remote Sensing of Environment*, vol. 233, pp. 111343, 2019, doi: 10.1016/j. rse.2019.111343
[12] Z.L. Na, H.M. Yao, H.Q. Chen, Y.M. Wei, K. Wen, Y. Huang, P.R. Liao, "Retrieval and evaluation of chlorophyll-A spatiotemporal variability using GF-1 imagery: Case study of Qinzhou Bay, China," *Sustainability*, vol. 13, pp. 4649, 2021, doi: 10.3390/su13094649
[13] J. Qun'ou, X. Lidan, S. Siyang, W. Meilin, X. Huijie, "Retrieval model for total nitrogen concentration based on UAV hyperspectral remote sensing data and machine learning algorithms – A case study in the Miyun Reservoir. China," *Ecological Indicators*, vol. 124, pp. 107356, 2021, doi: 10.1016/j.ecolind.2021.107356
[14] S. Lu, R. Deng, Y. Liang, L. Xiong, X. Ai, Y. Qin, "Remote sensing retrieval of total phosphorus in the pearl river channels based on the GF-1 remote sensing data," *Remote Sensing (Basel)*, vol. 12, pp. 1420, 2020, doi: 10.3390/RS12091420
[15] G. Dong, Z. Hu, X. Liu, Y. Fu, W. Zhang, "Spatio-temporal variation of total nitrogen and ammonia nitrogen in the water source of the middle route of the south-to-north water diversion project," *Water (Basel)*, vol. 12, pp. 2615, 2020, doi: 10.3390/w12092615
[16] J. Xu, C. Gao, Y. Wang, "Extraction of spatial and temporal patterns of concentrations of Chlorophyll-a and total suspended matter in poyang lake using GF-1 satellite data," *Remote Sensing (Basel)*, 12, 622, 2020, doi: 10.3390/rs12040622
[17] M. Papenfus, B. Schaeffer, A.I. Pollard, K. Loftin, "Exploring the potential value of satellite remote sensing to monitor chlorophyll-a for US lakes and reservoirs," *Environmental Monitoring and Assessment*, vol. 192, pp. 808, 2020, doi: 10.1007/s10661-020-08631-5
[18] S. Wang, J. Li, B. Zhang, Z. Lee, E. Spyrakos, C. Feng Liu, H. Zhao, Y. Wu, L. Zhu, L. Jia, W. Wan, F. Zhang, Q. Shen, E.N. Tyler, X. Zhang, "Changes of water clarity in large lakes and reservoirs across china observed from long-term MODIS," *Remote Sensing of Environment*, vol. 247, pp. 111949, 2020, doi: 10.1016/j.rse.2020.111949
[19] X. Wang, Y. Deng, Y. Tuo, R. Cao, Z. Zhou, Y. Xiao, "Study on the temporal and spatial distribution of chlorophyll a in Erhai Lake based on multispectral data from environmental satellites," *Ecological Informatics*, vol. 61, pp. 1574–9541, 2021, doi: 10.1016/j. ecoinf.2020.101201
[20] M. Saberioon, J. Brom, V. Nedbal, P. Souc˘ek, P. Cısar, "Chlorophyll-a and total suspended solids retrieval and mapping using Sentinel-2A and machine learning for inland waters," *Ecological Indicators*, vol. 113, pp. 106236, 2020, doi: 10.1016/j. ecolind.2020.10623
[21] E. Fantin Irudaya Raj, A. Mangalraj, "Smart water management system powered by the Internet of Things (IoT) for real-world applications." *In Internet of Things*, pp. 129–142, 2023.
[22] V. Sagan, K.T. Peterson, M. Maimaitijiang, P. Sidike, J. Sloan, B.A. Greeling, S. Maalouf, C. Adams, "Monitoring inland water quality using remote sensing: Potential and limitations of spectral indices, bio-optical simulations, machine learning, and cloud computing," *Earth Science Reviews*, vol. 205, pp. 103187, 2020, doi: 10.1016/j. earscirev.2020.103187
[23] B. Chen, X. Mu, P. Chen, B. Wang, J. Choi, H. Park, S. Xu, Y. Wu, H. Yang, "Machine learning-based inversion of water quality parameters in typical reach of the urban river by UAV multispectral data," *Ecological Indicators*, vol. 133, pp. 108434, 2021, doi: 10.1016/j.ecolind.2021.108434

[24] J. Pyo, S.M. Hong, J. Jang, S. Park, J. Park, J.H. Noh, K.H. Cho, "Drone-borne sensing of major and accessory pigments in algae using deep learning modelling," *GIscience and Remote Sensing*, vol. 59, pp. 310–332, 2022, doi: 10.1080/15481603.2022.2027120

[25] L. Wei, Z. Wang, C. Huang, Y. Zhang, Z. Wang, H. Xia, L. Cao, "Transparency estimation of narrow rivers by UAV-borne hyperspectral remote sensing imagery," *IEEE Access*, vol. 8, pp. 168137–168153, 2020, doi: 10.1109/ACCESS.2020.3023690

[26] E. Mantzouki, J. Campbell, E. Van Loon, P. Visser, I. Konstantinou, M. Antoniou, G. Gregory, A.G. Bravo, "A European multi lake survey dataset of environmental variables, phytoplankton pigments and cyanotoxins," *Scientific Data*, vol. 5, pp. 1–13, 2018, doi: 10.1038/sdata.2018.226

[27] B.A. Stauffer Matsoukis, H.A. Bowers, E. Buckley, T.W. Davis, T.H. Johengen, R. Kudela, H. Purcell, G.J. Smith, A.V. Woude, M.N. Tamburri, "Considerations in harmful algal bloom research and monitoring: Perspectives from a consensus-building workshop and technology testing," *Frontiers in Marine Science*, vol. 6, pp. 399, 2019, doi.10.3389/fmars.2019.00399

[28] G.G.K.W.M.S.I.R. Karunarathne, K.A.D.T. Kulawansa, M.F.M. Firdhous, "Wireless communication technologies in internet of things: A critical evaluation," *2018 International Conference on Intelligent and Innovative Computing Applications (ICONIC)*, pp. 1–5, 2018, doi: 10.1109/ICONIC.2018.8601226

[29] M.Z. Chowdhury, M. Shahjalal, M.K. Hasan, Y.M. Jang, "The role of optical wireless communication technologies in 5G/6G and IoT solutions: Prospects, directions, and challenges," *Applied Sciences*, vol. 9, pp. 4367, 2019, doi: 10.3390/app9204367

[30] D.R. Mishra, A. Kumar, L. Ramaswamy, V.K. Boddula, M.C. Das, B.P. Page, S.J. Weber, "CyanoTRACKER: A cloud-based integrated multi-platform architecture for global observation of cyanobacterial harmful algal blooms," *Harmful Algae*, vol. 96, pp. 101828, 2020, doi: 10.1016/j.hal.2020.101828

[31] J. Yang, A. Holbach, A. Wilhelms, Y. Qin, B. Zheng, H. Zou, G. B. Qin, Zhu, S. Norra, "Highly time-resolved analysis of seasonal water dynamics and algal kinetics based on in-situ multi-sensor-system monitoring data in Lake Taihu, China," *Science of the Total Environment*, vol. 660, pp. 329–339, 2019, doi: 10.1016/j.scitotenv.2019.01.044

[32] E. Batur, D. Maktav, "Assessment of surface water quality by using satellite images fusion based on PCA method in the Lake Gala, Turkey," *IEEE Transactions on Geoscience and Remote Sensing*, vol. 57, pp. 2983–2989, 2019, doi: 10.1109/TGRS.2018.2879024

[33] M. Masocha, T. Dube, T. Nhiwatiwa, D. Choruma, "Testing utility of Landsat 8 for remote assessment of water quality in two subtropical African reservoirs with contrasting trophic states," *Geocarto International*, vol. 33, pp. 667–680, 2018, doi: 10.1080/10106049.2017.1289561

[34] K.T. Peterson, V. Sagan, J.J. Sloan, "Deep learning-based water quality estimation and anomaly detection using Landsat-8/Sentinel-2 virtual constellation and cloud computing," *GIScience & Remote Sensing*, vol. 57, pp. 510–525, 2020, doi: 10.1080/15481603.2020.1738061

[35] Z. Lee, S. Shang, L. Qi, J. Yan, G. Lin, "A semi-analytical scheme to estimate Secchi-disk depth from Landsat-8 measurements," *Remote Sensing of Environment*, vol. 177, pp. 101–106, 2016, doi: 10.1016/j.rse.2016.02.033

[36] M. Govedarica, G. Jakovljevic, "Monitoring spatial and temporal variation of water quality parameters using time series of open multispectral data," *Proceedings of 7th International Conference Remote Sensing on Geoinformation of the Environment (RSCy2019)*, vol. 11174, pp. 298–307, 2019, doi: 10.1117/12.2533708

[37] K. Ismail, A. Boudhar, A. Abdelkrim, H. Mohammed, S. Mouatassime, A. Kamal, E. Driss, E. Idrissi, W. Nouaim, "Evaluating the potential of Sentinel-2 satellite images for water quality characterization of artificial reservoirs: The Bin El Ouidane Reservoir

case study (Morocco)," Meteorology Hydrology and Water Management. *Research and Operational Applications*, vol. 7, pp. 31–39, 2019, doi: 10.26491/mhwm/95087
[38] P.L. Brezonik, L.G. Olmanson, J.C. Finlay, M.E. Bauer, "Factors affecting the measurement of CDOM by remote sensing of optically complex inland waters," *Remote Sensing of Environment*, vol. 157, pp. 199–215, 2015, doi: 10.1016/j.rse.2014.04.033
[39] N.T.T. Ha, N.T.P. Thao, K. Koike, M.T. Nhuan, "Selecting the best band ratio to estimate chlorophyll-A concentration in a tropical freshwater lake using sentinel 2A images from a case study of lake babe (Northern Vietnam)," *ISPRS International Journal of Geo-Infermation*, vol. 6, pp. 290, 2017, doi: 10.3390/ijgi6090290
[40] W.G. Buma, S. Il Lee, "Evaluation of Sentinel-2 and Landsat 8 images for estimating chlorophyll-A concentrations in Lake Chad, Africa," *Remote Sensing*, vol. 12, pp. 2437, 2020, doi: 10.3390/rs12152437
[41] G. Hassan, M.E. Goher, M.E. Shaheen S.A. Taie, "Hybrid predictive model for water quality monitoring based on sentinel-2A L1C data," *IEEE Access*, vol. 9, pp. 65730–65749, 2021, doi: 10.1109/ACCESS.2021.3075849
[42] Y. Zhang, R. Ma, H. Duan, S. Loiselle, M. Zhang, J. Xu, "A novel MODIS algorithm to estimate chlorophyll a concentration in eutrophic turbid lakes," *Ecological Indicators*, vol. 69, pp. 138–151, 2016, doi: 10.1016/j.ecolind.2016.04.020
[43] J. Li, Y. Zhang, R. Ma, H. Duan, S. Loiselle, K. Xue, Q. Liang, "Satellite-based estimation of column-integrated algal biomass in nonalgae Bloom conditions: A case study of Lake Chaohu, China," *IEEE Journal of Selected Topics in Applied Earth Observations and Remote Sensing*, vol. 10, pp. 450–462, 2017, doi: 10.1109/JSTARS.2016.2601083
[44] J. Morón-López, M.C. Rodríguez-Sánchez, F. Carreño, J. Vaquero, A.G. Pompa-Pernía, M. Mateos-Fernández, J.A.P. Aguilar, "Implementation of smart buoys and satellite-based systems for the remote monitoring of harmful algae bloom in Inland Waters," *IEEE Sensors Journal*, vol. 21, pp. 6990–6997, 2021, doi: 10.1109/JSEN.2020.3040139
[45] D. Li, Z. Yang, Z. Zhu, M. Guo, W. Gao, Z. Sun, "Estimating the distribution of suspended sediment concentration in submerged vegetation flow based on gravitational theory," *Journal of Hydrology*, vol. 587, 2020, doi: 10.1016/j.jhydrol.2020.124921
[46] C.K.F. Lee, E. Nicholson, C. Duncan, N.J. Murray, "Estimating changes and trends in ecosystem extent with dense time-series satellite remote sensing," *Conservation Biology*, vol. 35, pp. 325–335, 2021, doi: 10.1111/cobi.13520
[47] J. Morón-López, M.C. Rodríguez-Sánchez, F. Carreño, J. Vaquero, A.G. Pompa-Pernía, M. Mateos-Fernández, J.A.P. Aguilar, "Implementation of smart buoys and satellite-based systems for the remote monitoring of harmful algae bloom in Inland Waters," *IEEE Sensors Journal*, vol. 21, pp. 6990–6997, 2020, doi: 10.1109/JSEN.2020.3040139
[48] N.A.P. Rostam, N.H.A.H. Malim, R. Abdullah, A.L. Ahmad, B.S. Ooi, D.J.C. Chan, "A complete proposed framework for coastal water quality monitoring system with algae predictive model," *IEEE Access*, vol. 9, pp. 108249–108265, 2021, doi: 10.1109/ACCESS.2021.3102044
[49] L. Kuang, P. Shi, C. Hua, B. Chen H. Zhu, "An enhanced extreme learning machine for dissolved oxygen prediction in wireless sensor networks," *IEEE Access*, vol. 8, pp. 198730–198739, 2020, doi: 10.1109/ACCESS.2020.3033455
[50] L. Manjakkal, S. Mitra, Y.R. Petillot, J. Shutler, E.M. Scott, M. Willander, R. Dahiya, "Connected sensors, innovative sensor deployment, and intelligent data analysis for online water quality monitoring," *IEEE Internet of Things Journal*, vol. 8, pp. 13805–13824, 2021, doi: 10.1109/JIOT.2021.3081772
[51] S.O. Olatinwo, T.-H. Joubert, "Enabling communication networks for water quality monitoring applications: A survey," *IEEE Access*, vol. 7, pp. 100332–100362, 2019, doi: 10.1109/ACCESS.2019.2904945

[52] M. Zeng, J. Peng, L. Jiang, J. Feng, "Temporal and spatial distribution of suspended sediment concentration in lakes based on satellite remote sensing and Internet of Things," *IEEE Access*, vol. 9, pp. 87849–87856, 2021, doi: 10.1109/ACCESS.2021.3089367
[53] R. Doerffer, P. Goryl, C. Brockmann, L. Bourg, "Algorithm Theoretical Bases Document (ATBD) for L2 processing of MERIS data of case 2 waters, 4th reprocessing," *Rapport Technique*, vol. 2, 2015.
[54] I.Y. Yeo, M. Lang, E. Vermote, "Improved Understanding of Suspended Sediment Transport Process Using Multi-Temporal Landsat Data: A Case Study from the Old Woman Creek Estuary (Ohio)," *IEEE Journal of Selected Topics in Applied Earth Observations and Remote Sensing*, vol. 7, pp. 636–647, 2014, doi: 10.1109/JSTARS.2013.2265191
[55] H.J. Nasiha, P. Shanmugam, "Estimating the bulk refractive index and related particulate properties of natural waters from remote-sensing data," *IEEE Journal of Selected Topics in Applied Earth Observations and Remote Sensing*, vol. 8, pp. 5324–5335, 2015, doi: 10.1109/JSTARS.2015.2439581
[56] Y. Li, C. Li, X. Li, "Remote sensing studies of suspended sediment concentration variations in a Coastal Bay during the passages of atmospheric cold fronts," *IEEE Journal of Selected Topics in Applied Earth Observations and Remote Sensing*, vol. 10, pp. 2608–2622, 2017, doi: 10.1109/JSTARS.2017.2655421
[57] X. Chen, L. Liu, X. Zhang, S. Xie, L. Lei, "A novel water change tracking algorithm for dynamic mapping of Inland water using time-series remote sensing imagery," *IEEE Journal of Selected Topics in Applied Earth Observations and Remote Sensing*, vol. 13, pp. 1661–1674, 2020, doi: 10.1109/JSTARS.2020. 2983729
[58] A.Y. Sun, B.R. Scanlon, "How can Big Data and machine learning benefit environment and water management: A survey of methods, applications, and future directions," *Environmental Research Letters*, vol. 14, pp. 073001, 2019, doi: 10.1088/1748-9326/ab1b7d
[59] P. Tahmasebi, S. Kamrava, T. Bai, M. Sahimi, "Machine learning in geo-and environmental sciences: From small to large scale," *Advances in Water Resources*, vol. 142, pp. 103619, 2020, doi: 10.1016/j.advwatres.2020.103619
[60] D. Ghai, S. L. Tripathi, S. Saxena, M. Chanda, M. Alazab, *Machine Learning Algorithms for Signal and Image Processing*, John Wiley & Sons, 2022.
[61] V. K. A. Somayajula, D. Ghai, S. Kumar, "Land Use/Land Cover Change Analysis using NDVI, PCA," In *2021 5th IEEE International Conference on Computing Methodologies and Communication*, pp. 849–855, 2021.
[62] V. K. A. Somayajula, D. Ghai, S. Kumar, S.L. Tripathi, C. Verma, C.O. Safirescu, T.C. Mihaltan, "Classification and validation of spatio-temporal changes in land use/land cover and land surface temperature of multitemporal images," *Sustainability*, vol. 14, no. 23, pp. 15677, 2022.
[63] C. Jayaram, G. Patidar, D. Swain, V.M. Chowdary, S. Bandyopadhyay, "Total suspended matter distribution in the Hooghly River Estuary and the Sundarbans: A remote sensing approach," *IEEE Journal of Selected Topics in Applied Earth Observations and Remote Sensing*, vol. 14, pp. 9064–9070, 2021, doi: 10.1109/JSTARS.2021.3076104
[64] S. Mohan Kumar, V. Geethalakshmi, S. Ramanathan, A. Senthil, K. Senthilraja, K. Bhuvaneswari, R. Gowtham, B. Kannan, S. Priyanka, "Action plan on rejuvenation of river Thamirabarani Pappankulam to Arumuganeri Stretch," *Tamilnadu Pollution Control Board, Sustainability*, vol. 14, pp. 14948, 2022, doi: 10.3390/su142214948

20 Less Complex U-Net (LCU-Net)

A Segmentation Module in Artificial Intelligence-Based Prediction Model of Breast Cancer

Mayank Kumar Singh, Indu Saini, and Neetu Sood
Dr B R Ambedkar National Institute of Technology, Jalandhar, India

20.1 INTRODUCTION

Artificial Intelligence (AI) has revolutionized the concept of automation in disease diagnosis [1]. With automated diagnosis [2, 3], we can have a system that is easily accessible, robust, free from human error, and sustainable. Designing a sustainable automated diagnosis system is a challenging task. Due to the sensitivity of the task, reliability becomes an essential factor [4]. The system must have the perfect accuracy for practice in real life. The diagnosis accuracy of the system depends upon the segmentation accuracy of the region of interest [5]. Large-scale research is being conducted around the globe to enhance the accuracy of segmentation [2, 6, 7]. Nowadays, almost every research involves the Convolutional Neural Network (CNN) instead of the classical segmentation techniques [8–10]. Because the classical techniques rely on a limited range of local features, CNN can extract a broader range of features independently and with better accuracy simultaneously. U-Net [11–13] is the most famous architecture of CNN used for segmentation. It uses cascaded encoder and decoder blocks with skip connections [14]. They can learn features of every scale because of the information sharing between layers. So, we have adopted a U-Net-based approach for our task. However, choosing the image to design the automated system is tricky.

Non-invasive image-based diagnosis is the most recommended method of diagnosis. It has been practiced for many diseases for quite some time. Today, almost every primary treatment is planned and done after observing the diagnostic images. There are multiple options for diagnosis like the X-ray [15], Ultrasound (UD) [16], Magnetic

DOI: 10.1201/9781003546382-20

Resonance Imaging (MRI) [17], and Computed Tomography (CT) scan [18]. They all involve unique radiation frequencies, hence different sets of transducers and diagnosis procedures. They all have unique advantages and characteristics; some are organ-specific. Although UD images are deficient [19], they are used far more than others. It can be used for any organ and any disease. It is because of its harmless radiation and most straightforward procedure. The level of radiation used in other diagnosis techniques harms humans [20]. That is why no one is allowed to have frequent exposure to them. Despite having a high-resolution output, they are always second to the UD. The transducer used for UD is the smallest device with the generator and receptor integrated into a single hand-held device [21]. For these reasons, UD is the only option to develop a sustainable system. The distortions in the UD have a granular structure [22], clearly visible in the image. The gradients of these structures are sometimes strong enough to suppress the gradient of nearby edges. Almost every image segmentation technique, one way or another, relies on these spatial gradients, so their output is highly affected by the distortion. Generally, the distortions are present in a large number around the true edges. It becomes nearly impossible for the segmentation technique to find the actual edges. A skilled expert can, however, quickly point out the true boundary, and their judgment is negligibly affected by the distortions because they search for patterns instead of local gradients. The tumors or any other structure in the UD have a unique pattern, which is expected of its class. No one can beat the efficiency of CNN in learning a pattern [23–25]. This is another reason why nearly every ongoing research in the automation field involves CNN.

The complexity of a model is a function of its depth. The deeper the network and the more the blocks count, the higher the complexity. Complex networks are instrumental in learning a complex task, such as the segmentation in noisy UD images. The only problem associated with the complex network is the high computation memory and data requirements. These parameters reduce the sustainability of the system. A shallow network can only learn a part of the task with marginal accuracy. However, the accuracy can be improved using a creative learning paradigm and an efficient pre-processing technique. Moreover, a new training paradigm is required because no large UD dataset is available to train and test a complex network. In this study, we have proposed a tumor segmentation technique using a Less Complex U-Net (LCU-Net) architecture. The LCU-Net learns to segment the tumor in the breast UD. We tested a unique learning paradigm using the skin cancer ISIC dataset [12, 23, 26, 27] in the study. The paradigm is designed to overcome the difference between the distribution of skin lesion images and a UD. The UD images are also processed uniquely before training of the LCU-Net. The efficacy of the proposed learning paradigm was validated with a large public dataset.

20.1.1 Research Highlights

Following are the highlights of the novelty of this chapter:

- A brief introduction to the recent U-Net network proposed for the segmentation of UD images.
- Unique training methodology to counter the data requirement of a deep network.

- Chain of processing steps for skin lesion images to train a network for breast UD image.
- The performance level of deep networks was dominated using a comparatively shallow network.

20.1.2 Chapter Organization

The chapter is organized as follows: Section 20.2 briefly discusses conventional segmentation techniques and learning-based segmentation techniques. Section 20.3 titled "Proposed Methodology," explains the processing of skin lesions and UD images in detail. In the same section, the architecture of the proposed LCU-Net is explained. The following section has more details regarding the image dataset used. Results and discussion are provided in Section 20.4, and our work is concluded in Section 20.5.

20.2 SEGMENTATION TECHNIQUES

20.2.1 Conventional Techniques

Conventional techniques like active contour, superpixel, graph cut, and thresholding have been used for segmentation in UD for decades [9, 18, 28, 29]. The thresholding technique is one of the premier techniques used for segmentation. A threshold value is obtained, minimizing each side's variance [30]. The technique is quite effective for identifying the foreground from the background. In the case of the UD image, the intensity histogram is majorly confined to a small range of dark intensities. Due to this narrow range of intensities, obtaining a threshold that can differentiate structures from their background is impossible. The noises in the UD also tend to misguide the threshold calculation. Superpixels, clusters of neighboring pixels, have proven useful in segmenting multiple diagnostic images [10]. Their application has also been extended to UD image segmentation [28]. In the initially proposed superpixel, the clusters were defined using iterative clustering of pixels based on their distance from the cluster center. Two distance parameters were defined: the spatial distance from the center and the intensity difference from the center. The distortion of the UD image makes it difficult to have a correct cluster center, and the technique is known for its over-segmentation output. It is most efficient if there are numerous objects in the image, but over-segmentation dominates images like UD. The graph cut algorithm converts the image into a graphical structure with nodes and connections. The pixels of the image become the nodes, and their relation with other pixels becomes the connections. The extent of correlation between the nodes decides the weight of the connection. Then, the algorithm toggles through the complete graph and keeps cutting the small weights. After removing the weak links, the image is divided into foreground and background. Some studies find this technique more efficient than thresholding [31].

Lesion Segmentation in a noisy environment still needs to be more efficient. Active contour, also known as the snake algorithm, is the most efficient among the conventional segmentation techniques. The boundary of a contour defined over the image is evolved to coincide with the underlying structure. The parameters that are used to evolve the boundaries are called force. Moreover, the forces are the interconnection of the boundary and the spatial gradients near the boundary. The evolution of the contour only stops when the forces stabilize each other, and the contour boundary becomes the segmentation output. The force equation and stopping condition of the contour evolution were the prime focus of the researchers. They believed that an ultimate segmentation could be achieved with a good combination. All these spatial techniques are used to dominate the field of segmentation. They were easy and effective in most of the cases. Nevertheless, they could have been more efficient in tackling distortions in the image. The requirement of user initialization has always been the bottleneck in their application. A fully automated system cannot be built using these semi-automatic techniques. So, they were quickly replaced by the learning-based techniques. The efficiency of CNN has completely overshadowed these conventional techniques [32].

20.2.2 Learning-Based Techniques

Recent years have seen exponential advancement in network architecture and ways of learning. Initial architectures like VGG-16 [33] proposed for classification on the Imagenet dataset started a revolution. Researchers started designing deeper linear networks in a structure like VGG-19 and AlexNet [34]. The concept was that building more profound architectures can improve efficiency. However, everything changed after a paper introduced residual connection [35]. The paper proved that there are better solutions than the increasing depth. The innovative idea of residual connection in a small network beats the deeper network in any task. Moreover, with time, different layers, connections, and training were introduced. Architectures like DenseNet had many layers interconnected using a web of skip connections [7, 36–38], which opened the pathway for many possibilities. Testing these technologies with unique combinations is quite famous among researchers.

The U-Net introduced [39] is now used primarily for segmentation tasks. It has a U-shaped architecture, a path connecting different types of blocks. The left half of the U-Net is called the encoder path, and the other is called the decoder. The input is provided to the encoder, which, after a series of convolution and pooling down samples to linear data. The data is then received by two fully connected layers and sent to the decoder. The decoder has multiple up-sampling blocks and convolution layers, which rebuild the resolution and have the segmentation output. The network learns a pixel-level classification, that is, classifying the pixels as boundary pixels. It is the fundamental architecture of the U-Net, which has evolved with time as per requirement. The paper [40] used a Neural Architecture Search network (NAS-net) concept to design its U-Net. The NAS-net is a state-of-the-art network used to engineer the best architecture for blocks in the CNN. The NAS-Net keeps the basic architecture intact, which was selected as the U-Net. The output network was comparatively more efficient than a regular CNN and had fewer coefficients. Residual Inception Channel Attention U-Net (RICU-Net) in [41] combines the attention mechanism and the inception module with the U-Net. The inception module lifts the filter size constraints, giving the network an architectural advantage. The study designed two different types of blocks to replace the convolution layer [42]. The encoder and decoder path introduced Ri and DC blocks, respectively. It achieved 80.80 Dice Similarity Coefficient (DSC) and 54.62 Jaccard Similarity Coefficient (JSC) on the Cancer Genomic Atlas dataset [43]. The U-Net has also successfully segmented the 2D and volumetric images [44]. To reduce the complexity of 3D architecture, fusion blocks are used to fuse the information of various slices. A single encoder path for each slice was used to extract information, but a single decoder path was used for the final output. The architecture needed to be simplified, and the encoder's coefficient evolution became tough to design due to multiple encoders. The Hierarchical Attention-Guided U-Net (HAU-Net) introduced in [45] incorporated transformer block. The transformer block enables the network ability to search for larger patterns. Attention blocks were added to increase the information sharing in the decoder path. ConvMixer, which uses depth-wise convolution and point-wise convolution, was used with DenseNet121. The study has two outputs: one is the classification score, and the second is a map for lesion detection. The outputs were combined for the final output. TBU-Net in [46] took the multilevel fusion concept to another level by combining the output of three blocks. The blocks were the high-frequency, low-frequency, and boundary extraction blocks. The boundary extraction block receives inputs from a U-Net, while the convolved output of the image is received as input to the low and high-frequency block. Another feature extraction block was added in skip connection to improve the information sharing between the encoder and decoder path. To reduce the number of parameters, the study in [47] used a G-S block in U-Net architecture. A Multi-Layer Perceptron (MLP) [48] block was added at the bottom of the network. The G-S block has a ghost module in combination with the SE module. A ghost block contains a couple of convolution blocks, and the SE block has a couple of fully connected layers. The features generated by the ghost blocks were arranged as tokens in the MLP training. The tokens of feature [49, 50] maps were shifted in both directions in height and depth. The network uses a unique block in the skip connection and names it as a ghost path. To further enhance the efficacy of the U-Net [51], it was proposed to connect the outputs of each encoder block to the fully connected block. The network was named Dynamic Hierarchical Multi-Scale (DHMS) fusion network. A unique fusion block with a multi-scale hierarchical structure was introduced. Very similar tokenized MPL blocks were used in the U-Net architecture.

20.3 PROPOSED METHODOLOGY

The proposed network is applied to the breast UD to segment the tumor. UD images are first pre-processed for training the network. The ISIC dataset also undergoes processing before training. The network was trained in many phases using the ISIC and UD datasets. Instead of using a pre-trained network, we proposed our training series. The training process guides the LCU-Net in learning to segment in a noisy environment. Initially, the network was trained four times using the modified skin images. In the end, the network was trained using the processed UD image for the final segmentation task. The pre-processing steps and the network architectures are explained below in detail.

20.3.1 LCU-Net

The architecture of the proposed network is in Figure 20.1. It has nine blocks, including the input and output layers as individual blocks and the bottom layers as one. The blocks are represented as black boxes (dash outline), which include multiple layers of convolutional filters, activation, and pooling. The left half of the architecture, also known as the encoder, includes Convolution filters. Meanwhile, the right half of the decoder part also includes a strided deconvolution (some of the studies may call it a transposed convolution) filter. In between, we have used a flattening layer [52], a fully connected layer [53], and an up-sampling layer. In the encoder path, the second block right after the input layer has 64 convolution filters of size 128 × 128. Then, we have an activation layer that implements the Relu activation function to the inputs [54]. The activation layer is followed by a MaxPool layer [55], which reduces the resolution of its input. The third and fourth block has 64 convolution filters, but of size 64 × 64 and 32 × 32, respectively, the rest are the same. The output of the block is converted into a single dimension using the flattening layer and given to the fully connected layer. The reshaping layer transforms the previous layer's output into a shape of 16 × 16. The deconvolution filter (of size 32 × 32) is used to increase the resolution of the inputs. Here, the stride of the convolution filter was set to 1, while the stride for the deconvolution filter was set to 2. A single deconvolution filter was then followed by 64 convolution filters of size 32 × 32 and an activation layer.

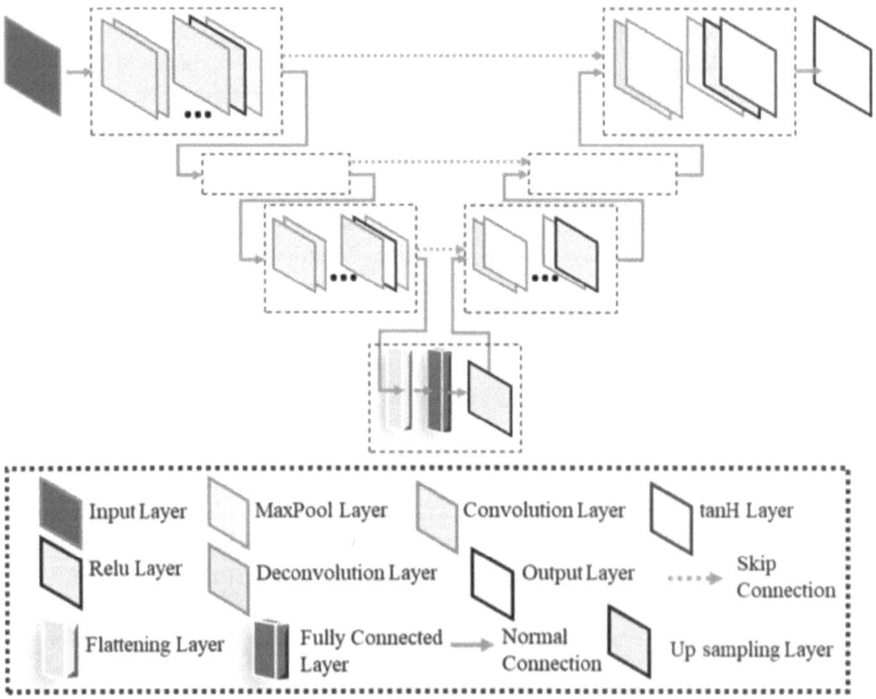

FIGURE 20.1 Proposed LCU-Net architecture.

The subsequent two blocks have the same pattern, only the size of the deconvolution filter becomes 32 × 32 and 64 × 64, and the convolution filter becomes 64 × 64 and 128 × 128. In the last decoder block, the output of the activation layer was passed through the tanh layer, and the output block is a convolution filter of size 1 × 1 × 3. The skip connections are concatenated with the inputs in the decoder path.

20.3.2 Pre-Processing of ISIC Dataset

The International Skin Imaging Collaboration (ISIC) is a famous dataset of skin lesions [56, 57]. It contains thousands of images of skin lesions of different classes of cancer. The dataset also contains the corresponding segmented masked images. We have used the dataset for the initial training of our U-Net. The images of the ISIC dataset were processed before the training procedure. First, the dataset was divided into training, testing, and validation groups. The images of each group were pre-processed, as given in Figure 20.2. The images were converted into a grayscale image. The first column of Figure 20.3 shows some sample images of the dataset, and the second column shows the corresponding grayscale image.

After the conversion, minimizing the difference between the intensity distribution of the obtained image and the UD images is needed. The distribution of the UD images was divided into two categories, namely, a Heavy Tail (HT) (Figure 20.4) and a Light Tail (LT) (Figure 20.5) distribution. A UD image with fewer high-intensity pixels was categorized as LT distribution and the rest as HT distribution. We considered integers between 0 and 255 as the range of intensity in a grayscale image, with 0 being the black and 255 being the white (as convention). For comparison, we calculated the total number of pixels having an intensity greater than 150 and empirically selected a threshold value. If the number of pixels is less than a threshold, then it is an LT distribution. Otherwise, it is HT. Then, we computed a unique average histogram for each HT (AHT) and LT (ALT) category (Figure 20.4(c) and Figure 20.5(c), respectively). The histograms of the converted skin images were then randomly matched to either ALT or AHT using the basic histogram matching technique. The last row of Figure 20.3 shows the output of histogram matching.

20.3.3 Pre-Training of LCU-Net

The next challenge is to train our LCU-Net such that the noise in UD images has a minor effect on its performance. To tackle the challenge, we used the concept of transfer learning and trained the network in different phases. After histogram matching, the images of the ISIC dataset were divided into four separate groups, the images of the first and the primary group were kept unchanged. Initially, we trained our network using this large dataset for skin lesion segmentation. Then, the second group of images was blurred using a zero-cantered Gaussian filter of variance 1 unit. The trained LCU-Net was again trained using these blurred images. In the third phase, the image group was corrupted using speckle noise. The fully-formed speckle, which has a Rayleigh-like distribution, was introduced in the image. Then, the LCU-Net undergoes another round of training to learn to segment lesions in the presence of speckle noise. In the end stage, the fourth group of images was used to train the

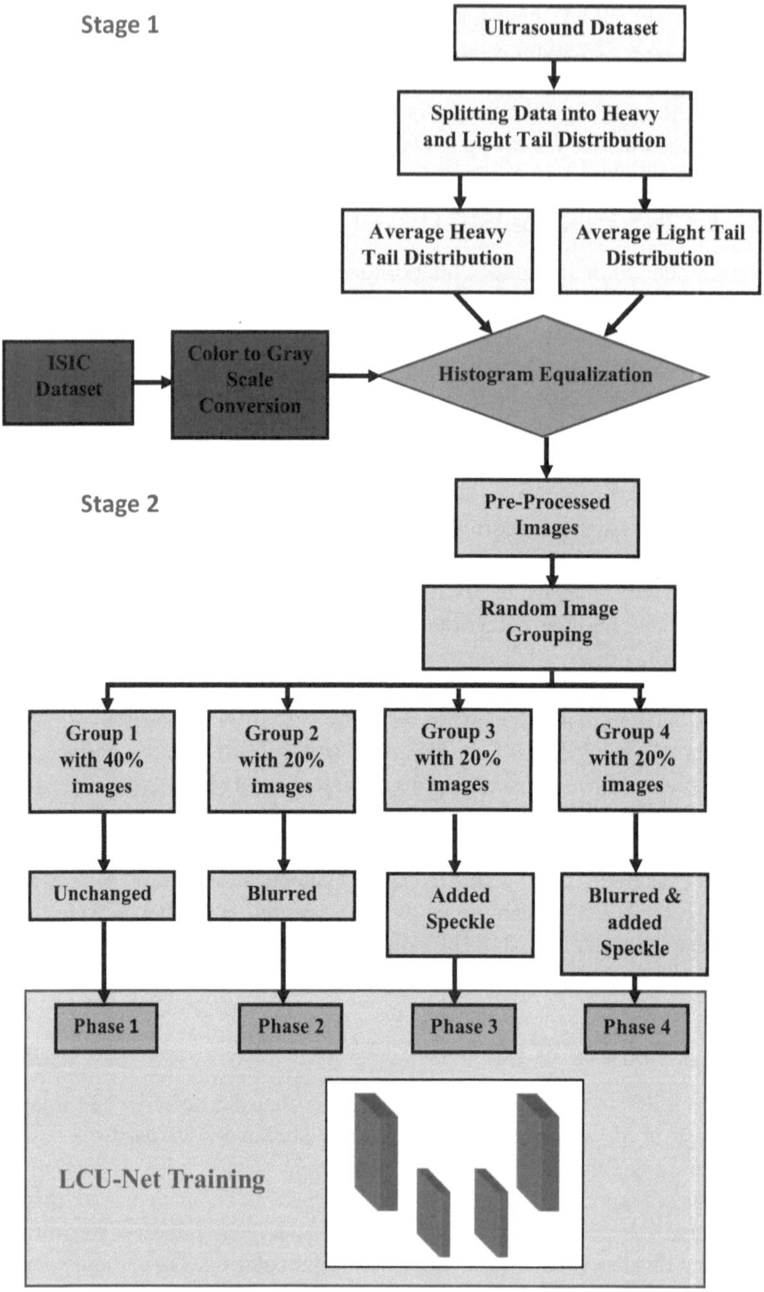

FIGURE 20.2 Flow diagram of pre-processing steps in skin image transformation and LCU-Net training.

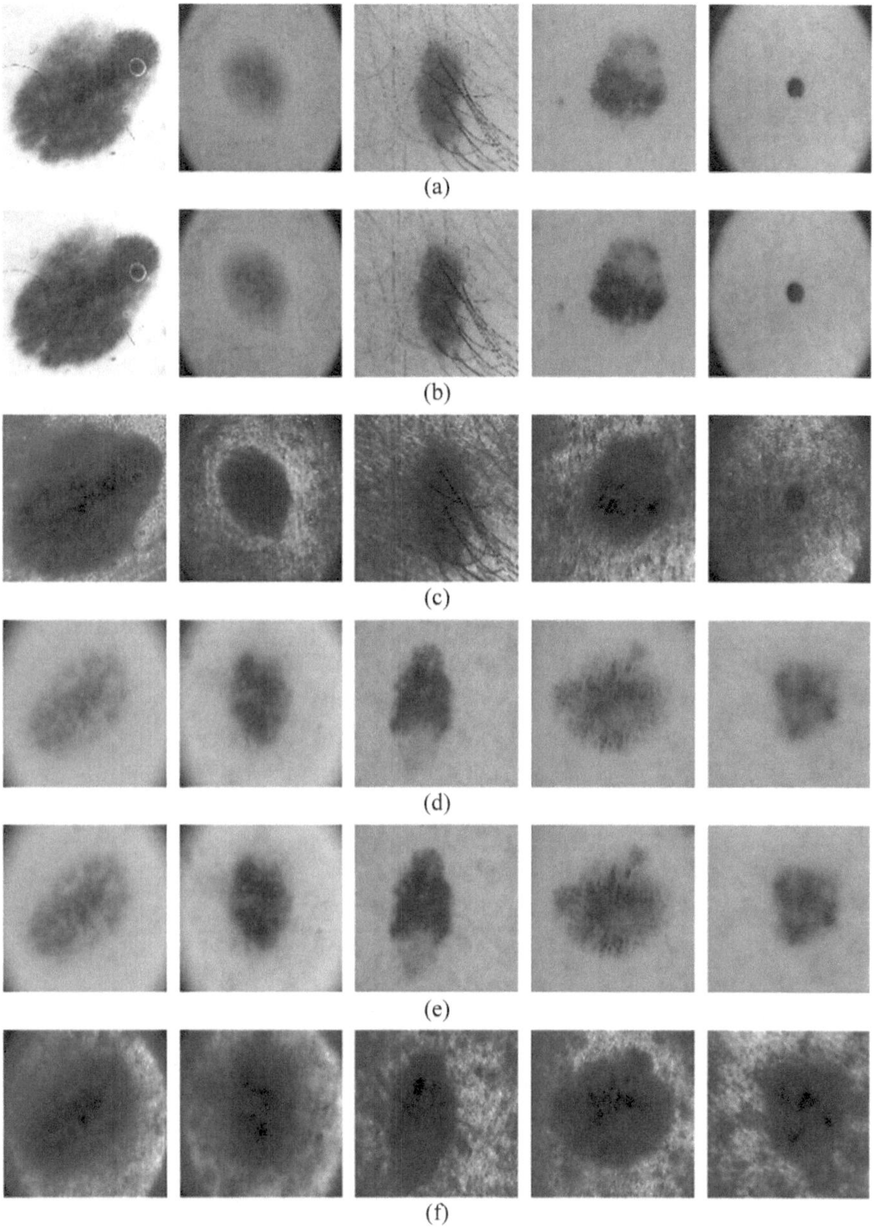

FIGURE 20.3 The grayscale converted images of (a) and (d) original ISIC images are in (b) and (e), respectively. The histogram matched the output of (a) and (d) in (c) and (f), respectively.

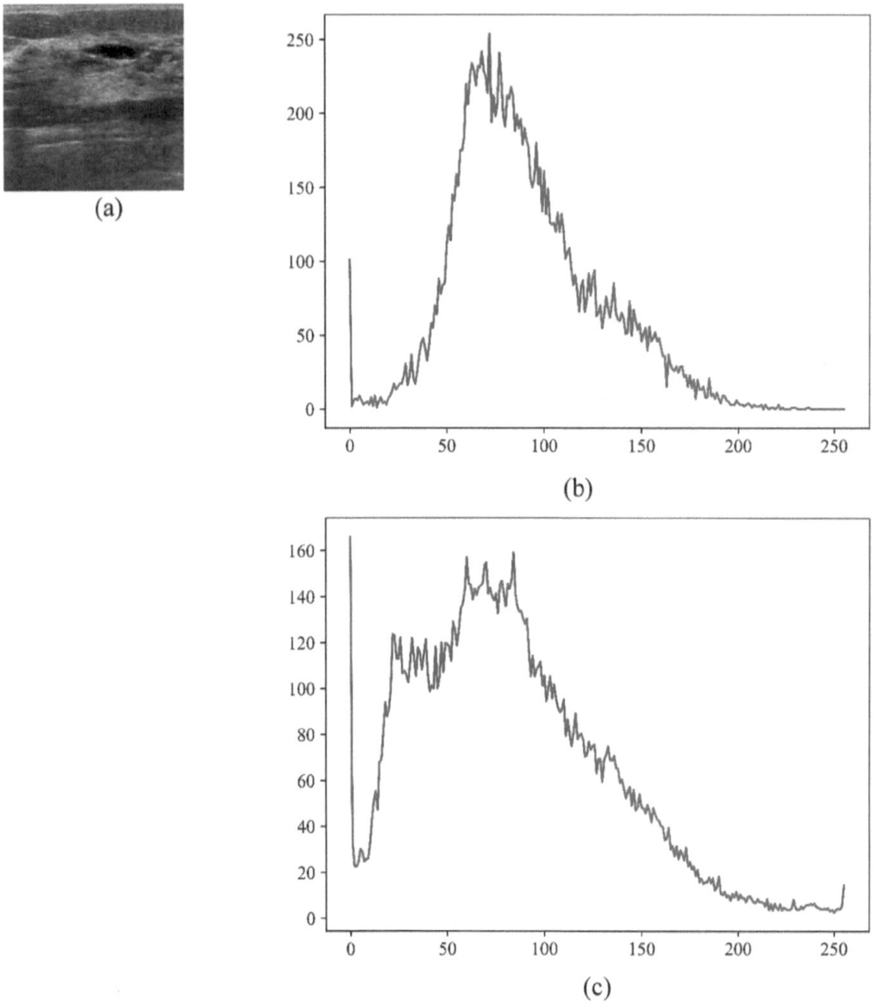

FIGURE 20.4 (a) A UD image with the histogram of (b) HT distribution type, and (c) the resultant AHT calculated across the dataset.

network obtained after individually training all the previous stages. Segmentation of the images of the fourth group is the toughest because the images of the fourth group were both blurred and corrupted by speckle noise. The pre-trained network learns to provide the most accurate segment in the worst-case scenario.

20.3.4 Pre-Processing of the UD Images

The distortions in the UD image pose a significant threat to the efficiency of the network. The distortions increase the intraclass variation, making the learning process very difficult. So, we have used a unique processing technique for UD before training

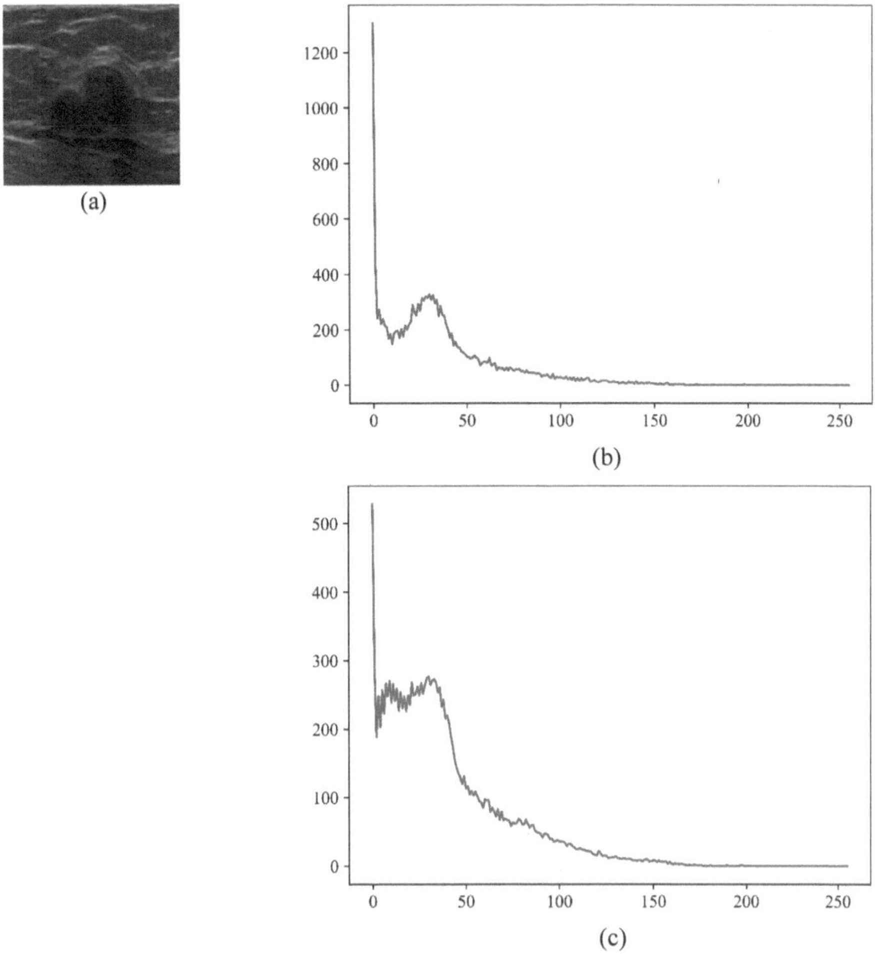

FIGURE 20.5 (a) A UD image with the histogram of (b) LT distribution type, and (c) the resultant ALT calculated across the dataset.

the network. The structures of noises in the UD are almost always granular, with intensity utterly different from the average intensity in its locality. The noises are observed to have a completely random structure, that is, no typical pattern. We have used this property of the noise to identify the corrupted pixels and then replace it with the average intensity of its 5 × 5 neighbors. To identify the corrupted pixels, we first calculated the first-order derivative of the image. A 3 × 3 differential filter, also known as the Sobel operator, was used. Then, we used a horizontally and vertically aligned differential filter pair to calculate the gradients in the respective direction. The horizontally aligned filter has the dimension of 3 × 7, and the vertically aligned filter has the dimension of 7 × 3. The combined output of the oriented filters will only have components with some associated pattern. The output of both filters was then subtracted from each other. The output of the subtraction will mostly have the distortion in the image. Their locations were identified, and the averaging operation suppressed the distortion.

20.4 RESULTS AND DISCUSSION

A large public dataset of UD is very rare to find. W. Al Dhabyani et al. in [58] provided a UD image dataset of female breasts. The dataset is famous for validating breast cancer classification or segmentation [59–62]. The dataset contains 780 images collected from breast cancer patients. It contains the masked output of each image. A medical expert outlined the mask image for the tumor. The expert-outlined boundaries are always considered the gold standard. To further increase image quantity and avoid overfitting, we applied image augmentation. After the augmentation [63], there were 3120 UD for training and testing our network. Another famous dataset used in our study is the ISIC [64]. The dataset was initially published as a challenge to design a classification module. The images are collected from various medical institutions for melanoma and non-melanoma cancers. We aim to use the data to train our network for segmentation, so the classification label is unimportant. Expert-outlined masked images are also provided with this dataset. We used the images of the ISIC from the years 2016, 2017, and 2018. Combined datasets of the challenges had 5873 images of skin lesions. We again applied the same image augmentation to the skin images and then had around 23,492 skin images. As mentioned in Figure 20.2, the data was divided into four groups. After the division, there were 9396 standard lesion images, 4698 blurred images, 4698 speckle images, and 4700 images both blurred and corrupted.

In this chapter, we implemented an automated segmentation technique in the UD image. The images of the ISIC dataset were processed prior to training the network. Figure 20.3 provides the output of the processing steps. The output in the third and last row explains why we have used the skin lesion dataset. After the histogram matching, the structure resembles the images of breast tumors in the UD image. The breast lesions also lie around the center portion of the UD image, with a unique shape. Some shapes of the lesion in the ISIC are close to a circle, some close to an ellipse [65], and the rest are random. That is precisely the case with the breast tumor. The boundaries of the breast tumor are also as vague as the skin lesions. Next, we introduced artificial noise in the skin images to mimic the noisy environment. Its training was divided into four phases to make the network efficient in a noisy environment. Some images were left unchanged for training and testing in each phase, and the rest were corrupted with different types of noises. The network was first trained to learn the segmentation of lesions in noise-free skin images. Then, the learning was shifted to segmenting a blurred boundary lesion. Next, the network's training targeted the boundaries corrupted by speckle noise (Figure 20.6). Ultimately, the network was trained and tested on images blurred and corrupted by speckles.

The segmentation accuracy at every testing phase is provided in Table 20.1. We used the Dice Similarity Coefficient (DSC) and Jaccard Similarity Coefficient (JSC) to judge the accuracy of segmentation. Details about the similarity coefficient and their calculation are given in the studies [66–70]. The Dice and Jaccard coefficients for the first, second, third, and fourth phases are 91.34, 84.05,89.26, 80.60, 89.10,

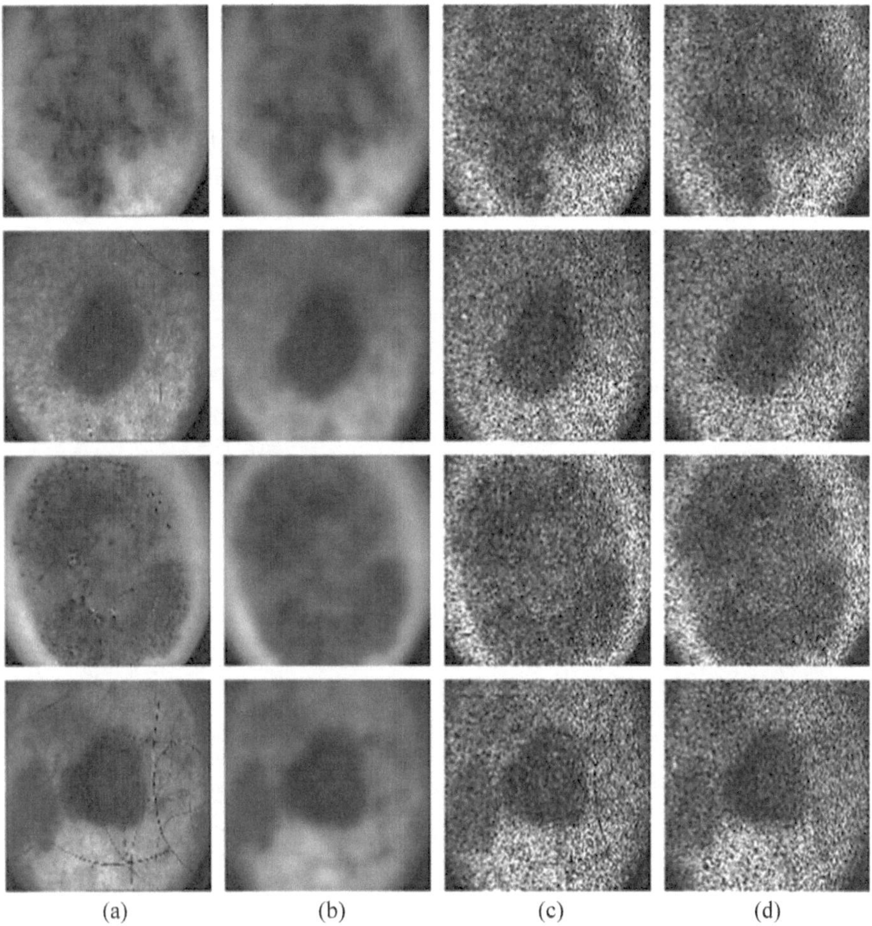

FIGURE 20.6 Distorted images of ISIC dataset: (a) Original images, (b) Blurred version, (c) Speckle added images, and (d) Blurred image corrupted by speckles.

TABLE 20.1
DSC and JSC Obtained at Different Phases of the Training

Phase	DSC	JSC
Phase 1	91.34	84.05
Phase 2	89.26	80.60
Phase 3	89.10	80.34
Phase 4	86.24	75.81

80.34, 86.24, and 75.8, respectively. From the values, one thing is to be noted: the blurring of edges has more impact on segmentation accuracy than the speckle.

After training and testing at different stages, the LCU-Net was trained using the public UD image dataset. Figure 20.7 shows the proposed processing for UD images in the dataset. Table 20.2 has the values of the average DSC and JSC for the proposed network and the most recent networks for the segmentation of images in the dataset.

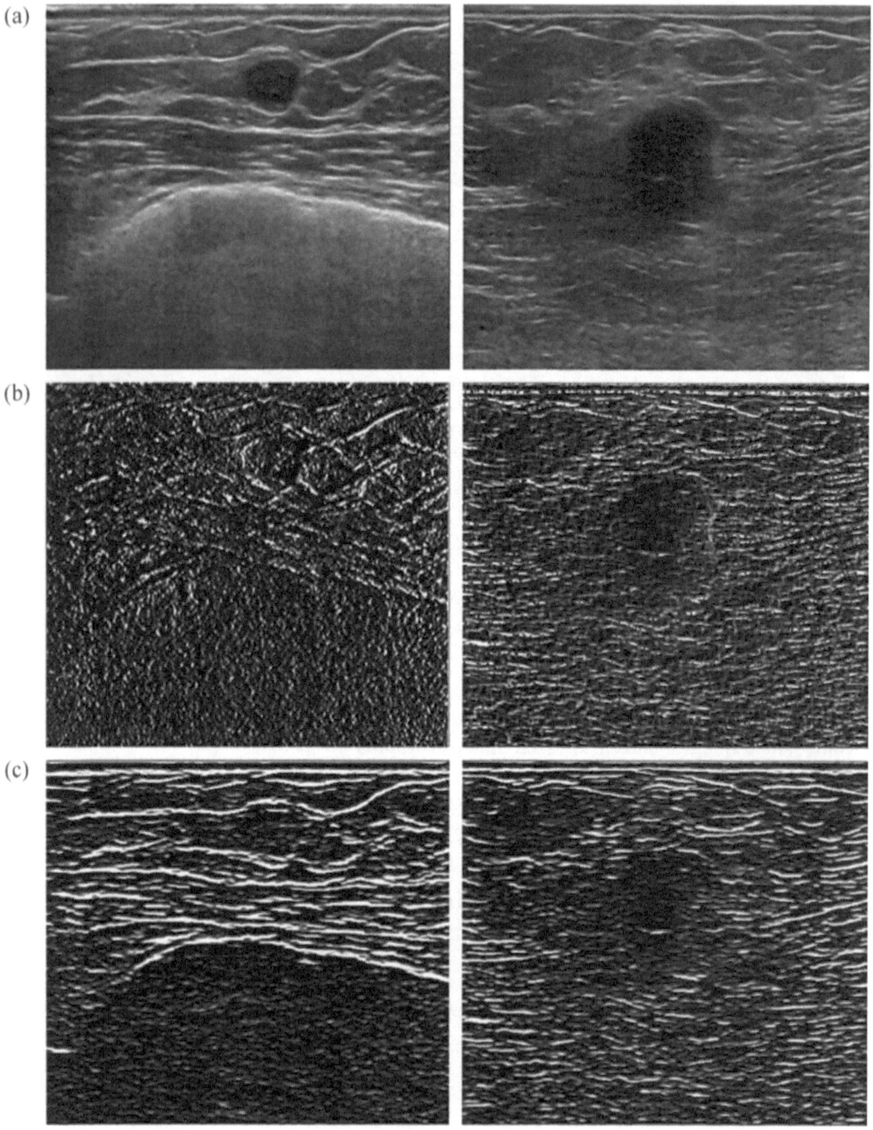

FIGURE 20.7 (a) Original UD image from ISIC dataset, (b) Output of Sobel operator, and (c) Combined output of two directional filter.

The networks used for comparison are described in the first section. These networks have the basic U-Net structure but involve other technologies. The networks have an extended encoder and decoder path with loads of interconnection. Within the encoder and decoder path, there are large numbers of blocks and interconnections. Even the blocks have many internal layers, and all these things make them a sizeable complex layer. The complex layers come at the cost of extensive data and memory requirements. The improvement in accuracy and the cost paid in terms of memory and data is not justifiable. Moreover, it is clear from Table 20.2 that increasing the number of blocks and increasing the information sharing could be more efficient. However, the proposed training paradigm has better segmentation accuracy than others with a small network depth. The proposed network has a DSC of 85.71 and a JSC of 74.99.

To show the performance of the conventional segmentation technique, their output for some randomly selected UD images is given in Figure 20.8. The first row in the image is the original image, and the second is the masked image provided in the dataset. The output of the Thresholding algorithm provided in the second last column has the least accuracy. The image in the third row completely misses the tumor region, and the rest has many surrounding pixels within the region of interest. The dark texture of the UD image and the slight difference between the tumor and its surroundings are hard to differentiate with a single threshold. Its output could be better for images with obvious tumor boundaries. A similar observation can be made about the output of the Graph cut algorithm (Fourth column in Figure 20.8). Although it has identified most of the tumor boundary, surrounding pixels with similar intensities are still a threat. On the other hand, the Segmentation through Active Contour has far better results than the Graph-cut and Thresholding. The local forces on the defined tumor boundary were good in finding the tumor boundary. Due to the connectivity constraint, it can produce more continuous regions. The UD in the third and last row of Figure 20.8 poses a unique challenge, as there are many very similar and very close to the intensities of the region of interest to confuse any algorithm. The active contour also feels for that, but it is better than the graph cut and threshold. The last column in the figure presents the output of the proposed LCU-Net. It has better results than conventional techniques. It has the masked image closest to the ground truth image. Even for the images in the third and fourth rows, the proposed network's output is far better than others.

TABLE 20.2
Comparison of the Proposed LCU-Net with Other Networks

Technique	DSC	JSC
ConvMixer	80.23	69.23
HAU-Net	83.11	71.1
TBU-Net	82.48	70.18
G-UNeXt	81.58	68.86
DHMS	82.80	70.65
Proposed (LCU-Net)	85.71	74.99

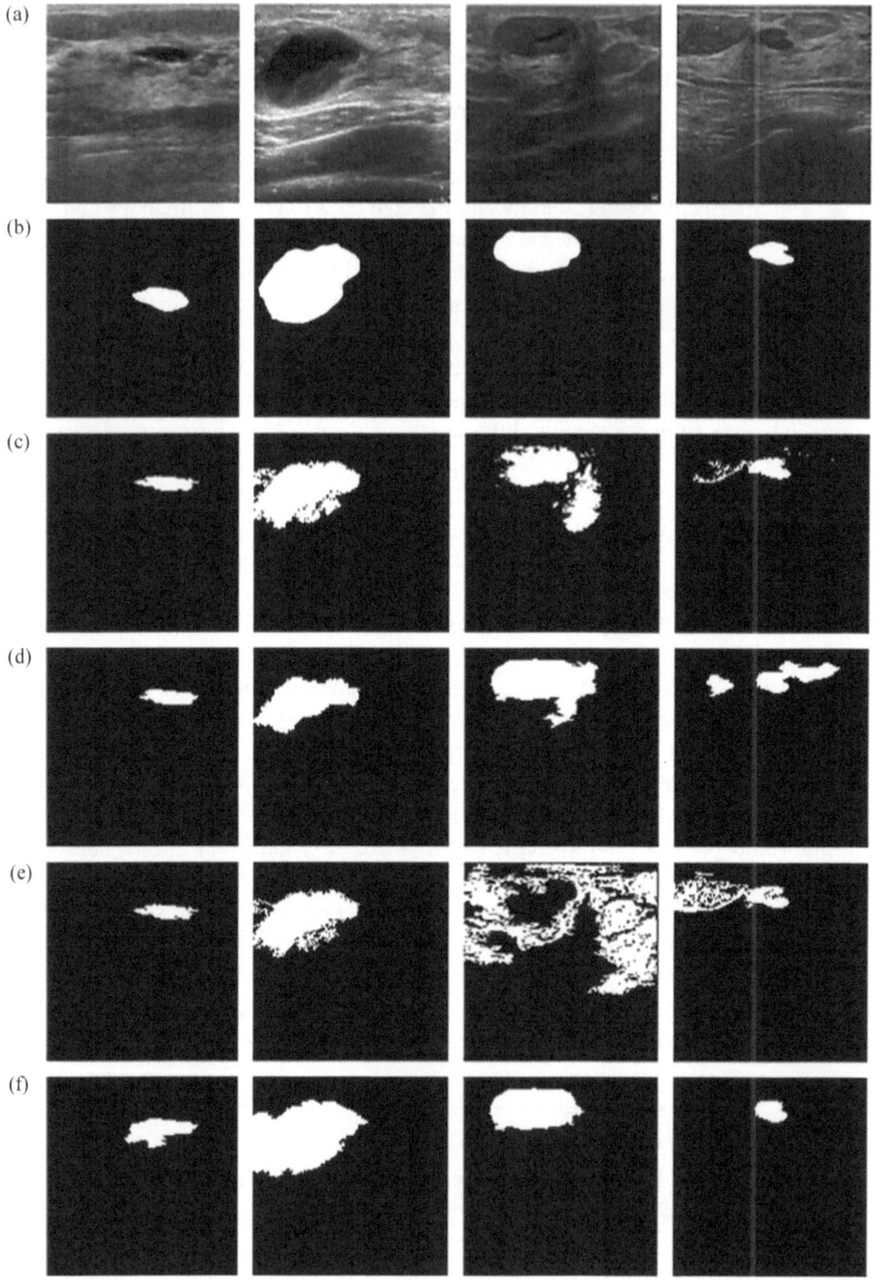

FIGURE 20.8 Some randomly selected: (a) UD image and their (b) Ground truth image (c), (d), (e), and (f) are the segmentation output (i.e., Active Contour, Graph-cut, Thresholding, and proposed LCU-Net, respectively).

20.5 CONCLUSION

This chapter proposes LCU-Net for segmentation in noisy UD. We tested a novel paradigm for training a network in data and memory scarcity. The network was trained using the ISIC's large skin lesion and breast UD image dataset in various phases. We applied the data augmentation to the datasets to overcome the overfitting situation. Before training, the skin lesion images were processed to match the distribution of a breast UD image. Then, four different groups of images were prepared for the network. Some images were blurred, and some were added with speckle noise. The groups were created entirely randomly, and no image was repeated in the other group. After four training phases with the ISIC images, the network was finally trained over the pre-processed UD image. The UD image was pre-processed using the directional filters. The filtering was done to suppress the distortions in the image and improve the segmentation result. The results were validated on an extensive public dataset and compared with the latest segmentation technique. With the accuracy of other complex networks, it was clear that increasing the number of layers and fusions has a minor impact on accuracy. With a new way of learning, the proposed network outperformed others and secured DSC and JSC values of 85.71 and 74.99, respectively.

REFERENCES

[1] K. Kumar, K. Chaudhury, and S. L. Tripathi, "Future of Machine Learning (ML) and Deep Learning (DL) in Healthcare Monitoring System," in *Machine Learning Algorithms for Signal and Image Processing*, 2022, pp. 293–313.

[2] A. Soni, K. Rawal, "Analyzing the effect of postural change on heart rate variability using multi-distance sample entropy (MDSE)," *Biomed. Signal Process. Cont.*, vol. 87, no. 2, 2024.

[3] A. E. Kavur, L. I. Kuncheva, and M. A. Selver, "Basic ensembles of vanilla-style deep learning models improve liver segmentation from ct images," in Saban Ozturk (Ed) *Convolutional Neural Networks for Medical Image Processing Applications*, CRC Press, 2022, pp. 52–74.

[4] M. Hassaballah and A. I. Awad, *Deep Learning in Computer Vision: Principles and Applications*. Mahmoud Hassaballah and Ali Ismail Awad (Eds.), CRC Press, 2020.

[5] J. S. Denker and C. C. J. Burges, "Image segmentation and recognition," in *The Mathematics of Generalization*, CRC Press, 2018, pp. 409–434.

[6] N. A. Shaharuddin and W. M. H. W. Mahmud, "Development of computer aided diagnosis system (CAD) for detection of kidney ultrasound images," in *2017 International Conference on Engineering Technology and Technopreneurship (ICE2T)*, 2017.

[7] S. Maqsood and R. Damaševičius, "Multiclass skin lesion localization and classification using deep learning based features fusion and selection framework for smart healthcare," *Neural Netw.*, vol. 160, pp. 238–258, 2023.

[8] Y. Nagaraj, A. Hema Sai Teja, and A. V. Narasimhadhan, "Automatic segmentation of intima media complex in carotid ultrasound images using support vector machine," *Arab. J. Sci. Eng.*, vol. 44, no. 4, pp. 3489–3496, 2019.

[9] Z. Tian, L. Liu, Z. Zhang, J. Xue, and B. Fei, "A supervoxel-based segmentation method for prostate MR images," *Med. Phys.*, vol. 44, no. 2, pp. 558–569, 2017.

[10] L. Zhao et al., "Automatic cytoplasm and nuclei segmentation for color cervical smear image using an efficient gap-search MRF," *Comput. Biol. Med.*, vol. 71, pp. 46–56, 2016.

[11] J. Zhang, Y. Zhang, Y. Jin, J. Xu, and X. Xu, "MDU-Net: Multi-scale densely connected U-Net for biomedical image segmentation," *Heal. Inf. Sci. Syst.*, vol. 11, no. 1, p. 13, 2023.

[12] B. Lei et al., "Skin lesion segmentation via generative adversarial networks with dual discriminators," *Med. Image Anal.*, vol. 64, p. 101716, 2020.

[13] F. Dubost et al., "GP-Unet: Lesion detection from weak labels with a 3D regression network BT - Medical image computing and computer assisted intervention – MICCAI 2017," 2017, pp. 214–221.

[14] H. Zang, L. Zhu, Z. Ding, X. Li, and S. Zhan, "Cascaded dense-UNet for image super-resolution," *J. Circuits, Syst. Comput.*, vol. 29, no. 08, p. 2050121, 2020.

[15] M. Kahani, A. Kamali-Asl, H. Ghadiri, and S. Hashemi, "A method for material decomposition in dual-energy contrast enhancement digital mammography," *Measurement*, vol. 88, pp. 87–95, 2016.

[16] J. Civale, J. Bamber, E. Harris, "Amplitude based segmentation of ultrasound echoes for attenuation coefficient estimation," *Ultrasonics*, vol. 111, pp. 106302, 2021.

[17] R. Mahmoudi, "Ventricular segmentation and modeling using topological watershed transformation and harmonic state model," *Int. J. Imaging Syst. Technol.*, vol. 33, no. 2, pp. 680–700, 2023.

[18] L. Gui, C. Li, and X. Yang, "Medical image segmentation based on level set and isoperimetric constraint," *Phys. Medica*, vol. 42, pp. 162–173, 2017.

[19] F. Adamo, G. Andria, F. Attivissimo, A. M. L. Lanzolla, and M. Spadavecchia, "A comparative study on mother wavelet selection in ultrasound image denoising," *Measurement*, vol. 46, no. 8, pp. 2447–2456, 2013.

[20] V. A. Karale, T. Singh, A. Sadhu, N. Khandelwal, and S. Mukhopadhyay, "Reduction of false positives in the screening CAD tool for microcalcification detection," *Sādhanā*, vol. 45, no. 1, p. 44, 2020.

[21] L. Shaddock and T. Smith, "Potential for use of portable ultrasound devices in rural and remote settings in Australia and other developed countries: A systematic review," *J. Multidiscip. Healthc.*, pp. 605–625, 2022.

[22] C.C. Shen and J.-E. Yang, "Estimation of ultrasound echogenicity map from B-mode images using convolutional neural network," *Sensors*, vol. 20, no. 17, 2020.

[23] F. Perez, C. Vasconcelos, S. Avila, and E. Valle, "Data Augmentation for Skin Lesion Analysis," in *OR 2.0 Context-Aware Operating Theaters, Computer Assisted Robotic Endoscopy, Clinical Image-Based Procedures, and Skin Image Analysis*, 2018, pp. 303–311.

[24] M. Altun, H. Gürüler, O. Özkaraca, F. Khan, J. Khan, and Y. Lee, "Monkeypox detection using CNN with transfer learning," *Sensors*, vol. 23, no. 4, 2023.

[25] M. M. Ahsan et al., "Deep transfer learning approaches for Monkeypox disease diagnosis," *Expert Syst. Appl.*, vol. 216, p. 119483, 2023.

[26] H. Wu, S. Chen, G. Chen, W. Wang, B. Lei, and Z. Wen, "FAT-Net: Feature adaptive transformers for automated skin lesion segmentation," *Med. Image Anal.*, vol. 76, p. 102327, 2022.

[27] H. C. Reis, V. Turk, K. Khoshelham, and S. Kaya, "InSiNet: A deep convolutional approach to skin cancer detection and segmentation," *Med. Biol. Eng. Comput.*, vol. 60, no. 3, pp. 643–662, 2022.

[28] A. E. Ilesanmi, O. P. Idowu, and S. S. Makhanov, "Multiscale superpixel method for segmentation of breast ultrasound," *Comput. Biol. Med.*, vol. 125, p. 103879, 2020.

[29] M. K. Sangole, S. T. Gandhe, and D. P. Patil, "Improved otsu algorithm for segmentation of malaria parasite images," *J. Med. Imaging Health Infor.*, 2022, pp. 179–194.

[30] J. Liao, Y. Wang, D. Zhu, Y. Zou, S. Zhang, and H. Zhou, "Automatic segmentation of crop/background based on luminance partition correction and adaptive threshold," *IEEE Access*, vol. 8, pp. 202611–202622, 2020.

[31] M. Hao, M. Zhou and L. Cai, "An improved graph-cut-based unsupervised change detection method for multispectral remote-sensing images," *Int. J. Remote Sens.*, vol. 42, no. 11, pp. 4005–4022, 2021.

[32] S. Rani, D. Ghai, and S. Kumar, "Reconstruction of simple and complex three dimensional images using pattern recognition algorithm," *J. Inf. Technol. Manag.*, vol. 14, no. Special Issue, pp. 235–247, 2022.

[33] J. Long, E. Shelhamer, and T. Darrell, "Fully convolutional networks for semantic segmentation," in *2015 IEEE Conference on Computer Vision and Pattern Recognition (CVPR)*, June 2015, pp. 3431–3440.

[34] S. Rani, D. Ghai, S. Kumar, M. V. V. P. Kantipudi, A. H. Alharbi, and M. A. Ullah, "Efficient 3D AlexNet architecture for object recognition using syntactic patterns from medical images," *Comput. Intell. Neurosci.*, vol. 2022, p. 7882924, 2022.

[35] K. He, X. Zhang, S. Ren, and J. Sun, "Deep residual learning for image recognition," in *2016 IEEE Conference on Computer Vision and Pattern Recognition (CVPR)*, 2016, pp. 770–778.

[36] S. Benyahia, B. Meftah, and O. Lézoray, "Multi-features extraction based on deep learning for skin lesion classification," *Tissue Cell*, vol. 74, p. 101701, 2022.

[37] Q. He, Q. Yang, and M. Xie, "HCTNet: A hybrid CNN-transformer network for breast ultrasound image segmentation," *Comput. Biol. Med.*, vol. 155, p. 106629, 2023.

[38] N. R. Rajalakshmi, R. Vidhyapriya, N. Elango, and N. Ramesh, "Deeply supervised U-Net for mass segmentation in digital mammograms," *Int. J. Imaging Syst. Technol.*, vol. 31, no. 1, pp. 59–71, 2021.

[39] O. Ronneberger, P. Fischer, and T. Brox, "U-Net: Convolutional networks for biomedical image segmentation," in *Medical Image Computing and Computer-Assisted Intervention – MICCAI 2015*, 2015, pp. 234–241.

[40] Y. Weng, T. Zhou, Y. Li, and X. Qiu, "NAS-Unet: Neural architecture search for medical image segmentation," *IEEE Access*, vol. 7, pp. 44247–44257, 2019.

[41] Z. Zeng, W. Xie, Y. Zhang, and Y. Lu, "RIC-Unet: An improved neural network based on unet for nuclei segmentation in histology images," *IEEE Access*, vol. 7, pp. 21420–21428, 2019.

[42] A. A. Abdelhamid et al., "Classification of monkeypox images based on transfer learning and the Al-Biruni earth radius optimization algorithm," *Mathematics*, vol. 10, no. 19, 2022.

[43] K. Tomczak, P. Czerwińska, and M. Wiznerowicz, "Review The Cancer Genome Atlas (TCGA): An immeasurable source of knowledge," *Contemp. Oncol. Onkol.*, vol. 2015, no. 1, pp. 68–77, 2015.

[44] X. Li, H. Chen, X. Qi, Q. Dou, C.-W. Fu, and P.-A. Heng, "H-DenseUNet: Hybrid densely connected UNet for liver and tumor segmentation from CT volumes," *IEEE Trans. Med. Imaging*, vol. 37, no. 12, pp. 2663–2674, 2018.

[45] H. Zhang et al., "HAU-Net: Hybrid CNN-transformer for breast ultrasound image segmentation," *Biomed. Signal Process. Control*, vol. 87, p. 105427, 2024.

[46] L. Chen, J. Li, and H. Ge, "TBUnet: A pure convolutional U-net capable of multifaceted feature extraction for medical image segmentation," *J. Med. Syst.*, vol. 47, no. 1, p. 122, 2023.

[47] X. Zhang, X. Cao, J. Wang, and L. Wan, "G-UNeXt: A lightweight MLP-based network for reducing semantic gap in medical image segmentation," *Multimed. Syst.*, vol. 29, no. 6, pp. 3431–3446, 2023.

[48] R. Yu, Y. Wang, Z. Zou, and L. Wang, "Convolutional neural networks with refined loss functions for the real-time crash risk analysis," *Transp. Res. Part C Emerg. Technol.*, vol. 119, p. 102740, 2020.

[49] Z. Wu, X. Zhang, F. Li, S. Wang, and L. Huang, "Multi-scale long-range interactive and regional attention network for stroke lesion segmentation," *Comput. Electr. Eng.*, vol. 103, p. 108345, 2022.

[50] X. Li et al., "ATTransUNet: An enhanced hybrid transformer architecture for ultrasound and histopathology image segmentation," *Comput. Biol. Med.*, vol. 152, p. 106365, 2023.

[51] Z. Cheng and L. Wang, "Dynamic hierarchical multi-scale fusion network with axial MLP for medical image segmentation," *Sci. Rep.*, vol. 13, no. 1, p. 6342, 2023.

[52] K. D. Miller, M. Fidler-Benaoudia, T. H. Keegan, H. S. Hipp, A. Jemal, and R. L. Siegel, "Cancer statistics for adolescents and young adults, 2020," *CA. Cancer J. Clin.*, vol. 70, no. 6, pp. 443–459, 2020.

[53] P. Pan, H. Chen, Y. Li, N. Cai, L. Cheng, and S. Wang, "Tumor segmentation in automated whole breast ultrasound using bidirectional LSTM neural network and attention mechanism," *Ultrasonics*, vol. 110, p. 106271, 2021.

[54] F. Alenezi, A. Armghan, and K. Polat, "Wavelet transform based deep residual neural network and ReLU based Extreme Learning Machine for skin lesion classification," *Expert Syst. Appl.*, vol. 213, p. 119064, 2023.

[55] D. Uzun Ozsahin, M. T. Mustapha, B. Uzun, B. Duwa, and I. Ozsahin, "Computer-aided detection and classification of monkeypox and chickenpox lesion in human subjects using deep learning framework," *Diagnostics*, vol. 13, no. 2, 2023.

[56] N. C. F. Codella et al., "Skin lesion analysis toward melanoma detection: {A} Challenge at the 2017 International Symposium on Biomedical Imaging (ISBI), Hosted by the International Skin Imaging Collaboration {(ISIC)}," *CoRR*, vol. abs/1710.0, 2017.

[57] N. C. F. Codella et al., "Skin Lesion Analysis Toward Melanoma Detection 2018: {A} Challenge Hosted by the International Skin Imaging Collaboration {(ISIC)}," *CoRR*, vol. abs/1902.0, 2019.

[58] W. Al-Dhabyani, M. Gomaa, H. Khaled, and A. Fahmy, "Dataset of breast ultrasound images," *Data Br.*, vol. 28, p. 104863, 2020.

[59] J. M. J. Valanarasu and V. M. Patel, "UNeXt: MLP-Based Rapid Medical Image Segmentation Network," in *Medical Image Computing and Computer Assisted Intervention -- MICCAI 2022*, 2022, pp. 23–33.

[60] M. A. Mazurowski, H. Dong, H. Gu, J. Yang, N. Konz, and Y. Zhang, "Segment anything model for medical image analysis: An experimental study," *Med. Image Anal.*, vol. 89, p. 102918, 2023.

[61] A. Ahila et al., "Meta-heuristic algorithm-tuned neural network for breast cancer diagnosis using ultrasound images," *Front. Oncol.*, vol. 12, 2022.

[62] J. Yang et al., "MedMNIST v2 - A large-scale lightweight benchmark for 2D and 3D biomedical image classification," *Sci. Data*, vol. 10, no. 1, p. 41, 2023.

[63] S. N. Ali et al., "Monkeypox skin lesion detection using deep learning models: A feasibility study," July 2022.

[64] N. Gessert, M. Nielsen, M. Shaikh, R. Werner, and A. Schlaefer, "Skin lesion classification using ensembles of multi-resolution EfficientNets with meta data," *MethodsX*, vol. 7, p. 100864, 2020.

[65] C. Liu, C. Hsu, Y. Chou, and C. Chen, "A multi-scale tumor detection algorithm in whole breast sonography incorporating breast anatomy and tissue morphological information," in *2014 IEEE Healthcare Innovation Conference (HIC)*, October 2014, pp. 193–196.

[66] N. M. Hussain Hassan, "Highly-efficient technique for automatic segmentation of X-ray bone images based on fuzzy logic and an edge detection technique," *Multidimens. Syst. Signal Process.*, vol. 31, no. 2, pp. 591–617, 2020.

[67] X. Zhu et al., "Comparative analysis of active contour and convolutional neural network in rapid left-ventricle volume quantification using echocardiographic imaging," *Comput. Methods Programs Biomed.*, vol. 199, p. 105914, 2021.

[68] D. Ghai, S.L. Tripathi, S. Saxena, M. Chanda, and M. Alazab, (Eds.), *Machine Learning Algorithms for Signal and Image Processing*, John Wiley & Sons, 2022.

[69] S.L. Tripathi, K. Dhir, D. Ghai, and S. Patil, (Eds.), *Health Informatics and Technological Solutions for Coronavirus (COVID-19)*, CRC Press, 2021.

[70] P. K. Shukla, J. K. Sandhu, A. Ahirwar, D. Ghai, P. Maheshwary, and P. K. Shukla. Multiobjective genetic algorithm and convolutional neural network based COVID-19 identification in chest X-ray images. *Math. Probl. Eng.*, vol. 2021, no. 1, pp. 1–9, 2021.

Index

Page numerals in *italics* refer to figures and those in **bold** to tables.

C

D

E

F

N

O

P

T

U